Canadian Essentials of Nursing Research

CARMEN G. LOISELLE, PhD, RN
Associate Professor and Director of Oncology Nursing
School of Nursing, Faculty of Medicine
McGill University

Senior Researcher
Lady Davis Institute and Centre for Nursing Research
Jewish General Hospital
Montreal, Quebec
Canada

JOANNE PROFETTO-McGRATH, PhD, RN
Professor
University of Alberta Faculty of Nursing
Edmonton, Alberta
Canada

DENISE F. POLIT, PhD
President
Humanalysis, Inc.
Saratoga Springs, New York

CHERYL TATANO BECK, DNSc, CNM, FAAN
Professor
University of Connecticut School of Nursing
Storrs, Connecticut

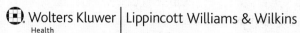
Wolters Kluwer | Lippincott Williams & Wilkins
Health
Philadelphia · Baltimore · New York · London
Buenos Aires · Hong Kong · Sydney · Tokyo

Acquisitions Editor: Hilarie Surrena
Product Manager: Helen Kogut
Vendor Manager: Beth Martz
Director of Nursing Production: Helen Ewan
Art Director, Design: Joan Wendt
Art Director, Illustration: Brett MacNaughton
Manufacturing Coordinator: Karin Duffield
Production Services: Aptara, Inc.

3rd Edition

9 8 7 6 5 4 3 2 1

Printed in China

Library of Congress Cataloging-in-Publication Data

Canadian essentials of nursing research / Carmen G. Loiselle . . . [et al.]. — 3rd ed.
   p. ; cm.
  Includes bibliographical references and index.
  ISBN 978-1-60547-729-9 (alk. paper)
  1. Nursing—Research—Methodology. 2. Nursing—Research—Canada. I.
Loiselle, Carmen G.
  [DNLM: 1. Nursing Research—methods—Canada. WY 20.5 C2115 2011]
  RT81.5.C355 2011
  610.73072—dc22

            2009035643

RRS0911

REVIEWERS

Ethel Bratt, RN, BSCN
Faculty
SIAST
Regina, Saskatchewan

Katharina Kovacs Burns, MSc, MHSA, PhD
Associate Director
Health Sciences
University of Alberta
Edmonton, Alberta

Helen Ewing, RN, BN, MN, DHSc
Assistant Professor
Athabasca University
Calgary, Alberta

Dolly Goldenberg, RN, BScN, MA(Eng), MScN, PhD
Professor and Chair of Graduate
  Programs in Nursing
University of Western Ontario
London, Ontario

Patricia Grainger, RN, BN, MN
Nurse Educator and Research Office
  Coordinator
Centre for Nursing Studies
St. John's, Newfoundland

Lyle G. Grant, BComm, LLB, BSN, MSN, PhD Student
Instructor
Douglas College
New Westminster, British Columbia

Kristen Gulbransen, RN, MN
Faculty
Red Deer College
Red Deer, Alberta

Claudette Kelly, RN, BScN, MA, PhD
Nurse Educator
Thompson Rivers University
Kamloops, British Columbia

Nicole Letourneau, PhD, MN, BN, RN
Professor and Canada Research Chair in
  Healthy Child Development
University of New Brunswick
Fredericton, New Brunswick

Tracey Rickards, BN, MN
Outreach/Research Nurse, Clinical
  Instructor, Course Instructor
University of New Brunswick
Fredericton, New Brunswick

Darlene Steven, BScN, BA, MHSA, PhD
Professor
Lakehead University
Thunder Bay, Ontario

Beverly Temple, RN, BScN, MN, PhD
Assistant Professor
University of Manitoba
Winnipeg, Manitoba

Cynthia Toman, RN, BScN, MScN, PhD
Assistant Professor
University of Ottawa
Ottawa, Ontario

Elizabeth VanDenKerkhof, RN, BScN, MSc, DrPH
Associate Professor
Queen's University
Kingston, Ontario

PREFACE

This third edition of *Canadian Essentials of Nursing Research* continues to feature state-of-the-art research undertaken by Canadian nurse researchers, as well as additional Canadian content relating to the history of nursing research, ethical considerations, models of nursing, and models of research utilization. At the same time, this edition contains all the innovative features that made the original award-winning text so popular. *Essentials of Nursing Research* is widely hailed by faculty, clinicians, and students alike for its up-to-date, clear, and "user-friendly" presentation.

Nursing research is the conduct of systematic studies to generate new knowledge pertaining to health and illness-related experiences. Nurse researchers are scientists who seek answers to pressing questions through systematic observation and recording of nursing-related phenomena. There is a growing expectation that nurses—especially those in clinical practice—will increasingly utilize the results of scientific studies as a basis for their practice. The need to apply new knowledge from research requires that we overcome the challenges related to accessing, reading, understanding, translating, and disseminating research findings into practice. One main purpose of this book is to assist beginning consumers of nursing research in evaluating the adequacy of research findings in terms of their scientific merit and potential for utilization.

The twenty-first century is a very exciting era for nursing research in Canada. Current nursing research agendas are more dynamic, more responsive to societal needs, and more closely aligned with innovation in health care delivery. In addition, the explosion of information technology has enabled clinicians, administrators, researchers, and other stakeholders to readily transcend geographical distances and time zones so that they may work together to answer important health care questions. In addition, an ever increasing critical mass of nursing research leaders make for a more visible, productive, and collaborative health-related research enterprise. A concerted effort to conduct transdisciplinary research also has stimulated new, innovative, and productive partnerships adding to a renewed body of knowledge. One challenge for the future, however, remains to diversify and increase communication channels so that the best nursing evidence becomes more accessible and more readily disseminated within and across disciplines and across relevant fields. Nursing research too often remains a well-kept secret.

Growing evidence indicates that the presentation of knowledge that is personally relevant to students contributes to optimal learning. Course evaluations and informal feedback from our students who have used the first or second edition clearly show that the timely exposure to examples of research conducted by Canadian nurse researchers enhances their understanding, appreciation of, and commitment to nursing research. This third edition should continue to stimulate students to become well-informed consumers of research and stay actively involved in the discovery of new nursing knowledge. We are honoured to have had the opportunity to update *Canadian Essentials of Nursing Research* during a most promising moment in the history of nursing research in Canada.

NEW TO THIS EDITION

➤ *Early introduction to evidence-based practice.* To enhance the reader's appreciation of requirements to conduct rigorous nursing research and highlight its relevance to practice, we have introduced the idea of evidence-based practice much earlier in the book. Chapter 1 provides concrete examples of nursing research in Canada that have led to innovative developments guiding EBP such as the creation of clinical practice guidelines.

> ✒ *Sustained emphasis throughout the chapters on the relevance of nursing research to evidence-based practice.* All chapters build on these notions to guide nurses in their evaluation of study quality and ensuing evidence in terms of rigour and potential use in practice.

> ✒ *New resources for students and instructors.* New resources based on this edition of *Canadian Essentials of Nursing Research* are available on thePoint, to enhance learning and instruction.

ORGANIZATION OF THE TEXT

The content of this edition is organized into six main parts.

> ✒ **Part 1**—*Overview of Nursing Research* serves as the overall introduction to fundamental concepts in nursing research. Chapter 1 introduces and summarizes the history and future of nursing research both in Canada and elsewhere, discusses the philosophical underpinnings of qualitative research versus quantitative research, and describes the major purposes of nursing research. Chapter 2 introduces readers to key terms, with new emphasis on terms related to the quality of research evidence. Chapter 3 presents an overview of the steps in the research process for both qualitative and quantitative studies. Chapter 4 provides an introduction to research reports—what they are and how to read them. Chapter 5 is devoted to a discussion of ethics in research studies.

> ✒ **Part 2**—*Preliminary Steps in the Research Process* includes three chapters and focuses on the steps that are taken in getting started on a research project. Chapter 6 focuses on the development of research questions and the formulation of research hypotheses. Chapter 7 discusses how to prepare and critique literature reviews. Chapter 8 presents information about theoretical and conceptual frameworks.

> ✒ **Part 3**—*Designs for Nursing Research* presents material relating to the design of qualitative and quantitative nursing studies. Chapter 9 describes some fundamental design principles and discusses many specific aspects of quantitative research design. Chapter 10 addresses the various research traditions that have contributed to the growth of naturalistic inquiry and qualitative research. Chapter 11 provides an introduction to some specific types of research (e.g., evaluations, surveys, secondary analyses, case studies), and also describes integrated qualitative/quantitative designs. Chapter 12 presents various designs for sampling of study participants.

> ✒ **Part 4**—*Data Collection* deals with the collection of research data. Chapter 13 discusses the full range of data collection options available to researchers, including both qualitative and quantitative approaches. Chapter 14, an especially important chapter for critiquing qualitative studies, explains methods for assessing data quality.

> ✒ **Part 5**—*Data Analysis* is devoted to the organization and analysis of research data. Chapter 15 reviews methods of quantitative analysis. The chapter assumes no prior instruction in statistics and focuses primarily on helping readers to understand why statistics are needed, what tests might be appropriate in a given research situation, and what statistical information in a research report means. Chapter 16 presents a discussion of qualitative analysis, greatly expanded and improved in this edition.

> ✒ **Part 6**—*Critical Appraisal and Utilization of Nursing Research* is intended to sharpen the critical awareness of consumers with respect to several key issues. Chapter 17 discusses the interpretation and appraisal of research reports. Chapter 18, the final chapter, offers guidance for research utilization and EBP.

KEY FEATURES

This third edition continues to place an emphasis on relevance and rigour of nursing studies. In addition, because research has shown that more personally relevant materials are better processed and recalled, we have made every effort to ensure that examples of nursing studies depict the work of various nurse researchers from across the country.

Research Examples and Critical Thinking Activities: Each chapter includes examples of studies in abstract style so that the gist is conveyed while providing the full citations so that students wanting more information can easily retrieve the journal articles. In addition, critical thinking activities are provided so that students can evaluate features of actual studies with full reports included in the appendices.

Tips: Each chapter contains numerous tips on what to expect in research reports vis-à-vis the topics that have been discussed in the chapter. In these tips, we pay special attention to help students read research reports, thus enabling them to translate the material presented in the textbook into meaningful concepts as they approach the research literature.

Guidelines for Critiquing Research Reports: Boxes containing guidelines for conducting a critique provide a list of questions that walk students through a study, drawing attention to various aspects that are amenable to appraisal by research consumers.

Learning Objectives: Learning objectives are identified at the outset of each chapter to focus students' attention to critical content.

Summary Points: A summary of key points is provided at the end of each chapter.

Methodologic and Theoretical References: A list of methodologic and theoretical references is provided at the end of the book to direct the student's further inquiry.

Teaching/Learning Package: A variety of teaching/learning resources is available for students and instructors who purchase *Canadian Essentials of Nursing Research, 3rd edition*. Visit the Point at http://thePoint.lww.com to learn about this exciting package.

Carmen G. Loiselle, PhD, RN
Joanne Profetto-McGrath, PhD, RN
Denise F. Polit, PhD
Cheryl Tatano Beck, DNSc, CNM, FAAN

IN APPRECIATION

With the continued success of *Canadian Essentials of Nursing Research*, we remained most committed to producing a third edition of the book. Many thanks go to our nursing colleagues from across Canada for so willingly sharing their research findings with us and for continuing to provide informative "behind the scenes" insights.

We are indebted to the Lippincott Williams & Wilkins team, Carol McGimpsey, Corey Wolfe, Barry Wight, Hilarie Surrena, and Helen Kogut, Product Manager, who remain great supporters of the "Canadianization" of *Essentials of Nursing Research*.

McGill University and the University of Alberta provided the authors with a most stimulating intellectual working environment. In addition, we thank our colleagues, from various institutions and affiliations, Drs. Nancy Feeley, Thomas Hack, Dorothy Forbes, Lesley Degner, and Lynne McVey, for their support and passion for research and clinical practice and for their pursuit of excellence in all realms of life. We acknowledge the significant contributions of Dr. Sylvie Lambert, Dr. Michelle Proulx, Kylie Hugo, and Okimi Peters who rigorously and diligently assisted us in finding the most relevant studies to be included in this new edition. We thank Kelly and Jamie Cassoff for their assistance in proof reading some chapters. We also acknowledge the precious assistance of medical librarian, Rachel Daly, MLIS, from the Centre for Nursing Research at the Jewish General Hospital in Montreal for her enthusiastic and dedicated work in cross-checking the numerous citations.

Finally, we acknowledge our respective spouses, Eric Gervais and Larry McGrath, our children, and our extended families and friends—for their love and support. They remained eagerly interested in the progress of our collaborative work.

To each of the above individuals we are indebted. Collectively, they made the production of this third edition a most pleasant, stimulating, and gratifying experience.

We dedicate this book to a recently deceased colleague—Dr. Chantal Caron, a wonderful human being and an accomplished nurse researcher at the Université de Sherbrooke in Québec. Dr. Caron died of cancer last year, at the age of 42.

CONTENTS

Overview of Nursing Research

1 Introducing Research and Its Relevance to Nursing Practice

LEARNING OBJECTIVES

On completing this chapter, you will be able to:

1. Describe why research is important to nursing and discuss evidence-based practice
2. Describe historical trends and future directions in nursing research
3. Describe alternate sources of evidence for nursing practice
4. Describe the main characteristics of the positivist and naturalistic paradigms, and discuss similarities and differences between quantitative and qualitative research
5. Identify several purposes of qualitative and quantitative research
6. Define new terms in the chapter

AN INTRODUCTION TO NURSING RESEARCH

It is an exciting time to be a nurse. Nurses are managing their clinical responsibilities at a time when the nursing profession and the larger health care system require an extraordinary range of skills and talents. Nurses are expected to deliver high-quality care, in a compassionate manner, with the added challenge of being cost-effective. To accomplish these goals, nurses must readily have access to and evaluate new evidence to decide whether to incorporate it into their practice. In today's world, *nurses are expected to be lifelong learners*, reflecting on, evaluating, and modifying their clinical practice based on the emerging scientific knowledge.

What Is Nursing Research?

Research is a systematic inquiry that uses rigorous methods to answer questions or solve problems. The ultimate goal of research is to develop, refine, and expand knowledge.

Nurses are increasingly engaged in studies that benefit the profession and the individuals it serves. As such, **nursing research** is designed to develop evidence about issues of importance to various stakeholders.

In this book, we emphasize clinical nursing research, that is, research designed to inform nursing practice and contribute to the well being and quality of life of individuals who are facing various challenges or health threats. Clinical nursing research typically begins with questions stemming from practice-related issues such as those that you may encounter in your practice.

Examples of nursing research questions

⇒ What types of musculoskeletal problems are older nurses most likely to experience (Cameron, Armstrong-Stassen, Kane, & Moro, 2008)?

⇒ What are the experiences of women with schizophrenia who had to negotiate support from formal and informal sources (Chernomas, Clarke, & Marchinko, 2008)?

The Importance of Research in Nursing

In Canada and elsewhere, nurses increasingly have been encouraged to get involved in research and adopt an **evidence-based practice** (EBP). EBP is broadly defined as the use of the best clinical evidence in making care decisions. Evidence can come from various sources, but there is general agreement that findings from rigorous studies constitute the best type of evidence for guiding nurses' decisions and actions. Nurses who incorporate high-quality evidence into their clinical practice are more likely to provide interventions that are appropriate, cost-effective, and promote optimal health outcomes.

Example of evidence-based practice

In Canada, nursing research has led to innovative developments guiding EBP such as the creation of clinical practice guidelines. Clinical practice guidelines include summaries of the best available evidence packaged in a format that readily guides clinical decision making. These guidelines can contribute to quality health care by promoting effective interventions based on solid evidence. A team in Ontario that includes Margaret B. Harrison (Professor, School of Nursing, Queen's University, Ontario), Marlene Mackey (Corporate Nursing quality coordinator, Ottawa Hospital, Ottawa), and collaborators in Eastern Ontario concerted their efforts toward the implementation of practice guideline recommendations related to the prevention of pressure ulcers. An evidence-based skin care program was developed and implemented by a transdisciplinary team of nurses, enterostomal therapists, clinical managers, clinical nurses, nurse educators, dieticians, a physiotherapist, occupational therapist, and a clinical director. In the implementation period, even though more than 25% of patients were considered at high risk for pressure ulcers, their prevalence decreased from 18% to 14%.

Various nurses associations such as the Registered Nurses Association of Ontario (RNAO) regularly publish evidence-based clinical practice guidelines: www.rnao.org.

Roles of Nurses in Research

With the current emphasis on EBP, it has become *every* nurse's responsibility to engage in one or more research activities along a continuum of participation. At one end of the continuum, nurses' involvement is indirect; they are considered research consumers as they read research reports to develop new skills and to keep up-to-date on findings that may affect their practice. At minimum, nurses are expected to maintain this level of involvement with research.

At the other end of the continuum, nurses actively engage in research activities. They participate in designing, refining, and implementing studies with a keen emphasis on producing new knowledge that will likely make a difference in the lives of patients.

Example of research by hospital-based nurses

Dean and Major (2008) each conducted an independent study on the use of humour in health care and compared their findings to identify common themes. Dean, a senior instructor at the University of Manitoba, observed and interviewed 15 health care providers from a palliative care unit. Major, a clinical nurse specialist at a health centre in Winnipeg, observed and interviewed 15 intensive care nurses. Common themes that emerged from their analysis included the value of humour for teamwork, emotion management, and maintaining human connections.

Between these two end points lies a variety of research-related activities that may be of great interest to nurses. These include the following:

➤ Participation in a **journal club**, which involves regular meetings among nurses to discuss and critique research articles

➤ Attendance to scientific presentations at conferences and professional meetings

➤ Review of a proposed study and reliance on clinical expertise to improve aspects of the study

➤ Assistance to researchers in participant recruitment and data collection

➤ Discussion of the implications and relevance of findings with various stake-holders (e.g., patients, clinicians, administrators)

Example of a study publicized in the mass media

Here is a headline about a study with more than 200 older adults living with advanced dementia in a nursing home in the Boston area which appeared in a Canadian newspaper in February 2008: *Antibiotics may be overused in nursing homes residents suffering from dementia.* Following 18 months of observation, the researchers found that 42% of these patients received antibiotics during this period. The closer they were to death, the more likely they were to receive antibiotics. Although withholding antibiotics to patients with advanced dementia may be considered unethical, the over-use of antibiotics contributes to the rise of "superbugs." Physicians are increasingly asked to consider the public health ramifications when prescribing antibiotics. What would you say if someone asked you about this study? Would you be able to comment on the relevance of the findings, based on your assessment of how rigorously the study was conducted? You should be able to do this after completing this course.

Within the aforementioned research-related activities, nurses with some research skills are better able to make informed contributions to nursing and to EBP than those without these skills. Having some knowledge of nursing research can expand the breadth and depth of every nurse's practice.

NURSING RESEARCH: PAST, PRESENT, AND FUTURE

Nursing research did not always have the prominence and importance it enjoys today. The interesting history of nursing research, however, portends a distinguished future. Table 1.1 summarizes some key events in the historical evolution of nursing research.

The Early Years: From Nightingale to the 1970s

Most would agree that nursing research began with Florence Nightingale. Based on her skilful analyses of factors affecting soldier mortality and morbidity during the Crimean War, she was successful in effecting changes in nursing care—and, more generally, in public health. Her landmark publication, *Notes on Nursing* (1859), describes her early research interest in environmental factors that promote physical and emotional well-being—an interest sustained by nurses 150 years later.

Many years after Nightingale's work, the nursing literature contained a paucity of research accounts. Studies in the early 1900s mainly focused on nursing education. As more nurses received university-based education, studies among nursing students in terms of their profile, characteristics, and challenges became popular. Later on, when hospital staffing patterns changed, researchers focused not only on the supply and demand of nurses but also on the amount of time required to perform certain nursing activities. During these years, nursing struggled with its professional identity, and nursing research took a twist toward studying nurses: what they did, how other groups perceived them, and who entered the profession.

In the 1950s, a number of forces combined to put nursing research on the upswing. More nurses with advanced academic preparation, government funding, and the establishment of the journal *Nursing Research* in the United States, and

TABLE 1.1 ▶	HISTORICAL LANDMARKS PERTAINING TO NURSING RESEARCH
YEAR	EVENT
1859	Florence Nightingale's *Notes on Nursing* is published
1900	*American Nursing Journal* begins publication
1923	Columbia University in New York establishes first doctoral program for nurses
1932	Weir report, jointly sponsored by the Canadian Nurses Association and the Canadian Medical Association, is published
1930s	*American Journal of Nursing* publishes clinical case studies
1952	The journal *Nursing Research* begins publication
1955	Inception of the American Nurses Foundation to sponsor nursing research
1957	Establishment of nursing research centre in the United States at Walter Reed Army Institute of Research
1959	First master's degree is nursing program established at the University of Western Ontario
1963	*International Journal of Nursing Studies* begins publication
1965	American Nurses Association (ANA) begins sponsoring nursing research conferences
1969	*Canadian Journal of Nursing Research* begins publication under the leadership of Dr. Moyra Allen
1971	ANA establishes a Commission on Research
1972	ANA establishes its Council of Nurse Researchers Canadian Helen Shore publishes first study on research–practice gap in nursing
1976	Stetler and Marram publish guidelines on assessing research for use in practice
1978	The journals *Research in Nursing & Health* and *Advances in Nursing Science* begin publication
1979	*Western Journal of Nursing Research* begins publication
1982	Alberta Heritage Foundation for Nursing Research is established and becomes first granting agency in Canada to exclusively fund nursing research The Conduct and Utilization of Research in Nursing (CURN) project publishes report
1983	*Annual Review of Nursing Research* begins publication
1986	National Center for Nursing Research (NCNR) is established within U.S. National Institutes of Health
1988	The journals *Applied Nursing Research* and *Nursing Science Quarterly* begin publication
1989	U.S. Agency for Health Care Policy and Research is established (renamed Agency for Healthcare Research and Quality, or AHRQ, in 1999)
1991	First fully funded nursing doctoral program established at the University of Alberta; second program established at University of British Columbia later in the year

(table continues on page 6)

TABLE 1.1	HISTORICAL LANDMARKS PERTAINING TO NURSING RESEARCH (continued)	
YEAR	EVENT
1992	The journal *Clinical Nursing Research* begins publication
1993	NCNR becomes a full NIH institute, the National Institute of Nursing Research (NINR) Cochrane Collaboration is established
1994	The journal *Qualitative Health Research* begins publication under the leadership of renowned nurse researcher Dr. Janice Morse
1997	Canadian Health Services Research Foundation is established with federal funding
1998	Sigma Theta Tau International, in cooperation with faculty at the University of Toronto, sponsors the first international conference on research utilization
1999	Canadian Government established $25 million Nursing Research Fund to be administered by the Canadian Health Services Research over a period of 10 years
2000	NINR issues funding priorities for 2000–2004; annual funding exceeds $100 million Canadian Institutes of Health Research (CIHR) is launched
2003	CIHR funds the first Strategic Training Initiatives in Health Research that are nursing led (PORT & FUTURE)
2004	The journal *Worldviews on Evidence-Based Nursing* is launched
2005	Sigma Theta Tau International publishes research priorities
2008	A first nursing research centre focusing on nursing intervention research is established. Funded by FRSQ, the centre is initially formed in Montreal (GRISIM, 2003) and then throughout Quebec (GRIISIQ, 2008)

upgraded research skills among nursing faculty are some of the forces that propelled nursing research.

In the 1960s, practice-oriented research began to emerge worldwide. The *International Journal of Nursing Studies* was first published in 1963, and the *Canadian Journal of Nursing Research* appeared in 1969. Also, the seeds for EBP were planted by the U.K.-based Royal College of Nursing Study of Nursing Care, which began assessing clinical effectiveness.

In the 1970s, nursing studies increased their emphasis on patients and health-related outcomes. In addition, theoretical and contextual issues that were arising led to the creation of journals that focused on these issues such as *Advances in Nursing Science*, *Research in Nursing & Health*, the *Western Journal of Nursing Research*, and the *Journal of Advanced Nursing*. Nurses also began to pay more attention to the utilization of research findings in nursing practice. A seminal article by Stetler and Marram (1976) offered guidance on assessing research for clinical application.

Nursing Research Since 1980

The 1980s brought nursing research to new levels. The first volume of the *Annual Review of Nursing Research* was published in 1983. These included reviews of evidence on selected areas of nursing practice and encouraged the use of research findings. In Canada, as elsewhere, the production and dissemination of nursing knowledge was dependent on the availability of funding. Federal funding for nursing research became available in Canada in the late 1980s through the National Health Research Development Program (NHRDP) and the Medical Research Council of Canada (MRC). Similarly, in the United States, the National Center for Nursing Research (NCNR) within the National Institutes of Health (NIH) was established in 1986. Also in the 1980s, new journals appeared such as *Applied Nursing Research* and the *Australian Journal of Nursing Research*.

In the late 1980s, forces within and external to nursing shaped the nursing research landscape. A group from McMaster University designed a clinical learning strategy called Evidence-Based Medicine (EBM). EBM held that research findings provided evidence that was far superior to tradition or opinions of authorities. This stand constituted a profound shift for medical practice and had a significant impact on all health care professions. In 1989, the U.S. government established an agency that is now known as the Agency for Healthcare Research and Quality (AHRQ), which supports research designed to improve the quality of health care, reduce health costs, and enhance patient safety. EBP in nursing also began to develop in the 1990s. In 1998, the University of Toronto and Sigma Theta Tau International held the first international research utilization conference.

In 1993 in the United States, nursing research was given more visibility and autonomy when the Center for Nursing Research was promoted to full institute status within the National Institutes of Health (NIH). The birth of the National Institute of Nursing Research (NINR) placed nursing research into the mainstream of research activities enjoyed by other health disciplines.

Funding opportunities for nursing research expanded in Canada as well in the late 1990s. The **Canadian Health Services Research Foundation** (CHSRF) was established in 1997 with an endowment from federal funds, and plans for the **Canadian Institutes of Health Research** (CIHR) were underway. Beginning in 1999, the CHSRF earmarked $25 million for nursing research conducted in the health services research domain. Likewise, CIHR became an important source of funding for nursing research. In addition, several CHSRF/CIHR Chair Awards were granted to key investigators within the nursing research community. These 10-year awards were established to promote knowledge generation and transfer in various research areas (e.g., oncology, community health, management). In addition to growth in funding opportunities for nursing research internationally, the 1990s witnessed the birth of several more journals for nurse researchers, including *Qualitative Health Research*, *Clinical Nursing Research*, and *Clinical Effectiveness*. Another major contribution to EBP was inaugurated in 1993: the Cochrane Collaboration, an international network of institutions and individuals that maintains and updates systematic reviews of hundreds of clinical interventions to facilitate EBP. Today, nursing research in Canada enjoys funding from several organizations and programs including The Canadian Health Services Research Foundation (CHSRF), The Canadian Institutes of Health Research (CIHR), Partnership Programs by CHSRF and CIHR, The Canadian Association for Nursing Research (CANR), The Canadian Nurses Foundation (CNF), and The Consortium for Nursing Research and Innovation (CNRI) to name a few.

Example of a CHSRF/CIHR Chair Award recipient

Dr. Nancy Edwards is a prominent nurse researcher who has conducted research on the design, evaluation, dissemination, and uptake of complex community health interventions and programs. Dr. Edwards has pioneered projects in sub-Saharan Africa, the Caribbean, China, and Canada. She is a professor in the School of Nursing, Faculty of Health Sciences and the Department of Epidemiology and Community Medicine at the University of Ottawa. Dr. Edwards is also the director of the Multiple Interventions for Community Health program and holds an appointment as Vice-Chair of the Advisory Board for the CIHR Institute of Public and Population Health. She and her colleagues have completed numerous studies, including an investigation on safety in home care (Lang, Edwards, & Fleiszer, 2008) and a study on the implementation of clinical guidelines (Ploeg, Davies, Edwards, Gifford, & Miller, 2007). Her program as a CHSRF/CIHR Chair is called *Multiple Interventions in Community Health Nursing Care*.

Directions for Nursing Research in the New Millennium

The new millennium witnessed many important increases in national, provincial, and local funding opportunities with several centres for nursing research created across Canada. In 2002, the Ontario Ministry of Health and Long Term Care awarded nearly $6 million to nursing research. In 2003, GRISIM (the *Groupe de recherche interuniversitaire en science infirmières de Montréal*) was established through provincial and private funding. In October 2008, GRISIM became GRI-ISIQ (Quebec Interuniversity Nursing Intervention Research Group) to include additional universities beyond Montreal (i.e., University of Sherbrooke and Laval University). In 2004, McMaster University and the University of Toronto collaborated to establish the Nursing Health Services Research Unit (NHSRU). The NHSRU has a multidisciplinary team of 46 co-investigators and more than 50 researchers representing nursing, business, labour studies, sociology, economics, health care policy, engineering, and anthropology. In 2007, the Knowledge Utilization Studies Program (KUSP) at the University of Alberta was established to focus on research utilization in nursing and other allied health professionals.

Nursing research continues to develop at a rapid pace and the impetus to provide evidence to guide advanced practice will undoubtedly lead to research collaborations flourishing in the years ahead. Certain trends for the 21st century are at the forefront:

⇒ *Heightened focus on EBP.* Efforts to translate research findings into practice continue even more vigorously. Nurses at all levels are encouraged to engage in evidence-based practice. In addition, involvement in translational research—the transfer of research findings to clinical settings—is of considerable interest.

⇒ *Stronger knowledge base through rigorous research and confirmatory methods.* Practicing nurses can only adopt new approaches based on corroborated or replicated findings. Corroboration can be achieved through **replication,** that is, repeating the same studies with different samples, contexts, or at different times to ensure that findings are robust.

⇒ *More emphasis on systematic reviews.* **Systematic reviews** gather and integrate research information on a given topic to draw conclusions about the quality of the evidence accumulated to date. Systematic reviews are central to EBP.

⇒ *Increased involvement in transdisciplinary research.* Research collaboration across disciplines continues to expand in the 21st century as researchers address fundamental health care problems from their complementary perspectives. CIHR has been supporting this trend through the funding of Strategic Training Initiative in Health Research (STIHR) where nurse researchers lead transdisciplinary groups of mentors and trainees (Loiselle, Sitaram, Hack, Bottorff, & Degner, 2008). For instance, a training initiative in cardiovascular nursing called FUTURE—Facilitating Unique Training Using Research and Education—and one in psychosocial oncology/oncology nursing, PORT—Psychosocial Oncology Research Training (Loiselle, Bottorff, Butler, & Degner, 2004) each have received 1.8 million over a period of 6 years to train the next generation of promising young researchers. PORT has been renewed for an additional six years and expanded to include trainees from Bangalore, India (Loiselle et al., 2008).

⇒ *Active dissemination of research findings.* The Internet and other modes of electronic communications have had a significant impact on the dissemination of research findings, which in turn help promote EBP. Through online publishing (e.g., the *Online Journal of Knowledge Synthesis for Nursing*); online resources such as Lippincott's NursingCenter.com; electronic document retrieval and delivery; e-mail; and electronic mailing lists, archived webcasts, information about innovations is accessed more widely and more quickly than ever before.

⇒ *Emphasis on the visibility of nursing research.* Efforts to increase the visibility of nursing research are expanding. Nurse researchers must bring forward their research to professional organizations, consumer organizations, government, the public, and the corporate world to garner support for their research.

⇒ *Enhanced focus on cultural and health disparity issues.* The topics of culturally sensitive care and health disparities have emerged as centre to nursing which, in turn, has stimulated discussion on the concept of ecologic validity. Ecologic validity refers to the extent to which the process and outcomes of research are relevant to various contexts, beliefs, behaviours, and values of diverse groups.

In terms of substantive areas, research priorities and goals for the future are also under discussion. The Think Tank on Nursing Science in Canada, a group of nurse researchers that sets the agenda for research goals and priorities, has identified two main goals: (1) minimizing barriers to the conduct of nursing research through more collaborative efforts between universities and teaching hospitals and (2) increasing designated funding for nursing research through formal research training programs at the master's and doctoral levels. In terms of research priorities, along with the Academy of Canadian Executive Nurses (ACEN), they have identified three main areas: (1) patient safety and quality-of-life issues, (2) nursing work environments and workload, and (3) evidence-based decision making.

SOURCES OF EVIDENCE FOR NURSING PRACTICE

As a nursing student, you are gaining skills on how to practice nursing and the process of learning about best-practice will continue throughout your career. Over a decade ago, Millenson (1997) estimated that 85% of health care practices were not scientifically supported. Although this percentage may have decreased since then, there is agreement that nursing practice should rely more heavily on solid evidence. Evidence hierarchies acknowledge certain sources of knowledge as superior to others. A brief description of these sources underscores how research-based knowledge is important.

Tradition and Authority

Within Western culture and within nursing, certain beliefs are accepted as truths—and certain practices are accepted as relevant—simply based on custom. However, tradition may undermine effective practices. Traditions may be so entrenched that their validity or usefulness is not questioned. There is growing concern that many nursing interventions are based on tradition rather than on sound evidence.

An additional source of knowledge is authority—for instance, a person recognized for their status or training. Reliance on authority is to some degree unavoidable; however, like tradition, authority as a knowledge source has its limitations. Authorities are not infallible (particularly if their expertise is based mainly on personal experience), yet their knowledge may at times go unchallenged.

Clinical Experience, Trial and Error, and Intuition

Clinical experience is a familiar source of knowledge. The ability to recognize regularities and to make predictions based on observations is a hallmark of the human mind. Nevertheless, personal experience has its own biases as each nurse's experience is typically too limited to generalize and therefore it cannot be readily transferred to other contexts. Likewise, sometimes we tackle problems by successively trying out alternative solutions. This approach may be practical, but it is often fallible and inefficient. Moreover, this approach tends to be haphazard, and the solutions are, in many instances, idiosyncratic.

Nurses sometimes rely on "intuition" in their practice. Intuition is a type of knowledge that cannot be accounted through reasoning or prior instruction. Although intuition undoubtedly plays a role in nursing practice—as it does in the conduct of research—it cannot serve as the basis for policies and practice guidelines for nurses.

Logical Reasoning

Inductive (from specific to more general) and deductive (from general to more specific) reasoning are useful strategies to understand the world around us but logical reasoning is highly dependant on the accuracy of the information that it is based upon.

Assembled Information

In making clinical decisions, health care professionals use information that has been assembled from various sources. For example, local, national, and international *bench-marking data* provide information on such issues as the rates of using various procedures (e.g., rates of caesarean deliveries) or rates of infection (e.g., rates of nosocomial pneumonia), which is useful in evaluating clinical practices. *Quality improvement and risk data*, such as medication error reports, can be used to assess practices and determine the need for practice change. Such sources, although offering useful information, do not provide direct information on whether improvement in patient outcomes is the result of their use.

Disciplined Research

Research conducted within a disciplined format is the most sophisticated method of acquiring evidence and also the most reliable. Current emphasis on evidence-based practice increasingly requires nurses to base their practice on research-based findings rather than on tradition, intuition, or personal experience. However, nursing will always remain a rich blend of art and science.

PARADIGMS AND METHODS FOR NURSING RESEARCH

A **paradigm** is a worldview, a general perspective on the complexities of the "real" world. Disciplined inquiry in the field of nursing is being conducted mainly (although not exclusively, as we discuss in Chapter 10) within two broad paradigms. This section describes the two paradigms and broadly outlines the research methods associated with them.

The Positivist/Postpositivist Paradigm

The paradigm that has dominated nursing for decades now is known as *positivism* (at times referred to as *logical positivism*). Positivism is rooted in 19th-century thought, guided by suchphilosophers as Comte, Newton, and Locke. Positivism is a reflection of a broader cultural phenomenon (*modernism*) that emphasizes the rational and the scientific.

As shown in Table 1.2, a fundamental assumption of positivists is that there is a reality *out there* that can be studied and known. Adherents of positivism assume that nature is basically ordered and regular and that an objective reality exists independent of human observation. In other words, the world is assumed not to be merely a creation of the human mind. The related assumption of **determinism**

TABLE 1.2	MAJOR ASSUMPTIONS OF THE POSITIVIST AND NATURALISTIC PARADIGMS	
TYPE OF ASSUMPTION	POSITIVIST PARADIGM	NATURALISTIC PARADIGM
The nature of reality	Reality exists; there is a real world driven by real natural causes	Reality is multiple, subjective, and mentally constructed by individuals
The relationship between the researcher and those being studied	The researcher is independent from those being researched	The researcher interacts with those being researched, and findings are the creation of the interaction
The role of values in the inquiry	Values are to be held in check; objectivity is sought	Subjectivity and values are inevitable and desirable
Best methods for obtaining evidence/ knowledge	⇒ Seeks generalizations ⇒ Emphasis on discrete concepts ⇒ Fixed design ⇒ Focus on the objective and quantifiable ⇒ Measured, quantitative information; statistical analysis ⇒ Control over context; decontextualized ⇒ Outsider knowledge—researcher as external ⇒ Verification of researcher's hunches ⇒ Focus on the product	⇒ Seeks patterns ⇒ Emphasis on the whole ⇒ Flexible design ⇒ Focus on the subjective and nonquantifiable ⇒ Narrative information; qualitative analysis ⇒ Context-bound; contextualized ⇒ Insider knowledge—researcher as internal ⇒ Emerging interpretations grounded in participants' experiences ⇒ Focus on product and process

refers to the positivists' belief that *phenomena* (observable facts and events) are not haphazard or random, but rather have antecedent causes. If a person develops lung cancer, the scientist in a positivist tradition assumes that there must be one or more reasons that can be potentially identified. Within the **positivist paradigm,** much research is aimed at understanding the underlying causes of natural phenomena.

Because of their belief in an objective reality, positivists seek to be objective. Their approach involves reliance on orderly, rigorous procedures with tight control over situations to test hunches about the nature of the phenomena being studied and relationships among them.

Strict positivist thinking has been challenged and few researchers adhere to the tenets of pure positivism. In the *postpositivist paradigm*, there is still a belief in reality and a desire to understand it, but postpositivists recognize the impossibility of total objectivity. They do, however, seek objectivity and strive to be as neutral as possible. Postpositivists also appreciate the challenges of knowing reality with certainty and therefore seek *probabilistic* evidence—that is, what the true state of a phenomenon *probably* is, with a high and ascertainable degree of likelihood. This modified positivist position remains a dominant force in nursing research. For the sake of simplicity, we refer to it as positivism.

The Naturalistic Paradigm

The **naturalistic paradigm** (also referred to as the *constructivist paradigm*) began as a countermovement to positivism with writers such as Weber and Kant. The naturalistic paradigm represents an important alternative approach for conducting nursing research. Table 1.2 compares four major assumptions of the positivist and naturalistic paradigms.

For the naturalistic inquirer, reality is not a fixed entity but rather a construction of the individuals participating in the research; reality exists within a context, and many constructions are possible. Naturalists thus take the position of relativism: if there are always multiple interpretations of reality that exist in people's minds, then there is no process by which the ultimate truth or falsity of the constructions can be determined.

The naturalistic paradigm assumes that knowledge is maximized when the distance between the inquirer and the participants in the study is minimized. The voices and interpretations of those under study are keys to understanding the phenomenon of interest, and subjective interactions are the primary way to access them. The findings from a naturalistic inquiry are the product of the interaction between the inquirer and the participants.

Paradigms and Methods: Quantitative and Qualitative Research

Research methods are the techniques researchers use to structure a study and to gather and analyze information relevant to the research question(s). The two alternative paradigms have strong implications for the choice of research methods. Methods typically differ according to whether one conducts **quantitative research,** which is most closely allied with the positivist paradigm, and **qualitative research,** which is most often associated with naturalistic inquiry. However, positivists sometimes undertake qualitative studies, and naturalistic researchers sometimes collect quantitative data. This section provides an overview of methods linked to the two paradigms.

The Scientific Method and Quantitative Research

The traditional, positivist **scientific method** is a general set of orderly, disciplined procedures used to acquire information. Quantitative researchers typically use deductive reasoning to generate predictions that are tested in the "real" world. They use a *systematic* approach, meaning that the investigators progress logically through a series of steps, according to a prespecified plan. The researchers use various "controls" to minimize biases and maximize precision and validity.

Empirical evidence is rigorously gathered (i.e., evidence collected directly or indirectly through the senses rather than through personal hunches). In the positivist paradigm, information is gathered systematically, using already tested means. Usually the information gathered is quantitative—that is, numeric information that is subsequently analyzed through statistical procedures. Scientists strive to go beyond the specifics of a research situation; the degree to which findings can be generalized is an agreed upon criterion for evaluating the quality and importance of quantitative studies.

Example of an internationally renowned Canadian nurse researcher who relies mainly on quantitative methods

Dr. Celeste Johnston is Professor in the School of Nursing at McGill University. She is also a James McGill Professor and Associate Director for Research at the School. Dr. Johnston is among the few nurses in Canada to have been a Fellow of The Canadian Academy of Health Sciences and received the one time CNA Centennial Award for her work on pain. During her term as president of the Canadian Pain Society, Dr. Johnston founded the Canadian Pain Coalition. In addition, she has jointly established the *Groupe de recherche interuniversitaire en interventions en sciences infirmières en Québec* (GRIISIQ) with her colleague Dr. Nicole Ricard. GRIISIQ is the first consortium of nurse researchers in Canada focusing on the design, implementation, and testing of nursing interventions. Dr. Johnston is at the forefront of pain research among preterm infants and her work has become the leading authority in pain assessment and management in this population. Some of her earlier works included contributing to the development of the Premature Infant Pain Profile (PIIP) (Stevens, Johnston, Petryshen, & Taddio, 1996) and leading studies examining the impact of sucrose analgesia on the pain response of preterm neonates (Johnston, Stremler, Horton, & Friedman, 1997; Stevens et al., 1999). More recently, Dr. Johnston has studied the impact of Kangaroo care as a nonpharmacological intervention to reduce infant pain during painful procedures (Johnston et al., 2003, 2008). These studies have all used quantitative methods.

The traditional scientific method used by quantitative researchers has enjoyed considerable recognition, and it has been used productively by nurse researchers studying a wide range of nursing problems. This is not to say, however, that this approach can solve all nursing problems such as certain moral or ethical issues. Therefore, nursing cannot rely exclusively on scientific information.

The scientific method also must contend with problems of *measurement*. In studying a phenomenon, scientists attempt to measure it—that is, to attach numeric values that express quantity. Physiologic phenomena such as blood pressure can be measured with accuracy and precision, however, the same cannot be said of some psychosocial phenomena. If the phenomenon of interest is an individual's hope in the face of a terminal illness, a researcher may be challenged in finding the most objective means to measure a patient's level of hope (e.g., high versus low). A final issue is that most nursing research focuses on human beings who are inherently complex and diverse. Within any given study, the scientific method focuses on a particular facet of the human experience (e.g., weight gain, chemical dependency). Sometimes this narrower focus can lead to a narrower or fragmented view of the world—one main criticism of the positivist paradigm.

Naturalistic Methods and Qualitative Research

Naturalistic methods of inquiry deal with human complexity by exploring it. Researchers in the naturalistic tradition acknowledge the inherent depth of humans, the ability of humans to shape and create their own experiences, and the idea that "truth" is a composite of realities. Naturalistic researchers tend to focus on the dynamic, holistic, and individual aspects of phenomena and attempt to capture those aspects in their entirety, within the context of those who are experiencing them. Consequently, naturalistic investigations emphasize *understanding* the human experience as it is lived, usually through the collection and analysis of qualitative materials that are narrative and subjective.

Flexible, evolving procedures are used to capitalize on findings that emerge in the course of the study. Naturalistic inquiry takes place in natural settings (in the *field*), frequently over extended periods of time. The collection of information and its analysis typically progress concurrently. Researchers sift through the existing information to gain insight with new questions emerging to be further explored. Through an inductive process, the researcher integrates the evidence to develop a framework that helps explain the phenomenon under study.

Example of an internationally renowned Canadian nurse researcher who relies mainly on qualitative methods

Dr. Sally Thorne is the Director of the School of Nursing at the University of British Columbia (UBC) and a nurse anthropologist. Dr. Thorne's program of research focuses on patient—health care professional communication patterns particularly within the context of a cancer diagnosis (e.g., Maheu & Thorne, 2008; Thorne, Hislop, Armstrong, & Oglov, 2008). She is the principal investigator of the Communication in Cancer Care research group at UBC. Dr. Thorne is an expert in the design and implementation of qualitative research methodologies. In addition to publishing the findings of her qualitative research in nationally and internationally renowned journals, she has published several position papers, book chapters, and an entire book on the topic of qualitative methodology (e.g., McPherson & Thorne, 2006; Thorne, 2004, 2008, 2009; Thorne, Kirkham, & O'Flynn-Magee, 2004).

Naturalistic studies yield rich, in-depth information that can potentially clarify the multiple dimensions of a complicated phenomenon (e.g., the process by which patients with a serious illness). The findings from in-depth qualitative research are typically grounded in the real-life experiences of people with first-hand knowledge of a phenomenon. The highly personal approach that enriches the analytic insights, however, can sometimes result in trivial or superficial findings by less skilful researchers.

TIP
Researchers usually are not explicit in the naming of the specific paradigm that underlies their studies. Qualitative researchers, however, are more likely to mention that the naturalistic paradigm guided their inquiry than quantitative researchers are to mention positivism.

Multiple Paradigms and Nursing Research

Paradigms are lenses that assist in sharpening the focus on a particular phenomenon; they should not be blinders that limit our intellectual curiosity. The emergence of divergent paradigms in research is a healthy and desirable trend. Nursing knowledge would be meagre, indeed, without a rich array of approaches and methods available within the two paradigms—methods that are often complementary in their strengths and limitations.

We have emphasized the differences between the positivist and naturalistic paradigms and their associated methods so that their distinctions would be easy to understand. Despite their differences, however, these paradigms have many features in common:

⇝ *Ultimate goal of gaining understanding.* Both quantitative and qualitative researchers seek to capture "the truth" about an aspect of the world in which they are interested, and both can make significant—and mutually beneficial—contributions to nursing.

⇝ *Empirical evidence.* Researchers in both traditions gather and analyze evidence empirically, that is, through their senses. Neither qualitative nor quantitative researchers are "armchair" analysts, relying on their own beliefs to generate knowledge.

⇝ *Reliance on human cooperation.* Evidence for nursing research comes primarily from humans, so the need for human cooperation is essential. To understand people's characteristics and experiences, researchers must encourage them to participate in research *and* to act and speak openly.

⇝ *Ethical constraints.* Research with human beings is guided by ethical principles that may compete with the goals of the inquiry (e.g., the investigation of a promising nursing intervention that is offered only to the experimental group). As discussed in Chapter 5, ethical dilemmas often confront researchers, regardless of paradigms or methods.

⇝ *Fallibility of research.* Virtually all studies—in either paradigm—have limitations. Every research question can be addressed in many different ways, and inevitably there are tradeoffs. No single study can ever definitively answer a research question. Each study adds to a body of accumulating evidence.

Thus, despite philosophical and methodological differences, researchers using the positivist or naturalistic method share overall goals and face many challenges. The selection of an appropriate method depends to some degree on the researcher's worldview and training but also on the nature of the research question. If a researcher asks, "What is the impact of a tailored approach to patient education on patients' psychosocial adjustment to illness?" the researcher may decide to rely on a quantitative approach if the research questions relate to the measurement of knowledge, anxiety, and well-being. Researchers may rely on qualitative methods if the goal is to document patients' experiences with the teaching approach under investigation.

In reading about the alternative paradigms for nursing research, you may be more attracted to one of the two paradigms—the paradigm that corresponds most closely to your view of the world and of reality. Learning about and respecting both approaches to disciplined inquiry, however, and recognizing the strengths and limitations of each are important. In this textbook, we provide an overview of the methods associated with both qualitative and quantitative research and offer guidance on how to understand, critique, and use findings from both.

> TIP
>
> How can you tell whether a study is qualitative or quantitative? As you progress through this book, you should be able to tell based on the title, or the terms appearing in the abstract at the beginning of the report. At this point, though, it may be easiest to distinguish the two types of studies based on whether *numbers* appear in the report, especially in tables. Qualitative studies may have no tables with numeric information, or only a single table with numbers describing participants' characteristics (e.g., how many males and females). Quantitative studies typically present several tables with numbers and statistical information. Qualitative studies, by contrast, may have "word tables" or diagrams illustrating processes inferred from the narrative information gathered.

PURPOSES OF NURSING RESEARCH

The general purpose of nursing research is to answer questions or solve problems of relevance to nursing. Sometimes a distinction is made between basic and applied nursing research. *Basic research* seeks to extend the knowledge base in a discipline. For example, the study of grieving may be undertaken without the *explicit* goal of modifying nursing practice. *Applied research* focuses on finding solutions to issues in nursing practice. A study on the effectiveness of a nursing intervention to facilitate the process of grieving, for instance, would be considered applied research.

> TIP
>
> Researchers rarely specify whether their intent is to address a clinical problem or to generate basic knowledge. The underlying orientation of a study (whether basic or applied) generally has to be inferred and, in some cases, it may be ambiguous.

The specific purposes of nursing research include identification, description, exploration, explanation, prediction, and control. Within each purpose, nurse researchers address various types of questions; certain questions are more amenable to qualitative than to quantitative inquiry, and vice versa.

Identification and Description

Qualitative research often focuses on phenomena that are poorly understood. In some cases, so little is known that the phenomenon has yet to be clearly identified—or has been inadequately defined or conceptualized. The in-depth, probing nature of qualitative research is well suited to answering such questions as, "What is this phenomenon?" and "What is its name?" (Table 1.3). In quantitative research, by contrast, researchers begin with a phenomenon that has been clearly defined, sometimes through a prior qualitative study. Thus, in quantitative research, identification typically precedes the inquiry.

TABLE 1.3	RESEARCH PURPOSES AND RESEARCH QUESTIONS	
PURPOSE	TYPES OF QUESTIONS: QUANTITATIVE RESEARCH	TYPES OF QUESTIONS: QUALITATIVE RESEARCH
Identification		What is this phenomenon? What is its name?
Description	How prevalent is the phenomenon? How often does the phenomenon occur? What are the characteristics of the phenomenon?	What are the dimensions of the phenomenon? What variations exist? What is important about the phenomenon?
Exploration	What factors are related to the phenomenon? What are the antecedents of the phenomenon?	What is the full nature of the phenomenon? What is really going on here? What is the process by which the phenomenon evolves or is experienced?
Explanation	What are the measurable associations between phenomena? What factors cause the phenomenon? Does the theory explain the phenomenon?	How does the phenomenon work? Why does the phenomenon exist? What is the meaning of the phenomenon? How did the phenomenon occur?
Prediction and control	What will happen if we alter a phenomenon or introduce an intervention? If phenomenon X occurs, will phenomenon Y follow? How can we make the phenomenon happen, or alter its nature or prevalence? Can the occurrence of the phenomenon be controlled?	

Qualitative example of identification

Pilkington and Kilpatrick (2008) conducted an in-depth study to explore the lived experience of suffering among 12 elderly persons residing in two long-term care facilities in Canada. The researchers identified three core concepts to describe the participants' experience with suffering: (1) unbounded desolation—knowing isolation, (2) resolute acquiescence—going on living in the face of suffering, and (3) benevolent affiliation—alliances with others to assist in living with suffering.

Description of phenomena is another important purpose of research. In descriptive studies, researchers observe, count, delineate, elucidate, and classify. Nurse researchers have described a wide variety of phenomena. Examples include patients' stress levels, health beliefs, and pain responses. Quantitative description focuses on the prevalence, size, and measurable attributes of phenomena. Qualitative description, on the other hand, relies on in-depth exploration to describe the dimensions, variations, and importance of phenomena. Table 1.3 compares descriptive questions posed by quantitative and qualitative inquiries.

Exploration

Similar to descriptive research, exploratory research begins with a phenomenon of interest, but goes beyond description by investigating the full nature of the phenomenon and factors related to it. For example, a *descriptive quantitative study* of preoperative stress might document the levels of stress experienced by patients and the percentage of patients who experienced high as opposed to low levels. An exploratory study might ask: What factors are related to a patient's stress level? Do a patient's clinical outcomes change in relation to the level of stress experienced? Exploratory qualitative research seeks to shed light on the various processes related to the manifestation of a particular phenomenon.

Quantitative example of description

Armstrong-Esther et al. (2008) undertook a study to describe gerontological nurses' knowledge of antipsychotic drugs, including their knowledge about dosing and side effects, and nurses' use of the medication such as the reasons for administering the antipsychotic drugs and length of time used.

Qualitative example of description

Woodgate (2008) undertook an in-depth study to describe the feelings of children and adolescents diagnosed with cancer as they relate to their cancer symptoms.

Quantitative example of exploration

Hall (2008) explored, through a quantitative survey, the career planning and development needs of registered nurses working in native reserves and in Inuit communities in rural and remote areas of Ontario.

Qualitative example of exploration

Maheu and Thorne (2008) interviewed 21 women with a past diagnosis of breast and/or ovarian cancer and a family history of cancer to explore ways in which they experienced and understood inconclusive BRCA 1/2 genetic test results.

Prediction and Control

Many phenomena defy explanation and it is difficult to understand their causes. Yet it is often possible to predict phenomena even without a complete understanding. For example, research has shown that the incidence of Down syndrome in infants increases with age of the mother. We can predict that a woman aged 40 years is at higher risk for bearing a child with Down syndrome than a woman aged 25. We can partially control the outcome by educating women about this risk and offering testing. Note, however, that in this example even though we can somewhat predict and control the phenomenon, it does not explain *why* older women are at higher risk.

Quantitative example of prediction

Semenic, Loiselle, and Gottlieb (2008) studied the potential influence of sociodemographic, psychosocial, and perinatal factors on the length of exclusive breastfeeding among 189 Canadian primiparous mothers. Breastfeeding self-efficacy, in-hospital formula supplementation, prenatal class attendance, and type of delivery independently predicted women's reliance on exclusive breastfeeding.

Explanation

The goals of explanatory research are to understand the underpinnings of natural phenomena and to explain systematic relationships among phenomena. Explanatory research is often linked to a *theory*, which represents a method of organizing and integrating ideas about the manner in which phenomena are manifested or interrelated. Whereas descriptive research provides new information, and exploratory research provides promising insights, explanatory research focuses on understanding the causes or full nature of a phenomenon.

In quantitative research, theories or prior findings are used deductively as the basis for generating explanations that are then tested empirically. That is, based on existing theory or a body of evidence, researchers make specific predictions that, if upheld by the findings, lend credibility to the explanation. In qualitative studies, researchers may search for explanations about how or why a phenomenon exists or what a phenomenon means as a basis for developing a theory that is grounded in rich, in-depth, experiential evidence.

Quantitative example of explanation
Godin, Bélanger-Gravel, and Nolin (2008) designed a study to explain how body mass index (BMI) might influence leisure-time physical activity. The researcher used the Theory of Planned Behavior to test possible relationships among the study variables. Findings pointed to the explanation as to why high BMI has a significant negative effect on leisure-time physical activity.

Qualitative example of explanation
Mordoch and Hall (2008) undertook a study to explain how children, between 6 and 16 years of age, managed their experiences of living with a parent with depression, schizophrenia, or bipolar disorder.

> **TIP**
>
> It is the researchers' responsibility to explain the purpose of the study, and this usually happens fairly early in a research report. Most nursing studies have multiple aims. Almost all studies have some descriptive intent. Some exploratory studies are undertaken with the expectation that the results will serve a predictive or control function. Pure explanatory studies are the least common in the nursing literature.

NURSING RESEARCH AND EBP

The nursing and medical literatures have treated the topic of evidence-based practice at some length (e.g., DiCenso et al., 1998, 2005; Estabrooks, 1998; Guyatt & Rennie, 2002; Melnyk & Fineout-Overholt, 2005). The types of studies providing evidence to guide practice have focused on etiology, screening, and detection; diagnosis and assessment; prognosis; treatment, therapy, and interventions; and meaning. The results of many of these studies have been instrumental in advancing EBP. Here are some examples of these contributions.

Assessment and Diagnosis

Nursing studies have increasingly focused on the development of tools to assess individuals and to measure important health-related clinical outcomes. The contribution of high-quality assessment tools is crucial for EBP.

Example of a study aimed at assessment
Gelinas, Fillion, and Puntillo (2009) conducted a study to test a promising instrument called C-POT aimed at assessing pain among non verbal patients.

Treatment, Therapy, or Intervention

Many nursing studies seek to evaluate particular treatment modalities or therapies as well as compare various types of nursing interventions and their impact on patient outcomes. Such intervention studies play a critical role in EBP.

Example of a study aimed at testing an intervention
Loiselle et al. (2009) are testing the impact of a multimedia patient education intervention on cancer knowledge, perceived competence, and support for autonomy among individuals with melanoma or colorectal cancer.

Meaning and Processes

Research that provides evidence on what health and illness mean to patients is important for EBP. A promising program of research by Dr. Virigina Lee in Quebec points to the various ways that patients can be supported through the process of making meaning through the experience of a serious illness.

Example of a study aimed at documenting meaning making in illness
Lee (2008) tested a nursing intervention aimed at enhancing meaning making in the context of a cancer diagnosis.

ASSISTANCE TO CONSUMERS OF NURSING RESEARCH

This book is designed to assist you in enhancing skills needed to review, evaluate, and use nursing studies (i.e., to become skilful consumers of nursing research). In each chapter, we present information related to the content and process of undertaking research and provide specific guidance in several ways. First, we offer tips on what you can expect to find in actual research reports according to the content of the particular chapters. These include tips that help you find concepts discussed in this book.

Second, we include guidelines for critiquing the aspects of a study covered in each chapter. The questions in Box 1.1 are designed to assist you in using the

---

BOX 1.1 QUESTIONS FOR A PRELIMINARY OVERVIEW OF A RESEARCH REPORT

1. How relevant is the research problem to the actual practice of nursing? Does the study focus on a topic that is considered a priority area for nursing research?
2. Is the research quantitative or qualitative?
3. What is the underlying purpose (or purposes) of the study—identification, description, exploration, explanation, or prediction and control?
4. What might be some clinical implications of this research? To what type of people and settings is the research most relevant? If the findings are accurate, how might the results of this study be used by *me*?

information in this chapter in an overall preliminary assessment of a research report. Last, the critical thinking activities at the end of each chapter guide you through appraisals of real research examples of both qualitative and quantitative studies (some of which are presented in their entirety in the appendices). These activities also challenge you to think about how the findings from these studies could be used in nursing practice.

TIP

The following websites are useful starting points for further information about nursing research and EBP:

- *Canadian Association for Nursing Research: http://www.canr.ca*
- *Canadian Association of Schools of Nursing: http://www.casn.ca*
- *Canadian Health Services Research Foundation (CHSRF): http://www/chsrf.ca*
- *Canadian-International Nurse Researcher Database: http://nurseresearcher.com*
- *Canadian Institutes of Health Research (CIHR): http://www.cihr-irsc.gc.ca*
- *Canadian Nurses Association: http://www.cna-nurses.ca*
- *Canadian Nurses Foundation: http://canadiannursesfoundation.ca*
- *Cochrane Collaboration: http:www.cochrane.org*
- *Lippincott's Nursing Center: http:www.nursingcenter.com*
- *National Centre for Knowledge Transfer: http://ckt-ctc.ca*
- *National Institute of Nursing Research: http://ninr.nih.gov/ninr*
- *Agency for Healthcare Research and Quality: http:www.ahrq.gov*
- *Sigma Theta Tau International: http:www.nursingsociety.org*

RESEARCH EXAMPLES AND CRITICAL THINKING ACTIVITIES

EXAMPLE 1 ■ Quantitative Research

Aspects of a quantitative nursing study, featuring terms, and concepts discussed in this chapter are presented below, followed by some questions to guide critical thinking.

Study

"Telehome monitoring in patients with cardiac disease who are at high risk of readmission" (Woodend et al., 2008)

Study Purpose

Individuals with chronic conditions, such as heart failure and angina, use many health care services repeatedly. The researchers tested the impact of a 3-month telehome monitoring intervention on hospital readmission, quality of life, and functional status among individuals with heart failure or angina.

Research Method

A randomized controlled study was undertaken with 249 participants with heart failure ($n = 121$) or angina ($n = 128$) who were randomly assigned to the intervention or usual care group. An equal number of participants with hearth failure or angina were assigned to the intervention ($n = 62$). The intervention consisted of 3 months of weekly video conferencing with a nurse, daily phone line transmission of weight and blood pressure readings as well as periodic communication of 12-lead electrocardiogram results. A technician visited participants' homes shortly following discharge from the hospital to install the home-monitoring system and provide training to the participants on its use.

Patient Outcomes

The outcomes variables selected by the researchers to evaluate the effectiveness of the intervention included (1) readmission, (2) health care resource use, (3) morbidity (symptoms and functional status), and (4) quality of life. Data were collected at 1 month, 3 months, and 1 year postdischarge.

Key Findings

- Telehome monitoring significantly reduced the number of hospital readmissions and days spent in the hospital for participants with angina.
- The intervention significantly improved quality of life and functional status in participants with heart failure or angina.
- Overall, participants found the technology easy to use and were satisfied with the intervention.

Conclusions

The researchers concluded that telehealth technologies are an appropriate way of providing home monitoring to patients with heart disease at high risk of hospital readmission.

CRITICAL THINKING SUGGESTIONS

1. Answer the questions from Box 1.1 (p. 19) regarding this study.
2. Also consider the following targeted questions, which may assist you in assessing aspects of the study's merit:
   a. Why do you think Woodend and colleagues (2008) decided to have a group of patients who received usual care?
   b. If you wanted to replicate this study to see whether the findings could be confirmed, what might you want to change to maximize the utility of the replication study? For example, what type of individuals would you recruit to participate?
   c. Could this study have been undertaken as a qualitative study? Why or why not?

EXAMPLE 2 ■ Qualitative Research

Aspects of a qualitative nursing study, featuring key terms, and concepts discussed in this chapter are presented below, followed by some questions to guide critical thinking.

Study

"Perinatal beliefs and practices of immigrant Punjabi women living in Canada" (Grewal, Bhagat, & Balneaves, 2008)

Study Purpose

Grewal et al. (2008) conducted an in-depth study to describe the knowledge and cultural traditions surrounding the new immigrant Punjabi women's perinatal experiences and the ways in which their traditional beliefs and practices are legitimized and incorporated into the Canadian health care context.

Research Method

Grewal et al. (2008) recruited 15 first-time mothers who had emigrated within the past 5 years to Canada from Punjab, India. Members of a South Asian women's advocacy group were contacted to ask them to discuss the study within the Punjabi community and health care professionals at a large urban centre in British Columbia and to invite eligible women to participate in the study. Participants took part in a face-to-face, individual interview conducted by an experienced female research assistant who was known to the community, had children, was originally from Punjab and who was fluent in both Punjabi and English. All interviews were conducted in Punjabi and lasted about 1.5 hours. Interviews were tape-recorded, translated into English, and transcribed for analysis. All transcripts were reviewed

(Research Examples and Critical Thinking Activities continues on page 22)

Research Examples and Critical Thinking Activities (continued)

by one of the authors who speaks Punjabi. In addition, five Punjabi health professionals who currently work with women in the immigrant Punjabi community in British Columbia were invited to participate in a focus group to review the preliminary study findings.

Key Findings

The women who participated in this study ranged in age from 21 to 31 years and had been residing in Canada for an average of 2 years. Three major categories emerged from the analysis of the transcripts: (1) the pervasiveness of traditional health beliefs and practices relating to the perinatal period, including diet, lifestyle (e.g., avoiding stress), and rituals (e.g., creating a positive energy); (2) the important role of family members in supporting women during the perinatal experiences such as obtaining help from their husband for transportation and obtaining advice from other family members; and (3) the positive and negative interactions women had with health professionals in the Canadian health care system.

Conclusions

The researchers concluded that to ensure culturally safe care to immigrant Punjabi women and their families during the perinatal period, change is required among health professionals (e.g., education to foster culturally sensitive care), the health care system (e.g., acknowledgement of the beliefs, values, and practices of Punjabi women), and the community (e.g., partnering with community leaders).

CRITICAL THINKING SUGGESTIONS

1. Answer the questions in Box 1.1 (p. 19) regarding this study.

2. Also consider the following targeted questions, which may assist you in assessing aspects of the study's merit:
   a. Why do you think Grewal et al. collected data from the participants in addition to consulting health professionals?
   b. Why do you think that the researchers audiotaped and transcribed their interviews and then reviewed them with study participants?
   c. Do you think it would have been appropriate for Grewal et al. to conduct this study using quantitative research methods? Why or why not?

EXAMPLE 3 ■ Quantitative Research

1. Read the abstract and the introduction from the study by Bryanton et al. (2008) ("Predictors of Early Parenting Self-Efficacy") in Appendix A of this book, and then answer the questions in Box 1.1 (p. 19).

2. Also consider the following targeted questions, which may further sharpen your critical thinking skills and assist you in assessing aspects of the study's merit:
   a. What gap in the existing body of research was the study designed to fill?
   b. Would you describe this study as applied or basic, based on information provided in the abstract?
   c. Could this study have been undertaken as a qualitative study? Why or why not?
   d. Who financially supported this research? (This information appears in a footnote at the end of the report.)

EXAMPLE 4 ■ Qualitative Research

1. Read the abstract and the introduction from the study by Woodgate, Ateah, and Secco (2008) ("Child with Autism") in Appendix B of this book, and then answer the questions in Box 1.1 (p. 19).

2. Also consider the following targeted questions, which may further sharpen your critical thinking skills and assist you in assessing aspects of the study's merit:
   a. What gap in the existing research was the study designed to fill?
   b. Was Woodgate's study conducted within the positivist paradigm or the naturalistic paradigm? Provide a rationale for your choice.

Summary Points

- ➢ **Nursing research** is a systematic inquiry to develop knowledge about issues of importance to nurses and serves to establish a base of knowledge for nursing practice.

- ➢ Nurses in various settings are pursuing an **evidence-based practice** (EBP) that incorporates research findings into their decisions and their interactions with clients.

- ➢ Knowledge of nursing **research methods** enhances the professional practice of all nurses, including both consumers of research (who read, evaluate, and use studies) and producers of research (who design and undertake studies).

- ➢ Nursing research began with Florence Nightingale but developed slowly until its rapid acceleration in the 1950s. Since the 1970s, nursing research has focused on problems related to clinical practice.

- ➢ The **Canadian Health Services Research Foundation** (CHSRF) has been funding a series of research chairs and related programs specific to nursing since 1999.

- ➢ Future emphases of nursing research are likely to include EBP and research utilization projects, **replications** of research, integrative reviews, transdisciplinary studies, expanded dissemination efforts, and outcomes research.

- ➢ Disciplined research is widely considered superior to other sources of evidence for nursing practice, such as tradition, authority, clinical experience, trial and error, and intuition.

- ➢ Disciplined inquiry in nursing is conducted mainly within two broad **paradigms,** or worldviews with underlying assumptions about the complexities of reality: the positivist paradigm and the naturalistic paradigm.

- ➢ Researchers in the **positivist paradigm** assume that there is an objective reality and that natural *phenomena* (observable facts and events) are regular and orderly. The related assumption of **determinism** refers to the belief that events are not haphazard but rather the result of prior causes. Pure positivism has been replaced with a *postpositivist* perspective that acknowledges the difficulty of making totally objective observations and knowing reality with certainty.

- ➢ Researchers in the **naturalistic paradigm** assume that reality is not a fixed entity but is rather a construction of human minds, and thus "truth" is a composite of multiple constructions of reality.

- ➢ The positivist paradigm is associated with **quantitative research**—the collection and analysis of numeric information. Quantitative research is typically conducted within the traditional **scientific method,** which is a systematic and controlled process. Quantitative researchers base their findings on **empirical evidence** (evidence collected by way of the human senses) and strive for generalizability of their findings beyond a single setting or situation.

- ➢ Researchers within the naturalistic paradigm emphasize understanding the human experience as it is lived through the collection and analysis of subjective, narrative materials using flexible procedures that evolve in the field; this paradigm is associated with **qualitative research.**

- ➢ Nursing research can be either *basic* (designed to provide information for the sake of knowledge) or *applied* (designed to solve specific problems). Research purposes include identification, description, exploration, explanation, prediction, and control.

STUDIES CITED IN CHAPTER 1*

*This reference list contains only those studies that were cited in this chapter. Citations pertaining to theoretical, methodological, or nonempirical work are included together in a separate section at the end of the book (beginning on page 399).

Armstrong-Esther, C., Hagen, B., Smith, C., & Snelgrove, S. (2008). An exploratory study of nurses' knowledge of antipsychotic drug use with older persons. *Quality in Ageing, 9*(1), 29–40.

Bryanton, J., Gagnon, A. J., Hatem, M., & Johnston, C. (2008). Predictors of early parenting self-efficacy: Results of a prospective cohort study. *Nursing Research, 57*(4), 252–259.

Cameron, S. J., Armstrong-Stassen, M., Kane, D., & Moro, F. B. P. (2008). Musculoskeletal problems experienced by older nurses in hospital settings. *Nursing Forum, 43*(2), 103–114.

Chernomas, W. M., Clarke, D. E., & Marchinko, S. (2008). Relationship-based support for women living with serious mental illness. *Issues in Mental Health Nursing, 29*(5), 437–453.

Dean, R. A. K., & Major, J. E. (2008). From critical care comfort: The sustaining value of humour. *Journal of Clinical Nursing, 17*(8), 1088–1095.

DiCenso, A., Cullum, N., & Ciliska, D. (1998). Implementing evidence-based nursing: Some misconceptions. *Evidence-Based Nursing, 1*(2), 38–40.

Estabrooks, C. A. (1998). Will evidence-based nursing practice make practice perfect? *Canadian Journal of Nursing Research, 30,* 15–36.

Gelinas, C., Fillion, L., & Puntillo, K. A. (2009). Item selection and content validity of the critical-care pain observation tool for non-verbal adults. *Journal of Advanced Nursing, 65*(1), 203–216.

Godin, G., Bélanger-Gravel, A., & Nolin, B. (2008). Mechanism by which BMI influences leisure-time physical activity behavior. *Obesity, 16*(6), 1314–1317.

Grewal, S. K., Bhagat, R., & Balneaves, L. G. (2008). Perinatal beliefs and practices of immigrant Punjabi women living in Canada. *Journal of Obstetric, Gynecologic, & Neonatal Nursing, 37*(3), 290–300.

Guyatt, G., & Rennie, D. (2002). Users' guide to the medical literature: Essentials of evidence-based clinical practice. Chicago: American Medical Association Press.

Hall, L. M. (2008). Career planning and development needs of rural and remote nurses. *Journal of Research in Nursing, 13,* 207–217.

Johnston, C. C., Filion, F., Campbell-Yeo, M., et al. (2008). Kangaroo mother care diminishes pain from heel lance in very preterm neonates: A crossover trial. *BMC Pediatrics, 8,* 13.

Johnston, C. C., Stevens, B., Pinelli, J., et al. (2003). Kangaroo care is effective in diminishing pain response in preterm neonates. *Archives of Pediatrics & Adolescent Medicine, 157,* 1084–1088.

Johnston, C. C., Stremler, R., Horton, L., & Friedman, A. (1997). Single versus triple dose of sucrose for pain in preterm neonates. *Biology of the Neonate, 75,* 160–166.

Johnston, C., Stremler, R., Stevens, B., & Horton, L. (1997). Effectiveness of oral sucrose and simulated rocking on pain response in preterm neonates. *Pain, 72*(1/2), 193–199.

Lang, A., Edwards, N., & Fleiszer A. (2008). Safety in home care: A broadened perspective of patient safety. *International Journal for Quality in Health Care, 20,* 130–135.

Lee, V. (2008). The existential plight of cancer: Meaning making as a concrete approach to the intangible search for meaning. *Support Care Cancer, 16,* 779–785.

Loiselle, C. G., Bottorff, J., Butler, L., & Degner, L. F. (2004). PORT—Psychosocial Oncology Research Training: A newly funded strategic initiative in health research. *Canadian Journal of Nursing Research (CJNR), 36*(1), 159–164.

Loiselle, C. G., Koerner, A., Wiljer, D., & Fitch, M. (2009). *Contributions of an innovative multimedia tool to patients' experiences with melanoma or colorectal cancer: A mixed method approach.* Unpublished grant proposal funded by the Canadian Partnership Against Cancer (CPAC).

Loiselle, C. G., Sitaram, B., Hack, T. H., Bottorff J., & Degner, L. F. (2008). Canada and India partnering to advance oncology nursing research. *Oncology Nursing Forum (ONF), 35*(4), 583–587.

Maheu, C., & Thorne, S. (2008). Receiving inconclusive genetic test results: An interpretive description of the BRCA1/2 experience. *Research in Nursing and Health, 31*(6), 553–562.

McPherson, G., & Thorne, S. (2006). Exploiting exceptions to enhance interpretive qualitative health research: Insights from a study of cancer communication. *International Journal of Qualitative Methodology, 5*(2), 1–11.

Melnyk, B. M., & Fineout-Overhold, E. (2005). *Evidence- based practice in nursing and healthcare: A guide to best practice.* Philadelphia: Lippincott Williams & Wilkins.

Millenson, M. L. (1997). *Demanding medical excellence: Doctors and accountability in the information age* (p. 469). London: University of Chicago Press.

Mordoch, E., & Hall, W. A. (2008). Children's perceptions of living with a parent with a mental illness: Finding the rhythm and maintaining the frame. *Qualitative Health Research, 18*(8), 1127–1144.

Pilkington, F. B., & Kilpatrick, D. (2008). The lived experience of suffering: A Parse research method study. *Nursing Science Quarterly, 21*(3), 228–237.

Ploeg J., Davies, B., Edwards, N., Gifford, W., & Miller, P. (2007). Factors influencing best-practice guideline implementation: Lessons learned from administrators, nursing staff and project leaders. *Worldviews Evidenced Based Nursing, 4*(4), 210–219.

Semenic, S., Loiselle, C., & Gottlieb, L. (2008). Predictors of the duration of exclusive breastfeeding among first-time mothers. *Research in Nursing and Health, 31*(5), 428–441.

Stetler, C. B., & Marram, G. (1976). Evaluating research findings for applicability in practice. *Nursing Outlook,* 24, 559–563.

Stevens, B., Johnston, C., Franck, L., Petryshen, P., Jack, A., & Foster, G. (1999). The efficacy of developmentally sensitive interventions and sucrose for relieving procedural pain in very low birth weight neonates. *Nursing research, 48*(1), 35–43.

Stevens, B., Johnston, C., Petryshen, P., & Taddio, A. (1996). Premature infant pain profile: Development and initial validation. *The Clinical Journal of Pain, 12*(1), 13–22.

Thorne, S. (2004). Qualitative secondary analysis. In M. Lewis-Beck, A. Bryman, & T. F. Liao (Eds.), *Encyclopedia of research methods for the social science* (Vol. 3, p. 1006). Thousand Oaks, CA: Sage.

Thorne, S. (2009). The role of qualitative research within an evidence-based context: Can meta-synthesis be the answer? *International Journal of Nursing Studies, 46*(4, 569–575).

Thorne, S., Kirkham, S. R., & O'Flynn-Magee, K. (2004). The analytic challenge in interpretive description. *International Journal of Qualitative Methods, 3*(1), 1–21.

Thorne, S. E. (2008). Meta-synthesis. In L. M. Given (Ed.), *The SAGE enclopedia of qualitative research methods* (pp. 510–513). Thousand Oaks, CA: Sage.

Thorne, S. E., Hislop, T. G., Armstrong, E.-A., & Oglov, V. (2008). Cancer care communication: The power to harm and the power to heal? *Patient Education and Counseling, 71,* 34–40.

Woodend, A., Sherrard, H., Fraser, M., Stuewe, L., Cheung, T., & Struthers, C. (2008). Telehome monitoring in patients with cardiac disease who are at high risk of readmission. *Heart & Lung: The Journal of Acute and Critical Care, 37*(1), 36–45.

Woodgate, R. L. (2008). Feeling states: A new approach to understanding how children and adolescents with cancer experience symptoms. *Cancer Nursing, 31*(3), 229–238.

Woodgate, R. L., Ateah, C., & Secco, L. (2008). Living in a world of our own: The experience of parents who have a child with autism. *Qualitative Health Research, 18*(8), 1075–1083.

2 Key Concepts in Qualitative and Quantitative Research

On completing this chapter, you will be able to:

1. Distinguish terms associated with quantitative and qualitative research

2. Describe similarities and differences between qualitative and quantitative research activities

THE BUILDING BLOCKS OF RESEARCH

Research, like any other discipline, has its own language and terminology—its own *jargon*. Some terms are used by both qualitative and quantitative researchers and other terms are used mainly by the former or the latter.

The Places and Faces of Research

When researchers address a problem or answer a question through a systematic investigation—regardless of whether it is qualitative or quantitative—they are doing a **study** (or a research project). When several investigators are working together to address a research problem, they are doing a collaborative study.

Example of a collaborative study

Wong et al., an interdisciplinary and international team (2008)—including two nurses, a physician, and a public administrative analyst—undertook a collaborative study to examine whether nursing students' perceptions of their educational experience, including peers, faculty, campus diversity, and overall experience were influenced by their ethnocultural background and the educational institution attended.

TIP

How can you tell whether an article appearing in a nursing journal is a *study*? In journals that specialize in research (e.g., the *Canadian Journal of Nursing Research, CJNR*), most articles are original research reports, but in specialty journals, there is usually a mix of research and nonresearch articles. Sometimes you can tell by the title, but sometimes you cannot. For example, Olson et al. (2008) from the Faculty of Nursing at the University of Alberta published an article entitled "Possible links between behavioural and physiological indices of tiredness, fatigue, and exhaustion in advanced cancer" in *Supportive Care in Cancer*. Although the title of the article suggests a possible study, it is not. The article presents a theoretical review on the potential links between behavioural and physiological indices of various forms of fatigue. If you look at the major headings of an article, and if there is no heading called "Method" or "Methodology" (the section that describes what a researcher *did*) and no heading called "Findings" or "Results" (the section that describes what a researcher *found*), then it is probably not an actual study.

TABLE 2.1 ⊙ KEY TERMS USED IN QUANTITATIVE AND QUALITATIVE RESEARCH		
CONCEPT	QUANTITATIVE TERM	QUALITATIVE TERM
Person contributing information	Study participant Respondent	Study participant Informant, key informant
Person undertaking the study	Researcher, investigator	Researcher, investigator
That which is being studied	Concepts Constructs Variables	Phenomena Concepts
Information gathered	Data (numeric values)	Data (narrative descriptions)
Links between concepts	Relationships (causal, functional)	Patterns
Logical reasoning processes	Deductive reasoning	Inductive reasoning
Quality of evidence	Reliability, validity, generalizability	Trustworthiness

Studies with humans involve two sets of people: those who conduct the study and those who provide the information. In a quantitative study, the people being studied are called the **study participants,** as shown in Table 2.1. (When participants provide information by answering questions, as in an interview, they may be called **respondents.**) In a qualitative study, the participants play an active role rather than a passive role and are called **informants, key informants,** or study participants. The person who conducts a study is the **researcher** or *investigator* (or sometimes—the *scientist*). Studies are sometimes undertaken by a single researcher, but more often they involve a research team.

Research can be undertaken in various *settings* (the specific places where information is gathered) and in one or more *sites*. Some studies take place in **naturalistic settings**—in the **field**—(e.g., in people's homes); others are performed in highly controlled **laboratory settings.** Qualitative researchers, especially, are likely to engage in **fieldwork** in natural settings because they are interested in the contexts of people's lives and experiences. A site is the overall location for the research—it could be an entire community (e.g., an Italian neighbourhood in Toronto) or an institution in a community (e.g., a clinic in Edmonton). Researchers sometimes engage in **multisite studies** because the use of multiple sites offers a larger or more diverse group of participants.

Phenomena, Concepts, and Constructs

Research involves abstract rather than tangible phenomena. For example, the terms *pain*, *resilience*, and *grief* are all abstractions of particular aspects of human behaviour and characteristics. These abstractions are referred to as **concepts** (or, in qualitative research, **phenomena**).

Researchers also use the term construct. Similar to a concept, a construct is a mental representation of some phenomenon. Kerlinger and Lee (2000) distinguish concepts from constructs by noting that **constructs** are abstractions that are deliberately and systematically invented (or constructed) by researchers for a specific purpose. For example, *self-care* in Orem's model of health maintenance is a construct. The terms *construct* and *concept* may be used interchangeably, although by convention, a construct refers to a more operational definition of a concept.

Theories, Models, and Frameworks

A **theory** is a systematic, abstract explanation of some aspect of reality. In a theory, concepts are knitted together into a system to explain some aspect of the world. Theories play a role in both qualitative and quantitative research.

In a quantitative study, researchers may start with a theory or a conceptual model or framework (the distinction is discussed in Chapter 8) and, using deductive reasoning, make predictions about how phenomena will behave *if the theory were "true."* The specific predictions are then tested through research, and the results are used to reject, modify, or lend support to the theory.

In qualitative research, theories may be used in various ways. Sometimes conceptual frameworks derived from various disciplines or qualitative research traditions (which we describe in Chapter 3) offer an orienting view with clear conceptual underpinnings. In some qualitative studies, however, theory is the *product* of the research. Information from participants is the starting point for the researcher's conceptualization that seeks to explain patterns and commonalities emerging from researcher–participant interactions. The goal is to develop a theory that explains a phenomenon as they emerge, not as they are preconceived. Theories generated in a qualitative study are sometimes subjected to subsequent testing through quantitative research.

Variables

In a quantitative study, concepts are referred to as **variables.** A variable, as the name implies, is something that varies. Weight, anxiety level, and body temperature are all variables (i.e., each of these properties varies from one person to another). In fact, nearly all aspects of human beings and their environment are variables. For example, if everyone weighed 60 kg, weight would not be a variable; it would be a *constant*. But it is precisely because people and conditions *do* vary that research is conducted. Most quantitative researchers seek to understand how or why things vary and to learn how differences in one variable are related to differences in another. For example, lung cancer research is concerned with the variable of lung cancer. It is a variable because not everyone has the disease. Researchers have studied variables that might be linked to lung cancer and have identified cigarette smoking. Smoking is also a variable because not everyone smokes. A variable, then, is any quality of a person, group, or situation that varies or takes on different values—typically, numeric values.

> **TIP**
>
> Every study focuses on one or more phenomena, concepts, or variables, but these terms *per se* are not necessarily used in research reports. For example, a report might say: "The purpose of this study is to examine the effect of a multimedia nursing intervention on patient satisfaction with care." Although the researcher has not explicitly used the term *concept*, the concepts (variables) under study are *type of nursing intervention* and *patient satisfaction with care*. Key concepts or variables are often indicated in the study title.

Variables are often inherent characteristics of people, such as age, blood type, or height. Sometimes, however, researchers *create* a variable. For example, if a researcher is testing the effectiveness of patient-controlled analgesia compared to intramuscular analgesia in relieving pain after surgery, some patients would be given patient-controlled analgesia and others would receive intramuscular analgesia. In the context of this study, method of pain management is a variable because different patients are given different analgesic methods.

Sometimes a variable can take on a range of different values that can be represented on a continuum (e.g., height or weight). Other variables take on only a few values; sometimes such variables convey quantitative information (e.g., number of children), but others simply involve placing people into categories (e.g., male, female).

Dependent Variables and Independent Variables

Many quantitative studies seek to determine the causes of a particular phenomenon. Does a nursing intervention *cause* improved patient outcomes? Does a certain procedure *cause* stress? The presumed cause is called the **independent variable,** and the presumed effect is called the **dependent variable.**

Variation in the dependent variable is presumed to *depend on* variation in the independent variable. For example, researchers investigate the extent to which lung cancer (the dependent variable) depends on or is caused by smoking (the independent variable). Or, researchers might examine the effect of tactile stimulation (the independent variable) on weight gain (the dependent variable) in premature infants. The dependent variable (sometimes called the **outcome variable**) is the one researchers want to understand, explain, or predict. In lung cancer/smoking research, it is the cancer that researchers are trying to explain and predict, not smoking.

Frequently, the terms *independent variable* and *dependent variable* are used to designate the *direction of influence* between variables rather than cause and effect. For example, suppose a researcher studied the mental health of caretakers caring for spouses with Alzheimer's disease and found better mental health outcomes for wives than for husbands' caregivers. The researcher might be unwilling to take the position that the caregivers' mental health was *caused* by gender. Yet the direction of influence clearly runs from gender to mental health: it makes *no* sense to suggest that mental health status influenced the caregivers's gender! Although in this example the researcher does not infer a cause-and-effect connection, it is appropriate to conceptualize mental health as the dependent variable and gender as the independent variable.

Many dependent variables have multiple causes or antecedents. If we were interested in studying influences on people's weight, for example, age, height, physical activity, and eating habits might be the independent variables. Two or more *dependent* variables also may be of interest to researchers. For example, suppose we wanted to compare the effectiveness of two methods of nursing care for children with cystic fibrosis. Several dependent variables could be designated as measures of treatment effectiveness, such as length of hospital stay, recurrence of respiratory infections, presence of cough, and so forth. It is common to design studies with multiple independent and dependent variables.

Variables are not *inherently* dependent or independent. A dependent variable in one study may be an independent variable in another study. For example, a study might examine the effect of nurses' contraceptive counselling (the independent variable) on unwanted births (the dependent variable). Another study might investigate the effect of unwanted births (the independent variable) on episodes of child abuse (the dependent variable). The role that a variable plays in a particular study determines whether it is an independent or a dependent variable.

The distinction between dependent and independent variables is often difficult for students. Do not be discouraged—the distinction becomes clearer with practice.

TIP

Few research reports *explicitly* label variables as dependent or independent, despite the importance of this distinction. Moreover, variables (especially independent variables) are sometimes not fully spelled out. Take the following research question: What is the effect of exercise on heart rate? In this example, heart rate is the dependent variable. Exercise, however, is not in itself a variable. Rather, exercise versus something else (e.g., no exercise) is a variable; "something else" is implied rather than stated in the research question. If exercise was not compared with something else (e.g., no exercise or different amounts of exercise), then exercise would not be a variable.

Conceptual and Operational Definitions

Concepts in a study need to be defined and explicated, and dictionary definitions are almost never adequate. Two types of definitions are of particular relevance in a study—conceptual and operational.

The concepts in which researchers are interested are abstractions of "observable" phenomena. A **conceptual definition** is the abstract, theoretical meaning of a concept being studied. Even seemingly straightforward terms need to be conceptually defined by researchers. Take the example of the concept of *spirituality*. Chiu et al. (2004) did a comprehensive review of how spirituality was conceptually defined in the research literature and found that current definitions revolve around four distinct themes: existential reality, transcendence, connectedness, and power/force/energy. Researchers undertaking studies of spirituality need to make clear which conceptual definition of spirituality they have adopted. In qualitative studies, conceptual definitions of key phenomena may be a major end product, reflecting the intent to have the meaning of concepts defined by the participants themselves.

In quantitative studies, however, researchers clarify and define research concepts at the outset because they must indicate how variables will be observed and measured. An **operational definition** specifies the operations that researchers must perform to collect the required information on a particular concept. Operational definitions should be in line with conceptual definitions.

Variables differ in the ease with which they can be operationalized. The variable weight, for example, is easy to define and measure. We might operationally define weight as follows: the amount that an object weighs in kilograms, to the nearest kilogram. Note that this definition designates that weight is determined by one measuring system (kilograms) rather than another (e.g., pounds). The operational definition might also specify that participants' weight will be measured to the nearest kilogram using a spring scale with participants fully undressed following a 10-hour fast. This operational definition clearly indicates what is meant by the variable *weight*.

Unfortunately, few variables of interest to nurses are as easily operationalized. There are multiple methods of measuring most variables, and researchers must choose the method that best captures the variables under study. Take, for example, *anxiety*, which can be defined in terms of either physiologic or psychological functioning. For researchers choosing to emphasize physiologic aspects of anxiety, the operational definition might involve measurement of extent of sweating through the Palmar Sweat Index. If, on the other hand, researchers conceptualize anxiety as a psychological state, the operational definition might involve a paper-and-pencil measure such as the State Anxiety Scale. Even if there may not be full agreement in the research or clinical community in terms of the chosen conceptual and operational definitions in a particular report, still, these definitions must be spelled out clearly in the report.

BOX 2.1 EXAMPLE OF QUANTITATIVE DATA

Question:	Thinking about the past week, how depressed would you say you have been on a scale from 0 to 10, where 0 means "not at all" and 10 means "the most possible?"
Data:	Participant 1: 9
	Participant 2: 0
	Participant 3: 4

TIP

Most research reports never use the term *operational definition* explicitly. Quantitative research reports do, however, provide information on how key variables were measured (i.e., they specify the operational definitions even if they do not use this label). This information is usually included in a section called "Measures" or "Instruments."

Data

Research **data** (datum is the singular noun) are the pieces of information obtained in a study. All pieces of data gathered in a study make up the **data set.**

In quantitative studies, researchers identify the variables of interest, develop operational definitions, and then collect relevant data from participants. The actual values of the variables constitute the study data. In quantitative studies, researchers collect primarily **quantitative data** (i.e., numeric information). For example, suppose we were conducting a quantitative study in which a key variable was *depression.* We would try to measure how depressed different participants were. We might ask, "Thinking about the past week, how depressed would you say you have been on a scale from 0 to 10, where 0 means 'not at all' and 10 means 'the most possible'?" Box 2.1 presents data from three fictitious respondents. Participants have provided a number corresponding to their degree of depression: 9 for participant 1 (a high level of depression), 0 for participant 2 (no depression), and 4 for participant 3 (very mild depression). The numeric values for all participants in the study, collectively, would constitute the data on the variable depression.

In qualitative studies, researchers collect primarily **qualitative data,** which are narrative descriptions. Narrative information can be obtained by having conversations with participants, by making notes about how participants behave in naturalistic settings, or by obtaining narrative records (e.g., diaries). Suppose we were studying depression qualitatively. Box 2.2 presents some qualitative data from three participants responding conversationally to the question, "Tell me about how you've been feeling lately. Have you felt sad or depressed at all, or have you generally been in good spirits?" Here, the data consist of rich narrative

BOX 2.2 EXAMPLE OF QUALITATIVE DATA

Question:	Tell me about how you have been feeling lately—have you felt sad or depressed at all, or have you generally been in good spirits?
Data:	*Participant 1:* "I've been pretty depressed lately, to tell you the truth. I wake up each morning and I can't seem to think of anything to look forward to. I mope around the house all day, kind of in despair. I just can't seem to shake the blues, and I've begun to think I need to go see a shrink."
	Participant 2: "I can't remember ever feeling better in my life. I just got promoted to a new job that makes me feel like I can really get ahead in my company. And I've just gotten engaged to a really great guy who is very special."
	Participant 3: "I've had a few ups and downs the past week, but basically things are on a pretty even keel. I don't have too many complaints."

descriptions of participants' emotional state. The analysis of such qualitative data is a particularly labour-intensive process.

Relationships

Researchers usually study phenomena in relation to other phenomena—they examine relationships. A **relationship** is a bond or connection between two or more phenomena; for example, researchers repeatedly have found that there is a *relationship* between cigarette smoking and lung cancer. Both qualitative and quantitative studies examine relationships, but in different ways.

In quantitative studies, researchers are primarily interested in the relationship between independent variables and dependent variables. Variation in the dependent variable is presumed to be systematically related to variation in the independent variable. Relationships are often explicitly expressed in quantitative terms, such as *more than*, *less than*, and so forth. For example, let us consider as a possible dependent variable a person's weight. What variables are related to a person's weight? Some possibilities include height, caloric intake, and exercise. For each of these three independent variables, we can make a prediction about its relationship to the dependent variable:

Height: Taller people weigh more than shorter people.

Caloric intake: People with higher caloric intake are heavier than those with lower caloric intake.

Exercise: The lower the amount of exercise, the greater the person's weight.

Each of these statements expresses a presumed relationship between weight (the dependent variable) and a measurable independent variable. Most quantitative research is conducted to determine whether relationships do or do not exist among variables, and often to quantify how strong the relationship is.

 TIP

Relationships are expressed in two basic forms, depending on what the variables are like. First, relationships can be expressed as "if more of variable X, then more (or less) of variable Y." For example, there is a relationship between height and weight: with more height, there tends to be more weight; that is, taller people tend to weigh more than shorter people. The second form is sometimes confusing to students because there is no explicit relational statement. The second form involves relationships expressed as group differences. For example, there is a *relationship* between gender and height: men tend to be taller than women.

Variables can be related to one another in different ways. One type of relationship is a **cause-and-effect** (or **causal**) **relationship.** Within the positivist paradigm, natural phenomena are assumed not to be haphazard; they have antecedent causes that are presumably discoverable. In our example about a person's weight, we might speculate that there is a causal relationship between caloric intake and weight: all else being equal, eating more calories causes weight gain.

Example of a study focusing on a causal relationship
Godin et al. (2008) studied whether the promotion of "safe sex" in a community-level programme in gay bars, saunas, and sex shops in Quebec city, Canada, would increase safe sex behaviour—the latter being defined as the use of condoms during intercourse.

Not all relationships between variables can be interpreted causally. There is a relationship, for example, between a person's pulmonary artery and tympanic temperatures: people with high readings on one have high readings on the other. We cannot say, however, that pulmonary artery temperature caused tympanic temperature, nor that tympanic temperature caused pulmonary artery temperature, despite the relationship between the two variables. This type of relationship is sometimes referred to as a *functional (or associative) relationship* rather than a causal one.

Example of a study focusing on a functional/associative relationship
Okoli, Richardson, and Johnson (2008) studied adolescents' initial smoking experience such as feeling dizzy, feeling sick, and coughing in relation to previous exposure to smoking from peers and family members (rated as high, moderate, low, and minimal).

TIP

How can you tell if a researcher is testing a causal relationship? Researchers are likely to ask whether the outcome variable is *caused by, affected by, resulted from,* or *influenced by* the independent variable. If researchers are not seeking to establish a causal relationship, they are more likely to ask whether the outcome variable is *related to, linked to,* or *associated with* the independent variable.

Qualitative researchers are not concerned with quantifying relationships, or in testing and confirming causal relationships. Rather, qualitative researchers seek patterns of association as a way of illuminating the underlying meaning and dimensionality of phenomena of interest. Patterns of interconnected themes and processes are identified as a means of understanding the whole.

Example of a qualitative study of patterns
Dubois and Loiselle (2008) explored the perceived role of informational support in relation to health care services use among women and men newly diagnosed with cancer (n = 20). They found that when participants felt satisfied with the informational support received, the cancer information was used to guide or support their use of health care services (e.g., ask questions to oncologists or nurses). Those participants reporting a negative experience with cancer information provided by health care professionals (e.g., information difficult to understand) felt paralysed or unsure about their subsequent health care services utilization.

CRITICAL CHALLENGE OF CONDUCTING RESEARCH

Researchers face numerous challenges in conducting research. For example, there are conceptual challenges (e.g., How should concepts be defined?), financial challenges (e.g., How will the study be paid for?), ethical challenges (e.g., Can the study achieve its goals without infringing on human rights?), and methodologic challenges (e.g., Will the adopted method yield results that can be trusted?). This book provides guidance relating to these issues and this section highlights key methodologic concepts while illustrating differences between qualitative and quantitative research. In reading this section, it is important to remember that the worth of a study for evidence-based practice (EBP) is based on how well researchers deal with these issues.

Reliability, Validity, and Trustworthiness

Researchers want their findings to genuinely reflect the issue or phenomenon being studied. Research users need to assess the quality of evidence in a study by evaluating the conceptual and methodologic decisions researchers made, and researchers strive to make the best decisions to produce evidence of the highest quality.

Quantitative researchers use several criteria to assess the quality of a study, sometimes referred to as its **scientific merit.** Two important criteria are reliability and validity. **Reliability** is the accuracy and consistency of information obtained in a study. The term is most often associated with the methods used to measure variables. For example, if a thermometer measures Henry's temperature as being 98.1°F one minute and 102.5°F the next minute, the reliability of the thermometer would be considered suspect. The concept of reliability is also important in interpreting statistical analyses. Statistical reliability refers to the probability that the same results would be obtained with a new sample of participants.

Validity is a more complex concept that concerns the *soundness* of the study's evidence—that is, whether the findings are cogent and well grounded. Validity is an important criterion for assessing the method of measuring variables. In this context, the validity question is whether there is evidence to support the assertion that the methods are really measuring the abstract concepts that they purport to measure. Is a paper-and-pencil measure of depression *really* measuring depression? Or is it measuring something else, such as loneliness or low self-esteem? The validity criterion underscores the importance of having solid conceptual and operational definitions of variables.

An additional aspect of validity concerns the quality of the researcher's evidence regarding the link between the independent variable and the dependent variable. Did a nursing intervention *really* bring improvements in patients' outcomes— or were other factors responsible the outcomes? Researchers make numerous methodologic decisions that can influence this type of validity.

Qualitative researchers use somewhat different criteria (and different terminology) in evaluating a study's quality. Generally, qualitative researchers discuss methods of enhancing the **trustworthiness** of the results (Lincoln & Guba, 1985). Trustworthiness encompasses several different dimensions, one of which is credibility.

Credibility, an especially important aspect of trustworthiness, is achieved to the extent that the research methods engender confidence in the "truth" of the data and their interpretation. Credibility can be enhanced through various strategies (see Chapter 14), but one in particular merits early discussion because it has implications for the design of studies, including quantitative ones. **Triangulation** is the use of multiple sources or referents to draw conclusions about what constitutes the "truth." In a quantitative study, this might mean having two different operational definitions of the dependent variable to determine whether results are consistent across both. In a qualitative study, triangulation might involve using multiple means of data collection to converge on the "truth" (e.g., having in-depth conversations with participants paired with observing them in natural settings). Triangulation can also be done across paradigms—that is, integrating both qualitative and quantitative approaches in a single study to offset the limitations of each.

Example of triangulation
McClement and Harlos (2008) studied the experiences of family members to reduced intake of food and fluid and weight loss of a terminally ill relative while hospitalized on an inpatient palliative care unit. Their study involved in-depth, face-to-face interviews with 23 family members. They also interviewed 13 patients and 11 health care providers. In addition, they used participant observation on the palliative care unit to add to the data.

Nurse researchers design their studies to minimize threats to the reliability, validity, and increase trustworthiness of their findings. Users of research must evaluate the extent to which the researchers were successful.

TIP

In reading and evaluating research reports, it is appropriate to assume a "show me" attitude—that is, to expect researchers to build and present a solid case for the merit of their findings. They do this by presenting evidence that the findings are reliable and valid or trustworthy.

Bias

Bias is a major concern in research because it can threaten the study's validity and trustworthiness. In general, a **bias** is an influence that produces a distortion in the study results. Bias can result from various factors, including study participants' lack of candour or desire to please, researchers' preconceptions, or faulty methods of collecting data.

To some extent, bias can never be avoided totally. Some bias is haphazard and affects only small segments of the data. For instance, a handful of study participants might fail to provide accurate information because they were tired at the time of data collection. Systematic bias results when the bias is consistent or uniform. For example, if a scale consistently measures people's weights as being 2 pounds heavier than their true weight, there is systematic bias. Rigorous research method aims to eliminate or minimize bias—or, at least, to detect its presence so it can be taken into account in interpreting the data.

Researchers adopt a variety of strategies to address bias. Triangulation is one such approach, the idea being that multiple sources of information help to counterbalance biases and offer avenues to identify them. In quantitative research, methods to combat bias often entail research control.

Research Control

Quantitative research typically involves efforts to control various aspects of the study. **Research control** involves holding constant other influences on the dependent variable so that the true relationship between the independent and dependent variables can be understood. In other words, research control attempts to eliminate contaminating factors that might distort the relationship between variables of interest.

The issue of confounding factors—**extraneous variables**—can best be illustrated with an example. Suppose we were interested in the question, does young maternal age affect infant birth weight? Existing studies have shown that teenagers more often have low-birth-weight babies than women in their 20s or 30s; the question here is whether maternal age itself (the independent variable) causes differences in birth weight (the dependent variable) or whether there are other mechanisms that account for the relationship between age and birth weight. We need to design a study that controls other influences on the dependent variable to clarify the effect of the independent variable.

Two possible extraneous variables are women's nutritional habits and their prenatal care. Teenagers tend to be less careful than older women about their eating patterns during pregnancy, and are also less likely to obtain prenatal care. Both nutrition and the amount of care could, in turn, affect birth weight. Thus, if these two factors are not controlled, then any observed relationship between mother's age and her baby's weight at birth could be caused by the mother's age itself, her diet, or her prenatal care. Without control, it would be impossible to know what the underlying cause really is.

These three possible explanations might be portrayed schematically as follows:

1. Mother's age → infant birth weight

2. Mother's age → adequacy of prenatal care → infant birth weight

3. Mother's age → nutritional adequacy → infant birth weight

The arrows here symbolize a causal mechanism or an influence. In examples 2 and 3, the effect of maternal age on infant birth weight is mediated by prenatal care and nutrition, respectively; these are **mediating variables** in these last two models. Some research is specifically designed to test paths of mediation, but in the present example, these variables are extraneous to the research question. Our task is to design a study so that the first explanation can be tested. Both nutrition and prenatal care must be controlled to learn whether explanation 1 is valid. If they are not controlled, they will confound the results.

How can we impose such control? There are a number of ways, as discussed in Chapter 9, but the general principle underlying each alternative is the same: *the extraneous variables of the study must be held constant*. The extraneous variables must be handled so that, *in the context of the study*, they are not related to the independent or dependent variable.

Research control is a fundamental feature of quantitative studies. The world is complex, and variables are interrelated in complicated ways. In quantitative studies, it is difficult to examine this complexity directly. Researchers analyze a few relationships at a time and put the pieces together like a jigsaw puzzle. That is why even simple quantitative studies can make contributions to knowledge. The extent of the contribution, however, is often related to how well a researcher controls confounding influences. In reading reports of quantitative studies, you will need to consider whether the researcher has, in fact, appropriately controlled extraneous variables.

Although research control in quantitative studies is viewed as a critical tool for managing bias and enhancing validity, there are situations in which too much control can introduce bias. For example, if researchers tightly control the ways in which key study variables can manifest themselves, it is possible that the true nature of those variables will be obscured. When key concepts are phenomena that are poorly understood, then an approach that allows some flexibility (as in a qualitative study) is better suited. Research rooted in the naturalistic paradigm does not impose controls. With their emphasis on holism and the individuality of human experience, qualitative researchers typically adhere to the view that to impose controls on a research setting is to remove meaning of reality.

Randomness and Reflexivity

For quantitative researchers, a powerful tool for eliminating bias involves the concept of **randomness**—having certain features of the study established by chance rather than by design or personal preference. When people in a community are selected at random to participate in a study, for example, each person in the community has an equal chance of being selected. This, in turn, means that there are no systematic biases in the makeup of the study group. Men are as likely to be selected as women, for example.

Qualitative researchers do not consider randomness a useful tool for understanding phenomena. Qualitative researchers tend to use information obtained early in the study in a purposeful (nonrandom) fashion to guide their inquiry and to pursue information-rich sources that can help them refine their conceptualizations. Researchers' judgments are viewed as indispensable vehicles for uncovering the complexities of the phenomena of interest. However, qualitative researchers often rely on reflexivity to guard against personal bias in making judgments. **Reflexivity** is the process of reflecting critically on the self, and of analyzing and making note of personal values that could affect data collection and interpretation.

Example of reflexivity
Dahlke and Phinney (2008) explored how nurses care for hospitalized older adults at risk of delirium and the challenges they faced in this work. Their study involved interviews with nurses working in a midsized regional hospital in western Canada. During the study, the researchers maintained a journal about observations and interpretations made during the interviews and recorded any salient points or thoughts that occurred while conducting the study.

Generalizability and Transferability

Nurses increasingly rely on evidence from research to guide their clinical practice. If study findings are totally unique to the people or circumstances of the original research, can they be used as a basis for changes in practice? The answer, clearly, is no.

As noted in Chapter 1, **generalizability** is the criterion used in a quantitative study to assess the extent to which study findings can be applied to other groups and settings. How do researchers enhance the generalizability of a study? First, they must design studies strong in reliability and validity. There is little point in wondering whether results are generalizable if they are not accurate or valid. In selecting participants, researchers must also give thought to the types of people to whom the results might be generalized. If a study is intended to have implications for male and female patients, then men and women should be included as participants. If an intervention is intended to benefit patients in urban and rural hospitals, then perhaps a multisite study is needed.

Qualitative researchers do not specifically seek to make their findings generalizable. Nevertheless, they often seek understandings that might be informative in other situations. Lincoln and Guba (1985), in their influential book on naturalistic inquiry, discuss the concept of **transferability,** the extent to which qualitative findings can be transferred to other settings, as an aspect of a study's trustworthiness. An important mechanism for promoting transferability is the amount of information provided about the contexts for the study. **Thick description,** a widely used term in qualitative research, refers to a rich and thorough description of the research setting and of observed processes. Both quantitative and qualitative reports need to thoroughly describe study participants and research settings so that the utility of the evidence for nursing practice can be assessed.

GENERAL QUESTIONS IN REVIEWING A STUDY

Most of the remaining chapters of this book contain guidelines to help you evaluate different aspects of a research report. Box 2.3 presents some further suggestions for performing a review of a research report, drawing on concepts explained in this chapter. These guidelines supplement those presented in Box 1.1 of Chapter 1.

BOX 2.3   ADDITIONAL QUESTIONS FOR A PRELIMINARY OVERVIEW OF A STUDY

1. What is the study all about? What are the main phenomena, concepts, or constructs under investigation?
2. If the study is quantitative, what are the independent and dependent variables?
3. Do the researchers examine relationships or patterns of association among variables or concepts? Does the report imply the possibility of a causal relationship?
4. Are key concepts clearly defined, both conceptually and operationally?
5. Are you able to discern any steps the researcher took to enhance the study's reliability, validity, and generalizability (quantitative research) or trustworthiness (qualitative research)?

EXAMPLE 1 ■ Quantitative Research

Aspects of a quantitative nursing study are presented below. Questions to guide critical thinking follow.

Study

"Do catheter washouts extend patency time in long-term urethral catheters? A randomized controlled trial of acidic washout solution, normal saline washout, or standard care" (Moore et al., 2009)

Study Purpose

The study tested the effectiveness of catheter washouts in preventing or reducing catheter blockage and in so doing reducing the number of catheter changes per month for individuals with long-term indwelling catheters. The intervention involved saline washout or washout with a commercially available acidic solution (Contisol™).

Research Method

A multisite randomized controlled trial conducted with three groups: control (usual care, no washout), saline washout, or commercially available acidic washout solution (Contisol™). A total of 73 adults residing in a long-term care setting or receiving home care with a long-term indwelling catheter (>30 days) that blocks on a regular basis (>1 a month) were randomly assigned to one of the three groups. Twenty-six participants were allocated to receive Contisol™, 21 participants were assigned to the saline washout group, and 26 received no intervention. A computer-generated list of random numbers determined group assignment. Outcome data were gathered at baseline and weekly thereafter for 8 weeks or until the end of three catheter changes or a reported UTI.

Outcome Variables

The primary outcome variable was mean time to first catheter change. Additionally, the researchers gathered information on the following secondary outcomes: mean urinary pH, incidence of microscopic hematuria and leukocytes, measurement of cross-section luminal area of used catheters, and incidence of symptomatic urinary track infection (UTI).

Key Findings

- Mean time to first catheter change did not differ among groups.
- There were no significant differences between any of the secondary outcome variables. Regardless of group assignments, all participants' urine was positive for microscopic hematuria and leukocytes. No adverse events were reported in either washout groups. No participant reported symptomatic UTI. The mean urinary pH did not correlate with incidence of blockage.
- Evidence remains insufficient to support whether catheter washout with saline or Contisol™ is more effective than usual care (no washout) in preventing blockage.

CRITICAL THINKING SUGGESTIONS

1. Answer questions 1, 2, 3, and 5 from Box 2.3 (p. 37) regarding this study.
2. Also consider the following targeted questions, which may assist you in assessing aspects of the study's merit:
   a. What are some of the extraneous variables the researchers would have wanted to control—what factors other than the treatment could have affected the outcomes?
   b. What is your perception of the validity of the outcome measures?
   c. How did the researchers reduce bias in forming the groups that were compared?
   d. Would it have been appropriate to address the research question using qualitative research methods? Why or why not?

3. If the results of this study are valid and generalizable, how can these findings be used in clinical practice?

EXAMPLE 2 ■ Qualitative Research

Aspects of a qualitative nursing study, featuring key terms and concepts discussed in this chapter, are presented below, followed by some questions to guide critical thinking.

Study

"Perspectives of survivors of traumatic brain injury and their caregivers on long-term social integration" (Lefebvre, Cloutier, & Levert, 2008)

Study Purpose

Lefebvre and her colleagues sought to document the repercussions of traumatic brain injury (TBI) on victim's long-term social integration (10 years posttrauma) and the determinants and barriers of social integration, and the impact of TBI on family caregivers.

Research Method

The researchers interviewed TBI survivors and their family caregivers to gain a better understanding of the barriers and facilitators to social integration following a TBI and the impact of the TBI on family caregivers. Twenty participants who had a moderate or severe TBI and 21 family caregivers were interviewed. The interviews, lasting an average of 90 minutes, were audiotaped and transcribed. The participants and their family caregivers were interviewed simultaneously in their homes. Questions asked of participants included: "Tell me about your activities of daily living." "What are the factors which facilitated their realization? Questions asked to the family caregivers were, for instance, "What changes have occurred in your life since the accident?" Transcripts were initially analysed to identify themes and then compared to identify commonalities and differences in the data. All of the researchers read and approved the verbatim transcriptions and data coding.

Key Findings

Approximately half of the TBI participants said they were satisfied with their current social integration. Determinants of social integration emerging from the analysis of participants interviews included the following:

- Receiving long-term follow-up services;
- Safeguarding or developing their family life (e.g., participating in household chores);
- Having a social life (e.g., attaining a recognized social status) and support from family caregivers; and
- Having a spiritual life.

In addition, participants identified being unable to return to work, having a depressive episode, abusing alcohol or other illicit substance, experiencing problems in relationships (e.g., divorce or separation), and TBI sequellae as barriers to social integration.

The family caregivers interviewed identified that the TBI affected their professional life or main occupation (e.g., taking leave from or giving up a fulfilling job to take care of their loved one), family relations (e.g., some TBI sequellae hard to live with), relations with people in their larger social network (e.g., not engaged in leisure activities), physical and emotional health (e.g., felt emotionally exhausted). Family caregivers reported that these difficulties were aggravated by the lack of resources for long-term care and follow-up.

CRITICAL THINKING SUGGESTIONS

1. Answer questions 1, 3, and 5 from Box 2.3 (p. 37) regarding this study.

2. Also consider the following targeted questions, which may assist you in assessing aspects of the study's merit:

    a. Lefebvre and her colleagues did not control extraneous variables, nor did they use randomness in this study. Would these decisions affect the quality of the study?

(Research Examples and Critical Thinking Activities continues on page 40)

Research Examples and Critical Thinking Activities (continued)

 b. Some actual data are presented in the summary—indicate what the data are.

 c. Would it have been appropriate to address the research question using quantitative research methods? Why or why not?

3. If the results of this study are trustworthy, how can these be used in clinical practice?

EXAMPLE 3 ■ Quantitative Research

1. Read the abstract and the introduction from the study by Bryanton and colleagues (2008) in Appendix A of this book and then answer questions 1 through 3 in Box 2.3 (p. 37).

2. Also consider the following targeted questions, which may further sharpen your critical thinking skills and assist you in assessing aspects of the study's merit:

 a. Did the researchers randomly assign participants to groups in this study?

 b. What are some of the extraneous variables that the researchers would have wanted to control in this study?

EXAMPLE 4 ■ Qualitative Research

1. Read the abstract, introduction, and literature review section of the study by Woodgate, Ateah, and Secco (2008) in Appendix B of this book (and skim the remainder of the report) and then answer the relevant questions in Box 2.3 (p. 37).

2. Also consider the following targeted questions, which may further sharpen your critical thinking skills and assist you in assessing aspects of the study's merit:

 a. Find an example of actual *data* in this study. (You will need to look at the first few paragraphs of the "Results" section of the report.)

 b. Does Woodgate's report discuss reflexivity?

 c. Would it have been appropriate for Woodgate and colleagues to conduct her study using quantitative research methods? Why or why not?

Summary Points

- A **study** (or *investigation*) is undertaken by one or more **researchers** (or *investigators*). The people who provide information in a study are the **study partici-pants** (in both quantitative and qualitative research) or **informants** (in qualitative research).

- **Collaborative research** involving a research team with both clinical and methodologic expertise is increasingly common in addressing problems of clinical relevance.

- The *site* is the overall location for the research; researchers sometimes engage in **multisite studies.** *Settings*—the more specific places where data collection occurs—range from **naturalistic (field) settings** to formal laboratories.

- Researchers investigate phenomena or **concepts** (or **constructs**), which are abstractions or mental representations inferred from behaviour or events.

- Concepts are the building blocks of **theories,** which are systematic explanations of some aspect of the world.

- In quantitative studies, concepts are called variables. A **variable** is a characteristic or quality that takes on different values (i.e., varies from one person to another).

➢ The **dependent** (or **outcome**) **variable** is the behaviour, characteristic, or outcome the researcher is interested in explaining, predicting, or affecting. The **independent variable** is the presumed cause of, antecedent to, or influence on the dependent variable.

➢ A **conceptual** definition clarifies the abstract or theoretical meaning of a concept being studied. An **operational definition** specifies the procedures and tools required to measure a variable.

➢ **Data**—the information collected during the course of a study—may take the form of narrative information (**qualitative data**) or numeric values (**quantitative data**).

➢ Researchers often focus on the relationship between two concepts. A **relationship** is a bond (or pattern of association) between two phenomena; when the independent variable causes or determines the dependent variable, it is a **causal** (or **cause-and-effect**) **relationship.**

➢ **Inductive reasoning** is the process of developing conclusions from specific observations, whereas **deductive reasoning** is the process of developing specific predictions from general principles.

➢ Researchers face numerous conceptual, practical, ethical, and methodologic challenges. The major methodologic challenge is designing studies that are reliable and valid (quantitative studies) or trustworthy (qualitative studies).

➢ **Reliability** refers to the accuracy and consistency of information obtained in a study. **Validity** is a more complex concept that concerns the *soundness* of the study's evidence—that is, whether the findings are cogent and well grounded.

➢ **Trustworthiness** in qualitative research encompasses several dimensions, including credibility. **Credibility** is achieved to the extent that the research methods engender confidence in the truth of the data and in the researchers' interpretations. **Triangulation,** the use of multiple sources or referents to draw conclusions about what constitutes the truth, is one approach to establishing credibility.

➢ A **bias** is an influence that distorts study results. In quantitative research, a powerful tool to eliminate bias concerns **randomness**—having features of the study established by chance rather than by design or preference.

➢ Qualitative researchers often keep personal biases in check through **reflexivity,** the process of reflecting critically on the self and noting personal values that could affect data collection and interpretation.

➢ Quantitative researchers use various methods of **research control** to hold constant confounding influences on the dependent variable so that its relationship to the independent variable can be better understood. The confounding influences are **extraneous variables**—extraneous to the purpose of the study.

➢ **Generalizability** is the criterion used in a quantitative study to assess the extent to which the findings can be applied to other groups and settings.

➢ A similar concept in qualitative studies is **transferability,** the extent to which qualitative findings can be transferred to other settings. A mechanism for promoting transferability is **thick description,** the rich, thorough description of the research context so that others can make inferences about contextual similarities.

STUDIES CITED IN CHAPTER 2*

This reference list contains only those studies that were cited in this chapter. Citations pertaining to theoretical, methodological, or nonempirical work are included together in a separate section at the end of the book (beginning on page 399).

Bryanton, J., Gagnon, A. J., Hatem, M., & Johnston, C. (2008). Predictors of early parenting self-efficacy: Results of a prospective cohort study. *Nursing Research, 57*(4), 252–259.

Dahlke, S., & Phinney, A. (2008). Caring for hospitalized older adults at risk for delirium: The silent, unspoken piece of nursing practice. *Journal of Gerontological Nursing*, *34*(6), 41–47.

Dubois, S., & Loiselle, C. G. (2008). Understanding the role of cancer informational support in relation to health care service use among newly diagnosed individuals. *Canadian Oncology Nursing Journal (CONJ)*, *18*(4), 193–198.

Fredericks, S., Sidani, S., & Shugurensky, D. (2008). The effect of anxiety on learning outcomes post-CABG. *Canadian Journal of Nursing Research (CJNR)*, *40*(15), 126–140.

Godin, G., Naccache, H., Côté, F., Leclerc, R., Fréchette, M., & Alary, M. (2008). Promotion of safe sex: Evaluation of a community-level intervention programme in gay bars, saunas, and sex shops. *Health Education Research*, *23*, 287–297.

Johnston, C., Gagnon, A., Rennick, J., et al. (2007). One-on-one coaching to improve pain assessment and management practices of pediatric nurses. *Journal of Pediatric Nursing*, *22*(6), 467–478.

Lefebvre, H., Cloutier, G., & Levert, M. J. (2008). Perspectives of survivors of traumatic brain injury and their caregivers on long-term social integration. *Brain Injury*, *22*(7), 535–543.

McClement, S., & Harlos, M. (2008). When advanced cancer patients won't eat: Family responses. *International Journal of Palliative Nursing*, *14*(4), 182–188.

Moore, K. N., Hunter, K. F., McGinnis, R. H., et al. (2009). Do catheter washouts extend patency time in long-term indwelling urethral catheters? A randomized controlled trial of acidic washout solution, normal saline washout, or standard care. *Journal of Wound Ostomy & Continence Nursing*, *36*(1), 82–90.

Okoli, C., Richardson, C., & Johnson, J. (2008). An examination of the relationship between adolescents' initial smoking experience and their exposure to peer and family member smoking. *Addictive Behaviors*, *33*(9), 1183–1191.

Olson, K., Hayduk, L., Cree, M., et al. (2008). The changing causal foundations of cancer-related symptom clustering during the final month of palliative care: A longitudinal study. *BMC Medical Research Methodology* *8*(36). doi:10.1186/1471-2288-8-36.

Wong, S., Seago, J., Keane, D., & Grumbach, K. (2008). College students' perceptions of their experiences: What do minority students think? *Journal of Nursing Education*, *47*(4), 190–195.

Woodgate, R. L., Ateah, C., & Secco, L. (2008). Living in a world of our own: The experience of parents who have a child with autism. *Qualitative Health Research*, *18*(8), 1075–1083.

3 Understanding the Research Process in Qualitative and Quantitative Studies

On completing this chapter, you will be able to:

1. Distinguish experimental and nonexperimental research

2. Identify the three main disciplinary traditions for qualitative nursing research

3. Describe the flow and sequence of activities in quantitative and qualitative research, and discuss why they differ

4. Define new terms presented in the chapter

Researchers usually decide early on whether to conduct a quantitative or qualitative study; they typically work within a paradigm that is consistent with their worldview and that gives rise to the types of question that excite their curiosity. After selecting a paradigm, researchers proceed to design and implement their study, but the progression of activities differs in qualitative and quantitative research. In this chapter, we discuss the flow of both types of study.

TIP

The flow of a research project is not transparent to those reading a research report. Researchers rarely articulate the progression of steps they took in initiating and completing a study. This chapter will help you better understand the research process. It is also intended to heighten your awareness of the many decisions that researchers make—decisions that have a strong bearing on study quality.

MAJOR CLASSES OF QUANTITATIVE AND QUALITATIVE RESEARCH

Before describing the evolution of a research project, we briefly describe broad categories of quantitative and qualitative research.

Quantitative Research: Experimental and Nonexperimental Studies

A basic distinction in quantitative studies is between experimental and nonexperimental research. In **experimental research,** researchers actively introduce an intervention or treatment. In **nonexperimental research,** on the other hand, researchers collect data without making changes or introducing treatments. For example, if a researcher gave bran flakes to one group of participants and prune juice to another to evaluate which method facilitated elimination more effectively, the study would be experimental because the researcher intervened in the normal course of things. If, on the other hand, a researcher compared elimination patterns of two groups of people whose regular eating patterns differed—for example, some normally took foods that stimulated bowel elimination and others did not—there is no intervention. Such a study, which focuses on existing attributes, is nonexperimental.

Experimental studies are explicitly designed to test causal relationships. Sometimes nonexperimental studies also seek to elucidate or detect causal relationships, but doing so is tricky and less conclusive. Experimental studies offer the possibility of greater control over extraneous variables than nonexperimental studies.

Example of experimental research

Fillion et al. (2008) tested the effectiveness of a stress/fatigue management program among breast cancer survivors. Participants were randomly assigned either to the intervention group, which involved four weekly group meetings and one short telephone session, or to the group that received usual care.

In this example, the researchers intervened by designating that some patients would receive the special support intervention and others would not. In other words, the researchers had control over the independent variable, which in this case was receipt or nonreceipt of the intervention.

Example of nonexperimental research

Bryanton et al. (2008) conducted a study among 652 women in the early postpartum period to determine predictors of their perceptions (positive or negative) of their childbirth experience.

In this nonexperimental study, the researchers did not intervene in any way. They merely measured the participants' perceptions. We will see in Chapter 9 why making causal inferences in nonexperimental studies is a difficult issue.

Qualitative Research: Disciplinary Traditions

Qualitative studies (which are nonexperimental) are often rooted in research traditions that originate in the disciplines of anthropology, sociology, and psychology. Three such traditions have had especially strong influences on qualitative nursing research and are briefly described in this chapter. Chapter 10 provides a fuller discussion of alternative research traditions and the methods associated with them.

The **grounded theory** tradition, which was developed in the 1960s by two sociologists, Glaser and Strauss (1967), seeks to describe and understand the key social–psychological and structural processes that occur in a social setting. Most grounded theory studies focus on an evolving social experience—the social and psychological stages and phases that characterize a particular event or episode. A major component of grounded theory is the discovery of a *core variable* (or *core category*) that is central in explaining what is going on in that social scene. Grounded theory researchers strive to generate comprehensive explanations of phenomena that are grounded in reality.

Example of a grounded theory study

Chiovitti (2008) uses grounded theory to develop a theory of caring from the perspective of nurses working with patients in three urban acute psychiatric hospital settings. Two in-depth face-to-face individual interviews were conducted with 17 nurses during their shift. The core variable found was called "protective empowering." Two antecedents to "protective empowering" were identified: (1) respecting the patient and (2) not taking the patient's behaviour personally. In addition, four categories were identified to represent the contexts through "protective empowering" occurred: (1) keeping the patient safe, (2) encouraging the patient's health, (3) authentic relating, and (4) interactive teaching.

Phenomenology, which has its disciplinary roots in both philosophy and psychology, is concerned with the lived experiences of humans. Phenomenology is an approach to thinking about what life experiences of people are like and what they mean. The phenomenological researcher asks: What is the *essence* of this phenomenon as experienced by these people? Or, What is the meaning of the phenomenon to those who experience it?

Example of a phenomenological study
Gantert et al. (2008) conducted a phenomenological study to describe seniors' perceptions of their relationships with in-home health care providers—specifically, their experience of the relationship-building process and associated facilitators and barriers.

Ethnography is the primary research tradition within anthropology, and provides a framework for studying the patterns and experiences of a defined cultural group in a holistic fashion. Ethnographers typically engage in extensive fieldwork, often participating to the extent possible, in the life of the culture of interest. The aim of ethnographers is to learn from (rather than to "study") members of a cultural group, to understand their worldview as they perceive and live it.

Example of an ethnographic study
Tang and Browne (2008) used ethnographic methods to study how *race* and *racialization* (the process of categorizing individuals or groups based on their race) operate within the context of health care service use among Aboriginal people. Aboriginal individuals described avoiding health care services, as they expected to be discriminated against and be treated differently.

MAIN STEPS IN A QUANTITATIVE STUDY

In quantitative studies, researchers move from a start point (posing a question) to an end point (getting an answer) in a fairly linear sequence. This section describes the progression of activities that is typical in a quantitative study; the next section describes how qualitative studies differ.

Phase 1: The Conceptual Phase

The early steps in a quantitative study typically involve activities with a strong conceptual element. During this phase, researchers call on such skills as creativity, deductive reasoning, and a firm grounding in previous research on the topic of interest.

Step 1: Formulating and Delimiting the Problem

The first step is to identify an interesting, significant research problem and to develop research questions. In developing research questions, nurse researchers need to consider substantive issues (Is the question significant?), clinical issues (Could the findings be useful in practice?), methodological issues (Can a study be designed to yield high-quality evidence?), practical issues (Are adequate resources available to do the study?), and ethical issues (Can this question be rigorously addressed without committing ethical transgressions?).

Step 2: Reviewing the Related Research Literature

Quantitative research is typically conducted within the context of previous knowledge. Quantitative researchers typically strive to understand what is already known about a topic by conducting a thorough **literature review** before any data are collected.

Step 3: Undertaking Clinical Fieldwork

Researchers embarking on a clinical nursing study often benefit from spending time in clinical settings, discussing the topic with clinicians and administrators, and observing current practices. Such clinical fieldwork can provide perspectives on recent clinical trends and health care delivery models; it can also help researchers better understand affected clients and the settings in which care is provided.

Step 4: Defining the Framework and Developing Conceptual Definitions

When quantitative research is performed within the context of a theoretical framework (i.e., when a theory is used as a basis for predictions that can be tested), the findings may have broader significance. Even when the research question is not embedded in a theory, researchers must have a clear sense of the concepts under study. Thus, an important early task is the development of conceptual definitions.

Step 5: Formulating Hypotheses

As noted in Chapter 2, hypotheses state researchers' expectations about relationships among study variables. The research question identifies the variables and asks how they might be related; a hypothesis is the predicted answer. For example, the research question might be: Is pre-eclamptic toxaemia in pregnant women related to stress experienced during pregnancy? This might lead to the following hypothesis: Pregnant women who report high levels of stress during pregnancy are more likely than women with lower levels of stress to develop pre-eclamptic toxaemia. Most quantitative studies test hypotheses.

Phase 2: The Design and Planning Phase

In the second major phase of a quantitative study, researchers make decisions about the methods to use to address the research question, and plan for the actual collection of data. As a consumer, you should be aware that the methodological decisions that researchers make during this phase affect the integrity, interpretability, and clinical utility of the results. Thus, you must be able to evaluate the decisions so that you can determine how much faith to put in the evidence. A major objective of this book is to help you evaluate methodological decisions.

Step 6: Selecting a Research Design

The **research design** is the overall plan for obtaining answers to the research questions and for addressing the challenges we described in Chapter 2. In quantitative studies, research designs tend to be highly structured and to include controls to reduce the effects of extraneous variables. There are a wide variety of experimental and nonexperimental research designs.

Step 7: Developing Protocols for the Intervention

In experimental research, researchers create the independent variable, which means that participants are exposed to two or more different treatments or conditions. An **intervention protocol** must be developed, specifying exactly what the intervention will entail (e.g., what it is, who will administer it, how frequently and over how long a period it will last, and so on) *and* what the alternative condition will be. The goal of well-articulated protocols is to have all participants in each group be treated in the same way. In nonexperimental research, of course, this step would not be necessary.

Step 8: Identifying the Population to be Studied

Quantitative researchers need to specify a population, indicating what attributes participants should possess, and thereby clarifying the group to which study results can be generalized. A **population** is *all* the individuals or objects with common, defining characteristics. For example, a researcher might specify that the study population consist of all licensed nurses residing in Canada.

Step 9: Designing the Sampling Plan

Researchers typically collect data from a **sample,** which is a subset of the population. Using samples is practical, but the risk is that the sample will not adequately reflect the population's traits. In a quantitative study, a sample's adequacy is assessed by the criterion of *representativeness*; that is, how typical, or representative, the sample is of the population. The **sampling plan** specifies in advance *how* the sample will be selected and *how many* study participants there will be.

Step 10: Specifying Methods to Measure Variables

Quantitative researchers must develop or borrow methods to measure study variables as accurately as possible. Based on the conceptual definitions, researchers select methods to operationalize the variables (i.e., to collect the data). A variety of quantitative data collection approaches exist; the most common methods are self-reports (e.g., interviews), observations, and biophysiologic measurements.

Step 11: Developing Methods to Protect Human/Animal Rights

Most nursing studies involve human subjects, although some involve animals. In either case, procedures need to be developed to ensure that the study adheres to ethical principles. Each aspect of the study plan needs to be reviewed to determine whether participants' rights have been adequately protected.

Step 12: Finalizing and Reviewing the Research Plan

Before collecting data, researchers often seek feedback from colleagues or advisers and perform "tests" to ensure that plans will work smoothly. For example, they may assess the *readability* of written materials to determine whether participants with low reading skills can comprehend them, or they may *pretest* their measuring instruments to assess their adequacy. If researchers have concerns about their study plans, they may undertake a **pilot study,** which is a small-scale version or trial run of the major study.

Example of a pilot study

Guirguis-Younger, Cappeliez, and Younger (2008) piloted a community-based behavioural intervention with six elderly participants who were depressed and were receiving home care for a variety of chronic or acute health conditions to evaluate the feasibility, effectiveness, and the key components of the intervention.

Phase 3: The Empirical Phase

The empirical phase of a quantitative study involves collecting data and preparing data for analysis. The empirical phase is often the most time-consuming part of the study.

Step 13: Collecting the Data

Data collection in a quantitative study normally proceeds according to a pre-established plan. The *data collection plan* specifies procedures for actually collecting the data (e.g., where, when, and how the data will be gathered), for recruiting the sample, and for training those who will collect the data.

Step 14: Preparing Data for Analysis

The data collected in a quantitative study are rarely amenable to direct analysis. One preliminary step is **coding,** which is the process of translating data into numeric form. For example, responses to a question about gender might be coded (1) for females and (2) for males. Another typical step involves transferring data from written forms to computer files for analysis.

Phase 4: The Analytic Phase

The quantitative data gathered in the empirical phase are not reported in *raw* form (i.e., as a mass of numbers). They are subjected to analysis and interpretation, which occurs in the fourth major phase of the project.

Step 15: Analyzing the Data

Research data must be processed and analyzed in an orderly fashion so that relationships can be discerned and hypotheses can be tested. Quantitative data are analyzed through **statistical analyses,** which include some simple procedures as well as complex methods.

Step 16: Interpreting the Results

Interpretation is the process of making sense of the results and examining their implications. In quantitative studies, researchers attempt to interpret study results in light of prior evidence and theory and in light of the rigour of the research methods. Interpretation also involves determining how the findings can best be used in clinical practice, or what further research is needed before utilization can be recommended.

Phase 5: The Dissemination Phase

In the analytic phase, the researcher comes full circle: the questions posed at the outset are answered. The researcher's job is not completed, however, until the study results are disseminated.

Step 17: Communicating the Findings

A study cannot contribute evidence to practice if the results are not communicated. Another—and often final—task of a research project is the preparation of a *research report* that can be shared with others. We discuss research reports in Chapter 4.

Step 18: Utilizing Research Evidence in Practice

Ideally, the concluding step of a good study is to plan for its use in practice settings. Although nurse researchers may not always be able to undertake a plan for utilizing research findings, they can contribute to the process by developing suggestions for how study findings could be incorporated into nursing practice and by vigorously pursuing opportunities to disseminate their findings to practicing nurses.

ACTIVITIES IN A QUALITATIVE STUDY

Quantitative research involves a fairly linear progression of tasks (i.e., researchers lay out in advance the steps to be taken to maximize the integrity of the study and then follow them as faithfully as possible). In a qualitative study, by contrast, the progression is closer to a circle than to a straight line—qualitative researchers are continually examining and interpreting data and making decisions about how to proceed based on what has already been discovered.

Because qualitative researchers have a flexible approach to collecting and analyzing data, it is impossible to define the flow of activities precisely—the flow varies from one study to another, and researchers themselves do not know ahead of time exactly how the study will unfold. We try to provide a sense of how a qualitative study is conducted, however, by describing some major activities and indicating how and when they might be performed.

Conceptualizing and Planning a Qualitative Study

Identifying a Research Problem

Qualitative researchers generally begin with a general topic area, often focusing on an aspect of a topic that is poorly understood and about which little is known. They therefore do not develop hypotheses or pose refined research questions at the outset. Qualitative researchers often proceed with a fairly broad question that allows the focus to be sharpened once they are in the field.

Performing a Literature Review

Not all qualitative researchers agree about the value of doing an upfront literature review. Some believe that the literature should not be consulted before collecting data. Their concern is that prior studies might unduly influence their conceptualization of the phenomenon under study. According to this view, the phenomenon should be elucidated based on participants' viewpoints rather than on prior information. Others believe that researchers should conduct at least a cursory literature review at the outset. In any event, qualitative researchers typically find a relatively small body of relevant literature because of the types of questions they ask.

Selecting and Gaining Entrée into Research Sites

Before going into the field, qualitative researchers must identify an appropriate site. For example, if the topic is the health care beliefs of the urban poor, a low-income inner-city neighbourhood must be identified. In many cases, researchers need to make preliminary contacts with key actors in the site to ensure cooperation and access to informants (i.e., researchers need to **gain entrée** into the site). Gaining entrée typically involves negotiations with *gatekeepers* (or *stakeholders*) who have the authority to permit entry into their world.

Designing Qualitative Studies

Quantitative researchers do not collect data before finalizing the research design. Qualitative researchers, by contrast, use an **emergent design**—a design that emerges during the course of data collection. Certain design features are guided by the study's qualitative tradition, but qualitative studies do not have a rigid structure that prohibits changes in the field.

Addressing Ethical Issues

Qualitative researchers, like quantitative researchers, must also develop plans for addressing ethical issues—and, indeed, there are special concerns in qualitative studies because of the more intimate nature of the relationship that typically develops between researchers and study participants.

Conducting a Qualitative Study

In qualitative studies, the activities of sampling, data collection, data analysis, and interpretation typically take place iteratively. Qualitative researchers begin by talking with or observing people who have first-hand experience with the phenomenon under study. The discussions and observations are loosely structured, allowing participants to express a full range of beliefs and behaviours. Analysis and interpretation are ongoing, concurrent activities, used to guide decisions about whom to sample next and what questions to ask or observations to make. The process of data analysis involves clustering together related types of narrative information into a coherent scheme.

As analysis and interpretation progress, the researcher begins to identify *themes* and categories, which are used to build a descriptive theory of the phenomenon. The kinds of data obtained become increasingly focused and purposeful as a theory emerges. Theory development and verification shape the sampling and data-gathering process—as the theory develops, the researcher seeks participants who can confirm and enrich the theoretical understandings as well as participants who can potentially challenge them and lead to further theoretical development.

Quantitative researchers decide in advance how many participants to include in the study, but qualitative researchers' sampling decisions are guided by the data themselves. Many qualitative researchers use the principle of **saturation,** which occurs when themes and categories in the data become repetitive and redundant, such that no new information can be gleaned by further data collection.

Quantitative researchers seek to collect high-quality data by using measuring instruments with demonstrated reliability and validity. Qualitative researchers, by contrast, *are* the main data collection instrument and must take steps to ensure the trustworthiness of the data. The central feature of these efforts is to confirm that the findings accurately reflect participants' experiences and viewpoints, rather than the researchers' perceptions. For example, one confirmatory activity involves going back to participants and sharing preliminary interpretations with them so that they can evaluate whether the researcher's thematic analysis is consistent with their experiences.

Disseminating Qualitative Findings

Quantitative reports almost never contain any **raw data**—data exactly in the form they were collected, which are numeric values. Qualitative reports, by contrast, are usually filled with rich verbatim passages directly from study participants. The excerpts are used in an evidential fashion to support or illustrate researchers' interpretations and thematic construction.

Example of raw data in a qualitative report

Goodridge et al. (2008) studied the perspectives of intensive care unit (ICU) health care professionals pertaining to potential obstacles in providing quality care to individuals with chronic obstructive pulmonary disease (COPD) at end-of-life. Three focus groups, ranging in size from four to seven participants, were conducted with a total of 17 clinicians, including 15 registered nurses and 2 respiratory therapists. Following each focus group, one participant from that group was interviewed individually to confirm the themes emerging from the discussion. One theme that emerged was *feelings of complicity in prolonging suffering* as illustrated by the focus group interaction: P1: . . . there's a lot of times that I see where we all are, we're all standing around thinking "Oh, my God, I can't believe we're going to intubate this patient. I can't believe we're going to do this." And, sure enough, a few months down the road, they die a horrible death in the ventilator in ICU . . . "I can't believe we are going to do this." P5: And that's were it becomes hard on our part, because, you know pretty well what's coming, and we're just simply prolonging [life], and at times [it] feels [like] that you're being abusive.

Like quantitative researchers, qualitative nurse researchers want to see their findings used by others. Qualitative findings can serve as the basis for formulating hypotheses that are tested by quantitative researchers, and for developing measuring instruments used for both research and clinical purposes. Qualitative findings can also provide a foundation for designing effective nursing interventions. Qualitative studies help to shape nurses' perceptions of a problem or situation, their conceptualization of potential solutions, and their understanding of patients' concerns and experiences.

RESEARCH EXAMPLES AND CRITICAL THINKING ACTIVITIES

EXAMPLE 1 ■ Quantitative Research

The progression of activities in a quantitative study by one of this book's authors (Beck) is summarized below, followed by some questions to guide critical thinking.

Study

"Further validation of the Postpartum Depression Screening Scale" (Beck & Gable, 2001)

Study Purpose

Beck and Gable (2001) undertook a study to evaluate the Postpartum Depression Screening Scale (PDSS), an instrument designed for use by clinicians and researchers to screen mothers for postpartum depression (PPD).

Phase 1. Conceptual Phase, 1 Month: This phase was the shortest because most of the conceptual work had been done earlier in developing the instrument (Beck & Gable, 2000). The literature had already been reviewed, so the review only needed to be updated. The same framework and conceptual definitions that had been used in the first study were used in the new study.

Phase 2. Design and Planning Phase, 6 Months: The second phase involved fine-tuning the research design, gaining entrée into the hospital where participants were recruited, and obtaining approval of the hospital's ethics review committee. During this period, Beck met with statistical consultants and an instrument development consultant to finalize the design.

Phase 3. Empirical Phase, 11 Months: The design called for administering the PDSS to 150 mothers who were 6 weeks postpartum, and then scheduling a psychiatric diagnostic interview for them to determine whether they were suffering from PPD. Recruitment of participants and data collection took nearly a year.

Phase 4. Analytic Phase, 3 Months: Statistical tests were performed to determine a cut-off score on the PDSS above which mothers would be identified as having screened positive for PPD. Data analysis also was undertaken to determine the accuracy of the PDSS in predicting diagnosed PPD.

Phase 5. Dissemination Phase, 18 Months: The researchers prepared a research report and submitted it to the journal *Nursing Research* for possible publication. It was accepted for publication within 4 months, but it was "in press" (awaiting publication) for 14 months. During this period, the authors presented their findings at conferences, and prepared a report for the agency that funded the research.

Key Findings

Beck and Gable found that the PDSS was a reliable and valid tool for screening mothers and considered that the scale was ready for routine use.

CRITICAL THINKING SUGGESTIONS

1. Answers questions 1 and 3 from Box 1.1 (Chapter 1, p. 19) regarding this study.
2. Also consider the following targeted questions, which may further sharpen your critical thinking skills and assist you in understanding this study:
   a. Was the study experimental or nonexperimental? What do you think the *population* for this study was?
   b. How would you evaluate Beck and Gable's dissemination plan?
   c. What are your thoughts about how time was allocated in this study; that is, how much time was spent in each phase?
   d. Would it have been appropriate for the researchers to address the research question using qualitative research methods? Why or why not?

(Research Examples and Critical Thinking Activities continues on page 52)

Research Examples and Critical Thinking Activities (continued)

3. If the results of this study are valid and generalizable, what are some of the uses to which the findings might be put in clinical practice?

EXAMPLE 2 ■ Qualitative Research

The progression of activities in a qualitative study is summarized below, followed by some questions to guide critical thinking.

Study

"An in-depth exploration of information-seeking behavior among individuals with cancer: Part 1. Understanding differential patterns of active information-seeking" (Lambert, Loiselle, & Macdonald, 2009a) and "An in-depth exploration of information-seeking behavior among individuals with cancer: Part 2. Understanding patterns of information disinterest and avoidance" (Lambert, Loiselle, & Macdonald, 2009b)

Study Purpose

Lambert and colleagues undertook a grounded theory to describe and explain the information-seeking behaviors patterns of individuals diagnosed with breast, prostate, or colorectal cancer.

Phase 1. Conceptual Phase, 5 months: Lambert became interested in the information-seeking behavior of individuals diagnosed with cancer when she became involved in Loiselle's (second author) program of research which focuses on cancer information needs and the use of information technology in proving tailored cancer information. Loiselle's previous studies revealed that individuals diagnosed with cancer vary in the type and amount of information they prefer. However, no study to date had systematically documented potential, differential cancer information-seeking behaviors. Lambert gained entry into chemotherapy and radiotherapy clinics by contacting the Nursing Director.

Phase 2. Design and Planning Phase, 7 months: Lambert and colleagues chose a grounded theory design because they wanted to explain differential preferences for type, amount, and sources of cancer information, as well as the various information management strategies used by individuals. The grounded theory developed was expected to identify the antecedents to each emerging information-seeking behavior pattern, describe its essential characteristics, and outcome. Lambert and colleagues discussed the best approach for recruiting participants and collecting the data (individual interviews versus focus groups). Once the design was finalized, the research proposal was submitted to ethics review committees. Following ethics approval, Lambert and colleagues met with the Nursing Director and the clinical nurse specialist to introduce and further discuss the overall study and participant recruitment strategies.

Phase 3. Empirical/Analytic Phases, 18 months: Data collection and data analysis occurred simultaneously in this study. Lambert and colleagues conducted in-depth, individual, face-to-face interviews with 30 individuals diagnosed with breast, prostate, or colorectal cancer and eight focus groups with an additional 30 participants. Some strategies used by Lambert and colleagues to enhance the trustworthiness of their findings included: (1) audiotaping all interviews and focus groups so that they would have verbatim transcripts for data analysis and (2) discussing the emerging theory with participants.

Phase 4. Dissemination Phase, 12 months: Lambert and colleagues submitted the two manuscripts to Cancer Nursing and the two papers were published in January 2009. Lambert and colleagues also presented the findings at national and international conferences.

Key Findings

The core variable identified was "playing my part and taking care of myself." Related to this core variable, five patterns of information-seeking behaviors emerged from the analysis:

intense information-seeking, complementary information-seeking, fortuitous information-seeking, minimal information-seeking, and guarded information-seeking.

CRITICAL THINKING SUGGESTIONS

1. Answers questions 1 and 3 from Box 1.1 (Chapter 1, p. 19) regarding this study.

2. Also consider the following targeted questions, which may further sharpen your critical thinking skills and assist you in understanding this study:
   a. What are your thoughts about how time was allocated for each phase of the study?
   b. Given the focus of the study, do you think that grounded theory was the appropriate research approach?
   c. Who were the "gatekeepers" in the hospital who helped Lambert and colleagues recruit the sample?
   d. Would it have been appropriate for Lambert and colleagues to address the research question using quantitative research methods? Why or why not?

3. If the results of this study are valid and generalizable, in what ways can the results be applied to clinical practice?

EXAMPLE 3 ■ Quantitative Research

The progression of activities in the study by Bryanton and colleagues (2008) in Appendix A is not spelled out in detail in the report (this is normal), but there are cues that provide some insights about scheduling. Answer the following questions regarding the timeframe of the study:

1. When was the study submitted to the journal for publication? (See the footnote at the end of the report.) How long did it take between acceptance and publication?

2. What is your estimate of how long the study took, from the time it was conceptualized (and an application was submitted for financial support) until the time when the report was published?

EXAMPLE 4 ■ Qualitative Research

The progression of activities in Woodgate's study in Appendix B is not spelled out in detail in the report, but there are cues that provide insights about scheduling. Answer the following questions regarding the timeframe of the study:

1. Over how long a period were the data for this study collected? Why do you think it took this long to collect the data?

2. Did Woodgate receive funding to complete her study? (Information regarding funding is usually found in a footnote.)

3. When was the study accepted for publication? (Is it specified?)

4. How long did it take between when the report was accepted for publication and when it was published? (Is it specified?)

5. What is your estimate of how long the study took; from the time it was conceptualized until the time when the report was published? (Does the report present this information?)

Summary Points

⇒ Quantitative studies are either experimental or nonexperimental. In **experimental research,** researchers actively introduce a treatment or intervention; in **nonexperimental research,** researchers make observations of existing characteristics and behaviour without intervening.

⇒ Qualitative nursing research often is rooted in research traditions from the disciplines of anthropology, sociology, and psychology. Three such traditions are ethnography, grounded theory, and phenomenology.

⇒ **Grounded theory** seeks to describe and understand key social–psychological processes that occur in social settings.

⇒ **Phenomenology** is concerned with lived experiences and is an approach to learning about what people's life experiences are like and what they mean.

⇒ **Ethnography** provides a framework for studying the meanings, patterns, and experiences of a defined cultural group in a holistic fashion.

⇒ In a quantitative study, researchers progress in a linear fashion from posing a research question to answering it in fairly standard steps.

⇒ The main phases in a quantitative study are the conceptual, planning, empirical, analytic, and dissemination phases.

⇒ The conceptual phase involves defining the problem to be studied, doing a **literature review** engaging in clinical fieldwork for clinical studies, developing a framework and conceptual definitions, and formulating hypotheses to be tested.

⇒ The design and planning phase entails selecting a **research design,** formulating the **intervention protocol** (in experimental research), specifying the **population,** developing a **sampling plan,** specifying methods to measure the research variables, designing procedures to protect subjects' rights, and finalizing the research plan (and, in some cases, conducting a **pilot study**).

⇒ The empirical phase involves collecting the data and preparing the data for analysis (e.g., **coding** the data).

⇒ The analytic phase involves analyzing the data through **statistical analysis** and interpreting the results.

⇒ The dissemination phase entails communicating the findings and promoting their utilization.

⇒ The flow of activities in a qualitative study is more flexible and less linear than in a quantitative study.

⇒ Qualitative researchers begin with a broad question that is narrowed through the actual process of data collection and analysis.

⇒ In the early phase of a qualitative study, researchers select a site and then take steps to **gain entrée** into it; gaining entrée typically involves enlisting the cooperation of *gatekeepers i stakeholders* within the site.

⇒ Qualitative studies typically involve an **emergent design:** researchers select informants, collect data, and then analyze and interpret them in an ongoing fashion. Field experiences help to shape the design of the study.

⇒ Early analysis leads to refinements in sampling and data collection, until **saturation** (redundancy of information) is achieved.

⇒ Qualitative researchers conclude by disseminating findings that can subsequently be used to guide further studies, to develop structured measuring tools, and to influence nurses' perceptions of a problem and their conceptualizations of potential solutions.

STUDIES CITED IN CHAPTER 3*

*This reference list contains only those studies that were cited in this chapter. Citations pertaining to theoretical, methodological, or nonempirical work are included together in a separate section at the end of the book (beginning on page 399).

Beck, C. T., & Gable, R. K. (2001). Further validation of the Postpartum Depression Screening Scale. *Nursing Research, 50,* 155–164.

Bryanton, J., Gagnon, A. J., Johnston, C., & Hatem, M. (2008). Predictors of women's perceptions of the childbirth experience. *Journal of Obstetric, Gynecologic, & Neonatal Nursing, 37*(1), 24–34.

Chiovitti, R. (2008). Nurses' meaning of caring with patients in acute psychiatric hospital settings: A grounded theory study. *International Journal of Nursing Studies, 45*(2), 203–223.

Fillion, L., Gagnon, P., Leblond, F., et al. (2008). A brief intervention for fatigue management in breast cancer survivors. *Cancer Nursing, 31*(2), 145–159.

Gantert, T. W., McWilliam, C. L., Ward-Griffin, C., & Allen, N. J. (2008). The key to me: Seniors' perceptions of relationship-building with in-home service providers. *Canadian Journal on Aging, 27*(1), 23–34.

Glaser, B. G., & Strauss, A. L. (1967). *The discovery of grounded theory: Strategies for Qualitative Research.* Chicago: Aldine.

Goodridge, D., Duggleby, W., Gjevre, J., & Rennie, D. (2008). Caring for critically ill patients with advanced COPD at the end of life: A qualitative study. *Intensive and Critical Care Nursing, 24*(3), 162–170.

Guirguis-Younger, M., Cappeliez, P., & Younger, A. (2008). A community-based intervention for treating depression in seniors. *The Canadian Journal of Nursing Research, 40*(1), 60–79.

Lambert, S. D., Loiselle, C. G., & Macdonald, M. E. (2009a). An in-depth exploration of information-seeking behavior among individuals with cancer: Part 1. Understanding differential patterns of active information-seeking. *Cancer Nursing, 32*(1), 11–25.

Lambert, S. D., Loiselle, C. G., & Macdonald, M. E. (2009b). An in-depth exploration of information-seeking behavior among individuals with cancer: Part 2. Understanding patterns of information disinterest and avoidance. *Cancer Nursing, 32*(1), 26–36.

Tang, S. Y., & Browne, A. J. (2008). "Race" matters: Racialization and egalitarian discourses involving Aboriginal people in the Canadian health care context. *Ethnicity & Health, 13*(2), 109–127.

4 Reading Research Reports

On completing this chapter, you will be able to:

1. Name types of research reports

2. Describe the major sections in a research journal article

3. Characterize the style used in quantitative and qualitative research reports

4. Distinguish research summaries and research critiques

5. Define new terms in the chapter

TYPES OF RESEARCH REPORTS

Evidence from nursing studies is communicated through *research reports* that describe what was studied, how it was studied, and what was found. Research reports—especially reports for quantitative studies—are often daunting to readers without research training. This chapter is designed to help make research reports more accessible.

Researchers communicate information about their studies in various ways. The most common types of research reports are theses and dissertations, books, presentations at conferences, and journal articles. You are most likely to be exposed to research results at professional conferences or in journals. However, there is a recent push across Canadian universities to disseminate research findings beyond traditional academic reports (part of the drive for evidence-based practice detailed later in Chapter 18), so chances are that you will see more research described in such venues as institutional newsletters.

Presentations at Professional Conferences

Research findings are presented at conferences as oral presentations or poster sessions.

➤ *Oral presentations* follow a format similar to that used in journal articles, which we discuss later in this chapter. The presenter of an oral report is typically allotted 10 to 20 minutes to describe the most important aspects of the study.

➤ In *poster sessions,* many researchers simultaneously present visual displays summarizing their studies, and conference attendees circulate around the room perusing these displays.

One attractive feature of conference presentations is that there may be less time elapsed between the completion of a study and the dissemination of findings than is the case with journal articles. Conferences also offer an opportunity for dialogue among researchers and conference attendees. The listeners at oral presentations and viewers of poster displays can ask questions to help them better understand how the study was done or what the findings mean; moreover, they can offer the researchers suggestions about the clinical implications of the study. Thus, professional conferences offer a particularly valuable forum for a clinical audience.

> **TIP**
>
> Conferences are immediate forums for researchers; preliminary findings on ongoing studies can be presented to obtain valuable feedback from colleagues. Research articles, by contrast, can take months or even years to produce. As a consumer of research, you should note not only the date of publication for the article, but also the date of acceptance to publish and the data collection period, which many journals now include.

Research Journal Articles

Research **journal articles** are reports that summarize studies in professional journals. Because competition for journal space is keen, the typical research article is brief—generally only 10 to 25 double-spaced manuscript pages. This means that researchers must condense a lot of information about the study purpose, research methods, findings, interpretation, and clinical significance into a short report.

Publication in journals is competitive; even the journals themselves are ranked in order from highest to lowest impact, calculated by the Institute for Scientific Information (ISI). A journal's impact factor is taken into consideration, along with other factors such as targeted audience, and when and where researchers choose to publish their work. Usually, research articles are reviewed, based on the journal's review guidelines, by two or more **peer reviewers** (other researchers doing work in the field) who make recommendations about whether the article should be accepted, rejected, or revised and re-reviewed. These are usually "**blind**" **reviews**—reviewers are not told researchers' names, and researchers are not told reviewers' names.

In major nursing research journals, the rate of acceptance is low—it can be as low as 5% of submitted manuscripts. Thus, consumers of research articles have some assurance that the reports have already been evaluated by other nurse researchers. Nevertheless, the publication of an article does not mean that the findings can be uncritically accepted. The validity of the findings and their utility for clinical practice depend on how the study was conducted. Research methods courses help consumers to evaluate the quality of research evidence reported in journal articles.

THE CONTENT OF RESEARCH JOURNAL ARTICLES

Research reports in journals tend to follow a certain format and are written in a particular style. Research reports begin with a title that succinctly conveys (typically in 15 or fewer words) the nature of the study. In qualitative studies, the title includes the central phenomenon and group under investigation; in quantitative studies, the title usually indicates the independent and dependent variables and the population. Because there is a steady increase in publishing results from pilot studies, most journals now also note this upfront in the title for reader clarity.

Quantitative reports—and many qualitative ones—typically follow a conventional format for organizing content: the **IMRAD format.** This format involves organizing material into four sections—the **I**ntroduction, **M**ethod, **R**esults, and **D**iscussion. The main text of the report is usually preceded by an abstract and followed by references.

The Abstract

The **abstract** is a brief description of the study placed at the beginning of the article. The abstract answers, in about 100 to 200 words, the following questions: What were the research questions? What methods were used to address those questions? What were the findings? and What are the implications for nursing practice? Readers can review an abstract to assess whether the report is of interest and should be read in its entirety.

Some journals have moved from having traditional abstracts—single paragraphs summarizing the main features of the study—to more informative, structured abstracts with specific headings. For example, abstracts in *Nursing Research* after 1997 present information about the study organized under the following headings: Background, Objectives, Method, Results, Conclusions, and Key Words. Although these headings may vary slightly according to journal preference, the same basic information is presented to standardize reporting for greater reader clarity and comparison between studies.

Box 4.1 presents abstracts from two actual studies. The first is a traditional abstract for a quantitative study entitled "Exploring the Technology Readiness of Nursing and Medical Students at a Canadian University" (Caison, Bulman, Pai, & Neville, 2008). The second is a "new style" abstract for a qualitative study

---

BOX 4.1   EXAMPLES OF ABSTRACTS FROM JOURNAL ARTICLES
  ▶

Quantitative Study

Technology readiness is a well-established construct that refers to individuals' ability to embrace and adopt new technology. Given the increasing use of advanced technologies in the delivery of health care, this study uses the Technology Readiness Index (Parasuraman, 2000) to explore the technology readiness of nursing and medical students from the fall 2006 cohort at Memorial University of Newfoundland. The three major findings from this study are that (i) rural nursing students are more insecure with technology than their urban counterparts, (ii) male medical students score higher on innovation than their female counterparts, and have higher overall technology readiness attitude than female medical students, and (iii) medical students who are older than 25 have a negative technology readiness score whereas those under 25 had a positive score. These findings suggest health care professional schools would be well served to implement curricular changes designed to support the needs of rural students, women, and those entering school at a nontraditional age. In addition, patterns such as those observed in this study highlight areas of emphasis for current practitioners as health care organizations develop continuing education offerings for staff (Caison, Bulman, Pai, & Neville, 2008).

Qualitative Study

Objective: To explore the unique experiences, challenges, and coping strategies of pregnant women diagnosed with thrombophilia and who are on daily heparin injections.
Design: A qualitative, descriptive approach with semistructured interviews was used.
Participants and Setting: Nine women from the thrombosis clinic of a large university-affiliated hospital in Montreal, Canada, participated in the study.
Data Analysis: Thematic analysis was used throughout the processes of interviewing, transcribing, and reviewing the data.
Results: Findings indicate that past pregnancy experiences influenced the meaning of diagnosis and treatment as well as the participants' experience of uncertainty. Participants expressed a need for increased professional support in health care decision making as well as increased information around injection technique. In facing these challenges, participants coped by taking control and maintaining perspective.
Conclusions: Coping with thrombophilia in pregnancy can be a stressful experience. However, the ensuing challenges are perceived as manageable discomforts in light of the outcome of a healthy baby (Martens & Emed, 2007).

entitled "The Experiences and Challenges of Pregnant Women Coping with Thrombophilia" (Martens & Emed, 2007). These two studies are used as illustrations throughout this chapter.

The Introduction

The introduction acquaints readers with the research problem and its context. The introduction usually describes the following:

➢ *The central phenomena, concepts, or variables under study.* The problem area under investigation is identified and key terms are defined.

➢ *The statement of purpose, research questions, and/or hypotheses to be tested.* Researchers explain what they set out to accomplish by conducting the study.

➢ *A review of the related literature.* Current knowledge relating to the study problem is briefly described so that readers can understand how the study fits in with previous findings and can assess the contribution of the new study.

➢ *The theoretical framework.* In theoretically driven studies, the framework is usually presented in the introduction.

➢ *The significance of and need for the study.* Most research reports include an explanation of why the study is important to nursing.

Thus, the introduction sets the stage for a description of what the researcher did and what was learned. The information in the introduction corresponds roughly to the activities undertaken in the conceptual phase of the project, as described in Chapter 3.

In the following example from an introductory paragraph, the researcher describes the background of the problem, the population of primary interest (pregnant women with thrombophilia) and the need for the study (to better understand the impact of this serious condition on the pregnancy experience).

Example from an introductory paragraph

"Thrombophilia is a serious hypercoagulability disorder that contributes to maternal mortality and has been associated with significant pregnancy complications including intrauterine growth restriction, preeclampsia, and recurrent fetal loss. The incidence of thrombophilia is approximately 15% in the general population (Greer, 2003) and recurrent fetal loss occurs in as many as 65% of pregnant women with thrombophilia (Kovalevsky, Gracia, Berlin, Sammel, & Barnhart, 2004; Kujovich, 2004; Rey, Kahn, David, & Shrier, 2003). At this time, there are no screening protocols in place, and thrombophilia often goes undiagnosed until several pregnancy complications have already occurred (Kujovich, 2004; Walker, Grieves, & Preston, 2001). This may lead to considerable emotional and psychological distress greatly impacting the experience of women with thrombophilia who desire to have children" (Martens & Emed, 2007, p. 55).

TIP

The introduction sections of many reports are not specifically labelled "Introduction." The report's introduction immediately follows the abstract.

The Method Section

The method section describes the methods the researcher used to answer the research questions. The method section tells readers about major methodologic decisions and may offer rationales for those decisions. For example, a report for a qualitative study may explain why a qualitative approach was considered to be appropriate and fruitful.

In a report for a quantitative study, the method section usually describes the following, which may be in specifically labelled subsections:

⇒ *The research design.* A description of the research design focuses on the overall plan for structuring the study, often including the steps the researcher took to minimize biases and control extraneous variables.

⇒ *The sample.* Quantitative research reports describe the population under study, specifying the criteria by which the researcher decided whether a person would be eligible for the study. The method section also describes the actual sample, indicating how people were selected and the number of subjects in the sample. Most journals now also request an indication of the data collection period, so readers can be aware of the "age" of the data.

⇒ *Measures and data collection.* Researchers describe the methods and procedures used to collect the data, including how the critical research variables were operationalized. They also present information about the quality of the measurement tools, such as the reported reliability of the instrument (discussed further in Chapter 14).

⇒ *Study procedures.* The method section contains a description of the procedures used to conduct the study, including a description of any intervention. The researcher's efforts to protect participants' rights may also be documented in this section.

Table 4.1 presents excerpts from the method section of the quantitative study by Caison et al. (2008), describing aspects of the research design, sample (i.e., participants), data collection strategies (i.e., instrument), and procedures (data collection).

TABLE 4.1   EXCERPTS FROM METHOD SECTION, QUANTITATIVE REPORT

METHODOLOGIC ELEMENT	EXCERPT FROM CAISON ET AL. (2008)
Research design	In order to explore the technology readiness of nursing and medical students, the fall 2006 cohorts of medical and nursing students at Memorial University of Newfoundland (MUN) were studied, using a cross-sectional survey approach. (p. 285)
Participants	MUN, the largest university in Atlantic Canada, is located in the provincial capital of St. John's, Newfoundland and Labrador. The School of Medicine offers an undergraduate medical education program leading to the M.D. degree, which prepares students for licensing as a physician. The School of Nursing offers three undergraduate programs. . . . Only the regular and fast track Bachelor of Nursing students were included in the study because the post-RN nursing students are considerably further along in their professional development. . . . (p. 285)
Instruments	The instrument utilized in this study was a 35-item survey designed to assess health professional attitudes toward technology, and was adapted from the work of Parasuraman (2000) and Parasuraman and Colby (2001). . . . Respondents were asked to rate their degree of agreement on a 5-point Likert scale for each item (i.e., 1 = strongly disagree, to 5 = strongly agree) and complete 9 demographic questions. (p. 286)
Data collection	Once approval of the Human Investigation Committee of Memorial University was granted, the research team approached the nursing and medical student societies to gain support for this study. . . . The research team then, with permission of the instructors, administered the instrument during a first-year course for each discipline. Students were advised they were not required to participate and that their responses were anonymous. . . . (p. 285)

TABLE 4.2	EXCERPTS FROM METHOD SECTION, QUALITATIVE REPORT
METHODOLOGIC ELEMENT	EXCERPT FROM MARTENS AND EMED (2007)
Recruitment	Eligible individuals were identified by the clinical nurse specialist or the attending physicians at the thrombosis clinic of a large university-affiliated hospital in Montreal, Canada. Ethical approval was obtained from the institutional review boards at both the hospital and the university. (p. 56)
Participants	Women diagnosed with acquired or inherited thrombophilia who were prescribed UFH or LMWH during pregnancy and who were pregnant at the time of the study or had been pregnant within the past 12 months were eligible. (p. 56)
Data collection	Data were collected via semistructured interviews conducted over 4 months. Participants were encouraged to tell their stories and were given freedom to expand on what they felt was most significant. Interviews were conducted by the first author, lasted approximately 45 minutes, and took place at a location most convenient for the participant, such as the hospital or the participant's home. (p. 56)
Data analysis	Thematic analysis was used throughout the process of interviewing, transcribing, and reviewing the data. Transcripts and field notes were examined line by line and key statements regarding participants' experiences highlighted and coded. Codes were then defined, categorized, and compiled into themes. Categories were reviewed for overlap, compared between subjects, and continually refined. Trustworthiness (Lincoln & Guba, 1985) was enhanced by audiotaping and transcribing each interview verbatim and by completing field notes within 24 hours of each interview. In addition, each step of the analysis was reviewed and validated by the coauthor. (p. 57)

Qualitative researchers discuss many of the same issues, but with different emphases. For example, reports for qualitative studies often provide more information about the research setting and the study context and less information on sampling. Also, because formal instruments are not used to collect qualitative data, there is little discussion about data collection methods, but there may be more information on data collection procedures. Qualitative reports increasingly are including descriptions of the researchers' efforts to ensure the trustworthiness of the data. Some qualitative reports also have a subsection on data analysis. There are fairly standard ways of analyzing quantitative data, but such standardization does not exist for qualitative data, so qualitative researchers may describe their analytic approach. Table 4.2 presents excerpts from the method section of the qualitative study by Martens and Emed (2007), describing aspects of their sample, data collection, and data analysis.

In quantitative studies, the method section describes decisions made during the design and planning phase of the study and implemented during the empirical phase (see Chapter 3). In qualitative studies, the methodologic decisions are made during the planning stage and also during the course of data collection and fieldwork.

The Results Section

The results section presents the research **findings** (i.e., the results obtained from data analysis). The text presents a narrative summary of the findings, often accompanied by tables or figures that highlight the most noteworthy results.

Results sections typically contain basic descriptive information, including a description of the participants (e.g., their average age). In quantitative studies, researchers also provide descriptive information about key variables. For example, in a study of the effect of prenatal drug exposure on birth outcomes, the results section might begin by describing the average birth weights and Apgar scores of the infants, or the percentage of infants with low birth weight (less than 2500 g).

In quantitative studies, the results section also reports the following information relating to the statistical analyses performed:

➤ *The name of statistical tests used.* A **statistical test** is a procedure for testing hypotheses and evaluating the believability of the findings. For example, if the percentage of low-birth-weight infants in the sample of drug-exposed infants is computed, how probable is it that the percentage is accurate? If the researcher finds that the average birth weight of drug-exposed infants in the sample is lower than the birth weight of infants who were not exposed to drugs, how probable is it that the same would be true for other infants not in the sample? That is, is the relationship between prenatal drug exposure and infant birth weight *real* and likely to be replicated with a new sample of infants? Statistical tests answer such questions. Statistical tests are based on common principles; you do not have to know the names of all statistical tests (there are dozens of them) to comprehend the findings.

➤ *The value of the calculated statistic.* Computers are used to compute a numeric value for the particular statistical test used. The value allows the researchers to draw conclusions about the meaning of the results. The *actual* numeric value of the statistic, however, is not inherently meaningful and need not concern you.

➤ *The significance.* The most important information is whether the results of the statistical tests were significant (not to be confused with important or clinically relevant). If the results were **statistically significant,** it means that, based on the statistical test, the findings are probably reliable and replicable with a new group of people. Research reports also indicate the **level of significance,** which is an index of how probable it is that the findings are reliable. For example, if a report indicates that a finding was significant at the .05 level, this means that only 5 times out of 100 (5/100 = .05) would the results be spurious. In other words, 95 times out of 100, similar results would be obtained with other samples from the same population. Readers can therefore have a high degree of confidence—but not total assurance—that the findings are accurate.

Example from the results section of a quantitative study

Independent sample *t*-tests were used to explore relationships between the technology readiness constructs and the various demographic variables in the study. When comparing nursing students and medical students on the four components of technology readiness, the researcher observed no significant differences. However, the insecurity subscale was observed to be significantly different between all students who intend to practice in a rural ($\mu = 3.5567$) versus urban ($\mu = 3.2889$) setting following graduation ($t = 2.00$, $df = 75$, $p \leq .0496$). Following Cohen's (1988) guidelines, this effect was found to be of a moderate size ($d = 0.5838$) (Caison et. al., 2008).

In this excerpt, Caison and her colleagues indicated that the study participants' mean score (represented by the symbol μ) on the measure of insecurity was significantly higher in the group that intended to practice rurally. In this case, the finding is fairly reliable; close to 5 times in 100 ($p = .05$) would the results have occurred as a fluke. Note that to comprehend this finding, you do not need to understand what the *t* statistic is, nor do you need to concern yourself with the degrees of freedom (*df*) measure. The additional Cohen test (represented by the symbol *d*) backs up this finding by showing that the observed difference matters.

Exploring this theme of interest further, Caison and colleagues go on to look specifically at nursing students in terms of their geographical background and technological readiness:

As shown in Table V, significant differences do emerge between the technology readiness of various demographic groups. It was observed that the rural nursing students indicated significantly greater insecurity with technology than did their urban counterparts. The associated Cohen's *d* of 0.83 reveals this to be a strong effect.

This time, the researchers found a significant difference in the insecurity subscale between nursing students who originate from rural versus urban backgrounds—supported very strongly by the additional Cohen test.

TIP

Be especially alert to the *p* values (probabilities) when reading statistical results. If a *p* value is greater than .05 (e.g., *p* = .08), the results are considered *not* to be statistically significant by conventional standards. Nonsignificant results are sometimes abbreviated NS. Also, be aware that the results are *more* reliable if the *p* value is smaller. For example, there is a higher probability that the results are accurate when *p* = .01 (only 1 in 100 chance of a false result) than when *p* = .05 (5 in 100 chances of a false result). Researchers sometimes report an exact probability estimate (e.g., *p* = .03), as in the above example, or a probability below conventional thresholds (e.g., *p* < .05, less than 5 in 100).

In qualitative reports, the researcher often organizes findings according to the major *themes* or categories that were identified in the data. The results section of qualitative reports sometimes has several subsections, with headings corresponding to the themes. Excerpts from the raw data are presented to support and provide a rich description of the thematic analysis. The results section of qualitative reports may also present the researcher's emerging theory about the phenomenon under study, although this may appear in the concluding section of the report.

Example from the results section of a qualitative study
As women faced the possibility of pregnancy complications, painful daily injections, and a perceived lack of professional support, they exemplified remarkable resourcefulness in taking control and taking steps to meet their needs. One woman expressed this succinctly: "When you want to have a baby . . . nothing will stop you" (Martens & Emed, 2007, p. 59).

In this excerpt, through the use of a direct quote from one study participant, the researchers illustrated the finding that taking control was a dominant coping strategy employed by these women.

The Discussion

In the discussion section, researchers draw conclusions about the meaning and implications of the findings. In this section, the researchers try to unravel what the results mean, why things turned out the way they did, and how the results can be used in practice. The discussion in both qualitative and quantitative reports may incorporate the following elements:

≈ *An interpretation of the results.* The interpretation involves the translation of findings into practical, conceptual, or theoretical meaning.

≈ *Implications.* Researchers often offer suggestions for how their findings could be used to support and/or improve nursing practice, and they may also make recommendations on how best to advance knowledge through additional research.

➤ *Study limitations.* The researcher is in the best position possible to discuss study limitations, such as sample deficiencies, design problems, and so forth. Reports that identify these limitations indicate to readers that the author was aware of these limitations and probably took them into account in interpreting the findings.

Example from the discussion section of a quantitative report

"This research study . . . adds to the knowledge base on this topic as few other studies have been conducted with this particular population. Furthermore, it points to possible policy and curricular adjustments that could improve the technology readiness of future health care practitioners. . . . Further research is planned with a larger sample size to confirm these results. Additionally, this study provided a snapshot of the technological readiness of medical and nursing students in the autumn of 2006, though the technology readiness of entering students may vary from year to year" (Caison et al., 2008, pp. 290–291).

As this example illustrates, researchers may speculate in the discussion section about what more can be achieved in this area.

References

Research journal articles conclude with a list of the books, reports, and journal articles that were referenced in the report. If you are interested in pursuing additional reading on a substantive topic, the reference list of a recent study is an excellent place to begin.

THE STYLE OF RESEARCH JOURNAL ARTICLES

Research reports tell a story. However, the style in which many journal articles are written—especially for quantitative studies—makes it difficult for beginning research consumers to become interested in the story. To unaccustomed audiences, research reports may seem pedantic or bewildering. Four factors contribute to this impression:

➤ *Compactness.* Journal space is limited, so authors compress many ideas and concepts into a short space. Interesting, personalized aspects of the investigation often cannot be reported. And, in qualitative studies, only a handful of supporting quotes can be included.

➤ *Jargon.* The authors of both qualitative and quantitative reports use research terms that are assumed to be part of the readers' vocabulary but that may be mystifying.

➤ *Objectivity.* Quantitative researchers often avoid any impression of subjectivity, and so their research stories are told in a way that makes them sound impersonal. For example, most quantitative research reports are written in the passive voice (i.e., personal pronouns are avoided). Use of the passive voice makes a report less lively than use of the active voice, and it tends to give the impression that the researcher did not play an active role in conducting the study. Qualitative reports, by contrast, are more subjective and personal and are written in a more conversational style.

➤ *Statistical information.* In quantitative reports, numbers may intimidate readers who do not have strong mathematic interest or training.

A goal of this textbook is to assist you in understanding the content of research reports and in overcoming anxieties about jargon and statistical information.

READING, SUMMARIZING, AND CRITIQUING RESEARCH REPORTS

Nurses who want to develop and support an evidence-based practice must be able to read and critically appraise research reports. This section offers some general guidance on reading nursing research reports.

Reading and Summarizing Research Reports

The skills involved in critical appraisal take time to develop. The first step in being able to use research findings in practice is to understand research reports. Your first few attempts to read research reports might be overwhelming, and you may wonder whether being able to understand, let alone appraise, them is a realistic goal. As you progress through this textbook, you will acquire skills to help you evaluate these reports. Some preliminary tips on digesting research reports follow:

➢ Grow accustomed to the style of research reports by reading them frequently, even though you may not yet understand all the technical points. Try to keep the underlying rationale for the style of research reports in mind as you read.

➢ Initially, read from a hard copy of an on-line article so that you can use a highlighter; write notes in the margins, and so forth.

➢ Read journal articles slowly. It may be useful to skim the article first to get the major points and then to read the article more carefully a second time.

➢ On the second or later reading of a journal article, train yourself to become an *active* reader. Reading actively involves constantly monitoring yourself to determine whether you understand what you are reading. If you have comprehension problems, go back and reread difficult passages or make notes about your confusion so that you can ask someone for clarification. Usually, that "someone" will be your research instructor or a faculty member, but also consider contacting the researchers themselves. The postal and e-mail addresses of the researchers are usually included in the journal article, and researchers are generally more than willing to discuss their research with others.

➢ Keep this textbook with you as a reference while you read articles initially, so that you can look up unfamiliar terms in the glossary or the index.

➢ Try not to get bogged down in (or scared away by) statistical information. Try to grasp the gist of the story without letting symbols and numbers frustrate you.

➢ Until you become accustomed to the style and jargon of research journal articles, you may want to "translate" them mentally or in writing. You can do this by expanding compact paragraphs into looser constructions, by translating jargon into more familiar terms, by recasting sentences into an active voice, and by summarizing findings with words rather than with numbers. As an example, Box 4.2 presents a summary of a fictitious study about the psychological consequences of having an abortion, written in the style typically found in research journal articles. Terms that can be looked up in the glossary of this book are underlined, and bolded marginal notes indicate the type of information the author is communicating. Box 4.3 presents a "translation" of this summary, recasting the research information into language that is more digestible.

When you attain a reasonable level of comprehension of a research report, a useful next step is to write a brief (1- to 2-page) synopsis. A synopsis summarizes the study's purpose, research questions, methods, findings, interpretation of the findings, and implications for practice. You do not need to be concerned at this point about critiquing the study's strengths and weaknesses, but rather about succinctly and objectively presenting a summary of what was done and what was

BOX 4.2 SUMMARY OF A FICTITIOUS STUDY FOR TRANSLATION

Purpose of the study	The potentially negative sequelae of having an abortion on the psychological adjustment of adolescents have not been adequately studied. The present study sought to determine whether alternative pregnancy resolution decisions have different long-term effects on the psychological functioning of young women.	**Need for the study**
Research design	Three groups of low-income pregnant teenagers attending an inner-city clinic were the subjects in this study: those who delivered and kept the baby; those who delivered and relinquished the baby for adoption; and those who had an abortion. There were 25 subjects in each group. The study instruments included a self-administered questionnaire and a battery of psychological tests measuring depression, anxiety, and psychosomatic symptoms. The instruments were administered upon entry into the study (when the subjects first came to the clinic) and then 1 year after termination of the pregnancy.	**Study population**
Research instruments		**Research sample**
Data analysis procedure	The data were analyzed using analysis of variance (ANOVA). The ANOVA tests indicated that the three groups did not differ significantly in terms of depression, anxiety, or psychosomatic symptoms at the initial testing. At the posttest, however, the abortion group had significantly higher scores on the depression scale, and these girls were significantly more likely than the two delivery groups to report severe tension headaches. There were no significant differences on any of the dependent variables for the two delivery groups.	**Results**
Implications	The results of this study suggest that young women who elect to have an abortion may experience a number of long-term negative consequences. It would appear that appropriate efforts should be made to follow abortion patients to determine their need for suitable treatment.	**Interpretation**

learned. By preparing a synopsis, you will become more aware of aspects of the study that you did not understand.

Critiquing Research Reports

A written research **critique** is different from a research summary or synopsis. A research critique is a careful, critical appraisal of a study's strengths and limitations.

BOX 4.3 TRANSLATED VERSION OF FICTITIOUS RESEARCH STUDY

As researchers, we wondered whether young women who had an abortion had any emotional problems in the long run. It seemed to us that not enough research had been done to know whether any psychological harm resulted from an abortion.

We decided to study this question ourselves by comparing the experiences of three types of teenagers who became pregnant—first, girls who delivered and kept their babies; second, those who delivered the babies but gave them up for adoption; and third, those who elected to have an abortion. All teenagers in our sample were poor, and all were patients at an inner-city clinic. Altogether, we studied 75 girls—25 in each of the three groups. We evaluated the teenagers' emotional states by asking them to fill out a questionnaire and to take several psychological tests. These tests allowed us to assess things such as the girls' degree of depression and anxiety and whether they had any complaints of a psychosomatic nature. We asked them to fill out the forms twice: once when they came into the clinic, and then again a year after the abortion or the delivery.

We learned that the three groups of teenagers looked pretty much alike in terms of their emotional states when they first filled out the forms. But when we compared how the three groups looked a year later, we found that the teenagers who had abortions were more depressed and were more likely to say they had severe tension headaches than teenagers in the other two groups. The teenagers who kept their babies and those who gave their babies up for adoption looked pretty similar 1 year after their babies were born, at least in terms of depression, anxiety, and psychosomatic complaints.

Thus, it seems that we might be right in having some concerns about the emotional effects of having an abortion. Nurses should be aware of these long-term emotional effects, and it even may be advisable to institute some type of follow-up procedure to find out if these young women need additional help.

Critiques usually conclude with the reviewer's summary of the study's merits, recommendations about the value of the evidence, and suggestions for improving the study or the report.

Research critiques of individual studies are prepared for various reasons, and they differ in scope, depending on their purpose. Peer reviewers who are asked to prepare a written critique of a manuscript for a journal editor before acceptance for publication generally critique the following aspects of the study:

≫ *Substantive*—Was the research problem significant to nursing?

≫ *Theoretical*—Were the theoretical underpinnings sound?

≫ *Methodologic*—Were the methods rigorous and appropriate?

≫ *Ethical*—Were the rights of study participants protected?

≫ *Interpretive*—Did the researcher properly interpret data and develop reasonable conclusions?

≫ *Stylistic*—Is the report clearly written, grammatical, and well organized?

In short, peer reviewers provide comprehensive feedback to the researchers and to journal editors about the merit of both the study and the report, and typically offer suggestions for improvements (e.g., for redoing some analyses).

By contrast, critiques designed to guide decisions for evidence-based practice need not be as comprehensive. For example, it is of little significance to practicing nurses that a research report is ungrammatical. A critique on the clinical utility of a study focuses on whether the findings are accurate and clinically meaningful. If the findings cannot be trusted, it makes little sense to incorporate them into practice.

By understanding research methods, you will be in a position to critique the rigor of studies, and this is a primary aim of this book. Most chapters offer guidelines for evaluating various research decisions that will help you to make an overall appraisal of a study. Chapter 17 provides extra guidance on undertaking a critique.

Competent consumers of research must be able to critique not only single, independent studies but also a body of studies on a topic of clinical interest. We describe literature reviews in Chapter 7 and discuss integrative reviews in Chapter 18.

▶ RESEARCH EXAMPLES AND CRITICAL THINKING ACTIVITIES

EXAMPLE 1 ■ Quantitative Research

An abstract for a quantitative nursing study is presented below, followed by some questions to guide critical thinking.

Study
"Predictors of job satisfaction for rural acute care registered nurses in Canada" (Penz, Stewart, D'Arcy, & Morgan, 2008)

Abstract
"This study examines the predictors of job satisfaction among rural acute care registered nurses. The data are from a cross-sectional national survey, which was part of a larger project, The Nature of Nursing Practice in Rural and Remote Canada. This analysis suggests that a combination of individual, workplace, and community characteristics are interrelated predictors of job satisfaction for rural acute care nurses. There were nine variables that accounted for 38% of the total variance in job satisfaction. Four variables alone (available and up-to-date equipment and supplies, satisfaction with scheduling and shifts, lower psychological job demands, and home community satisfaction) explained 33% of the variance. Recruitment and retention strategies in rural areas must acknowledge that rural

(Research Examples and Critical Thinking Activities continues on page 68)

Research Examples and Critical Thinking Activities (continued)

nurses' work lives and community lives are inextricably intertwined. Attention to these issues will help ensure high-quality working environments and a continued commitment to quality nursing care in the rural hospital settings in Canada" (p. 785).

CRITICAL THINKING SUGGESTIONS

1. "Translate" the abstract into a summary that is more consumer friendly. Underline any technical terms and look them up in the glossary.

2. Also consider the following targeted questions:
   a. What were the independent variables in this study? How were they operationalized?
   b. What was the dependent variable in this study? How was it operationalized?
   c. Was the study experimental or nonexperimental?
   d. Were any of the findings statistically significant?
   e. Would it have been appropriate for the researchers to address the research question using qualitative research methods? Why or why not?

3. If the results of this study are valid and generalizable, what are some of the uses to which the research evidence might be put into clinical practice?

EXAMPLE 2 ■ Qualitative Research

An abstract for a qualitative nursing study is presented below, followed by some questions to guide critical thinking.

Study

"Daughters caring for dying parents: A process of relinquishing" (Read & Wuest, 2007)

Abstract

"Caring for elderly, dying parents is challenging for daughters as they try to balance other obligations and responsibilities. The purpose of this grounded theory study was to explain the domain of daughters' caregiving experiences in Newfoundland and Labrador, Canada. The primary author interviewed 12 women whose parents had died. Three types of turmoil (emotional, relational, and societal) emerged as the central issue for these women. The authors discovered a substantive theory of Relinquishing with interdependent processes of Keeping Vigil, Navigating Systems, Facing Loss, and an end process of Coming to Terms. In moving through the process of Relinquishing, social conditions of personal ideas, family expectations, and societal demands determine strategies employed by any one daughter to manage her turmoil. The findings fill a gap in knowledge related to daughters' caregiving for dying parents by contributing a theoretical framework that will inform women, health care providers, researchers, and health policy makers" (p. 932).

CRITICAL THINKING SUGGESTIONS

1. "Translate" the abstract into a summary that is more consumer friendly. Underline any technical terms and look them up in the glossary.

2. Also consider the following targeted questions:
   a. What was the phenomenon under investigation in this study?
   b. What qualitative research tradition did the authors use in this study? Based on what you have learned thus far about qualitative research traditions, does the selected tradition appear to be appropriate to address the research question?
   c. In this traditional abstract, what main features of the study were summarized?
   d. Would it have been appropriate for the researcher to address the research question using quantitative research methods? Why or why not?

3. If the results of this study are trustworthy, what are some of the uses to which the research evidence might be put into clinical practice?

EXAMPLE 3 ■ Quantitative Research

Read the abstract for the study by Moore and colleagues found in Appendix C of this book. "Translate" the abstract into a summary that is more consumer friendly.

EXAMPLE 4 ■ Qualitative Research

Read the abstract for the study by Bottorff and colleagues found in Appendix D of this book. "Translate" the abstract into a summary that is more consumer friendly.

Summary Points
· ·

- ⇝ The most common types of research reports are theses and dissertations, books, conference presentations (including oral reports and poster sessions), and, especially, journal articles.

- ⇝ Research **journal articles** provide brief descriptions of studies and are designed to communicate the contribution the study has made to knowledge.

- ⇝ Quantitative journal articles (and many qualitative ones) typically follow the **IMRAD format** with the following sections: introduction (explanation of the study problem and its context), method section (the strategies used to address the research problem), results (the actual study **findings**), and discussion (the interpretation of the findings).

- ⇝ Journal articles typically begin with a structured **abstract** (a brief synopsis of the study) and conclude with references (a list of works cited in the report).

- ⇝ Research reports are often difficult to read because they are dense, concise, and may contain a lot of jargon.

- ⇝ Qualitative research reports are written in a more inviting and conversational style than quantitative ones, which are more impersonal and include information on statistical tests.

- ⇝ **Statistical tests** are procedures for testing research hypotheses and evaluating the believability of the findings. Findings that are **statistically significant** are ones that have a high probability (p) of being accurate.

- ⇝ The ultimate goal of this book is to help students to prepare a research **critique,** which is a careful, critical appraisal of the strengths and limitations of a piece of research, often for the purpose of considering the worth of its evidence for nursing practice.

STUDIES CITED IN CHAPTER 4*

This reference list contains only those studies that were cited in this chapter. Citations pertaining to theoretical, methodological, or nonempirical work are included together in a separate section at the end of the book (beginning on page 399).

Caison, A. L., Bulman, D., Pai, S., & Neville, D. (2008). Exploring the technology readiness of nursing and medical students at a Canadian University. *Journal of Interprofessional Care, 22*(3), 283–294.

Martens, T. Z., & Emed, J. D. (2007). The experiences and challenges of pregnant women coping with thrombophilia. *Journal of Obstetric, Gynecologic, & Neonatal Nursing, 36*(1), 55–62.

Penz, K., Stewart, N. J., D'Arcy, C., & Morgan, D. (2008). Predictors of job satisfaction for rural acute care registered nurses in Canada. *Western Journal of Nursing Research, 30*(7), 785–800.

Read, T., & Wuest, J. (2007). Daughters caring for dying parents: A process of relinquishing. *Qualitative Health Research, 17*(7), 932–944.

CHAPTER

5 | Reviewing the Ethical Aspects of a Nursing Study

▶ LEARNING OBJECTIVES

On completing this chapter, you will be able to:

1. Discuss the historical background that led to the creation of various codes of ethics

2. Understand the potential for ethical dilemmas stemming from conflicts between ethics and requirements for high-quality research evidence

3. Identify the eight primary ethical principles articulated in the Tri-Council Policy Statement on research ethics and identify procedures for adhering to them

4. Given sufficient information, evaluate the ethical dimensions of a research report

5. Define new terms in the chapter

ETHICS AND RESEARCH
▶

Nurses face many ethical issues in their practice. The prolongation of life by artificial means is but one example of situations that have led to discussions about ethics in health care practice. Similarly, the expansion of nursing research has led to ethical concerns about the rights of study participants. Ethics can create particular challenges for nurse researchers because ethical requirements sometimes conflict with the need to produce the highest possible quality evidence for practice. This chapter discusses some of the major ethical principles that should be considered in reviewing studies.

Historical Background

As modern, civilized people, we might like to think that systematic violations of moral principles by researchers occurred centuries ago rather than in recent times, but this is not the case. The Nazi medical experiments of the 1930s and 1940s are the most famous example of recent disregard for ethical conduct. The Nazi program of research involved the use of prisoners of war and racial "enemies" in experiments designed to test the limits of human endurance and human reaction to diseases and untested drugs. The studies were unethical not only because they exposed these people to physical harm and even death but also because the participants could not refuse participation.

There are recent examples from other Western countries. For instance, between 1932 and 1972, a study known as the Tuskegee Syphilis Study, sponsored by the U.S. Public Health Service, investigated the effects of syphilis on 400 men from a poor black community. Medical treatment was deliberately withheld to study the course of the untreated disease. Similarly, Dr. Herbert Green of the National Women's Hospital in Auckland, New Zealand, studied women with cervical cancer in the 1980s; patients with carcinoma *in situ* were not given treatment so that researchers could study the natural progression of the disease. Another well-known case of unethical research involved the injection of live cancer cells into elderly patients at the Jewish Chronic Disease Hospital in Brooklyn in the 1960s without the consent of those patients. There are examples from Canada, too. A world-renowned Canadian psychiatrist attempted to wipe out his patients' memories and insert new thoughts (i.e., to "brain wash" them). Many other examples of studies with ethical transgressions—often less obvious than these examples—have emerged to give ethical concerns the high visibility they have today.

Codes of Ethics

In response to human rights violations, various codes of ethics have been developed. One of the first internationally recognized sets of ethical standards is the **Nuremberg Code,** developed in 1949 after the Nazi atrocities were made public in the Nuremberg trials. Another notable set of international standards is the **Declaration of Helsinki,** which was adopted in 1964 by the World Medical Assembly and most recently revised in 2000 (*http://www.wma.net/e/policy/b3.htm*).

Most disciplines have established their own **codes of ethics.** In Canada, the Canadian Nurses Association (CNA) first published a document entitled *Ethical Guidelines for Nurses in Research Involving Human Participants* in 1983 (revised in 1994 and 2002). The goal of this document is to provide nurses in all areas of professional practice with guidelines relating to research activities. These guidelines complement the broader *Code of Ethics for Registered Nurses* developed in 2002 and recently revised in a Centennial Edition (CNA, 2008). Some nurse ethicists have called for an international code of ethics for nursing research, but nurses in most countries have developed their own professional codes or follow the codes established by their governments. The International Council of Nurses, however, has developed a *Code for Nurses*, which was most recently updated in 2006 (*http://www.icn.ch/icncode.pdf*).

Government Regulations for Protecting Study Participants

Governments throughout the world fund research and establish rules for how such research must be conducted to adhere to ethical principles. Health Canada adopted the *Good Clinical Practice: Consolidated Guidelines* (GCP) in 1997 as the guidelines for certain types of research, namely clinical trial research involving human participants. In addition, the government of Canada specified the *Tri-Council Policy Statement: Ethical Conduct for Research Involving Humans* (TCPS) in 1998 with 2000, 2002, and 2005 amendments, as the guidelines to protect human subjects in all types of research (*http://www.pre.ethics.gc.ca/english/policystatement/policystatement.cfm*). The TCPS was jointly adopted by the major Canadian research agencies—the Canadian Institutes of Health Research (CIHR), Natural Sciences and Engineering Research Council (NSERC), and Social Sciences and Humanities Research Council (SSHRC). A revised version of the TCPS is expected in 2009.

The TCPS articulates eight guiding ethical principles on which standards of ethical conduct in research are based. These principles were based on several sources, including past guidelines of the Councils, statements by other Canadian agencies, and input from the international community. An essential component of the GCP and the TCPS is that a research ethics committee, formally known in Canada as a Research Ethics Board (REB), should first review and approve each study that involves human subjects.

TIP

In addition to those provided above, the following websites offer information about various professional codes of ethics and ethical requirements for government-sponsored research:

➤ Introductory Tutorial for the Tri-Council Policy Statement: Ethical Conduct for Research Involving Humans: *http://www.pre.ethics.gc.ca/english/tutorial/*
➤ Canadian Nurses Association: *http://www.cna-aiic.ca/CNA/practice/ethics/code/default_e.aspx*
➤ American Nurses Association: *http://www.ana.org/ethics*
➤ Policies from the U.S. National Institutes of Health, Office of Human Subjects Research (OHSR): *http://ohsr.od.nih.gov*
➤ Featured column with relevant tutorials and publications at the Office of Research Integrity (U.S. Department of Health and Human Services): *http://www.ori.dhhs.gov/*

Ethical Dilemmas in Conducting Research

Research that violates ethical principles is rarely done to be cruel but more typically occurs out of a conviction that knowledge is important and beneficial in the long run. There are situations in which the rights of participants and the demands of the study are put in direct conflict, creating **ethical dilemmas** for researchers. In reading research reports, you need to be aware of such dilemmas. Here are some examples of research questions in which the desire for strong evidence conflicts with ethical considerations:

1. *Research question:* Are nurses equally empathic in their treatment of male and female patients in intensive care units?

   Ethical dilemma: Ethics require that participants be aware of their role in a study. Yet if the researcher informs the nurses in this study that their empathy in treating male and female patients will be scrutinized, will the nurses' behaviour continue to reflect their usual practice? If the nurses alter their behaviour because they know research observers are watching, the findings will not be valid.

2. *Research question:* What are the coping mechanisms of parents whose children have a terminal illness?

   Ethical dilemma: To answer this question, the researcher may need to probe into the psychological state of the parents at a vulnerable time in their lives. Such probing could be disturbing, yet knowledge of the parents' coping mechanisms might lead to more effective ways of dealing with parents' grief.

3. *Research question:* Does a new medication prolong life in cancer patients?

   Ethical dilemma: The best way to test the effectiveness of an intervention is to administer the intervention to some participants but withhold it from others to see whether differences between the groups emerge. However, if a new drug is untested, the group receiving it may be exposed to potentially hazardous side effects. On the other hand, the group *not* receiving it may be denied a beneficial treatment.

4. *Research question:* What is the process by which adult children adapt to the day-to-day stresses of caring for a parent with Alzheimer's disease?

   Ethical dilemma: In a qualitative study, which would be appropriate for this research question, the researcher sometimes becomes so closely involved with participants that they become willing to share "secrets" or privileged information with the researcher. Interviews can become confessions—sometimes of unseemly or illegal behaviour. In this example, suppose a woman admitted to abusing her mother physically—how does the researcher respond to that information without undermining a pledge of confidentiality? And, if the researcher reveals the information to appropriate authorities, how can a pledge of confidentiality be given in good faith to other participants?

As these examples suggest, researchers are sometimes in a bind: their goal is to advance knowledge, using the best methods possible, but they must also adhere to the dictates of ethical rules that have been developed to protect participants' rights.

ETHICAL PRINCIPLES FOR PROTECTING STUDY PARTICIPANTS

The ethical framework established by the TCPS (1998) is based on a desire to balance the need for research—which is viewed as a fundamental moral commitment to advance human welfare—with the imperative of respecting human dignity. The underlying ethic involves two responsibilities—to establish ethically acceptable research goals and to use suitable means of reaching those goals. The policy statement articulates eight guiding ethical principles: respect for human dignity, respect for free and informed consent, respect for vulnerable persons, respect for privacy and confidentiality, respect of justice and inclusiveness, balancing harms and benefits, minimizing harm, and maximizing benefit. These fundamental principles are briefly described next, followed by a discussion of procedures researchers use to uphold them.

Respect for Human Dignity

A fundamental principle of modern research ethics is respect for human dignity. This principle aspires to protect the interests of study participants, in terms of bodily, psychological, and cultural integrity. The principle of respect for human dignity encompasses the right to self-determination and the right to full disclosure.

Humans are viewed as autonomous agents, capable of controlling their own activities. The principle of **self-determination** means that prospective participants have the right to decide voluntarily whether to participate in a study, without the risk of incurring adverse consequences. It also means that participants have the right to ask questions, to refuse to give information, and to withdraw from the study.

A person's right to self-determination includes freedom from coercion. **Coercion** involves explicit or implicit threats of penalty for failing to participate in a study or excessive rewards for agreeing to participate. The obligation to protect potential participants from coercion requires careful consideration when researchers are in a position of authority or influence over potential participants, as might be the case in a nurse–patient relationship. Coercion can in some cases be subtle. For example, a generous monetary incentive (or **stipend**) offered to encourage the participation of an economically disadvantaged group (e.g., the homeless) might be mildly coercive because such incentives could place undue pressure on prospective participants.

The principle of respect for human dignity also includes people's right to make informed, voluntary decisions about study participation, which requires full disclosure. **Full disclosure** means that the researcher has fully described the nature of the study, the person's right to refuse participation, the researcher's responsibilities, and the likely risks and benefits that would be incurred.

Respect for Free and Informed Consent

The TCPS stipulates that people are generally presumed to have the ability—and the right—to make free and informed decisions. Thus, respect for human dignity implies respect for participants' right to individual consent. **Informed consent** means that participants have adequate information about the research;

comprehend the information; and have the power of free choice, that is, to consent voluntarily to participate in the research or to decline participation.

Informed consent is based on the right to self-determination and full disclosure, but in certain circumstances, participants' right to self-determination poses challenges. An important issue concerns some people's inability to make well-informed judgments about the costs and benefits of participation (e.g., children). We discuss the issue of special classes of research participants in the next section.

Adherence to the principle of full disclosure may also be problematic. Full disclosure can sometimes result in two types of biases: (1) biases resulting from inaccurate data and (2) biases stemming from difficulty recruiting a good sample. Suppose we were testing the hypothesis that high school students with a high rate of absenteeism are more likely to be substance abusers than students with good attendance. If we approached potential participants and fully explained the study purpose, some students likely would refuse to participate. Nonparticipation would be selective; in fact, we would expect that those least likely to volunteer would be students who are substance abusers—the group of primary interest. Moreover, by knowing the specific research question, those who do participate might not give candid responses. It might be argued that full disclosure would totally undermine the study.

One technique that researchers sometimes use in such situations is **covert data collection,** or *concealment*—the collection of information without participants' knowledge and thus without their consent. This might happen, for example, if a researcher wanted to observe people's behaviour in a real-world setting and was concerned that doing so openly would change the very behaviour of interest. Researchers might choose to obtain information through concealed methods, such as by observing through a one-way mirror, videotaping participants through hidden equipment, or observing while pretending to be engaged in other activities.

A second, and more controversial, technique is the use of deception. *Deception* can involve either deliberately withholding information about the study or providing participants with false information. For example, we might describe the study of high school students' use of drugs as research on students' health practices, which is a mild form of misinformation.

Deception and concealment are problematic ethically because they interfere with the participants' right to make a truly informed decision about the personal costs and benefits of participation. Some people argue that the use of deception or concealment is never justified. Others, however, believe that if the study involves low risk to participants and if there are anticipated benefits to science and society, deception or concealment may be justified to enhance the validity of the findings.

Another issue relating to full disclosure has emerged recently concerning the collection of data from people over the Internet (e.g., analyzing the content of messages posted to chat rooms, discussion boards, or on listserves). The issue is whether such messages can be used as data without the authors' consent. Some researchers believe that anything posted electronically is in the public domain and therefore can be used without consent for purposes of research. Others, however, feel that the same ethical standards must apply in cyberspace research and that electronic researchers must carefully protect the rights of individuals who are involved in "virtual" communities. Researchers at the University of Toronto have developed useful guidelines for addressing ethical dilemmas arising in research on Internet communities (Flicker, Hans, & Skinner, 2004), and the forthcoming updated TCPS will address this issue in detail.

Respect for Vulnerable Persons

Ethical obligations are heightened when the people under study are deemed to be a vulnerable group. **Vulnerable subjects** (a term often used to refer to at-risk study participants) are people with diminished competence or decision-making ability. The TCPS instructs researchers to afford vulnerable groups special protections against exploitation or discrimination.

Groups that are considered to be vulnerable because of diminished competence include children, mentally or emotionally disabled people, and others who are unable to understand information or appreciate the consequences of participation (e.g., comatose patients). The TCPS specifically notes that, in studying such vulnerable groups, researchers must seek to balance two considerations—the vulnerability that arises from their incompetence and the injustice that would arise from excluding them from the study.

Special protections and procedures may also be needed for other groups who do not necessarily lack competence. These include physically disabled people (e.g., the deaf); people who may be at higher-than-average risk of unintended side effects because of their circumstances (e.g., pregnant women); or institutionalized people who may have *diminished autonomy* (e.g., prisoners).

TIP

Some terms introduced in this chapter are rarely used explicitly in research reports. For example, a report almost never calls to the readers' attention that the study participants were *vulnerable subjects*. You need to be sensitive to the special needs of groups that may be unable to act as their own advocates or to assess the costs and benefits of participating in a study.

Respect for Privacy and Confidentiality

Researchers demonstrate their respect for human dignity by placing a high value on study participants' privacy. Virtually all research with humans constitutes an intrusion into personal lives, but researchers should ensure that their research is not more intrusive than it needs to be and that participants' privacy is maintained throughout the study. The right to privacy is an internationally recognized ethical principle and has also been enshrined in Canadian law as a constitutional right protected in both federal and provincial statutes.

Participants also have the right to expect that any data they provide will be kept in strictest confidence. The principle of respect for privacy and confidentiality protects access to personal information. When study participants confide personal information to the researchers, or when their behaviour is observed, researchers have an obligation not to share the information with others (even family members or care providers) without the subjects' consent. A promise of **confidentiality** to participants is a pledge that any information they provide will not be publicly reported or made accessible to parties not involved in the research.

Respect for Justice and Inclusiveness

Justice connotes fairness and equality, and so one aspect of the justice principle concerns the equitable distribution of benefits and burdens of research. The selection of study participants should be based on research requirements and not on the vulnerability or compromised position of certain people. Historically, subject selection has been a key ethical concern, with many researchers selecting groups deemed to have lower social standing (e.g., socially disadvantaged people, prisoners, slaves, the mentally impaired) as study participants. The principle of justice imposes particular obligations toward individuals who are unable to protect their own interests (e.g., dying patients) to ensure that they are not exploited for the advancement of knowledge.

Distributive justice also imposes duties to neither neglect nor discriminate against individuals and groups who may benefit from advances in research. During the 1980s and early 1990s, there was growing evidence that women, ethnic or racial minorities, and the elderly were being unfairly excluded from many clinical studies. Section 5 of the TCPS specifically deals with issues of inclusion in research, and section 6 focuses on research involving Aboriginal people. For example, the TCPS stipulates (Article 5.1) that ". . . researchers shall not exclude prospective or actual research subjects on the basis of such attributes as culture, religion, race, mental or physical disability, sexual orientation, ethnicity, sex or age, unless there is a valid reason for doing so" (CIHR, NSERC, & SSHRC, 1998, p. 5.2).

The principle of fair treatment covers issues other than subject selection. For example, the right to fair treatment means that researchers must treat people who decline to participate in a study (or who withdraw from the study after agreeing to participate) in a nonprejudicial manner; that they must honour all agreements made with participants (including the payment of any promised stipends); that they demonstrate sensitivity to and respect for the beliefs, habits, and lifestyles of people from different cultures; that they afford participants courteous treatment at all times; and that they avoid situations in which there is a conflict of interest.

Balancing Harms and Benefits

The ethical conduct of research with humans requires a careful analysis of the balance and distribution of harms and benefits of the research. The TCPS indicates that, "Modern research ethics . . . require a favourable harms-benefit balance— that is, that the foreseeable harms should not outweigh anticipated benefits" (CIHR, NSERC, & SSHRC, 1998, p. i.6).

Research is often undertaken under conditions of uncertainty—research involves advancing the frontiers of knowledge, and so it may not be possible to anticipate all possible harms and benefits of participation. This fact imposes special ethical burdens on researchers to undertake studies that address important questions, use methodologically sound methods, and are conducted with sensitivity and diligence.

One principle related to a balanced distribution of harms and benefits is that of **beneficence,** which imposes a duty on researchers to maximize net benefits. Human research should be intended to produce benefits for subjects themselves or—a situation that is more common—for other individuals or society as a whole. In most research, the primary benefit concerns the advancement of knowledge, which can be used to promote human health and welfare in the long run.

Another related principle is **nonmaleficence**—researchers' duty to avoid or minimize harm to participants. Participants must not be subjected to unnecessary risks of harm or discomfort, and their participation in a study must be essential to achieving scientifically and societally important aims that could not otherwise be realized. In research with humans, *harm* and *discomfort* can take many forms; they can be physical, emotional, social, or financial. Ethical researchers must use strategies to minimize all types of harms and discomforts, even ones that are temporary.

Clearly, exposing study participants to experiences that result in serious or permanent harm is unacceptable. Ethical researchers must be prepared to terminate their research if they suspect that continuation would result in injury, death, or undue distress to study participants. Although protecting human beings from physical harm may be reasonably straightforward, the psychological consequences of participating in a study are usually subtle and thus require close attention. For example, participants may be asked questions about their personal views, weaknesses, or fears. Such queries might lead people to reveal sensitive personal information. The point is not that researchers should refrain from asking questions but rather that they need to be aware of the nature and scope of the intrusion on people's psyches.

The need for sensitivity may be even greater in qualitative studies, which often involve in-depth exploration into highly personal areas. In-depth probing may expose deep-seated worries and anxieties that study participants had previously repressed. Qualitative researchers, regardless of the underlying research tradition, must thus be especially vigilant in monitoring such problems.

Nonmaleficence also involves ensuring freedom from exploitation. Involvement in a study should not place participants at a disadvantage or expose them to situations for which they have not been prepared. Participants need to be assured that their participation, or information they might provide, will not be used against them. For example, a woman divulging her income should not fear losing public health benefits; a person reporting drug abuse should not fear exposure to criminal authorities.

Study participants enter into a special relationship with researchers, and this relationship should not be exploited. Exploitation might be overt and malicious (e.g., sexual exploitation, use of participants' identification to create a mailing list), but it might also be less flagrant (e.g., getting participants to provide more information in a 1-year follow-up interview, without having warned them of this possibility at the outset). Because nurse researchers may have a nurse–client (in addition to a researcher–participant) relationship, special care may be needed to avoid exploiting that bond. Patients' consent to participate in a study may result from their understanding of the researcher's role as *nurse*, not as *researcher*.

In qualitative research, the risk of exploitation may be especially acute because the psychological distance between investigators and participants typically declines as the study progresses. The emergence of a pseudotherapeutic relationship between researchers and participants is not uncommon, and this imposes additional responsibilities on researchers—and additional risks that exploitation could inadvertently occur. On the other hand, qualitative researchers are typically in a better position than quantitative researchers to do good, rather than just to avoid doing any harm, because of the close relationships they often develop with participants.

Further Considerations Specific to Aboriginal People

In May 2007, CIHR released research ethics guidelines specific to Aboriginal people. The *CIHR Guidelines for Health Research Involving Aboriginal People* is a precursor to the revised section on Aboriginal health research in the updated TCPS expected in 2009. It captures the unique needs of this population, taking into account the historical context and Aboriginal perspective on western scientific approaches. Further ethical considerations focus on developing and maintaining respectful partnerships with Aboriginal communities, in a *participatory-research approach*. The Guidelines suggest 15 basic principles, including the need for research of mutual benefit; the role of elders in community consent; and responsibilities of the researcher to understand and protect sacred knowledge.

PROCEDURES FOR PROTECTING STUDY PARTICIPANTS

Now that you are familiar with fundamental ethical principles for conducting research, you need to understand the procedures researchers follow to adhere to them. These procedures should be evaluated in critiquing the ethical aspects of a study.

TIP

When information about ethical considerations is presented in research reports, it almost always appears in the method section, typically in the subsection devoted to data collection procedures but sometimes in a subsection describing the sample.

BOX 5.1 POTENTIAL BENEFITS AND RISKS OF RESEARCH TO PARTICIPANTS

Major Potential Benefits to Participants

- Access to an intervention that might otherwise be unavailable to them
- Comfort in being able to discuss their situation or problem with a friendly, objective person
- Increased knowledge about themselves or their conditions, either through opportunity for introspection and self-reflection or through direct interaction with researchers
- Escape from a normal routine, excitement of being part of a study
- Satisfaction that information they provide may help others with similar problems or conditions
- Direct monetary or material gain through stipends or other incentives

Major Potential Risks to Participants

- Physical harm, including unanticipated side effects
- Physical discomfort, fatigue, or boredom
- Psychological or emotional distress resulting from self-disclosure, introspection, fear of the unknown, discomfort with strangers, fear of eventual repercussions, anger or embarrassment at the type of questions being asked
- Social risks, such as the risk of stigma, adverse effects on personal relationships, loss of status
- Loss of privacy
- Loss of time
- Monetary costs (e.g., for transportation, child care, time lost from work)

Risk/Benefit Assessments

One of the strategies that researchers use to protect study participants—and that you as a reviewer can use to assess the ethical aspects of a study—is to conduct a **risk/benefit assessment.** Such an assessment is designed to determine whether the benefits of participating in a study are in line with the costs, be they financial, physical, emotional, or social—that is, whether the *risk/benefit* ratio is acceptable. Box 5.1 summarizes major costs and benefits of research participation.

TIP

In your evaluation of the risk/benefit ratio of a study, you might consider whether you yourself would have felt comfortable being a study participant.

The risk/benefit ratio should also be considered in terms of whether the risks to research participants are commensurate with the benefit to society and to nursing. The degree of risk to be taken by participants should never exceed the potential humanitarian benefits of the knowledge to be gained. Thus, an important question in assessing the overall risk/benefit ratio is whether the study focuses on a significant topic that has the potential to improve patient care.

All research involves some risks, but in many cases, the risk is minimal. **Minimal risk** is defined as risks anticipated to be no greater than those ordinarily encountered in daily life or during routine tests or procedures. When the risks are not minimal, researchers must proceed with caution, taking every step possible to reduce risks and maximize benefits.

Example of risk/benefit assessment

Read and Wuest (2007) studied the life challenges faced by daughters' caring for dying parents. Here is how they described the risk and benefits: "The primary author explained that participation in our study might not benefit the participants, and they were advised they could withdraw from the study at any time; none did. All of the women were eager to help advance the 'system' as they experienced it and disclosed their hope that their participation might lead to improvements for future daughter caregivers . . . The primary author remained cognizant of the emotional responses that discussion about recalling the caregiving experience might evoke and made follow-up phone calls to the women a few days after the interview. A social worker was available to the women if there was need for further follow-up, but none availed of this opportunity" (p. 935).

Informed Consent

A particularly important procedure for safeguarding human subjects and protecting their right to self-determination involves obtaining evidence of their informed consent. Researchers usually document the informed consent process by having participants sign a **consent form,** an example of which is shown in Figure 5.1. This form includes information about the study purpose, specific expectations regarding participation (e.g., how much time will be involved), the voluntary nature of participation, and potential costs and benefits.

> **TIP**
>
> When preparing a consent form, most Research Ethics Boards have standard templates, which researchers can use. The recommended reading level is Grade 8, and this can be checked using software such as Microsoft *Word* (see under Word Options/Proofing/Readability Statistics) or *RightWriter*.

Researchers rarely obtain written informed consent when the primary means of data collection is through self-administered questionnaires. Researchers generally assume **implied consent** (i.e., that the return of the completed questionnaire reflects respondents' voluntary consent to participate). This assumption, however, is not always warranted (e.g., if patients feel that their treatment might be affected by failure to cooperate).

In some qualitative studies, especially those requiring repeated contact with participants, it is difficult to obtain a meaningful informed consent at the outset. Qualitative researchers do not always know in advance how the study will evolve. Because the research design emerges during data collection and analysis, researchers may not know the exact nature of the data to be collected, what the risks and benefits will be, nor how much of a time commitment will be required. Thus, in a qualitative study, consent may be viewed as an ongoing, transactional process, referred to as **process consent.** In process consent, researchers continuously renegotiate the consent, allowing participants to play a collaborative role in the decision-making process regarding their ongoing participation.

Example of informed consent in a quantitative study

Lobchuk and Bokhari (2008) conducted a pilot study exploring the relationships among empathic responding by informal caregivers and the physical symptom experiences and psychological distress (i.e., anxiety and depression) reported by patients with ovarian cancer. After the relevant ethics permissions were obtained, "eligible patients received a written invitation from either the clinic clerk or the social worker to speak to the researchers about their interest in the study . . . If the patient agreed to speak to the research nurse, the patient was contacted by telephone, the study was explained, and the patient was invited to participate. If the patient agreed to participate, she was asked to sign and mail the consent form" (p. 810).

Confidentiality Procedures

Participants' right to privacy is protected either through anonymity or through other confidentiality procedures. **Anonymity** occurs when even the researcher cannot link a participant with his or her data. For example, if a researcher distributed

I, _____ agree to take part in a nursing study about the use of research findings in postoperative pain management. I understand that participation in the study may involve one or two interviews with a researcher, which will be tape recorded, and that the recording will be typed into a written record. I will be answering questions about:

- My experiences with and beliefs about pain management
- My experiences using research evidence
- Factors that I believe make it easier or more difficult to use current research or to follow current pain management practices
- factors that I think influence pain management practices in a unit and a hospital

I may also be completing short questions and scales (e.g., answering questions using ratings of 1 to 5 or more) about research use and factors thought to influence it. Alternatively I may only be completing scales and questionnaires.

I have been told that the interviews will take about 30 to 60 minutes and occur at a convenient time and place in my off-duty hours or with the unit manager's agreement during work hours.

I have been told that I may refuse to answer questions, stop the interview at any time, or withdraw from the study. I do not have to answer any questions or discuss any subject in the interview if I do not want to. My name will not appear on the questionnaires, and my specific answers will remain confidential. I will not be identified in any report or presentation that may arise from the study. Taking part in this study or dropping out will not affect my employment.

While I may not benefit directly from the study, the information gained may assist nurses with both research use and pain management for postoperative patients.

I have been told that the data (typed records of interviews, taped interviews, observations, results or questionnaires) will be preserved using record management standards that protect the privacy of the participants in the project and that guard against the disclosure of individual information. It has also been explained to me that the data may be used for other research studies in the future. If this is done, proper ethical review will be obtained to ensure that the same practices of confidentiality are observed as within this study.

The above research procedures have been explained to me. Any questions have been answered to my satisfaction. I have been given a copy of this form to keep.

_____	_____	_____
(Signature of Participant)	(Date)	(Printed Name)
_____	_____	_____
(Signature of Witness)	(Date)	(Printed Name)

If you have any questions about this study please contact:

Dr. Carole Estabrooks (Principal Investigator) or   **Telephone:** (780) 555-1234
Dr. Profetto-McGrath (Research Associate)   **Telephone:** (780) 555-4321

FIGURE 5.1   Sample consent form.

questionnaires to a group of nursing home residents and asked that they be returned without any identifying information, the responses would be anonymous. As another example, if a researcher reviewed hospital records from which all identifying information (e.g., name, address, and so forth) had been expunged, anonymity would again protect people's right to privacy.

Example of anonymity

Baxter and Boblin (2008) studied the kinds of decisions that baccalaureate students make in the clinical setting and the influences on their decision making, with the view to better understand and teach this critical skill. They state: "Students were encouraged to drop off the signed consent form into a marked box located in the school of nursing. Students were assured that their anonymity would be maintained and that their decision not to participate, to participate, or to later drop out of the study would not affect their standing at the university" (p. 346).

In situations in which anonymity is impossible, researchers implement other confidentiality procedures. These include securing individual confidentiality assurances from everyone involved in collecting or analyzing research data; maintaining identifying information in locked files to which few people have access; substituting **identification (ID) numbers** for participants' names on study records and computer files to prevent any accidental *breach of confidentiality*; and reporting only aggregate data for groups of participants or taking steps to disguise a person's identity in a research report.

Extra precautions are often needed to safeguard participants' privacy in qualitative studies. Anonymity is rarely possible in qualitative research because researchers usually meet with participants personally. Moreover, because of the in-depth nature of many qualitative studies, there may be a greater invasion of privacy than is true in quantitative research. Researchers who spend time in participants' homes may, for example, have difficulty segregating the public behaviours participants are willing to share from the private behaviours that unfold unwittingly during data collection. A final issue is adequately disguising participants in research reports to avoid a breach of confidentiality. Because the number of respondents is small and because rich descriptive information is presented in research reports, qualitative researchers need to take extra precautions to safeguard participants' identities. This may mean more than simply using a fictitious name—it may also mean withholding information about the characteristics of the informant, such as age and occupation.

Example of confidentiality procedures in a qualitative study

Spiers (2006) described expressing and acknowledging pain and stoicism within interpersonal contexts between home care nurses and their patients. Her qualitative study was based on an analysis of 31 videotaped home visits and participant interviews. The video portion of the tapes was not altered, as the researcher wanted to analyze facial expressions. However, any audio containing names or other identifying information was removed in dubbed tapes. Pseudonyms were used in the transcripts.

TIP

As a means of enhancing both personal and institutional privacy, research reports frequently avoid giving explicit information about the locale of the study. For example, the report might state that data were collected in a 200-bed, private, for-profit nursing home, without mentioning its name or location.

Debriefings and Referrals

Researchers can often show their respect for study participants—and proactively minimize emotional risks—by carefully attending to the nature of the interactions they have with them. For example, researchers should always be gracious and polite, should phrase questions tactfully, and should be sensitive to cultural and linguistic diversity.

There are also more formal strategies that researchers can use to communicate their respect and concern for participants' well-being. For example, it is sometimes advisable to offer **debriefing** sessions after data collection is completed to permit participants to ask questions or air complaints. Debriefing is especially important when the data collection has been stressful or when ethical guidelines had to be "bent" (e.g., if any deception was used in explaining the study). Researchers can also demonstrate their interest in participants by offering to share findings with them once the data have been analyzed (e.g., by mailing them a summary or advising them of an appropriate website). Finally, in some situations, researchers may need to assist study participants by making referrals to appropriate health, social, or psychological services.

Treatment of Vulnerable Groups

Adherence to ethical standards is often straightforward. The rights of special vulnerable groups, however, often need to be protected through additional procedures and heightened sensitivity. You should pay particular attention to the ethical dimensions of a study when people who are vulnerable are involved. Some safeguards that can be used with vulnerable groups include the following:

⇝ *Children.* Legally and ethically, children do not have the competence to give their informed consent; therefore, the informed consent of children's parents or legal guardians should be obtained. However, it is advisable—especially if the child is at least 7 years old—to obtain the child's assent as well. **Assent** refers to the child's affirmative agreement to participate. If the child is mature enough to understand the basic information in an informed consent form (e.g., a 13-year-old), researchers should obtain written consent from the child as well, as evidence of respect for the child's right to self-determination.

⇝ *Mentally or emotionally disabled people.* People whose disability makes it impossible for them to make an informed decision about participation (e.g., people affected by cognitive impairment or mental illness) also cannot provide informed consent. In such cases, researchers obtain written consent from the person's legal guardian, but informed consent from prospective participants should be sought as a supplement to consent from guardians whenever possible.

⇝ *Physically disabled people.* For certain physical disabilities, special procedures for obtaining consent may be required. For example, with deaf people, the entire consent process may need to be in writing. For people who cannot read or write or who have a physical impairment preventing them from writing, alternative procedures for documenting informed consent (e.g., videotaping the consent proceedings) can be used.

⇝ *Terminally ill people.* Terminally ill people who participate in a study can seldom expect to benefit personally from the research, and thus the risk/benefit ratio needs to be carefully evaluated. Researchers must also take steps to ensure that if terminally ill people participate in the study, their health care and comfort are not compromised.

⇝ *Institutionalized people.* Nurses often conduct studies with hospitalized or institutionalized people, who may feel pressured into participating or may believe that their treatment would be jeopardized by failure to cooperate. Prison inmates, who have lost their autonomy in many spheres of activity, may similarly feel constrained in their ability to give free consent. Researchers studying institutionalized groups need to place special emphasis on the voluntary nature of participation.

⋟ *Pregnant and breastfeeding women.* The TCPS notes that when researchers are contemplating research with pregnant women, they must take into consideration the benefits and harms not only for the pregnant woman but also for her embryo or foetus, and similar concerns arise in connection with breastfeeding mothers and their infants. Special care should be taken in research with pregnant women or new mothers, who might be at heightened physical and psychological risk.

Example of research with a vulnerable group

Spagrud et al. (2008) studied pain and distress from needles in children undergoing blood sampling relative to the parent–child interaction and the type of venous access. Patients were enrolled in the study arms based on the central venous device in place. All parents provided written consent for both themselves and their children to participate, and all children gave verbal assent.

Research Ethics Boards and External Reviews

It is sometimes hard for researchers to be objective in assessing risks and benefits or in developing procedures to protect human rights. Researchers' commitment to a topic area or their desire to conduct a rigorous study may cloud their judgment. Because of this possibility, the ethical dimension of a study is usually subjected to external review.

Canada, like most other Western countries, has developed a model of ethics review for research using human subjects. The model involves the review of proposed research plans, using the ethical guidelines outlined in the TCPS, by independent **Research Ethics Boards (REBs)** before the study gets underway. REBs are established in the institutions where research is conducted, such as in hospitals and universities, or even in the community itself as some Aboriginal communities have their own REBs and/or community research protocols.

The REBs are mandated to reject, propose modifications to, or terminate any research conducted within the institution or by members affiliated with it, if ethical transgressions are noted. The guidelines in the TCPS are considered a *minimum* standard for the ethical conduct of research. Each REB must consist of at least five members, and at least one person must be unaffiliated with the institution where the REB is housed. Studies that involve more invasive measures such as the collection of blood or the administration of drugs are highly scrutinized. Non-invasive studies such as chart reviews or behavioural interventions can be subject to *expedited review*, which means that they are able to be approved more quickly if deemed minimal risk. Researchers are sometimes called to appear before the REB in person to further explain/justify their approach to the research. Ethical approval for an ongoing study must be renewed annually, requiring researchers to detail the progress made and any changes to the study protocol.

Not all studies are reviewed by REBs or other formal committees. Nevertheless, researchers have a responsibility to ensure that their research plans are ethically acceptable, and it is a good practice for researchers to solicit external advice even when they are not required to do so.

TIP

Research reports may use alternate terms such as ethical review by *human subjects committees* or *Institutional Review Boards (IRB)*.

OTHER ETHICAL ISSUES

When critiquing the ethical dimensions of a study, a prime consideration is the researcher's treatment of human study participants. Two other ethical issues also deserve mention: the treatment of animals in research and research misconduct.

Ethical Issues in Using Animals in Research

A small but growing number of nurse researchers use animals rather than human beings as their subjects, typically focusing on biophysiologic phenomena. Despite some opposition to such research by animal rights activists, researchers in health fields likely will continue to use animals to explore basic physiologic mechanisms and to test experimental interventions that could pose risks (as well as offer benefits) to humans.

Ethical considerations are clearly different for animals and humans (e.g., the concept of *informed consent* is not relevant for animals). In Canada, researchers who use animals in their studies must adhere to the policies and guidelines of the Canadian Council on Animal Care (CCAC). The CCAC guidelines, articulated in the two-volume *Guide to the Care and Use of Experimental Animals* (*http://www.ccac.ca/*), establish principles for the proper care and treatment of animals used in biomedical and behavioural research. These principles cover such issues as the transport of animals, alternatives to using animals, pain and distress in animal subjects, researcher qualifications, the use of appropriate anaesthesia, and euthanizing animals under certain conditions during or after the study.

Holtzclaw and Hanneman (2002), in discussing the use of animals in nursing research, noted several important considerations. First, there must be a compelling reason to use an animal model—not simply convenience or novelty. Second, the study procedures should be humane, well planned, and well funded. They noted that animal studies require serious ethical and scientific consideration to justify their use.

Explicit instances of animal cruelty in health care research are rare but have been reported. For example, during the 1980s, a physiologist at the University of Western Ontario was accused of cruelty in a study in which a baboon was kept for several months in a restraining chair. The study was supported by the Canadian Medical Research Council (now the CIHR).

Example of animal research

McCullough and Bartfay (2007) conducted a study, using a murine model, to explore specific mechanisms by which chronic iron overload damages the liver. Twenty mice were housed in cages (five per cage) in a temperature- and humidity-controlled room with 12-hour light–dark cycles and given access to food and water. The researchers specifically noted that the study had institutional approval and that it conformed to the standards for animal treatment issued by the CCAC and by the Province of Ontario, particularly in terms of calculating the sample size required since this was a "terminal investigation" (the animal dies in the process of the investigation).

Research Misconduct

Millions of movie-goers watched breathlessly as Dr. Richard Kimble (Harrison Ford) exposed the fraudulent scheme of a medical researcher in the film *The Fugitive*. This film reminds us that ethics in research involves not only the protection of the rights of human and animal subjects but also protection of the public trust.

The issue of **research misconduct** (or *scientific misconduct*) has received increasing attention in recent years as incidents of researcher fraud and misrepresentation have come to light. In Canada, the three major federal funding sources (CIHR, NSERC, and SSHRC) have issued a TCPS on integrity in research and scholarship, updated in 2007 (*http://www.nserc.gc.ca/sf_e.asp?nav=sfnav&lbi=p9*).

The agencies hold researchers accountable for adhering to five principles, which cover issues such as conflicts of interest, proper acknowledgment of scholarly contributions, and obtaining permissions for use of information (*http://www.sshrc.ca/web/apply/policies/integrity_e.asp*). The policy statement articulates three fundamental aspects of research integrity: (1) *truthfulness* in describing the manner is which data are collected, analyzed, and reported; (2) *scrupulousness* in crediting sources of original research concepts and information; and (3) *probity* in the use of research funds.

Definitions of research misconduct, including that offered by the TCPS, usually include transgressions such as fabrication, falsification, and plagiarism. *Fabrication* involves making up study results and reporting them. *Falsification* involves manipulating research materials, equipment, or processes; it also involves changing or omitting data, or distorting results such that the research is not accurately represented in research reports. *Plagiarism* involves the appropriation of someone's ideas or results without giving due credit. In addition to these three main forms, research misconduct covers many other issues, such as improprieties of authorship, poor data management, conflicts of interest, inappropriate financial arrangements, failure to comply with governmental regulations, and unauthorized use of confidential information. The TCPS notes that misconduct does *not* include honest error or honest differences in interpretations or judgments of data. Unlike the United States, Canada does not have a national agency to deal with reported research misconduct. However, CIHR does have an Ethics Office with a Research Integrity Committee (RIC) mandated to address any allegations involving CIHR-funded researchers. The RIC recently provided an indication of the extent of allegations—a total of 67 allegations from April 2000 to March 2008 (*http://www.cihr-irsc.gc.ca/e/29073.html*).

Example of research misconduct

A well-publicized Canadian case involved Dr. Ranjit Kumar Chandra, an international expert in nutrition and immunology at Memorial University in Newfoundland. He was found to have published falsified data on studies involving hypoallergenic baby formula. It was his clinical nurse, Marilyn Harvey, who first exposed Dr. Chandra, when she came across published papers in reputable journals like the *British Medical Journal*, which she realised were reporting studies still underway. When pushed by the university to share his data in 2002, Dr. Chandra failed to locate it and soon retired. Only one of his studies has been retracted from the scientific literature, even though his research results over the last 20 years are now in question.

In reading research reports, you are not likely to be able to detect research misconduct. Awareness of this issue is, however, critical to being an astute consumer of research.

CRITIQUING THE ETHICS OF RESEARCH STUDIES

Guidelines for critiquing the ethical aspects of a study are presented in Box 5.2. A person serving on an REB or similar committee should be provided with sufficient information to answer all these questions. Research reports, however, do not always include detailed information about ethical procedures because of space constraints in journals. Thus, it may not always be possible to critique researchers' adherence to ethical guidelines. Nevertheless, we offer a few suggestions for considering the ethical aspects of a study.

Many research reports do acknowledge that the study procedures were reviewed by an REB or a human subjects committee of the institution with which the researchers are affiliated. When a research report specifically mentions a formal external review, it is generally safe to assume that a panel of concerned people thoroughly reviewed the ethical issues raised by the study.

BOX 5.2   QUESTIONS FOR CRITIQUING THE ETHICAL ASPECTS OF A STUDY

1. Was the study approved and monitored by a Research Ethics Board or other similar ethics review committees?

2. Were study participants subjected to any physical harm, discomfort, or psychological distress? Did the researchers take appropriate steps to remove or prevent harm?

3. Did the benefits to participants outweigh any potential risks or actual discomfort they experienced? Did the benefits to society outweigh the costs to participants?

4. Was any type of coercion or undue influence used to recruit participants? Did they have the right to refuse to participate or to withdraw without penalty?

5. Were participants deceived in any way? Were they fully aware of participating in a study, and did they understand the purpose and nature of the research?

6. Were appropriate informed consent procedures used with all participants? If not, were there valid and justifiable reasons?

7. Were adequate steps taken to safeguard the privacy of participants? How were the data kept anonymous or confidential?

8. Were vulnerable groups involved in the research? If yes, were special precautions instituted because of their vulnerable status?

9. Were groups omitted from the inquiry without a justifiable rationale (e.g., women, minorities)?

You can also come to some conclusions based on a description of the study methods. There may be sufficient information to judge, for example, whether study participants were subjected to physical or psychological harm or discomfort. Reports do not always specifically state whether informed consent was secured, but you should be alert to situations in which the data might have been gathered without explicit consent (e.g., if data were gathered unobtrusively).

In thinking about the ethical aspects of a study, you should also consider who the study participants were. For example, if the study involved vulnerable groups, there should be more information about protective procedures. You might also need to attend to who the study participants were *not*. For example, there has been considerable concern about the omission of certain groups (e.g., minorities) from clinical research.

It is often especially difficult to determine whether the participants' privacy was safeguarded unless the researcher specifically mentions pledges of confidentiality or anonymity. A situation requiring special scrutiny arises when data are collected from two people simultaneously (e.g., a husband and wife who are jointly interviewed) or when interviews in participants' homes occur with other family members present.

TIP

Consumers, like researchers, face the issue of ethical dilemmas. As a reviewer assessing the quality of research evidence for nursing practice, you must be critical of methodologic weaknesses—yet some weaknesses may reflect the researcher's need to conduct research ethically.

RESEARCH EXAMPLES AND CRITICAL THINKING ACTIVITIES

EXAMPLE 1 ■ Quantitative Research

Aspects of a quantitative nursing study, featuring key terms and ethical concepts discussed in this chapter, are presented below, followed by some questions to guide critical thinking.

Study

"Cervical cancer screening practices among university women" (Duffett-Leger, Letourneau, & Croll, 2008)

Study Purpose

The purpose of the study was to examine predictors of young university women's intentions to be screened for cervical cancer.

Research Method

Female students (aged <25 years) from an Eastern-Canadian university were invited to participate in an online survey through their university e-mail account. The survey was developed by the authors based on the Theory of Planned Behavior. A total of 1041 submitted their completed survey (approximately 36% of the eligible population).

Ethics-Related Procedures

The e-mail addresses of these women "were sorted by the Registrar's Office and then uploaded to WebCT by the system administrator. Thus, only those [students] who met the inclusion criteria were granted access to the secured site. WebCT also effectively prevents members of the sampled population from submitting a duplicate survey. A letter of invitation was sent to the study population via e-mail listserv created by a member of the university's information technology staff (ITS) for the sole purpose of this study. The e-mail invitation included information about the survey and a universal resource locator (URL) or web-address for the survey on Web Course Tools (WebCT), which could be accessed simply by double-clicking the hyperlink. Eligible women received two e-mail reminders and a final message highlighting the study findings" (p. 574).

Key Findings

- Social norms (perceptions about whether or not significant others think Pap screening is important) and perceived behavioural control (perceptions about resources or barriers to obtaining a Pap test) were significantly related to young women's intentions to be screened.

- Young women are more likely to learn about Pap tests from friends and family, rather than from health care professionals.

CRITICAL THINKING SUGGESTIONS

1. Answer questions 1 through 8 from Box 5.2 (p. 86) regarding this study.
2. This study utilises a web-based data collection method. What unique ethical considerations does this type of research pose?
3. If the results of this study are valid and reliable, what are some of the uses to which the findings might be put into clinical practice?

EXAMPLE 2 ■ Qualitative Research

Aspects of a qualitative nursing study by Woodgate, Ateah, and Secco (2008) found in Appendix B, featuring key terms and ethical concepts discussed in this chapter, are presented below, followed by some questions to guide critical thinking.

Study

"Living in a world of our own: The experience of parents who have a child with autism" (Woodgate, Ateah, & Secco, 2008)

Study Purpose

This hermeneutic phenomenological study explored parents' experiences having a child with autism.

(Research Examples and Critical Thinking Activities continues on page 88)

Research Examples and Critical Thinking Activities (continued)

Research Methods

Study participants were recruited through an autism support group in a Western Canadian city. A total of 21 parents (16 mothers and 5 fathers), aged between 30 and 40 years, were interviewed either individually or with their spouse. The in-depth, open-ended interviews were audiotaped and lasted between 1.5 and 3 hours. Three mothers required a second interview. Interviewer field notes were made to describe further the context of each interview.

Ethics-Related Procedures

Woodgate and her colleagues obtained university-based ethical approval for the study. They state that "ethical standards were maintained throughout the course of the project by careful attention to issues of recruitment, written consent, confidentiality, anonymity, potential vulnerability, and sensitivity" (p. 1078).

Key Findings

- Parents described their experiences as isolating or "living in a world of our own," mainly due to the lack of external resources.
- Trying to overcome this sense of isolation was a constant challenge represented by the themes of "vigilant parenting," "sustaining the self and family," and "fighting all the way."

CRITICAL THINKING SUGGESTIONS

1. Answer questions 1 through 8 from Box 5.2 (p. 86) regarding this study.

2. Also consider the following targeted questions, which may assist you in further assessing the ethical aspects of the study:
   a. Why do you think the researchers offered parents the option to be interviewed alone or jointly with their spouse?
   b. Why do you think the researchers thought it is necessary to ask the study transcriptionist to sign a confidentiality agreement? What do you think this kind of document would contain?
   c. If you had a child with autism, how would you feel about participating in the study?

3. If the results of this study are trustworthy, what are some of the uses to which the findings might be put into clinical practice?

Summary Points

- Because research has not always been conducted ethically, and because of the **ethical dilemmas** researchers often face in designing studies that are both ethical and methodologically rigorous, **codes of ethics** have been developed to guide researchers.

- In Canada, the Tri-Council Policy Statement on ethical conduct for research with humans set forth eight key ethical principles: respect for human dignity, respect for free and informed consent, respect for vulnerable persons, respect for privacy and confidentiality, respect of justice and inclusiveness, balancing harms and benefits, minimizing harm, and maximizing benefit.

- *Respect for human dignity* includes the participants' right to **self-determination,** which means participants have the freedom to control their own actions, including the right to refuse to participate in the study or to answer certain questions.

≈ **Informed consent** is intended to provide prospective participants with information needed to make a reasoned and voluntary decision about participation in a study.

≈ **Full disclosure** means researchers have fully described the study, including risks and benefits, to prospective participants. When full disclosure poses the risk of biased results, researchers sometimes use **covert data collection** or *concealment* (the collection of data without the participants' knowledge or consent) or *deception* (withholding information from participants or providing false information).

≈ **Vulnerable subjects** require additional protection as participants. They may be vulnerable because they are not able to make a truly informed decision about study participation (e.g., children); because of diminished autonomy (e.g., prisoners); or because their circumstances heighten the risk of physical or psychological harm (e.g., pregnant women).

≈ The principle of *justice* includes the right to fair and equitable treatment and to an inclusionary approach to recruitment of participants.

≈ **Beneficence** involves the performance of some good, and the protection of participants from harm and exploitation (**nonmaleficence**).

≈ Various procedures have been developed to safeguard study participants' rights, including the performance of a risk/benefit assessment, implementation of informed consent procedures, and efforts to safeguard participants' confidentiality.

≈ In a **risk/benefit assessment,** the individual benefits of participation in a study (and societal benefits of the research) are weighed against the costs to individuals.

≈ Informed consent normally involves the signing of a **consent form** to document voluntary and informed participation. In qualitative studies, consent may need to be continually renegotiated with participants as the study evolves, through **process consent** procedures.

≈ Privacy can be maintained through **anonymity** (wherein not even researchers know the participants' identity) or through formal **confidentiality** procedures that safeguard the information participants provide.

≈ Researchers sometimes offer **debriefing** sessions after data collection to provide participants with more information or an opportunity to air complaints.

≈ External review of the ethical aspects of a study by a **Research Ethics Board (REB)** or other human subjects committee is highly desirable and may be required by either the agency funding the research or the organization from which participants are recruited.

≈ Ethical conduct in research involves not only protection of the rights of human and animal subjects but also efforts to maintain high standards of integrity and avoid such forms of **research misconduct** as plagiarism, fabrication of results, or falsification of data.

STUDIES CITED IN CHAPTER 5*

This reference list contains only those studies that were cited in this chapter. Citations pertaining to theoretical, methodological, or nonempirical work are included together in a separate section at the end of the book (beginning on page 399).

Baxter, P. E., & Boblin, S. (2008). Decision making by baccalaureate nursing students in the clinical setting. *Journal of Nursing Education, 47*(8), 345–350.

Duffett-Leger, L. A., Letourneau, N. L., & Croll, J. C. (2008). Cervical cancer screening practices among university women. *Journal of Obstetric, Gynecologic, & Neonatal Nursing, 37*(5), 572–581.

Flicker, S., Haans, D., & Skinner, H. (2004). Ethical dilemmas in research on internet communities. *Qualitative Health Research, 14*(1), 124–134.

Holtzclaw, B. J., & Hanneman, S. K. (2002). Use of non-human biobehavioral models in critical care nursing research. *Critical Care Nursing Quarterly, 24*(4), 30–40.

Lobchuk, M. M., & Bokhari, S. A. (2008). Linkages among empathic behaviors, physical symptoms, and psychological distress in patients with ovarian cancer: A pilot study. *Oncology Nursing Forum, 35*(5), 808–814.

McCullough, K. D., & Bartfay, W. J. (2007). The dose-dependent effects of chronic iron overload in the production of oxygen free radicals and vitamin E concentrations in the liver of a murine model. *Biological Research for Nursing, 8*(4), 300–304.

Read, T., & Wuest, J. (2007). Daughters caring for dying parents: A process of relinquishing. *Qualitative Health Research, 17*(7), 932–944.

Spagrud, L. J., von Baeyer, C. L., Ali, K., et al. (2008). Pain, distress, and adult-child interaction during venipuncture in pediatric oncology: An examination of three types of venous access. *Journal of Pain and Symptom Management, 36*(2), 173–184.

Spiers, J. (2006). Expressing and responding to pain and stoicism in home-care nurse-patient interactions. *Scandinavian Journal of Caring Sciences, 20*, 293–301.

Woodgate, R. L., Ateah, C., & Secco, L. (2008). Living in a world of our own: The experience of parents who have a child with autism. *Qualitative Health Research, 18*(8), 1075–1083.

Preliminary Steps in the Research Process

CHAPTER

6 Scrutinizing Research Problems, Research Questions, and Hypotheses

On completing this chapter, you will be able to:

1. Describe the process of developing and refining a research problem

2. Distinguish statements of purpose and research questions for quantitative and qualitative studies

3. Describe the function and characteristics of research hypotheses and distinguish different types of hypotheses

4. Critique statements of purpose, research questions, and hypotheses in research reports with respect to their placement, clarity, wording, and significance

5. Define new terms in the chapter

RESEARCH PROBLEMS AND RESEARCH QUESTIONS

A study begins as a problem that a researcher would like to solve or as a question that he or she would like to answer. In this chapter we discuss the formulation and evaluation of research problems, research questions, and hypotheses. We begin by clarifying some related terms.

Basic Terms Relating to Research Problems

At the most general level, researchers select a *topic* or a phenomenon on which to focus. Patient compliance, coping with disability, and pain management are examples of research topics. Within these broad topic areas are many potential research problems. In this section, we illustrate various terms as we define them using the topic *side effects in patients undergoing chemotherapy*.

A **research problem** is a perplexing or troubling condition. Both qualitative and quantitative researchers identify a research problem within a broad topic area of interest. The purpose of disciplined research is to "solve" the problem—or to contribute to its solution—by accumulating relevant information. A **problem statement** articulates the problem to be addressed. Table 6.1 presents a problem statement related to the topic of side effects in chemotherapy patients.

Research questions are the specific queries researchers want to answer in addressing a research problem. Research questions guide the types of data to be collected in the study. Researchers who make specific predictions regarding the

TABLE 6.1   EXAMPLE OF TERMS RELATING TO RESEARCH PROBLEMS

TERM	EXAMPLE
Topic/focus	Side effects of chemotherapy
Research problem	Nausea and vomiting are common side effects among patients on chemotherapy, and interventions to date have been only moderately successful in reducing these effects. New interventions that can reduce or prevent these side effects need to be identified.
Statement of purpose	The purpose of the study is to test an intervention to reduce chemotherapy-induced side effects—specifically, to compare the effectiveness of patient-controlled and nurse-administered antiemetic therapy for controlling nausea and vomiting in patients on chemotherapy.
Research question	What is the relative effectiveness of patient-controlled antiemetic therapy versus nurse-controlled antiemetic therapy with regard to (a) medication consumption and (b) control of nausea and vomiting in patients on chemotherapy?
Hypotheses	(1) Participants receiving antiemetic therapy by a patient-controlled pump report less nausea than participants receiving the therapy by nurse administration; (2) participants receiving antiemetic therapy by a patient-controlled pump vomit less than participants receiving the therapy by nurse administration; (3) participants receiving antiemetic therapy by a patient-controlled pump consume less medication than participants receiving the therapy by nurse administration.
Aims/objectives	This study has as its aim the following objectives: (1) to develop and implement two alternative procedures for administering antiemetic therapy for patients receiving moderate emetogenic chemotherapy (patient controlled versus nurse controlled); (2) to test three hypotheses concerning the relative effectiveness of the alternative procedures on medication consumption and control of side effects; and (3) to use the findings to develop recommendations for possible changes to therapeutic procedures.

answers to research questions pose **hypotheses** that are tested empirically. Examples of both research questions and hypotheses are presented in Table 6.1.

In a research report, you might also encounter other related terms. For example, many reports include a **statement of purpose** (or purpose statement), which is the researcher's summary of the overall goal. A researcher might also identify several specific *research aims* or *objectives*—the specific accomplishments the researcher hopes to achieve by conducting the study. The objectives include obtaining answers to research questions but may also encompass some broader aims (e.g., developing recommendations for changes to nursing practice based on the study results), as illustrated in Table 6.1.

Research Problems and Paradigms

Some research problems are better suited for studies using qualitative versus quantitative methods. Quantitative studies usually involve concepts that are well developed, about which there is an existing body of literature, and for which reliable methods of measurement have been developed. For example, a quantitative study might be undertaken to determine whether postpartum depression is higher among women who return to work 6 months after delivery than among those who stay home with their babies. There are relatively accurate measures of postpartum depression that would yield quantitative information about the level of depression in a sample of employed and unemployed postpartum women.

Qualitative studies are often undertaken because some aspect of a phenomenon is poorly understood, and the researcher wants to develop a rich, comprehensive, and context-bound understanding of it. In the example of postpartum depression, qualitative methods would not be well suited to comparing levels of depression among two groups of women, but they would be ideal for exploring, for example, the *meaning* of postpartum depression among new mothers. In evaluating a research report, an important consideration is whether the research problem fits the chosen paradigm and its associated methods. It is important to note, however, that there is room for a combined methodologic approach, and the benefits and challenges of multimethod (mixed method) research are explained in Chapter 11.

Sources of Research Problems

Where do ideas for research problems come from? At a basic level, research topics originate with researchers' interests. Because research is a time-consuming enterprise, curiosity about and interest in a topic are essential to the success of the project.

Research reports rarely indicate the source of a researcher's inspiration for a study, but a variety of sources can fuel a researcher's curiosity, including the following:

≽ *Clinical experience.* The nurse's everyday experience is a rich source of ideas for research topics. Problems that need immediate solution have high potential for clinical significance.

≽ *Nursing literature.* Ideas for studies often come from reading the nursing literature. Research reports may suggest problem areas indirectly by stimulating the reader's imagination and directly by explicitly stating what additional research is needed.

≽ *Social issues.* Topics are sometimes suggested by global social or political issues of relevance to the health care community. For example, the feminist movement has raised questions about such topics as gender equity and domestic violence.

≽ *Theories.* Theories from nursing and other related disciplines are another source of research problems. Researchers ask, If this theory is correct, what would I predict about people's behaviours, states, or feelings? The predictions can then be tested through research.

≽ *Ideas from external sources.* External sources and direct suggestions can sometimes provide the impetus for a research idea. For example, ideas for studies may emerge from reviewing a funding agency's research priorities or from brainstorming with other nurses.

It should be noted that researchers who have developed a program of research on a topic area may get inspiration for "next steps" from their own findings, or from a discussion of those findings with others.

Example of a problem source for a research study

Dr. Greta Cummings has established a program of research from a problem source that she experienced personally as a nurse manager of more than 20 years. Her CLEAR (Connecting Leadership, Education and Research) Outcomes Research Program explores the effects of leadership on nursing and the Canadian health care system. Having gone through major hospital restructuring in the 1990s which laid-off thousands of nurses in Alberta, Dr. Cummings could see first-hand the stress on those who remained. She was determined to find ways to alleviate these negative effects. As a manager herself, Dr. Cummings saw promise in the pursuit of optimal nursing leadership styles—first to identify best approaches and then effectively train others. Ultimately, she hopes this form of intervention will have far reaching outcomes on nurse retention and better patient care.

Development and Refinement of Research Problems

The development of a research problem is a creative process. Researchers often begin with interests in a broad topic area, and then develop the topic into a more specific researchable problem. For example, suppose a nurse working on a medical unit begins to wonder why some patients complain about having to wait for pain medication when certain nurses are assigned to them. The general topic is discrepancy in patient complaints about pain medications administered by different nurses. The nurse might ask, What accounts for this discrepancy? This broad question may lead to other questions, such as How do the two groups of nurses differ? or What characteristics do the complaining patients share? At this point, the nurse may observe that the cultural or ethnic background of the patients and nurses could be a relevant factor. This may direct the nurse to a review of the literature for studies concerning ethnic groups and their relationship to nursing behaviours, or it may provoke a discussion of these observations with peers. These efforts may result in several research questions, such as the following:

⇝ What is the essence of patient complaints among patients of different ethnic backgrounds?

⇝ How are complaints by patients of different ethnic backgrounds expressed by patients and perceived by nurses?

⇝ Is the ethnic background of nurses related to the frequency with which they dispense pain medication?

⇝ Is the ethnic background of patients related to the frequency and intensity of their complaints of having to wait for pain medication?

⇝ Does the number of patient complaints increase when the patients are of dissimilar ethnic backgrounds as opposed to when they are of the same ethnic background as the nurse?

⇝ Do nurses' dispensing behaviours change as a function of the similarity between their own ethnic background and that of patients?

These questions stem from the same general problem, yet each would be studied differently; for example, some suggest a qualitative approach, and others suggest a quantitative one. A quantitative researcher might become curious about nurses' dispensing behaviours, based on some evidence in the literature regarding ethnic differences. Both ethnicity and nurses' dispensing behaviours are variables that can be reliably measured. A qualitative researcher who noticed differences in patient complaints would likely be more interested in understanding the *essence* of the complaints, the patients' *experience* of frustration, the *process* by which the problem was resolved, or the full *nature* of the nurse–patient interactions regarding the dispensing of medications. These are aspects of the research problem that would be difficult to measure quantitatively. Researchers choose a problem to study based on several factors, including its inherent interest to them and its fit with a paradigm of preference. Nurse researchers today also have the option (and are often encouraged) to join interprofessional health care teams to explore the problem from multiple viewpoints in a multimethod and/or multidisciplinary (possibly even interdisciplinary) study.

COMMUNICATING THE RESEARCH PROBLEM, PURPOSE, AND QUESTIONS

Researchers communicate their objectives in various ways in research reports. This section focuses on the wording and placement of problem statements, statements of purpose, and research questions.

Problem Statements

A problem statement is an expression of a dilemma or disturbing situation that needs investigation. A problem statement identifies the nature of the problem that is being addressed in the study and, typically, its context and significance. Generally, the problem statement should be broad enough to include central concerns but narrow enough in scope to serve as a guide to study design.

Example of a problem statement from a quantitative study

"Globally, there is an increasing shortage of registered nurses (RNs). This crisis is not expected to be resolved soon. Canadian Nurses Association (CNA 2002) reported Canada alone is predicted to have a projected shortfall of 113,000 RNs by 2016. . . . Retention of knowledgeable and experienced RNs, as well as retaining and promoting the continuing development of less-experienced RNs, are necessary to stabilize the workforce and to ensure an adequate supply of RNs over the upcoming years. . . . Job satisfaction has been shown to be a significant predictor of retention . . . job satisfaction may be perceived differently across the multigenerational RN workforce. Consequently, understanding job satisfaction within each generational group may lead to increasing clarity about strategies that could be implemented to promote RN retention for each generation of RNs in the current workforce" (Wilson, Squires, Widger, Cranley, & Tourangeau, 2008, pp. 716–717).

In this example, the general topic is nursing retention, but the investigators narrowed the focus of their inquiry to studying job satisfaction within generational groups. This problem statement asserted the nature of the problem (increasing the retention of RNs across all generational groups) and its significance (a projected shortfall of Canadian nurses within the next few years).

The problem statement for a qualitative study similarly expresses the nature of the problem, its context, and its significance. Qualitative studies that are embedded in a particular research tradition generally incorporate terms and concepts in their problem statements that foreshadow their tradition of inquiry. For example, the problem statement in a grounded theory study might refer to the need to develop deeper understandings of social processes. A problem statement for a phenomenological study might note the need to know more about people's experiences or the meanings they attribute to those experiences. And an ethnographer might indicate the desire to describe how cultural forces affect people's behaviour.

> **TIP**
>
> How can you tell a problem statement? Problem statements appear in the introduction to a research report—indeed, the first sentence of a research report is often the starting point of a problem statement. However, problem statements are often interwoven with a review of the literature, which provides context by documenting knowledge gaps. Problem statements are rarely explicitly labelled as such and must therefore be ferreted out. To help you, look for statements such as, "findings are inconsistent" or "there is a lack of research."

Statements of Purpose

Many researchers first articulate their goals as a broad statement of purpose, worded declaratively. The purpose statement captures, in a sentence or two, the essence of the study and establishes the general direction of the inquiry. The word *purpose* or *goal* usually appears in a purpose statement (e.g., "The purpose of this study was . . ." or "The goal of this study was . . ."), but sometimes the word *intent*, *aim*, or *objective* is used instead.

In a quantitative study, a well-worded statement of purpose identifies the key study variables and their possible interrelationships as well as the population of interest.

Example of a statement of purpose from a quantitative study

"Given the diverse attitudes of nurses of different generations, it is vital to explore how overall job satisfaction and satisfaction with specific aspects of work are similar and different across the generations. Therefore, we explored how RNs across the three youngest generations (1) rated their overall job satisfaction, (2) rated their specific components of job satisfaction, and (3) differed in their evaluations of overall job satisfaction and the specific components of job satisfaction" (Wilson et al., 2008, p. 718).

This statement identifies the population of interest (multigenerational RNs) and the three specific study objectives used to investigate the problem.

In qualitative studies, the statement of purpose indicates the nature of the inquiry, the key phenomenon under investigation, and the group or community under study.

Example of a statement of purpose from a qualitative study
"If the lack of culturally appropriate services is a barrier to Aboriginal women accessing HIV testing, and the number of positive tests among women within the Aboriginal community is increasing, then research to define *culturally appropriate HIV counseling and testing* for Aboriginal women is urgently required. Therefore, the purpose of this study was to identify Aboriginal women's perspectives on the characteristics of culturally appropriate HIV counseling and testing" (Bucharski, Reutter, & Ogilvie, 2006, p. 725).

This statement indicates that the phenomenon of interest is culturally appropriate HIV counselling and testing as defined by Canadian Aboriginal women.

Researchers typically use verbs in their statements of purpose that suggest how they sought to solve the problem, or what the state of knowledge on the topic is. A study whose purpose is to *explore* or *describe* a phenomenon is likely to focus on a little-researched topic, often involving a qualitative approach. A statement of purpose for a qualitative study may also imply a flexible design through the use of verbs such as *understand* or *discover*. Creswell (1998) notes that qualitative researchers often "encode" the tradition of inquiry not only through their choice of verbs but also through the use of certain terms or "buzz words" associated with those traditions, as follows:

⇒ *Grounded theory:* Processes, social structures, social interactions

⇒ *Phenomenological studies:* Experience, lived experience, meaning, essence

⇒ *Ethnographic studies:* Culture, roles, myths, cultural behaviour

Quantitative researchers also suggest the nature of the inquiry through their selection of verbs. A purpose statement indicating that the purpose is to *test* the effectiveness of an intervention or to *compare* two alternative nursing strategies suggests a study with a more established knowledge base, using a design with tight controls. Note that researchers' choice of verbs in a statement of purpose should connote a certain degree of objectivity. A statement of purpose indicating that the intent of the study was to *prove, demonstrate,* or *show* something suggests a bias.

Research Questions

Research questions are, in some cases, direct rewordings of statements of purpose, phrased interrogatively rather than declaratively. The research questions for the examples cited in the previous section might be as follows:

⇒ Do job satisfaction generational differences in nurses exist?

⇒ What are Canadian Aboriginal women's perspectives on culturally appropriate HIV counselling and testing?

Questions that are simple and direct invite an answer and help to focus attention on the kinds of data needed to provide that answer. Some research reports thus omit a statement of purpose and state only the research question. Other researchers use a set of research questions to clarify or amplify the purpose statement.

In a quantitative study, research questions identify the key variables (most often, the independent and dependent variables), the relationships among them, and the population under study.

Example of a research question from a quantitative study

In a research study which examined children (aged between 3 and 18 years) undergoing routine blood tests for cancer management, the first of two research questions was: Do these children experience differing pain and distress in response to three different types of venous access? (Spagrud, et al., 2008)

In this example, the independent variable is the needle group to which the child was routinely allocated; the dependent variables are the pain ratings and rate of child distress (measured by validated scales).

Researchers in the various qualitative traditions differ in the types of questions they believe to be important. Grounded theory researchers are likely to ask *process* questions, phenomenologists tend to ask *meaning* questions, and ethnographers generally ask *descriptive* questions about cultures. The terms associated with the various traditions, discussed earlier in connection with purpose statements, may also be incorporated into the research questions.

Example of a research question from a hermeneutic phenomenological study

What is the lived experience of parents who have a child with autism (Woodgate, Ateah, & Secco, 2008)?

Not all qualitative studies are rooted in specific research traditions, however. Many researchers use naturalistic methods to describe or explore phenomena without focusing on cultures, meaning, or social processes.

In qualitative studies, research questions sometimes evolve over the course of the study. Researchers begin with a *focus* that defines the general boundaries of the inquiry, but the boundaries are not cast in stone—they "can be altered and, in the typical naturalistic inquiry, will be" (Lincoln & Guba, 1985, p. 228). Naturalists thus begin with a research question in mind but are sufficiently flexible that the question can be modified as new information makes it relevant to do so.

TIP

Researchers most often state their purpose or research questions at the end of the introduction or immediately after the review of the literature. Sometimes, a separate section of a research report—typically located just before the method section—is devoted to stating the research problem formally and might be labelled "Purpose," "Statement of Purpose," "Research Questions," or, in quantitative studies, "Hypotheses."

RESEARCH HYPOTHESES IN QUANTITATIVE RESEARCH

In quantitative studies, researchers may present a statement of purpose and then one or more hypotheses. A hypothesis is a tentative prediction about the relationship between two or more variables in the population under study. In a qualitative study, the researcher does not begin with a hypothesis, in part because there is generally too little known about the topic to justify a hypothesis and, in part, because qualitative researchers want their inquiry to be guided by participants' viewpoints rather than by their own *a priori* hunches (although findings from qualitative studies may *lead to* the formulation of hypotheses). Thus, our discussion here focuses on hypotheses in quantitative research.

Function of Hypotheses in Quantitative Research

A hypothesis translates a research question into a statement of expected outcomes. For instance, the research question might ask, Does therapeutic touch affect patients' muscle tension levels? The researcher might hypothesize as follows: The muscle tension levels of patients treated with therapeutic touch is lower than the muscle tension levels of patients treated with physical touch.

Hypotheses sometimes emerge from a theory. Scientists reason from theories to hypotheses and test those hypotheses in the real world. The validity of a theory is never examined directly, but it can be evaluated through hypothesis testing. For example, the theory of reinforcement maintains that behaviour that is positively reinforced (rewarded) tends to be learned (repeated). The theory is too abstract to test, but hypotheses based on the theory can be tested. For instance, the following hypotheses are deduced from reinforcement theory:

⇒ Elderly patients who are praised (reinforced) for self-feeding require less assistance in feeding than patients who are not praised.

⇒ Paediatric patients who are given a reward (e.g., permission to watch television) when they cooperate during nursing procedures are more compliant during those procedures than nonrewarded peers.

Both of these propositions can be tested in the real world. The theory gains support if the hypotheses are confirmed. Even in the absence of a theory, hypotheses can offer direction and suggest explanations. For example, suppose we hypothesized that widowers experience more psychological distress in the 6 months after the death of their spouse than widows. This prediction could be based on theory (e.g., role expectation theory), earlier studies, or personal observations. The development of predictions in and of itself forces researchers to think logically, to exercise critical judgment, and to tie together earlier findings.

Now let us suppose that the above hypothesis is not confirmed by the evidence collected; that is, we find that men and women experience comparable levels of emotional distress in the 6 months after their spouses' death. The failure of data to support a prediction forces investigators to analyze theory or previous research critically, to review limitations of the study's method carefully, and to explore alternative explanations for the findings. The use of hypotheses in quantitative studies tends to induce critical thinking and, hence, to facilitate interpretation of the data.

To further illustrate the utility of hypotheses, suppose the researcher conducted a study guided only by the research question, *Is there a relationship between a person's gender and the degree of distress experienced after losing a spouse?* Investigators without a hypothesis are, apparently, prepared to accept any results. The problem is that it is almost always possible to explain something superficially after the fact, no matter what the findings are. Hypotheses guard against superficiality and minimize the possibility that spurious results will be misconstrued.

TIP

Some quantitative research reports explicitly state the hypotheses that guided the study, but most do not. The absence of a hypothesis sometimes is appropriate, but it often is an indication that researchers have failed to consider critically the implications of theory or existing knowledge or have failed to disclose the hunches that may have influenced their methodologic decisions.

Characteristics of Testable Hypotheses

Testable research hypotheses state the expected relationship between the independent variable (the presumed cause or antecedent) and the dependent variable (the presumed effect) within a population.

Example of a research hypothesis
"Less smoking cessation by the [lung cancer] patient leads to greater judgements of responsibility, anger, and less helping behaviour by the [primary] caregiver" (Lobchuk, McClement, McPherson, & Cheang, 2008, p. 683).

In this example, the independent variable is the patients' smoking behaviour, and the dependent variables are the caregivers' illness attribution reactions and helping behaviours. The hypothesis predicts that these variables are related—it is expected that caregivers will blame or feel anger toward patients with lung cancer who still smoke, and this decreases their helping behaviour.

Unfortunately, researchers sometimes state hypotheses that fail to make a relational statement, and such hypotheses are not testable. Consider, for example, the following prediction: "Pregnant women who receive prenatal instruction by a nurse regarding postpartum experiences are not likely to experience postpartum depression." This statement expresses no anticipated relationship; in fact, there is only one variable (postpartum depression), and a relationship by definition requires at least two variables.

When a hypothesis does not state an anticipated relationship, it cannot be tested. In our example, how would we know if the hypothesis was supported—what absolute standard could be used to decide whether to accept or reject the hypothesis? To illustrate more concretely, suppose we asked a group of mothers who received prenatal instruction the following question 2 months after delivery: Overall, how depressed have you been since you gave birth? Would you say (1) extremely depressed, (2) moderately depressed, (3) somewhat depressed, or (4) not at all depressed?

Based on responses to this question, how could we compare the actual outcome with the predicted outcome? Would *all* the women in the sample have to say they were "not at all depressed?" Would the prediction be supported if 51% of the women said they were "not at all depressed" *or* "somewhat depressed?" There is no adequate way of testing the accuracy of the prediction.

A test is simple, however, if we modify the prediction to the following: Pregnant women who receive prenatal instruction are less likely to experience postpartum depression than pregnant women with no prenatal instruction. Here, the dependent variable is the women's depression and the independent variable is their receipt or nonreceipt of prenatal instruction. The relational aspect of the prediction is embodied in the phrase *less . . . than*. If a hypothesis lacks a phrase such as *more than, less than, greater than, different from, related to, associated with*, or something similar, it is not amenable to testing in a quantitative study. To test this revised hypothesis, we could ask two groups of women with different prenatal instruction experiences to respond to the question on depression and then compare the groups' responses. The absolute degree of depression of either group would not be at issue.

Hypotheses should be based on justifiable rationales. The most defensible hypotheses follow from previous research findings or are deduced from a theory. When a relatively new area is being investigated, researchers may have to turn to logical reasoning or personal experience to justify predictions.

TIP

Hypotheses are typically fairly easy to identify because researchers make statements such as "The study tested the hypothesis that . . ." or "It was predicted that . . . ."

Wording Hypotheses

A hypothesis can predict the relationship between a single independent variable and a single dependent variable (a *simple hypothesis*), or it can predict a relationship between two or more independent variables or two or more dependent variables (a *complex hypothesis*). In the following examples, independent variables are indicated as IVs and dependent variables are identified as DVs:

Example of a simple hypothesis
Self-reported job satisfaction (IV) predicts intentions expressed about working as a U.K. nurse (DV) (Murrells, Robinson, & Griffiths, 2008).

Example of a complex hypothesis
Self-reported job satisfaction at earlier time-points (6 months, 18 months) (IVs) predicts working as a U.K. nurse at 18 months and 3 years after qualification (DVs) (Murrells, Robinson, & Griffiths, 2008).

Hypotheses can be stated in various ways as long as the researcher specifies or implies the relationship that will be tested. Here is an example about the effect of postpartum exercise:

1. Low levels of exercise are associated with greater weight retention than high levels of exercise.
2. There is a relationship between level of exercise and weight retention.
3. The greater the level of exercise, the lower the weight retention.
4. Women with different levels of exercise differ with regard to weight retention.
5. Weight retention decreases as the woman's level of exercise increases.
6. Women who exercise have lower weight retention than women who do not.

Other variations are also possible. The important point to remember is that the hypothesis specifies the independent variable (here, level of exercise postpartum), the dependent variable (weight retention), and the anticipated relationship between them.

Hypotheses usually should be worded in the present tense. Researchers make a prediction about a relationship in the population—not just about a relationship that will be revealed in a particular sample of study participants.

Hypotheses can be either directional or nondirectional. A **directional hypothesis** is one that specifies not only the existence but also the expected direction of the relationship between variables. In the six versions of the hypothesis above, versions 1, 3, 5, and 6 are directional because there is an explicit prediction that women who do not exercise postpartum are at greater risk of weight retention than women who do. A **nondirectional hypothesis,** by contrast, does not stipulate the direction of the relationship, as illustrated in versions 2 and 4. These hypotheses predict that a woman's level of exercise and weight retention are related, but they do not stipulate whether the researcher thinks that exercise is related to more weight retention, or less.

Hypotheses based on theory are usually directional because theories provide a rationale for expecting variables to relate in certain ways. Existing studies also offer a basis for specifying directional hypotheses. When there is no theory or related research, when findings from prior studies are contradictory, or when researchers' own experience leads to ambivalent expectations, nondirectional hypotheses may be appropriate. Some people argue, in fact, that nondirectional hypotheses are preferable because they connote impartiality. Directional hypotheses, it is said, imply that researchers are intellectually committed to certain outcomes, and such commitment might lead to bias. This argument fails to recognize that researchers typically *do* have hunches about the outcomes, whether they state those expectations explicitly or not. We prefer directional hypotheses—when there is a reasonable basis for them—because they clarify the study's framework and demonstrate that researchers have thought critically about the phenomena under study.

Another distinction is the difference between research and null hypotheses. **Research hypotheses** (also referred to as *substantive hypotheses*) are statements of actual expected relationships between variables. All hypotheses presented thus far are research hypotheses that indicate researchers' true expectations.

For statistical analyses, the logic of statistical inference requires that hypotheses be expressed as though no relationship were expected. **Null hypotheses** (or *statistical hypotheses*) state that there is no relationship between the independent variables and dependent variables. The null form of the hypothesis used in our preceding example would be: Mothers' exercise levels postpartum are unrelated to their weight retention. A null hypothesis might be compared to the assumption of innocence of an accused criminal in the Canadian justice system; the variables are assumed to be "innocent" of any relationship until they can be shown to be "guilty" through statistical procedures. The null hypothesis is the formal statement of this presumed innocence.

Research reports typically present research rather than null hypotheses. When statistical tests are performed, the underlying null hypotheses are assumed without being stated. If the researcher's actual research hypothesis is that no relationship among variables exists, the hypothesis cannot be adequately tested using traditional statistical procedures. This issue is explained in Chapter 15.

> **TIP**
>
> When researchers use statistical tests (and this is almost always the case in quantitative studies), it means that there were underlying hypotheses—*whether the researchers explicitly stated them or not*—because statistical tests are designed to test hypotheses.

Hypothesis Testing and Proof

Hypotheses are never *proved* (or *disproved*) through hypothesis testing; rather, they are *accepted* or *rejected*. Findings are always tentative. Certainly, if the same results are replicated in numerous studies, greater confidence can be placed in the conclusions. Hypotheses come to be increasingly supported with mounting evidence.

Let us look more closely at why this is so. Suppose we hypothesized that height and weight are related—which, indeed, they are in a general population. We predict that, on average, tall people weigh more than short people. We would then obtain height and weight measurements from a sample and analyze the data. Now suppose we happened by chance to choose a sample that consisted of short, fat people, and tall, thin people. Our results might indicate that there was no significant relationship between a person's height and weight. Would we then be justified in stating that this study *proved* or *demonstrated* that height and weight are unrelated?

As another example, suppose we hypothesized that tall people are better nurses than short people. This hypothesis is used here only to illustrate a point because, in reality, we would expect no relationship between height and a nurse's job performance. Now suppose that, by chance again, we draw a sample of nurses in which tall nurses received better job evaluations than short ones. Can we conclude definitively that height is related to nursing performance? These two examples demonstrate the difficulty of using observations from a sample to generalize to the population from which a sample has been drawn. Other problems, such as the accuracy of the measures, prohibit researchers from concluding with finality that hypotheses are proved.

CRITIQUING RESEARCH PROBLEMS, RESEARCH QUESTIONS, AND HYPOTHESES

In critiquing research reports, you will need to evaluate whether researchers have adequately communicated their research problem. The researchers' description of the problem, statement of purpose, research questions, and hypotheses set the stage for the description of what was done and what was learned. Ideally, you should not have to dig too deeply to decipher the research problem or to discover the questions.

Critiquing the Substance of a Research Problem

A critique of the research problem involves multiple dimensions. Substantively, you need to consider whether the problem has significance for nursing. The following issues are relevant in considering the significance of a study problem:

1. *Implications for nursing practice.* A primary consideration in evaluating the significance of a research problem is whether it has the potential to produce evidence for improving nursing practice: Are there practical applications that might stem from research on the problem? Will more knowledge about the problem improve nursing practice? Will the findings challenge (or lend support to) assumptions about nursing? If the answer to such questions is no, the significance of the problem is bound to be low.

2. *Extension of knowledge base.* Studies that build in a meaningful way on the existing knowledge base are well poised to make contributions to evidence-based nursing practice. Researchers, who develop a systematic *program of research* building on their own earlier findings, are especially likely to make significant contributions. For example, Beck's series of studies relating to postpartum depression (e.g., Beck, 1992, 1995, 1998, 2001, 2006; Beck & Gable, 2003) has influenced women's health care worldwide, most recently in her review of the state of the science in this area (Beck, 2008a, 2008b). As another example, Estabrooks developed a program of research in knowledge translation specific to nursing (Estabrooks, 1998, 1999a, 1999b; Estabrooks, Chong, Brigidear, & Profetto-McGrath, 2005; Estabrooks et al., 2005, 2008; Estabrooks, Midodzi, Cummings, & Wallin, 2007).

3. *Promotion of theory development.* Studies that test or develop a theory often have a better chance of contributing to knowledge than studies that do not have a conceptual context. For example, Marilyn Ford-Gilboe and colleagues have undertaken numerous studies to develop, refine, and test the Developmental Model of Health and Nursing, which we will describe in Chapter 8 (e.g., Black & Ford-Gilboe, 2004; Bluvol & Ford-Gilboe, 2004; Fulford & Ford-Gilboe, 2004).

4. *Correspondence to research priorities.* Research priorities have been established by research scholars, agencies that fund nursing research (such as the CIHR), and professional nursing organizations. Research problems stemming from

such priorities have a high likelihood of yielding important new evidence for nurses because they reflect expert opinion about areas of needed research. As an example, Loiselle, Semenic, and Côté (2005) conducted a systematic research dissemination project based on findings relating to breastfeeding information and support offered by hospitals and community health centers in the Montreal region. This project corresponds to a research and public health priority identified by the Ministry of Health and Social Services and the Conseil Québecois de la Recherche Sociale (CQRS).

When critiquing a study, you need to consider whether the research problem was meaningfully based on prior research, has a relationship to a theoretical context, addresses a current research priority, and, most importantly, can contribute useful evidence for nursing practice.

Critiquing Other Aspects of Research Problems

Another dimension in critiquing the research problem concerns methodologic issues—in particular, whether the research problem is compatible with the chosen research paradigm and its associated methods. You should also evaluate whether the statement of purpose or research questions have been properly worded and lend themselves to empirical inquiry.

In a quantitative study, if the research report does not contain explicit hypotheses, you need to consider whether their absence is justified. If there are hypotheses, you should evaluate whether the hypotheses are logically connected to the research problem and whether they are consistent with available knowledge or relevant theory. The wording of the hypothesis should also be assessed. The hypothesis is a valid guidepost to scientific inquiry only if it is testable. To be testable, the hypothesis must contain a prediction about the relationship between two or more measurable variables.

Specific guidelines for critiquing research problems, research questions, and hypotheses are presented in Box 6.1.

BOX 6.1   GUIDELINES FOR CRITIQUING RESEARCH PROBLEMS, RESEARCH QUESTIONS, AND HYPOTHESES

▶

1. What is the research problem? Is it easy to locate and clearly stated?

2. Does the problem have significance for nursing? How might the research contribute to nursing practice, administration, education, or policy?

3. Is there a good fit between the research problem and the paradigm within which the research was conducted? Is there a good fit with the qualitative research tradition? Or is there a good fit with the quantitative research tradition?

4. Does the report formally present a statement of purpose, research question, and/or hypotheses? Is this information communicated clearly and concisely, and is it placed in a logical and useful location?

5. Are purpose statements or questions worded appropriately? (For example, are key concepts/variables identified and the population of interest specified? Are verbs used appropriately to suggest the nature of the inquiry and/or the research tradition?)

6. If there are no formal hypotheses, is their absence justified? Are statistical tests used in analyzing the data despite the absence of stated hypotheses?

7. Do hypotheses (if any) flow from a theory or previous research? Is there a justifiable basis for the predictions?

8. Are hypotheses (if any) properly worded—do they state a predicted relationship between two or more variables? Are they directional or nondirectional, and is there a rationale for how they were stated? Are they presented as research or as null hypotheses?

▶ RESEARCH EXAMPLES AND CRITICAL THINKING ACTIVITIES

EXAMPLE 1 ■ Quantitative Research

Aspects of a quantitative nursing study, featuring terms and concepts discussed in this chapter, are presented below, followed by some questions to guide critical thinking.

Study

"Chronic pain in women survivors of intimate partner violence" (Wuest et al., 2008)

Research Problem

"In Canada, 18% of women over the age of 12 experience chronic pain . . . [it] is one of the many serious long-term health consequences of intimate partner violence (IPV). IPV is a pattern of physical, sexual, and/or emotional violence by an intimate partner in the context of coercive control . . . higher rates of chronic pain have been found in women who have experienced IPV than in those who have not. Disability related to chronic pain also is more likely in women with a history of IPV than in those without . . . . Despite the evidence that chronic pain is a serious problem that interferes with health and well-being in women with a history of abuse, little is known about the actual severity and patterns of chronic pain in community samples of women abuse survivors" (pp. 1–2).

Study Aims

There were four main aims of the study: (1) to describe the pattern of severity of chronic pain in a community sample of women in the early years after leaving abusive partners, as measured by the Chronic Pain Grade scale; (2) to illustrate the variation in site, frequency, and interference of pain reported as problematic in the past month by chronic pain severity; (3) to describe the relationships between chronic pain severity as indicated by disability category (high/low) and women's abuse histories, selected health indicators, health service use, and selected demographic variables; and (4) to document the pattern of use of selected medications by chronic pain severity.

Method

Data for the study were collected by structured interview with a community sample of 292 women who had separated from their abusive partners on average 20 months previously, as part of an ongoing longitudinal prospective investigation called the Women's Health Effects Study.

Key Findings

- More than one third of these women experienced high disability pain as measured by the Chronic Pain Grade scale.

- Beyond the usual pain locations associated with abuse, 43.2% reported swollen/painful joints.

- More interference in daily life was attributed to joint pain than to back, head, stomach, pelvic, or bowel pain.

- Women with high disability pain were more likely to have experienced child abuse, adult sexual assault, more severe spousal abuse, lifetime abuse-related injuries, symptoms of depression and posttraumatic stress disorder, lifetime suicide attempts, difficulty sleeping, and unemployment.

- High disability pain also was associated with visits to a family doctor and psychiatrist and use of medication in more than prescribed dosages. Less than 25% of women with high disability pain were taking opioids, or prescription nonsteroidal anti-inflammatory medications.

- High disability pain was not related to smoking, use of street drugs, potential for alcohol dependence, age, income, or education.

(Research Examples and Critical Thinking Activities continues on page 106)

Research Examples and Critical Thinking Activities (continued)

CRITICAL THINKING SUGGESTIONS

1. Answer questions 2 to 5 and 8 from Box 6.1 (p. 104) regarding this study.
2. Also consider the following targeted questions, which may assist you in further assessing aspects of the study:
   a. Do you think the researchers could have presented the study aims as hypotheses? If so, what would they be?
   b. What clues does the summary give you that this study is quantitative?
   c. Develop a research question for a phenomenological or grounded theory study (or both) relating to the same general topic area as this study.
3. If the results of this study are valid and reliable, what are some of the uses to which the findings might be put into clinical practice?

EXAMPLE 2 ■ Qualitative Research

Aspects of a qualitative nursing study, featuring terms and concepts discussed in this chapter, are presented below, followed by some questions to guide critical thinking.

Study

"Learning from stories of people with chronic kidney disease" (Molzahn, Bruce, & Sheilds, 2008)

Research Problem

"As a result of advances in science and technology, many people with chronic kidney disease (CKD) live longer and healthier lives. Nevertheless, the outcomes of treatment are not certain and the experience of living in-between a promise of treatment and prolonged life and the threat of death is not well understood. The experience of what happens for people in this in-between or liminal space and the impact of this experience remains unexplored" (p. 13).

Statement of Purpose

The purpose of the study was to explore how people with CKD describe/story experiences of liminality associated with CKD and its treatment.

Research Objectives

The researchers identified three specific research objectives: (1) define liminal spaces, (2) relate the need for awareness of liminal spaces to nursing care, and (3) summarize the research findings regarding the stories of patients with CKD about their experience with living in and managing liminal spaces.

Method

A qualitative design [narrative inquiry] was used to study the liminal experiences of people with CKD. A constructionist perspective frames the study (Gergen, 2004) and is founded on a premise that individuals, groups, and cultures create understandings of realities and sustain these perspectives through the stories they tell (Gergen). Accepting that experience happens narratively (Clandinin & Connelly, 2000), stories are individuals' constructions and perceptions of events, and, as such, can be a window into how individuals understand and make sense of what is happening to them (Salkalys, 2003, p. 15).

Key Findings

The people relating the stories described a number of liminal spaces, including living/not living, independence/dependence, restrictions/freedom, normal/not normal, worse off/better off, and alone/connected. Awareness of the liminal spaces can help nurses provide care that addresses the complexity of CKD.

CRITICAL THINKING SUGGESTIONS

1. Answer questions 2 to 6 from Box 6.1 (p. 104) regarding this study.

2. Also consider the following targeted questions, which may assist you in further assessing aspects of the study:
   a. Where in the research report do you think the researchers placed the statement of purpose and research questions?
   b. What clues does the summary give you that this study is qualitative?
   c. Could the findings from this study be used to generate hypotheses?
3. If the results of this study are trustworthy, what are some of the uses to which the findings might be put into clinical practice?

EXAMPLE 3 ■ Quantitative Research

1. Read the abstract and the introduction from the study by Bryanton and colleagues found in Appendix A of this book, and then answer the relevant questions in Box 6.1 (p. 104).
2. Also consider the following targeted questions, which may further sharpen your critical thinking skills and assist you in assessing aspects of the study:
   a. Would you describe the hypotheses in this study as simple or complex?
   b. State the researchers' research hypotheses as null hypotheses.

EXAMPLE 4 ■ Qualitative Research

1. Read the abstract and the introduction from the study by Woodgate and colleagues found in Appendix B of this book, and then answer the relevant questions in Box 6.1 (p. 104).
2. Also consider the following targeted questions, which may further sharpen your critical thinking skills and assist you in assessing aspects of the study:
   a. Do you think that Woodgate and her colleagues provided sufficient rationale for the significance of their research problem?
   b. Do you think that Woodgate et al. needed to include research questions in their report, or was the purpose statement clear enough to stand alone?

Summary Points

⇒ **A research problem** is a perplexing or enigmatic situation that a researcher wants to address through disciplined inquiry. Sources of ideas for nursing research problems include clinical experience, relevant literature, social issues, and theory.

⇒ Researchers usually identify a broad topic or focus, then narrow the scope of the problem and identify questions consistent with a paradigm of choice.

⇒ A **statement of purpose** summarizes the overall goal of the study; in both qualitative and quantitative studies, the purpose statement identifies the key concepts (variables) and the study group or population.

⇒ A **research question** states the specific query the researcher wants to answer to address the research problem.

⇒ A **hypothesis** is a statement of a predicted relationship between two or more variables. A testable hypothesis states the anticipated association between one or more independent and one or more dependent variables.

⇒ A **directional hypothesis** specifies the expected direction or nature of a hypothesized relationship; **nondirectional hypotheses** predict a relationship but do not stipulate the form that the relationship will take.

⇒ **Research hypotheses** predict the existence of relationships; **null hypotheses** express the absence of any relationship.

⇒ Hypotheses are never proved nor disproved in an ultimate sense—they are accepted or rejected, supported or not supported by the data.

STUDIES CITED IN CHAPTER 6*

This reference list contains only those studies that were cited in this chapter. Citations pertaining to theoretical, methodologic, or nonempirical work are included together in a separate section at the end of the book (beginning on page 399).

Beck, C. T. (2008a). State of the science on postpartum depression: What nurse researchers have contributed—Part 1. *The American Journal of Maternal Child Nursing, 33*(2), 121–126.

Beck, C. T. (2008b). State of the science on postpartum depression: What nurse researchers have contributed—Part 2. *The American Journal of Maternal Child Nursing, 33*(3), 151–158.

Beck, C. T. (1992). The lived experience of postpartum depression: a phenomenological study. *Nursing Research, 41*(3), 166–70.

Beck, C. T. (1995). Perceptions of nurses' caring by mothers experiencing postpartum depression. *Journal of Obstetrical and Gynecological Neonatal Nursing, 24*(9), 819–25.

Beck, C. T. (2001). Predictors of postpartum depression: an update. *Nursing Research, 50*(5), 275–85.

Beck, C. T. (2006). Postpartum depression: it isn't just the blues. *American Journal of Nursing, 106*(5), 40–50.

Beck, C. T., & Gable, R. K. (2003). Postpartum depression screening scale: Spanish version. *Nursing Research, 52*(5), 296–306.

Black, C., & Ford-Gilboe, M. (2004). Adolescent mothers: resilience, family health work and health-promoting practices. *Journal of Advanced Nursing, 48*(4), 351–60.

Bluvol, A., & Ford-Gilboe, M. (2004). Hope, health work and quality of life in families of stroke survivors. *Journal of Advanced Nursing, 48*(4), 322–32.

Bucharski, D., Reutter, L. I., & Ogilvie, L. (2006). "You need to know where we're coming from": Canadian aboriginal women's perspectives on culturally appropriate HIV counseling and testing. *Health Care for Women International, 27*, 723–747.

Creswell, J. W. (1998). *Qualitative inquiry and research design: Choosing among five traditions.* Thousand Oaks, CA: Sage.

Estabrooks, C. A. (1998). Will evidence-based nursing practice make practice perfect? *Canadian Journal of Nursing Research, 30*(1), 15–36.

Estabrooks, C. A. (1999a). The conceptual structure of research utilization. *Research in Nursing & Health, 22*(3), 203–216.

Estabrooks, C. A. (1999b). Modeling the individual determinants of research utilization. *Western Journal of Nursing Research, 21*(6), 758–772.

Estabrooks, C. A., Chong, H., Brigidear, K., & Profetto-McGrath, J. (2005). Profiling Canadian nurses' preferred knowledge sources for clinical practice. *Canadian Journal of Nursing Research, 37*(2), 118–140.

Estabrooks, C. A., Midodzi, W. K., Cummings, G. G., & Wallin, L. (2007). Predicting research use in nursing organizations: A multilevel analysis. *Nursing Research, 56*(4, Suppl.), S7–S23.

Estabrooks, C. A., Rutakumwa, W., O'Leary, K. A., et al. (2005). Sources of practice knowledge among nurses. *Qualitative Health Research, 15*(4), 460–476.

Estabrooks, C. A., Scott, S., Squires, J. E., et al. (2008). Patterns of research utilization on patient care units. *Implementation Science, 3*, 31.

Fulford, A., & Ford-Gilboe, M. (2004). An exploration of the relationships between health promotion practices, health work, and felt stigma in families headed by adolescent mothers. *Canadian Journal of Nursing Research, 36*(4), 46–72.

Lincoln, Y. S., & Guba, E. G. (1985). *Naturalistic inquiry.* Newbury Park, CA: Sage.

Lobchuk, M. M., McClement, S. E., McPherson, C., & Cheang, M. (2008). Does blaming the patient with lung cancer affect the helping behavior of primary caregivers? *Oncology Nursing Forum, 35*(4), 681–689.

Loiselle, C. G., Semenic, S., & Côté, B. (2005). Sharing empirical knowledge to improve breast-feeding promotion and support: description of a research dissemination project. *Worldviews Evidence Based Nursing, 2*(1), 25–32.

Molzahn, A. E., Bruce, A., & Sheilds, L. (2008). Learning from stories of people with chronic kidney disease. *Nephrology Nursing Journal, 35*(1), 13–20.

Murrells, T., Robinson, S., & Griffiths, P. (2008). Is satisfaction a direct predictor of nursing turnover? Modelling the relationship between satisfaction, expressed intention and behaviour in a longitudinal cohort study. *Human Resources for Health, 6*(1), 22.

Spagrud, L. J., von Baeyer, C. L., Ali K., et al. (2008). Pain, distress, and adult-child interaction during venipuncture in pediatric oncology: an examination of three types of venous access. *Journal of Pain Symptom Management, 36*(2), 173–84.

Wilson, B., Squires, M., Widger, K., Cranley, L., & Tourangeau, A. (2008). Job satisfaction among a multigenerational nursing workforce. *Journal of Nursing Management, 16*(6), 716–723.

Woodgate, R. L., Ateah, C., & Secco, L. (2008). Living in a world of our own: The experience of parents who have a child with autism. *Qualitative Health Research, 18*(8), 1075–1083.

Wuest, J., Merritt-Gray, M., Ford-Gilboe, M., Lent, B., Varcoe, C., & Campbell, J. C. (2008). Chronic pain in women survivors of intimate partner violence. *The Journal of Pain, 9*(11), 1049–1057.

7 Finding and Reviewing Studies in the Literature

On completing this chapter, you will be able to:

1. Describe several purposes of a research literature review
2. Identify bibliographic aids for retrieving nursing research reports, and locate references for a research topic
3. Identify appropriate information to include in a research literature review
4. Understand the steps involved in writing a literature review
5. Evaluate the style, content, and organization of a traditional literature review
6. Define new terms in the chapter

PURPOSES AND USES OF LITERATURE REVIEWS

Literature reviews serve a number of important functions in the research process—and they also play a critical role for nurses seeking to develop an evidence-based practice. This chapter presents information on locating research reports, organizing and preparing a written review, and critiquing reviews prepared by others.

Researchers and Literature Reviews

For researchers, familiarity with relevant research literature can help in various ways, such as the following:

➢ Identifying a research problem and refining research questions or hypotheses
➢ Getting oriented to what is and is not known about a topic, to learn what research can best make a contribution
➢ Determining gaps or inconsistencies in a body of research
➢ Identifying relevant theoretical or conceptual frameworks (or suitable research methods) for a research problem
➢ Gaining insights for interpreting study findings and developing implications

Literature reviews can inspire new research ideas and help to lay the foundation for studies. A literature review is a crucial early task for most quantitative researchers. As previously noted, however, qualitative researchers have varying opinions about literature reviews, with some deliberately avoiding a literature search before entering the field. Some viewpoints are associated with qualitative research traditions. In grounded theory studies, researchers typically begin to collect data before examining the literature. As the data are analyzed and the grounded theory takes shape, researchers then turn to the literature, seeking to relate prior findings to the theory. Phenomenologists, by contrast, often undertake a search for relevant materials at the outset of a study. Although Ethnographers often do not perform a thorough up-front literature review, they often do review the literature to help shape their choice of a cultural problem before going into the field.

Researchers usually summarize relevant literature in the introduction to research reports, regardless of when they perform the literature search. The literature review provides readers with a background for understanding current knowledge on a topic and illuminates the significance of the new study. Written reviews thus serve an integrative function and facilitate the accumulation of evidence on a problem.

Nonresearchers and Literature Reviews

Research reviews are not prepared solely in the context of doing a study. Nursing students and nurses in a variety of roles also review and synthesize evidence on a topic. The specific purpose of the review varies depending on the reviewer's role. Here are a few examples:

❧ Acquiring knowledge on a topic

❧ Evaluating current practices and making recommendations for change

❧ Developing evidence-based clinical protocols and interventions to improve clinical practice

❧ Developing or revising nursing curricula

❧ Elaborating policy statements and practice guidelines

Thus, both consumers and producers of nursing research require skills for preparing and critiquing the literature on a particular topic.

LOCATING RELEVANT LITERATURE
FOR A RESEARCH REVIEW

The ability to identify and locate documents on a topic of research is an important skill. Such skill requires adaptability—rapid technologic changes, such as the expanding use of the Internet, are making manual methods of finding information obsolete and more sophisticated methods are periodically being introduced. We urge you to consult with medical librarians at your institution for updated guidance.

TIP

Locating all relevant information on a research question is like being a detective. The various electronic and print literature retrieval tools are a tremendous aid, but there inevitably needs to be some digging for, and a lot of sifting and sorting of knowledge on a topic. Be prepared for sleuthing!

You may be tempted to perform a literature search through an Internet search engine, such as Yahoo or Google. This search might yield a lot of information, such as summaries for lay persons, press releases, connections to advocacy groups, and so forth. These quick Internet searches, however, are unlikely to give you comprehensive bibliographic information on the *research* literature on your topic—and you might become frustrated with searching through the vast number of informational sources now available.

Electronic Literature Searches

Almost all university libraries offer the tools to perform one's own searches of **electronic databases.** These databases can be accessed either through an **online search** (i.e., by directly communicating with a host computer over the Internet) or by CD-ROM (compact discs that store the bibliographic information). Their programs are user-friendly—they are menu driven with on-screen support, and retrieval usually can proceed with minimal instruction.

Major electronic databases that contain references on nursing studies include the following:

≋ CINAHL (**C**umulative **I**ndex to **N**ursing and **A**llied **H**ealth **L**iterature)

≋ MEDLINE (**Med**ical Literature On-**Line**)

≋ Cochrane Database

≋ EMBASE (the **E**xcerpta **M**edica data**base**)

≋ PsycINFO (**Psyc**hology **Info**rmation)

Most nursing faculty/school libraries subscribe to CINAHL, one of the most useful databases for nurses. The **CINAHL database** (*http://www.cinahl.com/*) is described more fully in the next section. The MEDLINE database, perhaps the second most important database for nurse researchers, can be accessed free of charge through PubMed (*http://www.ncbi.nlm.nih.gov/PubMed*).

Several other types of electronic resources should be mentioned. First, books and other holdings of libraries can almost always be scanned electronically using *online catalogue systems*, and the catalogue holdings of libraries across the country can be reviewed over the Internet. Second, it may be useful to search through Sigma Theta Tau International's Registry of Nursing Research on the Internet at *http://www.stti.iupui.edu/VirginiaHendersonLibrary/*. This registry is an electronic research database with more than 12,000 studies that can be searched by key words, variables, and researchers' names. The registry provides access to studies that have not yet been published. Electronic publishing is expanding at a rapid pace and medical librarians should be consulted for the latest updates.

TIP

It is rarely possible to identify all relevant studies exclusively through literature retrieval mechanisms. An excellent method of identifying additional references is to find recently published studies and examine their reference list. Researchers usually cite relevant and recent studies to provide context for their own work.

The CINAHL Database

This section illustrates some of the features of an electronic search, through the use of the CINAHL database. Our illustrated example relied on the online Ovid Search, but similar features are available through other software programs.

The CINAHL database covers references to more than 1200 English- and foreign-language nursing journals, as well as to books, dissertations, and selected conference proceedings in nursing and allied health fields. The database covers materials dating from 1982 to the present and has about 1 million records. In addition to providing bibliographic information (i.e., the author, title, journal, year of publication, volume, and page numbers of a reference), abstracts are available for almost 1000 journals.

Most searches are likely to begin with a **subject search**—a search for references relating to a specific topic. For this type of search, you would type in a word or phrase that captures the essence of the topic. Fortunately, through *mapping* capabilities, most retrieval software translates (maps) the topic you type into the most plausible CINAHL subject heading. An important alternative to a subject search is a **textword search** that looks for your specific words in text fields of each record, including the title and the abstract. (If you know the name of a researcher who has worked on a specific research topic, an **author search** might be productive.)

TIP

If you want to identify all major research reports on a topic, you need to be flexible and to think broadly about the key words and subject headings that could be related to your topic. For example, if you are interested in anorexia nervosa, you should search for anorexia, eating disorders, and weight loss, and perhaps appetite, eating behaviour, nutrition, bulimia, body weight changes, and body image.

After you have typed in your topic, the computer will tell you how many "hits" there are in the database (i.e., matches against your topic). In most cases, the number of hits initially will be large, and you will want to constrain the search to ensure that you retrieve only the most relevant references. You can limit your search in a number of ways. For example, you might want only references published in nursing journals, only those that are for studies, only those published in certain years (e.g., 2000 or later), or only those with participants in certain age groups (e.g., infants).

To illustrate with a concrete example, suppose we were interested in recent research on postoperative pain, which is the term we enter in a subject search. Here is an example of how many hits we could obtain on successive restrictions to the search for studies on therapies for postoperative pain, using the CINAHL database:

Search Topic/Restriction	*Hits*
Postoperative pain	2164
Restrict to therapy subheadings	1249
Limit to research reports with abstracts in English-language journals	391
Limit to core nursing journals	107
Limit to 2000 to 2004 publications	43

This narrowing of the search—from 2164 initial references on postoperative pain to 43 references for recent nursing research reports on postoperative pain therapies—took less than a minute to perform. Next, we would display the 43 references on the monitor, and we could then print full bibliographic information for the ones that appeared especially promising. An example of an abridged CINAHL record entry for a study identified through this search on postoperative pain is presented in Figure 7.1, a study by Forchuk and colleagues. The entry shows an accession number—the unique identifier for each record in the database—that can be used to order the full text of the report. The authors, their contact information, and the title of the study are then displayed, followed by source information. The source indicates the following:

Name of the journal (*Cancer Nursing*)
Volume (27)
Issue (1)

Accession Number
2004052949

Authors
Forchuk C, Baruth P, Prendergast M, Holliday R, Bareham R, Brimner S, Schulz V, Chan YCI, Yammine N.

Institution
University of Western Ontario; *cforchuk@uwo.ca*

Title
Postoperative arm massage: A support for women with lymph node dissection

Source
Cancer Nursing, *27*(1):25–33, 2004 Jan–Feb, (34 ref.)

CINAHL Subject Headings

Adult	Health Care Costs / ev [Evaluation]
Aged	Health Services / ut [Utilization]
Arm Circumference / ev [Evaluation]	Interrater Reliability
*Breast Neoplasms / su [Surgery]	Interviews
Cancer Patients	*Lymph Node Excision
Checklists	Lymphedema
Clinical Assessment Tools	*Massage
Clinical Trials	Middle Age
Coefficient Alpha	Pain Measurement
Convenience Sample	*Postoperative Care
Descriptive Statistics	*Postoperative Pain / th [Therapy]
Family Relations	Purposive Sample
Female	Range of Motion / ev [Evaluation]
Functional Assessment	Significant Other
	Stress Psychological / ev [Evaluation]
	T-Tests

Instrumentation
Shoulder Pain and Disability Index (SPADI)

Abstract
Purpose/objective: To evaluate the usefulness of arm massage from a significant other following lymph node dissection surgery. **Design:** Randomized clinical trial with a pretest-posttest design. Data were collected before surgery, within 24 hours after surgery, within 10 to 14 days post surgery, and 4 months after surgery. **Sample:** 59 women aged 21 to 78 years undergoing lymph node dissection surgery who had a significant other with them during the postoperative period. **Methods:** Subjects were randomly assigned to intervention and control groups. Subjects' significant others in the intervention group were first taught, then performed arm massage as a postoperative support measure. **Research main variables:** Variables included postoperative pain, family strengths and stressors, range of motion, and health related costs. **Findings:** Participants reported a reduction in pain in the immediate postoperative period and better shoulder function. **Conclusion:** Arm massage decreased pain and discomfort related to surgery, and promoted a sense of closeness and support amongst subjects and their significant other. **Implication for nursing practice:** Postoperative message therapy for women with lymph node dissection provided therapeutic benefits for patients and their significant other. Nurses can offer effective alternative interventions along with standard procedures in promoting optimal health.

ISSN
0162-220X

Language
English

FIGURE 7.1 Example of a printout from a CINAHL search.

Page numbers (25–33)
Year and month of publication (2004, Jan–Feb)
Number of cited references (34 ref.)

The printout shows all the CINAHL subject headings for this entry, any one of which could have been used to retrieve this reference through a subject search. Note that the subject headings include substantive topics (e.g., breast neoplasms, postoperative pain), methodologic topics (e.g., descriptive statistics, interviews), and headings relating to the group under study (e.g., female). Next, any formal instruments used in the study are noted under Instrumentation; in this case, the Shoulder Pain and Disability Index, or SPADI, is cited. Then the study abstract is presented. Based on the abstract, you would decide whether this study was pertinent to your literature review; if so, the full research report could be obtained. Reports in the CINAHL database can be ordered by mail or fax; therefore, it is not necessary for your library to subscribe to the referenced journal. Moreover, many of the retrieval service providers, such as Ovid, offer *full-text* online services, which would enable you to download documents from certain journals.

TIP

If your topic includes independent and dependent variables, you may need to do searches for each. For example, if you are interested in learning about the effect of stress on the health beliefs among individuals with acquired immunodeficiency syndrome (AIDS), you might want to read about the effects of stress (in general) and about people's health beliefs (in general). Moreover, you might also want to learn something about patients with AIDS and their problems. If you are searching for references electronically, you can combine searches, so that the references for two independent searches can be linked (e.g., the computer can identify those references that have both stress and health beliefs as subject headings or textwords).

Example of a literature search

Bourbonnais and Ducharme (2008) published a literature review on the act of screaming among elderly persons with dementia, including factors contributing to screaming and related interventions. They conducted computerized searches of the MEDLINE, CINAHL, EMBASE, PsycINFO, and Biological Abstracts databases, using the following key words: scream, screaming, vocally disruptive, disruptive behaviour, agitation, and vocalization alone or combined with dementia and/or intervention.

PREPARING WRITTEN REVIEWS OF RESEARCH EVIDENCE

Identifying references, using the guidelines and tools described in the previous section, is an early step in preparing a written review of research literature. Subsequent steps are summarized in Figure 7.2.

Retrieving and Screening References

As Figure 7.2 shows, after identifying promising references, you need to retrieve the full reports. In addition to obtaining reports through your library or through CINAHL, or other electronic databases, many nursing journals (e.g., *CJNR*) are now available online.

The next step is to screen reports for relevance and appropriateness. The report's *relevance*, which concerns whether it really focuses on the topic of interest, usually can be judged quickly by reading the introduction. *Appropriateness* concerns the nature of the information in the report. The most important information for a research review comes from reports that describe study findings. You should rely primarily on **primary source** research reports, which are descriptions of studies written by the researchers who conducted them. **Secondary source** research articles are descriptions of studies prepared by someone other than the original researcher, e.g., literature review articles. Recent review articles are a good place to begin a literature search because they

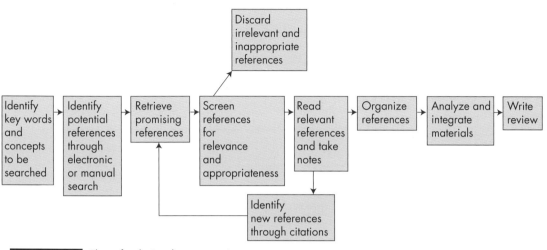

Flow of tasks in a literature review.

summarize current knowledge, and the reference lists are helpful. However, secondary descriptions of studies should not be considered substitutes for primary sources.

Examples of primary and secondary sources on breast cancer
Primary source—an original study based on data from 515 registered nurses working in oncology settings across Canada that developed and tested a model of work environment factors affecting oncology nurses' job satisfaction (Cummings et al., 2008).
   Secondary source—a review of articles on stress among individuals diagnosed with lung cancer (Hansen & Sawatzky, 2008).

For some literature reviews, it may be important to find references from the conceptual literature (i.e., references on a theory or conceptual model). In the conceptual literature, a primary source is a description of a theory written by the theory's developer, and a secondary source is a discussion or critique of the theory.

In addition to empirical and conceptual references, you may encounter various nonresearch references, including opinion articles, case reports, anecdotes, and clinical descriptions. Such materials may serve to broaden understanding of a research problem, demonstrate a need for research, or describe aspects of clinical practice. They may thus play important roles in formulating research ideas, but they have limited utility in written research reviews because they do not address the central question: What is the current state of *knowledge* on this problem?

Abstracting and Recording Notes

Once you judge a reference to be relevant and appropriate, you should read the entire report carefully and critically, using guidelines that are provided throughout this book. It is useful to work with photocopied articles, so that you can highlight or underline critical information. Even with a copied article, we recommend taking notes or writing a summary of the study's strengths and limitations. A formal protocol, such as the one presented in Figure 7.3, is sometimes helpful for recording information in a systematic fashion. Although many of the terms on this protocol are probably not familiar to you at this point, you will learn their meaning as you progress through this book.

Citation: Authors: _____
Title: _____
Journal: _____
Year: _____ Volume: _____ Issue: _____ Pages: _____

Type of Study: ☐ Quantitative ☐ Qualitative ☐ Both

Location/setting: _____

Key Concepts/ Concepts: _____
Variables: Intervention/Independent Variable: _____
Dependent Variable: _____
Controlled Variables: _____

Design Type: ☐ Experimental ☐ Quasi-experimental ☐ Preexperimental ☐ Nonexperimental
Specific Design: _____
Descrip. of Intervention: _____
_____

☐ Longitudinal/prospective ☐ Cross-sectional No. of data collection points: _____
Comparison group(s): _____

Qual. Tradition: ☐ Grounded theory ☐ Phenomenology ☐ Ethnography ☐ Other: _____

Sample: Size: _____ Sampling method: _____
Sample characteristics: _____

Data Sources: Type: ☐ Self-report ☐ Observational ☐ Biophysiologic ☐ Other: _____
Description of measures: _____
Data Quality: _____

Statistical Tests: Bivariate: ☐ *t* test ☐ ANOVA ☐ Chi-square ☐ Pearson's *r* ☐ Other: _____
Multivariate: ☐ Multiple regression ☐ MANOVA ☐ ANCOVA ☐ Other: _____

Findings: _____
_____
_____

Recommendations: _____
_____

Strengths: _____
_____

Weaknesses: _____
_____

FIGURE 7.3 Example of a literature review protocol.

Organizing the Evidence

Organization is crucial in preparing a written review. When literature on a topic is extensive, it is useful to summarize information in a table. The table could include columns with headings such as Author, Sample, Design, Data Collection Approach, and Key Findings. Such a table provides a quick overview that allows you to make sense of a mass of information.

Example of tabular organization

Neufeld and Newburn-Cook (2008) reviewed the literature relating to the risk factors for postoperative nausea and vomiting following neurosurgical procedures. Their review included several tables that summarized research related to this topic. For example, their first table summarized 13 studies, and the column headings were: Location of Study, Target Population, Study Design, Sample Size, Length of Study, Inclusion Criteria, and Exclusion Criteria.

Most writers find it helpful to work from an outline—a written one if the review is lengthy and complex or a mental one for short reviews. The important point is to work out a structure before starting to write so that the review has a meaningful flow. Although the specifics of the organization differ from topic to topic, the overall goal is to structure the review in such a way that the presentation is logical, demonstrates meaningful integration, and leads to a conclusion of what is known and not known about the topic.

After the organization of topics has been determined, you should review your notes or protocols. This not only helps refresh your memory about material read earlier but also lays the groundwork for decisions about where a particular reference fits in the outline. If certain references do not seem to fit anywhere, they may need to be put aside; remember that the number of references is less important than their relevance and the overall organization of the review.

TIP

An important principle in organizing a review is to figure out a way to cluster and compare studies. For example, you could contrast studies that have similar findings with studies that have conflicting or inconclusive findings, making sure to analyze why discrepancies may have occurred. Other reviews might have sample characteristics as an organizing scheme if findings vary according to such characteristics (e.g., if results differ for male and female participants). Doing a research review is a bit like doing a qualitative study—you must search for important *themes* in the findings.

Writing a Literature Review

Research reviews tend to be written in a particular style and typically include specific types of information.

Content of a Research Review

A written research review should provide a thorough, objective summary of the current state of evidence on a topic. A literature review should be neither a series of quotes nor a series of abstracts. The key tasks are to summarize and evaluate the evidence so as to reveal the state-of-the-art of knowledge of a topic—not simply to describe what researchers have done. The review should point out both consistencies and contradictions in the literature and offer possible explanations for inconsistencies (e.g., different conceptualizations or data collection methods).

Although important studies should be described in some detail, it is not necessary to provide extensive coverage for every reference. Reports with similar findings sometimes can be summarized together.

The literature should be summarized in your own words. The review should demonstrate that consideration has been given to the cumulative significance of the body of research. Stringing together quotes from various documents fails to show that previous research on the topic has been assimilated and understood.

Reviews should be as objective as possible. Studies that conflict with personal values or hunches should not be omitted. Also, the review should not deliberately ignore a study because its findings contradict other studies. Inconsistent results should be analyzed and the supporting evidence evaluated objectively.

The literature review should conclude with a critical summary that recaps key study findings and indicates how credible they are; it should also make note of gaps in the research. The summary thus requires critical judgment about the extensiveness and dependability of evidence on a topic.

As you progress through this book, you will become increasingly proficient in critically evaluating research reports. We hope you will understand the mechanics of writing a research review when you have completed this chapter, but we do not expect that you will be in a position to write a state-of-the-art review until you have acquired more research method skills.

Style of a Research Review

Students preparing their first written research review often have trouble adjusting to the standard style of research reviews. One issue is that students sometimes accept research results without criticism or reservation, reflecting a common misunderstanding about the conclusiveness of research. You should keep in mind that no hypothesis or theory can be proved or disproved by empirical testing, and no research question can be definitely answered in a single study. The problem is partly a semantic one: hypotheses are not proved, they are supported by research findings; theories are not verified, but they may be tentatively accepted if a substantial body of evidence demonstrates their legitimacy. When describing study findings, you should generally use phrases indicating tentativeness of the results, such as the following:

➤ Several studies have *found* . . .

➤ Findings thus far *suggest* . . .

➤ Results from a landmark study *indicated* . . .

➤ The data *supported* the hypothesis . . .

➤ There *appears* to be strong evidence that . . .

A related stylistic problem among novice reviewers is an inclination to intersperse opinions (their own or someone else's) into the review. The review should include opinions sparingly and should be explicit about their source. Your own opinions do not belong in a review, except for assessments of study quality.

The left-hand column of Table 7.1 presents examples of stylistic flaws. The right-hand column offers recommendations for rewording the sentences to conform to a more acceptable form for a research literature review. Many alternative wordings are possible.

Length of a Research Review

There are no formulas for how long a review should be. The length depends on several factors, including the complexity of the research question, the extent of prior

TABLE 7.1 ▶ EXAMPLES OF STYLISTIC DIFFICULTIES FOR RESEARCH REVIEWS

INAPPROPRIATE STYLE OR WORDING	RECOMMENDED CHANGE
1. It is known that unmet expectations engender stress.	Dr. A. Cassard, an expert on stress and anxiety, has found that unmet expectations engender stress (Cassard, 2008).
2. Women who do not participate in childbirth preparation classes tend to manifest a high degree of stress during labour.	Studies have found that women who participate in preparation for childbirth classes manifest less stress during labour than those who do not (Klotz, 2003; McTygue, 2008; Weller, 2004).
3. Studies have proved that doctors and nurses do not fully understand the psychobiologic dynamics of recovery from a myocardial infarction.	Studies by Lowe (2009) and Martin (2003) suggest that doctors and nurses do not fully understand the psychobiologic dynamics of recovery from a myocardial infarction.
4. Attitudes cannot be changed quickly.	Attitudes have been found to be relatively enduring attributes that cannot be changed quickly (Casey, 2009; Geair, 2008).

NOTE: All references in this table are fictitious.

research, and the purpose for which the review is being prepared. Literature reviews prepared for proposals (e.g., proposals to undertake a study or to test a clinical innovation) tend to be fairly comprehensive. Reviews in theses and dissertations are also lengthy. In these cases, the literature review serves both to summarize knowledge and to document the reviewer's capability.

Because of space limitations in journal articles, literature reviews that appear within research reports are concise. Literature reviews in the introduction to research reports demonstrate the need for the new study and provide a context for the research questions. The literature review sections of qualitative reports tend to be especially brief. However, there are stand-alone research reviews in nursing journals that are more extensive than those appearing in the introductions of research reports. We discuss such reviews next.

READING AND USING EXISTING RESEARCH REVIEWS

Most of this chapter provides guidance on how to conduct a literature review—how to locate and screen references, what type of information to seek, and how to organize and write a review. However, practicing nurses may not need to perform a full-fledged review if a comprehensive and recent literature review on the topic of interest has been published. Several different types of *integrative reviews* that can be used to support evidence-based nursing practice are briefly described in this section. Further information about conducting and critiquing integrative reviews is provided in Chapter 18.

Traditional Narrative Reviews

A traditional narrative literature review synthesizes and summarizes, in a narrative fashion, a body of research literature. The information offered in this chapter has been designed to help you prepare such a review.

Narrative integrative reviews are frequently published in nursing journals, especially in nursing specialty journals. These reviews may have a number of different purposes, including providing practitioners with state-of-the-art research-based information; providing a foundation for the development of innovations for clinical practice; and developing an agenda for further research.

Meta-Analysis

Meta-analysis is a technique for integrating quantitative research findings statistically. Meta-analysis treats the findings from a study as one piece of datum. The findings from multiple studies on the same topic are then combined to create a data set that can be analyzed in a manner similar to that obtained from individual studies. Thus, instead of study participants being the **unit of analysis** (the most basic entity on which the analysis focuses), individual studies are the unit of analysis in a meta-analysis. Typically, the meta-analyst takes information about the strength of the relationship between the independent and dependent variables from each study, quantifies that information, and then essentially takes an average across all studies.

Traditional narrative research reviews have some shortcomings that make meta-analyses appealing. For example, if there are many studies and results are inconsistent, it may be difficult to draw conclusions in a narrative review. Furthermore, integration in narrative reviews can be subject to reviewer biases. Another advantage of meta-analysis is that it can take into account the quality of the studies being combined. Meta-analysis provides a convenient and objective method of integrating a large body of findings and of observing patterns and relationships that might otherwise have gone undetected. Meta-analysis can thus serve as an important tool in evidence-based practice. Because of this fact, we discuss meta-analyses at greater length in the final chapter.

Qualitative Metasynthesis

A qualitative **metasynthesis** involves integrating qualitative research findings on a specific topic that are themselves interpretive syntheses of data (Sandelowski & Barroso, 2003). A metasynthesis is more than just a summary of findings—it involves interpretation of those findings, and this is where a metasynthesis differs from a meta-analysis. A metasynthesis is less about reducing data and more about amplifying and interpreting data. Sandelowski, Docherty, and Emden (1997) warn researchers that qualitative metasynthesis is a complex process that involves "carefully peeling away the surface layers of studies to find their hearts and souls in a way that does the least damage to them" (p. 370).

Various methods have been used to synthesize qualitative findings, but to date, no firm guidelines exist.

Example of a qualitative metasynthesis
Howard, Balneaves, and Bottorff (2007) conducted a metasynthesis of studies of the experience of breast cancer among women from diverse ethnocultural groups. Their metasynthesis used findings from a book and 14 published qualitative studies from the nursing, allied health, psychology, and medical literature from 1994 and 2005. The studies focused on women from four ethnocultural groups: Asian American, African American, Hispanic, and Aboriginal women. Five major themes emerged from their analysis: (1) the "othered" experience of a breast cancer diagnosis, (2) the treatment experience as "other," (3) losses associated with breast cancer, (4) the family context of breast cancer experience, and (5) coping with breast cancer through spirituality and community involvement.

Critiquing Research Reviews

Some nurses never prepare a written research review, and perhaps you will never be required to do one. Most nurses, however, do *read* research reviews (including the literature review sections of research reports), and should be prepared to evaluate such reviews critically. You may find it difficult to critique a research review because you are probably a lot less familiar with the topic than the writer. You may thus not be able to judge whether the author has included all relevant literature and has adequately summarized knowledge on that topic. Many aspects of a research review, however, are amenable to evaluation by readers who are not experts on the topic. Some suggestions for critiquing written research reviews are presented in Box 7.1. Additionally, when a literature review—whether it be a traditional review, a meta-analysis, or a metasynthesis—is published as a stand-alone article, it should include information that will help you understand its scope and evaluate its thoroughness. This is discussed in more detail in Chapter 18.

In assessing a written literature review, the overarching question is whether the review adequately summarizes the current state of research evidence. If the review is written as part of an original research report, an equally important question is whether the review lays a solid foundation for the new study.

BOX 7.1 GUIDELINES FOR CRITIQUING LITERATURE REVIEWS
▶

1. Does the review seem thorough—does it include all or most of the major studies on the topic? Does it include recent research? Are studies from other related disciplines included, if appropriate?

2. Does the review rely on appropriate materials (e.g., mainly on research reports, using primary sources)?

3. Is the review merely a summary of existing work, or does it critically appraise and compare key studies? Does the review identify important gaps in the literature?

4. Is the review well organized? Is the development of ideas clear?

5. Does the review use appropriate language, suggesting the tentativeness of prior findings? Is the review objective? Does the author paraphrase, or is there an overreliance on quotes from original sources?

6. If the review is part of a research report for a new study, does the review support the need for the study? If it is a critical integrative review designed to summarize evidence for clinical practice, does the review draw appropriate conclusions about practice implications?

EXAMPLE 1 ■ Quantitative Research

Aspects of a quantitative nursing study, featuring terms and concepts discussed in this chapter, are presented below, followed by some questions to guide critical thinking.

Study

"The effects and expense of augmenting usual care cancer clinic care with telephone problem-solving counselling" (Downe-Wamboldt et al., 2007)

Statement of Purpose

The purpose of the study was to determine the effect of a series of individualized, telephone-based problem-solving counselling sessions provided by a nurse during a 3-month interval on the onset of depression among individuals diagnosed with breast, lung, or prostate cancer. In addition, the researchers were interested in determining for whom the intervention was most acceptable, effective, and efficient.

Method

One hundred and seventy-five individuals diagnosed with breast, lung, or prostate cancer were randomly assigned to one of two groups: the intervention group (received the telephone-based counselling) or the usual care group (did not receive the intervention). Coping skills, depression, and adjustment were measured at baseline, prior to randomization, and 8 months later.

Literature Review From the Report (Excerpt)

"Reviews (Anderson, 1992; Bottomley, 1997) and meta-analyses (Devine & Westlake, 1995; Meyer & Mark, 1995; Sheard & Maguire, 1999) support the value of psychosocial intervention to enhance the quality of life of cancer patients. Some meta-analyses have distinguished the moderate effect of preventive psychosocial interventions compared with those for clinically depressed persons (Sheard & Maguire, 1999).

Individualized problem-solving therapy (counselling) is a cognitive-behavioral psychosocial intervention aimed at developing social competence, learned resourcefulness, and problem-solving skill in coping with everyday stresses and problems (Book, Dooley, & Catalano, 1991; D'Zurilla, 1986; Meichenbaum, 1985; Rosenbaum, 1990; Wasik, Bryant, & Lyons, 1990). This type of intervention has been shown to be effective and efficient with patients with chronic illness who are not adjusting well, live alone, and have ineffective coping methods whether offered in person (Roberts, Browne, & Streiner, 1995) or over the telephone (Hoxby, Roberts, Browne, Pallister, Gafni, & Streiner, 1997). It has not been tested over the telephone as a prevention treatment for persons not depressed nor poorly adjusted and recently beginning treatment of cancer (Gotay & Bottomley, 1998).

The first randomized trial of telephone support and/or problem-solving appeared in 1985 (Frasure-Smith & Prince, 1985). The effect of telephone support on the uptake of routine screening practices was not included in this analysis (Luckmann, Savageau, Clemow, Stoddard, & Costanza, 2003; Vogt, Glass, Glasgow, La Chance, & Lichtenstein, 2003). Specialized nurses, social workers, or trained lay personnel provided the telephone intervention for a variety of purposes and for various lengths of time. Only one (Roberts, Browne, & Streiner, 1995) of these nine trials (Evans, Halar, & Smith, 1985; Frasure-Smith & Prince, 1985; Roberts, Browne, & Streiner, 1995; Frasure-Smith & Prince, 1989; Hagopian & Rubenstein, 1990; Heller, Thompson, Tureba, Hogg, & Vlachos-Weber, 1991; Howelss, Wilson, Skinner, Newton, Morris, & Greene, 2002; Infante-Rivard, Krieger, Petitclerc, & Baumgarten, 1988; Parkerson, Michener, Wu, et al., 1989; Rene, Weinberg, Mazzuca, Brandt, & Katz, 1992; Wasson, Gaudette, Whaley, Sauvigne, Baribeau, & Welch, 1992; Weinberg, Tierney, Booher, & Katz, 1989; Weinberg, Tierney, Booher, & Katz, 1991; Kim & Oh, 2003) met the criteria for the highest level of quality evidence such as the rigor of concealed randomization (Guyatt & Rennie,

2002). It supports the value of the telephone on improved outcomes for distressed or at risk chronically ill patients at no further expenditures from a societal perspective for use of all health and social services including telephone intervention" (pp. 441–442).

Key Findings

■ The participants in the intervention group demonstrated, after 8 months, a maintenance of confrontive, optimistic, and supportant coping, and improvement in self-reliant coping. Whereas the participants in the control group exhibited a significant decline in the use of confrontive, optimism, and supportant coping.

■ Although not statistically significant, the intervention prevented a clinically important increase in the mean level of depressive symptoms.

■ There were no statistically significant group differences with respect to adjustment.

CRITICAL THINKING SUGGESTIONS

1. Answer the questions from Box 7.1 (p. 121) regarding this study.
2. Also consider the following targeted questions, which may assist you in further assessing aspects of the study:
   a. What was the independent variable in this study? Did the literature review cover findings from prior studies about this variable?
   b. What were the dependent variables in this study? Did the literature review cover findings from prior studies about these variables and their relationships with the independent variable?
   c. In performing the literature review, what key words might Downe-Wamboldt and colleagues have used to search for prior studies?
   d. Using the key words, perform a computerized search to see if you can find recent relevant studies to add to the literature review.
3. If the results of this study are valid and reliable, how can they be transferred to clinical practice?

EXAMPLE 2 ■ Qualitative Research

Aspects of a qualitative nursing study, featuring terms and concepts discussed in this chapter, are presented below, followed by some questions to guide critical thinking.

Study

"Factors influencing family caregivers' ability to cope with providing end-of-life cancer care at home" (Stajduhar, Martin, Barwich, & Fyles, 2008)

Statement of Purpose

The purpose of this qualitative study was to describe factors related to family caregivers' ability to cope with providing end-of-life cancer care at home.

Method

Data were collected as part of a larger ongoing mixed-method, multisite study examining family caregiver coping in end-of-life cancer care. The study involved in-depth interviews with 29 family members between 40 and 85 years of age providing care to a loved one diagnosed with advanced cancer for whom the primary goal of treatment was palliative and had a life expectancy of 6 months or less. Purposive sampling was used to obtain the sample for the study.

Literature Review From the Report (Excerpt, here references to relevant articles are in the form of numbers corresponding to each reference entry)

"One consistently reported predictor of having a dying person be cared for at home is the availability of a family caregiver.[8,9] Family caregivers are typically responsible for providing

(Research Examples and Critical Thinking Activities continues on page 124)

Research Examples and Critical Thinking Activities (continued)

most of the physical and emotional care of the patient, for managing complex symptoms in the home, and for organizing and coordinating health services on behalf of the dying person.[10,11] Often referred to as the 'hidden patients,'[12] family caregivers are expected to take on more and more of the care that was one provided by nurses in the home,[13] sometimes feeling pressured to do so[14] and ambivalent about it.[15]

It is well established that caregiving places considerable burdens on family caregivers.[16–18] A recent review of literature highlighted the nature and extent of physical and psychosocial morbidity and economic disadvantage that home-based palliative caregivers experience as a direct result of their caregiving role.[19] Many caregivers experience moderate to severe sleep problems.[20] (…) The economic cost associated with home-based care are also substantial. (…) In Canada, estimates suggest that family caregivers contribute about Can $6,000 of unpaid caregiving labor in the final 4 weeks of a patient's life.[26] (…)

As more and more the responsibility for care of the dying is placed on family caregivers, there is growing concern about their ability to cope with the demands of caregiving.[27,28] Some research has examined the strategies that family caregivers of patients with cancer use to cope with such demands. (…) Although these studies provide an understanding of the coping strategies used, only 1 was found that focused specifically on factors that influence caregivers' ability to cope with providing end-of-life cancer at home."

Key Findings

The findings suggest five factors that influenced the caregivers' ability to cope: (1) the caregivers' approach to life, (2) the patient's illness experience, (3) the patient's recognition of the caregivers' contribution to his or her care, (4) the quality of the relationship between the caregiver and the dying person, and (5) the caregiver's sense of security.

CRITICAL THINKING SUGGESTIONS

1. Answer the questions from Box 7.1 (p. 121) regarding this study.

2. Also consider the following targeted questions, which may assist you in further assessing aspects of the study:
   a. What was the central phenomenon that the researchers focused on in this study? Was that phenomenon adequately covered in the literature review?
   b. In performing the literature review, what key words might the researchers have used to search for prior studies?
   c. Using the key words, perform a computerized search to see if you can find a recent relevant study to add to the review.

3. If the findings of this study are trustworthy, what are some of the clinical uses pertaining to the findings?

EXAMPLE 3 ■ Quantitative Research

1. Read the introduction from the study by Bryanton and colleagues (2008) in Appendix A of this book and then answer the questions in Box 7.1 (p. 121).

2. Also consider the following targeted questions, which may further sharpen your critical thinking skills and assist you in assessing aspects of the study:
   a. What were the independent variables and the dependent variables in this study? Did the literature review cover findings from prior studies about these variables and their interrelationships?
   b. In performing the literature review, what key words might have been used to search for prior studies?
   c. Using the key words, perform a computerized search to see if you can find a recent relevant study to augment the review.

EXAMPLE 4 ■ Qualitative Research

1. Read the abstract and the introduction to Woodgate's study (Woodgate, Ateah, & Secco, 2008) in Appendix B of this book and then answer the relevant questions in Box 7.1 (p. 121).

2. Also consider the following targeted questions, which may further sharpen your critical thinking skills and assist you in assessing aspects of the study:

   a. What was the central phenomenon that Woodgate focused on in this study? Was that phenomenon adequately covered in the literature review?

   b. In what sections of the report did Woodgate discuss prior research?

   c. In performing their literature review, what key words might Woodgate et al. have used to search for prior studies?

   d. Using the key words, perform a computerized search to see if you can find a recent relevant study to add to the review.

Summary Points

⟫ A research **literature review** is a written summary of the state of knowledge on a research problem.

⟫ Researchers undertake literature reviews to determine knowledge on a topic of interest, to provide a context for a study, and to justify the need for a study; consumers review and synthesize evidence-based information to gain knowledge and improve nursing practice.

⟫ **Electronic databases,** which are important tools for locating references, usually can be accessed through an **online search** or by way of CD-ROM. For nurses, the **CINAHL database** is especially useful.

⟫ Most database searches begin with a **subject search,** but a **textword search** and an **author search** are other possibilities.

⟫ In writing a research review, reviewers should carefully organize the relevant materials, which should consist primarily of **primary source** research reports.

⟫ The role of reviewers is to point out what has been studied to date, how adequate and dependable those studies are, and what gaps exist in the body of research.

⟫ Nurses need to have skills in using and critiquing research reviews prepared by others, including traditional narrative reviews, **meta-analyses** (the integration of study findings using statistical procedures), and qualitative **metasyntheses** (integrations of qualitative research findings that produce new interpretations.)

STUDIES CITED IN CHAPTER 7*

This reference list contains only those studies that were cited in this chapter. Citations pertaining to theoretical, methodologic, or nonempirical work are included together in a separate section at the end of the book (beginning on page 399).

Bourbonnais, A., & Ducharme, F. (2008). Screaming in elderly persons with dementia: A critical review of the literature. *Dementia*, 7(2), 205–225.

Boyles, C. M., Bailey, P. H., & Mossey, S. (2008). Representations of disability in nursing and healthcare literature: An integrative review. *Journal of Advanced Nursing*, 62(4), 428–437.

Bryanton, J., Gagnon, A. J., Hatem, M., & Johnston, C. (2008). Predictors of early parenting self-efficacy: Results of a prospective cohort study. *Nursing Research*, 57(4), 252–259.

Cummings, G. G., Olson, K., Hayduk, L., et al. (2008). The relationship between nursing leadership and nurses' job satisfaction in Canadian oncology work environments. *Journal of Nursing Management, 16*(5), 508–518.

Dennis, C., & Kingston, D. (2008). A systematic review of telephone support for women during pregnancy and the early postpartum period. *Journal of Obstetric, Gynecologic, & Neonatal Nursing, 37*(3), 301–314.

Downe-Wamboldt, B. L. P., Butler, L. J., Melanson, P. M., et al. (2007). The effects and expense of augmenting usual cancer clinic care with telephone problem-solving counseling. *Cancer Nursing, 30*(6), 441–453.

Forchuk, C., Baruth, P., Prendergast, M., et al. (2004). Postoperative arm message: A support for women with lymph node dissection. *Cancer Nursing, 27*, 25–33.

Fraser, K. D., & Estabrooks, C. (2008). What factors influence case managers' resource allocation decisions? A systematic review of the literature. *Medical Decision Making, 28*(3), 394–410.

Hansen, F., & Sawatzky, J. V. (2008). Stress in patients with lung cancer: A human response to illness. *Oncology Nursing Forum, 35*(2), 217–223.

Howard, A. F., Balneaves, L. G., & Bottorff, J. L. (2007). Ethnocultural women's experiences of breast cancer: A qualitative meta-study. *Cancer Nursing, 30*(4), E27–E35.

Neufeld, S., & Newburn-Cook, C. (2008). What are the risk factors for nausea and vomiting after neurosurgery? A systematic review. *Canadian Journal of Neuroscience Nursing, 30*(1), 23–34.

Stajduhar, K. I., Martin, W. L., Barwich, D., & Fyles, G. (2008). Factors influencing family caregivers' ability to cope with providing end-of-life cancer care at home. *Cancer Nursing, 31*(1), 77–85.

Woodgate, R. L., Ateah, C., Secco, L. (2008). Living in a world of our own: The experience of parents who have a child with autism. *Qualitative Health Research, 18*(8), 1075–1083.

8 Examining the Conceptual/Theoretical Basis of a Study

On completing this chapter, you will be able to:

1. Identify the major characteristics of theories, conceptual models, and frameworks

2. Identify several conceptual models of nursing and other models used by nurse researchers

3. Describe how theory and research are linked in quantitative and qualitative studies

4. Critique the appropriateness of a theoretical framework—or its absence—in a study

5. Define new terms in the chapter

THEORIES, MODELS, AND FRAMEWORKS

Theories and conceptual models are the primary mechanisms by which researchers organize findings into a broader conceptual context. Different terms are associated with conceptual contexts for research, including *theories*, *models*, *frameworks*, *schemes*, and *maps*. There is overlap in how these terms are used, partly because they are used differently by different writers. We provide guidance in distinguishing them but note that our definitions are not universal.

Theories

Classically, **theory** is defined as an abstract generalization that offers a systematic explanation about how phenomena are interrelated. Traditionally, a theory embodies at least two concepts that are related in a manner that the theory purports to explain. As classically defined, theories consist of concepts and a set of propositions that form a logically interrelated system, providing a mechanism for deducing new statements from original propositions. To illustrate, consider the theory of reinforcement, which posits that behaviour that is reinforced (i.e., rewarded) tends to be repeated and learned. This theory consists of concepts (reinforcement and learning) and a proposition stating the relationship between them. The proposition lends itself to hypothesis generation. For example, we could deduce that hyperactive children who are praised when they are engaged in quiet play exhibit less acting-out behaviours than similar children who are not praised. This prediction, as well as many others based on the theory of reinforcement, could then be tested in a study.

Others use the term *theory* less restrictively to refer to a broad characterization of a phenomenon. Some authors specifically refer to this type of theory as **descriptive theory**—a theory that accounts for (i.e., thoroughly describes) a single phenomenon. Descriptive theories are inductive, empirically driven abstractions that "describe or classify specific dimensions or characteristics of individuals, groups, situations, or events by summarizing commonalities found in discrete observations" (Fawcett, 1999, p. 15). Such theories play an especially important role in qualitative studies.

Both classical and descriptive theories serve to make research findings meaningful and interpretable. Theories allow researchers to knit together observations into an orderly system. Theories also serve to explain research findings; theory may guide researchers' understanding not only of the *what* of natural phenomena but also of the *why* of their occurrence. Finally, theories help to stimulate research and the extension of knowledge by providing both direction and impetus.

Theories are abstractions that are created and invented by humans—they are not just *out there* waiting to be discovered. Theory development depends not only on observable facts but also on the theorist's ingenuity in pulling those facts together and making sense of them. Because theories are created, it follows that they are tentative. A theory can never be proved—a theory simply represents a theorist's best efforts to describe and explain phenomena. Through research, theories evolve and are sometimes discarded.

Theories are sometimes classified by their level of generality. **Grand theories** (or **macro-theories**) purport to explain large segments of the human experience. Some sociologists, such as Talcott Parsons, developed general theoretical systems to account for broad classes of social functioning. Within nursing, theories are more restricted in scope, focusing on a narrow range of phenomena. Theories that explain a portion of the human experience are sometimes referred to as **middle-range theories.** For example, there are middle-range theories to explain such phenomena as stress and infant attachment.

Models

A **conceptual model** deals with abstractions (concepts) that are assembled because of their relevance to a common theme. Conceptual models provide a perspective about interrelated phenomena, but they are more loosely structured than theories and do not link concepts in a logically derived deductive system. A conceptual model broadly presents an understanding of a phenomenon and reflects the philosophical views of the model's designer. There are many conceptual models of nursing that offer broad explanations of the nursing process. Conceptual models can draw on more than one theory and are an attempt to apply or specify the phenomenon to a particular setting. Conceptual models are not directly testable by researchers in the same way that theories are, but like theories, conceptual models can serve as springboards for generating hypotheses.

Some writers use the term **model** for mechanisms representing phenomena with a minimal use of words. Words that define a concept can convey different meanings to different people; thus, a visual or symbolic representation of a phenomenon can sometimes express abstract ideas in a more understandable form. Two types of models that are used in research contexts are schematic models and statistical models.

Statistical models, not elaborated on here, are mathematic equations that express the nature and magnitude of relationships among a set of variables. These models are tested using sophisticated statistical methods. A **schematic model** (or **conceptual map**) represents a phenomenon of interest in a diagram. Concepts and the linkages between them are represented through boxes, arrows, or other symbols, as in Figure 8.1. This model is the Developmental Model of Health and Nursing, or DMHN (Ford-Gilboe, 2002). The DMHN is a strengths-oriented model that focuses on how families and their members develop strategies needed to support a healthy lifestyle, with an emphasis on the family's role in shaping patterns of

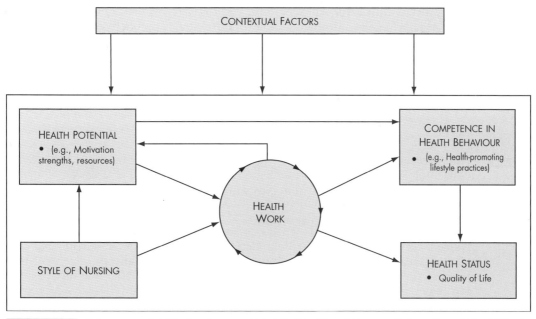

FIGURE 8.1 Schematic model: The Developmental Model of Health and Nursing. (Adapted from Fulford & Ford-Gilboe, 2004; Landenbach & Ford-Gilboe, 2004; Sgarbossa & Ford-Gilboe, 2004.)

response to health situations. According to the model, a person's health status (and quality of life) is affected by a multiplicity of factors, including contextual factors, nursing actions, and individual and family behaviours. The central concept in the DMHN is *health work*, which is a process through which families learn to manage health situations, problem-solve, and develop growth-seeking behaviours.

Frameworks

A **framework** is the overall conceptual underpinnings of a study. Not every study is based on a theory or model, but every study has a framework—a theoretical rationale. In a study based on a theory, the framework is the **theoretical framework;** in a study rooted in a specified conceptual model, the framework is often called the **conceptual framework** (although the terms *conceptual framework, conceptual model,* and *theoretical framework* are often used interchangeably).

The framework for a study is often implicit (i.e., not formally acknowledged or described). Worldviews and views on nursing shape how concepts are defined and operationalized. As noted in Chapter 2, researchers undertaking a study should make clear the conceptual definition of their key variables, thereby providing information about the study's framework.

Example of conceptual and operational definitions
As previously noted, the central concept in the Developmental Model of Health and Nursing is *health work*. Ford-Gilboe and her colleagues have developed both conceptual and operational definitions of this construct:

Conceptual definition: Health work is a universal process whereby families develop or learn ways of coping with health situations and using strengths and resources to achieve goals for healthy individual and family development (Ford-Gilboe, 2002).

Operational definition: Health work is observed in the problem-solving (coping) and goal attainment activities of the family. The construct is measured using a 21-question rating scale that was developed to measure the degree to which families engage in health work, the Health Options Scale, or HOS (Ford-Gilboe, 2002; Laudenbach & Ford-Gilboe, 2004).

In most qualitative studies, the frameworks are part of the research tradition within which the study is embedded. For example, ethnographers generally begin their work within a theory of culture. *Grounded theory* researchers incorporate sociologic principles into their framework and their approach to looking at phenomena. The questions that most qualitative researchers ask and the methods they use to address those questions inherently reflect certain theoretical formulations.

CONCEPTUAL MODELS AND THEORIES USED BY NURSE RESEARCHERS

Nurse researchers have used both nursing and nonnursing frameworks to provide conceptual contexts for their studies. This section briefly discusses some of the more prominent frameworks that have appeared in nursing research studies.

Conceptual Models of Nursing

Nurse theorists have developed a number of conceptual models of nursing that constitute formal explanations of what nursing is. Four concepts are central to models of nursing: person, environment, health, and nursing (Fawcett, 2004). The various nursing models define these concepts differently and link them in diverse ways. Moreover, the various models emphasize different processes as being central to nursing. For example, Sister Callista Roy's Adaptation Model identifies adaptation of patients as a critical phenomenon (Roy, in press). Martha Rogers (1986), by contrast, emphasizes the centrality of the individual as a unified whole, and her model views nursing as a process in which individuals are aided in achieving maximum well-being within their potential. The conceptual models were not developed primarily as a base for nursing research. Nevertheless, nurse researchers have turned to these conceptual frameworks for inspiration in formulating research questions and hypotheses.

In Canada, nursing education, practice, and research have been especially influenced by Moyra Allen's model of nursing, which has come to be known as the **McGill Model of Nursing** (Allen & Warner, 2002). This model focuses on the health-promoting interactions of nurses with individuals and families. The goal of nursing is to work with and actively promote patient and family strengths toward achievement of life goals. Health promotion is viewed as a collaborative process in which nurses help families explore health issues and develop healthy lives. In the McGill Model, the goal of nursing is to acknowledge the capabilities and strengths that clients and their families possess and to actively work with them to maintain, strengthen, and develop their health potential.

The previously discussed Developmental Model of Health and Nursing (Figure 8.1) represents a theoretical extension and refinement of the McGill Model of Nursing. In the model, family health work is supported by the family's health potential—the strengths, motivation, and resources of the family unit and its members. Health potential can, in turn, be affected by nursing actions. Although little research has been conducted to explore the relationship between nursing care and family health work, other aspects of the model have been subjected to formal testing, and results are promising.

Example of a study using the DMHN
Bluvol and Ford-Gilboe (2004) used the DMHN as the conceptual framework for a study exploring health promotion behaviours in families of stroke survivors living with a disability. They examined the relationships between hope, health, work, and quality of life in these families. Of the four hypotheses tested, positive relationships were found for stroke survivors, however, the model was less useful in explaining spouses' experiences.

Table 8.1 lists several other conceptual models of nursing, together with a study for each that claimed the model as its framework.

TABLE 8.1 SELECTED CONCEPTUAL MODELS OF NURSING USED BY NURSE RESEARCHERS

THEORIST	NAME OF MODEL/THEORY	KEY THESIS OF MODEL	RESEARCH EXAMPLE	FURTHER READINGS
F. Moyra Allen, 2002	McGill Model of Nursing	Nursing is the science of health-promoting interactions. Health promotion is a process of helping people cope and develop; the goal of nursing is to actively promote patient and family strengths and the achievement of life goals.	Gottlieb & Gottlieb (2007) proposed the Developmental/Health Framework within the McGill Model of Nursing, "to provide the substantive knowledge underlying whole person care" (p. E54).	
Madeline Leininger, 1991	Theory of Culture Care Diversity	Caring is a universal phenomenon but varies transculturally.	Porrett & Cox (2008) incorporated Leininger's theory into an ethnographic study of coping and help-seeking behaviour among English women with pelvic floor dysfunction.	
Betty Neuman, 2002	Health Care Systems Model	Each person is a complete system; the goal of nursing is to assist in maintaining client system stability.	Racher & Annis (2008) proposed the Community Health Action Model informed by Neuman's Model.	A Neuman Systems Model Perspective on Nursing in 2050 by Betty Neuman & Karen Reed, in Nursing Science Quarterly (2007). Imagining Nursing Practice: The Neuman Systems Model in 2050 by Lowry, Beckman, Gehrling & Fawcett, in Nursing Science Quarterly (2007).
Dorothea Orem, 2003	Self-Care Deficit Theory	Self-care activities are what people do on their own behalf to maintain health and well-being; the goal of nursing is to help people meet their own therapeutic self-care demands.	Aline Arrais Sampaio, de Souza Aquino, Leite de Araújo, et al. (2007) applied Orem's Self-Care Model to the study of ostomy patient care in Brazil.	Dead poets, nursing theorists and contemporary nursing practice by Person, in International Journal of Nursing Practice (2008).

(table continues on page 132)

	SELECTED CONCEPTUAL MODELS OF NURSING USED BY NURSE RESEARCHERS (continued)			
TABLE 8.1 ▶				
THEORIST	NAME OF MODEL/THEORY	KEY THESIS OF MODEL	RESEARCH EXAMPLE	FURTHER READINGS
Rosemary Rizzo Parse, 1999	Theory of Human Becoming	Health and meaning are co-created by indivisible humans and their environment; nursing involves having clients share views about meanings.	Pilkington & Kilpatrick (2008) studied the lived experience of suffering as an aspect of human becoming (Parse's theory) among older persons residing in long-term care facilities	The human becoming school of thought in 2050 by Rosemarie Rizzo Parse, in Nursing Science Quarterly (2007). A review of research related to Parse's theory of human becoming by Doucet & Bournes in Nursing Science Quarterly (2007).
Martha Rogers, 1986	Science of Unitary Human Beings	The individual is a unified whole in constant interaction with the environment; nursing helps individuals achieve maximum well-being within their potential.	Sook Kim, Sook Park, & Ae Kim (2008) studied the relationship of power and well-being to chakra meditation in Korean adults using Rogers' theory.	Imagining nursing practice in the year 2050: Looking through a Rogerian looking glass, by Todaro-Franceschi, in Nursing Science Quarterly (2007). The evolution of Rogers' science of unitary human beings: 21st century reflections, by Barbara W. Wright, in Nursing Science Quarterly (2007).
Sr. Callista Roy, 1999	Adaptation Model	Humans are adaptive systems that cope with change through adaptation; nursing helps to promote client adaptation during health and illness.	In a randomized, controlled trial, Bakan & Durmaz Akyol (2007) applied Roy's Adaptation Model to an education, exercise, and social support intervention programme to promote adaptation in Turkish patients with heart failure.	Imagining nursing practice: The Roy adaptation model in 2050, by Sato & Senesac, in Nursing Science Quarterly (2007).

Other Models Developed by Nurses

In addition to conceptual models that describe and characterize the nursing process, nurses have developed other models and theories that focus on specific phenomena of interest to nurses. One example is Nola Pender's Health Promotion Model (2006), which is designed to explain participation in health-promoting behaviours. According to this model, a person's decision to engage in health-promoting behaviours is affected by a number of cognitive/perceptual factors (e.g., the person's beliefs about the importance of health) and is modified indirectly by other factors (e.g., gender).

Another example is Mishel's Uncertainty in Illness Theory (1988, 1990), which focuses on the concept of uncertainty—the inability of a person to determine the meaning of illness-related events. According to this theory, a situation appraised as uncertain will mobilize individuals to use their resources to adapt to the situation. Mishel's conceptualization of uncertainty has been used as a framework for both qualitative and quantitative studies.

Example of a study based on uncertainty theory
Guided by Mishel's Uncertainty in Illness Theory, McCormick, Naimark, and Tate (2006) studied uncertainty, symptom distress, anxiety, and functional status in patients awaiting coronary artery bypass surgery.

Other Models Used by Nurse Researchers

Many concepts of interest to nurse researchers are not unique to nurses, and therefore nursing studies are sometimes linked to frameworks outside the nursing profession. Four conceptual models that have been used frequently in nursing studies are as follows:

❧ *Lazarus and Folkman's Theory of Stress and Coping.* This theory, which explains methods of dealing with stress, posits that coping strategies are learned, deliberate responses to stressors and are used to adapt to or change the stressors. According to this theory, people's perception of mental and physical health is related to the ways they evaluate and cope with life stress (Folkman, 1997; Lazarus & Folkman, 1984). An example of a Canadian nursing study that used this theory as its framework is the randomized controlled trial by Fillion et al. (2008), which verified the effectiveness of a group intervention designed to reduce fatigue in breast cancer survivors.

❧ *Azjen's Theory of Planned Behavior* (TPB). An extension of a theory called the Theory of Reasoned Action (TRA) (Azjen & Fishbein, 1980), the TPB provides a framework for understanding the relationships among a person's attitudes, intentions, and behaviours (Azjen, 2005). According to the TPB, behavioural intentions are the best predictor of a person's actual behaviour, and behavioural intentions are a function of attitude toward performing the behaviour, perceived control over the behaviour, and subjective norms—the person's belief in whether others think the behaviour should be performed. The TPB and TRA have been used in many Canadian nursing studies, including a study to understand the physical activity intentions of obese adults (Boudreau & Godin, 2007) and a study of nurses' intentions to provide continuous labour support to women with and without epidural analgesia (Payant, Davies, Graham, Peterson, & Clinch, 2008), which is described in greater detail at the end of this chapter.

❧ *Bandura's Social Cognitive Theory.* Social Cognitive Theory (Bandura, 1997) offers an explanation of human behaviour using the concepts of self-efficacy, outcome expectations, and incentives. Self-efficacy expectations involve people's belief in their own capacity to carry out particular behaviours (e.g., smoking cessation).

Self-efficacy expectations determine the behaviours a person chooses to perform, their degree of perseverance, and the quality of the performance. Many nurses have applied this theory to their research, including O'Farrell and Zou (2008), who studied nurses' values and perceptions of best-practice guidelines and a validated assessement tool related to the neurological assessment of patients with stroke.

➤ *Becker's Health Belief Model* (HBM). The HBM is a framework for explaining health-related behaviour, such as health care use and compliance with a medical regimen. According to the model, health-related behaviour is influenced by a person's perception of a threat posed by a health problem as well as by the value associated with actions aimed at reducing the threat (Becker, 1974). A revised HBM incorporates the concept of self-efficacy (Rosenstock, Strecher, & Becker, 1988). The study by Barata, Mai, Howlett, Gagliardi, and Stewart, 2008 is an interesting example which applies the HBM to explore women's beliefs about self-sampling for human papillomavirus (HPV), rather than conventional Pap testing.

The use of theories and conceptual models from other disciplines such as psychology (**borrowed theories**) has not been without controversy; some commentators advocate the development of unique nursing theories. However, nursing research is likely to continue on its current path of conducting studies within a multidisciplinary and multitheoretical perspective. Moreover, when a borrowed theory is tested and found to be empirically adequate in health-relevant situations of interest to nurses, it becomes **shared theory.**

TIP

Among nursing studies that are linked to a conceptual model or theory, about half are based on borrowed or shared theories. Among the models of nursing, those of Allen, Roy, Orem, and Rogers are especially likely to be used as the basis for research.

TESTING, USING, AND DEVELOPING THEORY THROUGH RESEARCH

The relationship between theory and research is a reciprocal one. Theories and models are built inductively from observations, and research findings provide an important source of observations. Concepts and relations that are validated in studies can be the foundation for theory development. The theory, in turn, must be tested by subjecting deductions from it (hypotheses) to further empirical inquiry. Thus, research plays a dual and continuing role in theory building and testing— qualitative methodology often associated with the former and quantitative with the latter. Theory can guide and generate ideas for research; research can assess the worth of the theory and provide a foundation for new ones.

Theories and Qualitative Research

Qualitative research traditions provide researchers with an overarching framework and theoretical grounding, although different traditions involve theory in different ways. Morse (2004) has developed a useful paper that discusses the derivation and kinds of concepts that qualitative inquiry generates.

Sandelowski (1993) makes a distinction between **substantive theory** (inductively derived conceptualizations of the target phenomena under study) and theory that reflects a conceptualization of human inquiry. Some qualitative researchers insist on an atheoretical stance regarding the phenomenon of interest, with the goal of suspending *a priori* conceptualizations (substantive theories) that might bias their collection and analysis of data. For example, phenomenologists are generally committed to theoretical naïveté, and explicitly try to hold preconceived views of the phenomenon in check. Nevertheless, phenomenologists are guided in their inquiries by a framework or philosophy that focuses their analysis on certain aspects of a person's lifeworld. That framework is based on the premise that human experience is an inherent property of the experience itself, not constructed by an outside observer.

Ethnographers bring a strong cultural perspective to their studies, and this perspective shapes their initial fieldwork. Fetterman (1998) has observed that most ethnographers adopt one of two cultural theories: *ideational theories*, which suggest that cultural conditions and adaptation stem from mental activity and ideas, or *materialistic theories*, which view material conditions (e.g., resources, money, production) as the source of cultural developments.

The theoretical underpinning of grounded theory studies is *symbolic interactionism*, which stresses that behaviour is developed through ongoing processes of negotiation within human interactions. Similar to phenomenologists, however, grounded theory researchers attempt to hold prior substantive theory (existing conceptualizations about the phenomenon) in abeyance until their own substantive theory emerges. Once the theory takes shape, grounded theorists use previous literature for comparison with the emerging categories of the theory. The goal of grounded theory is to use the data, grounded in reality, to provide an explanation of events as they occur in reality—not as they have been conceptualized in preexisting theories. Grounded theory methods are designed to facilitate the generation of theory that is *conceptually dense*, that is, has many conceptual patterns and relationships.

Example of theory in a grounded theory study

In her doctoral work, Boychuk Duchscher (2007) examined the first 12 months of transitioning for new nursing graduates moving into acute care practice. She used grounded theory, which "allowed for, facilitated and encouraged a deep and rich representation of the transition experience, and ultimately allowed for the creation of a set of models for transition that are informed by and grounded in the ongoing theoretical, conceptual and evidence-based knowledge of the researcher" (p. 8). Based on questionnaires, in-depth interviews, focus groups, and reflective journaling, Boychuk Duchscher developed the models of *Transition Shock* and *Stages of Transition* to apply in education and workplace programs for effective newly graduated registered nurses' professional socialization (Boychuk Duchscher, 2009).

In grounded theory studies, substantive theory is produced "from the inside," but theory can also enter a qualitative study "from the outside." Some qualitative researchers use existing theory or models as an interpretive framework. For example, a number of qualitative nurse researchers acknowledge that the philosophical roots of their studies lie in conceptual models of nursing such as those developed by Neuman, Parse, and Rogers.

Example of existing theory as an interpretive framework in a qualitative study

Pilkington and Kilpatrick (2008) studied the structure of the experience of suffering as an aspect of human becoming (Parse's theory) among older persons residing in long-term care facilities.

Another strategy that can lead to theory development involves an integrative review of qualitative studies on a specific topic, that is, a metasynthesis. In such integrative reviews, qualitative studies are combined to identify their essential elements. Findings from different sources are then used for theory building. Perrett (2007), for example, used the findings from a review of 35 years of qualitative studies applying Roy's Adaptation Model to highlight the concepts of *time* and *perception* as potential areas for further theoretical development.

Theories and Quantitative Research

Quantitative researchers, like qualitative researchers, link research to theory or models in several ways. The classic approach is to test hypotheses deduced from an existing theory. The process of theory testing begins when a researcher extrapolates the implications of the theory or conceptual model for a problem of interest. The researcher asks: If this theory or model is correct, what kinds of behaviour or outcomes would I expect to find in specified situations? Through such questioning, the researcher deduces implications of the theory in the form of research hypotheses, that is, predictions about how variables would be related if the theory were correct. For example, a researcher might conjecture that, if Orem's Self-Care Deficit theory (2003) is valid, nursing effectiveness could be enhanced in environments more conducive to self-care (e.g., a birthing room versus a delivery room). Comparisons between the observed outcomes of research and the relationship predicted by the hypotheses are the focus of the testing process. Studies that have tested the DMNH provide examples of this type of theory-research link. These studies involved the development of specific hypotheses derived from the model, the collection of data using measures that operationalized the key constructs of the model, and formal testing of the hypotheses using statistical procedures (e.g., Black & Ford-Gilboe, 2004; Bluvol & Ford-Gilboe, 2004; Sgarbossa & Ford-Gilboe, 2004).

Researchers sometimes base a new study on a theory or model in an effort to explain findings from previous research. For example, suppose that several researchers discovered that nursing home patients demonstrate greater levels of depression and noncompliance with nursing staff around bedtime than at other times. These descriptive findings are provocative, but they shed no light on the cause of the problem and consequently suggest no way to improve it. Several explanations, rooted in models such as Lazarus and Folkman's model or one of the models of nursing, may be relevant in explaining the behaviour and moods of the nursing home patients. By directly testing the theory in a new study (i.e., deducing hypotheses derived from the theory), a researcher could gain some understanding of why bedtime is a vulnerable period for the elderly in nursing homes.

TIP

When a quantitative study is based on a theory or conceptual model, the research report usually states this fact fairly early—often in the first paragraph, or even in the title. Many studies also have a subsection of the introduction called "Conceptual Framework" or "Theoretical Framework." The report usually includes a brief overview of the theory so that even readers with no background in the theory can understand, in a general way, the conceptual context of the study.

Tests of a theory sometimes take the form of testing a theory-based intervention. If a theory is correct, it has implications for strategies to influence people's attitudes or behaviours, including health-related ones. The impetus for an intervention may be a theory developed in a qualitative study. The actual tests of the effectiveness of the intervention—which are also indirect tests of the theory—are done in structured quantitative research.

Example of using theory in an intervention study

Fillion et al. (2008) developed an intervention designed to reduce fatigue and improve energy level, quality of life (both mental and physical), fitness, and emotional distress in breast cancer survivors. The 4-week intervention combined stress management and physical activity approaches, based on concepts from Lazarus and Folkman's theory of stress, as well as Salmon's unifying theory of physical activity in which "the biological effects of physical activity partially explain the beneficial psychological effects of exercise, which, in turn, reinforce adherence and, ultimately, contribute to stress adaptation processes" (p. 147).

A few nurse researchers have begun to adopt a useful strategy for furthering knowledge through the direct testing of two competing theories in a single study. Almost all phenomena can be explained in alternative ways. Researchers who directly test alternative explanations, using a single sample of participants, are in a position to make powerful comparisons about the utility of the competing theories.

It should also be noted that many researchers who cite a theory or model as their framework are not directly *testing* the theory. Silva (1986), in her analysis of 62 studies that used five nursing models, found that only 9 were direct and explicit tests of the models cited by the researchers. She found that the most common use of nursing models in empirical studies was to provide an organizing structure. In such an approach, researchers begin with a broad conceptualization of nursing (or stress, uncertainty, and so forth) that is consistent with that of the model. The researchers *assume* that the models they espouse are valid, and then use the model's constructs to provide a broad organizational or interpretive context. Using models in this fashion can serve a valuable organizing purpose, but such studies offer little evidence about the validity of the theory itself. To our knowledge, Silva's comprehensive review has not been replicated with a more recent sample of studies, although a 1993 review of Orem's Self-Care Deficit theory revealed little change in use (Spearman, Duldt, & Brown, 1993), while a recent update by Biggs (2008) noted a general increase in Orem-based research with 32 out of 335 studies specifically analyzing and developing theory. However, our sense is that, even today, many quantitative studies that cite models and theories are using them primarily as organizational or interpretive tools.

Example of using a model as an organizing structure

Godin, Roy, Haley, Leclerc, and Boivin (2008) undertook a study designed to identify factors associated with the maintenance of a high intention of avoiding initiation into drug injection among street youths in Montreal, Canada. Their study was theoretically grounded in (but did not test) Ajzen's theory of planned behaviour.

CRITIQUING CONCEPTUAL AND THEORETICAL FRAMEWORKS

You will find references to theories and conceptual frameworks in some of the studies you read. It is often challenging to critique the theoretical context of a published research report (or the absence of one), but we offer a few suggestions.

In a qualitative study in which a grounded theory is presented, you will not be given enough information to refute the proposed descriptive theory; only evidence supporting the theory is presented. However, you can determine whether the theory seems logical, whether the conceptualization is insightful, and whether the evidence is solid and convincing. In a phenomenological study, you should look to see whether the researcher addresses the philosophical underpinnings of the study. The researcher should briefly discuss the philosophy of phenomenology on which the study was based.

Critiquing a theoretical framework in a quantitative report is also difficult because most of you are not likely to be familiar with the cited models. Some suggestions for evaluating the conceptual basis of a quantitative study are offered in the following discussion and in Box 8.1.

The first task is to determine whether the study does, in fact, have a theoretical or conceptual framework. If there is no mention of a theory or conceptual model, you should consider whether the study's contribution to knowledge is diminished by the absence of such a framework. Nursing has been criticized for producing many pieces of isolated research that are difficult to integrate because

---

BOX 8.1 GUIDELINES FOR CRITIQUING THEORETICAL AND CONCEPTUAL FRAMEWORKS

1. Does the report describe an explicit theoretical or conceptual framework for the study? If not, does the absence of a framework detract from the usefulness or significance of the research?

2. Does the report adequately describe the major features of the theory or model so that readers can understand the conceptual basis of the study?

3. Is the theory or model appropriate for the research problem? Would a different framework have been more fitting?

4. Is the theory or model used as the basis for generating hypotheses that were tested, or is it used as an organizational or interpretive framework? Was this appropriate?

5. Do the research problem and hypotheses (if any) naturally flow from the framework, or does the purported link between the problem and the framework seem contrived? Are deductions from the theory logical?

6. Are the concepts adequately defined in a way that is consistent with the theory?

7. Is the framework based on a conceptual model of nursing or on a model developed by nurses? If it is borrowed from another discipline, is there adequate justification for its use?

8. Did the framework guide the study methods? For example, was the appropriate research tradition used if the study was qualitative? If quantitative, do the operational definitions correspond to the conceptual definitions? Were hypotheses tested statistically?

9. Does the researcher tie the findings of the study back to the framework at the end of the report? How do the findings support or undermine the framework? Are the findings interpreted within the context of the framework?

---

of the absence of a theoretical foundation, but sometimes the research is so pragmatic that it does not need a theory to enhance its utility. For example, research designed to determine the optimal frequency of turning patients has a utilitarian goal; it is difficult to see how a theory would enhance the value of the findings.

TIP

In most quantitative nursing studies, the research problem is *not* linked to a specific theory or conceptual model. Thus, students may read many studies before finding a study with an explicit theoretical underpinning.

If the study does involve an explicit framework, you would then ask whether the particular framework is appropriate. You may not be able to challenge the researcher's use of a specific theory or to recommend an alternative because that would require theoretical grounding. However, you can evaluate the logic of using a particular theory and assess whether the link between the problem and the theory is genuine. Does the researcher present a convincing rationale for the framework used? Do the hypotheses flow from the theory? Will the findings contribute to the validation of the theory? Does the researcher interpret the findings within the context of the framework? If the answer to such questions is no, you may have grounds for criticizing the study's framework, even though you may not be in a position to articulate how the conceptual basis of the study could be improved.

TIP

Some studies (in nursing as in any other discipline) claim theoretical linkages that are not justified. This is most likely to occur when researchers first formulate the research problem and then find a theoretical context to fit it. An after-the-fact linkage of theory to a research question *may* prove useful, but it is usually problematic because the researcher will not have taken the nuances of the theory into consideration in designing the study. If a research problem is truly linked to a conceptual framework, then the design of the study, the measurement of key constructs, and the analysis and interpretation of data will flow from that conceptualization.

RESEARCH EXAMPLES AND CRITICAL THINKING ACTIVITIES

EXAMPLE 1 ■ Quantitative Research

Aspects of a quantitative nursing study, featuring key terms and concepts discussed in this chapter, are presented below, followed by some questions to guide critical thinking.

Study

"Nurses' intentions to provide continuous labour support to women" (Payant et al., 2008)

Statement of Purpose

The purpose of the study was to examine the determinants of nurses' intentions to practice continuous, rather than intermittent, labour support for women with and without epidural analgesia (EA), as well as the organizational factors influencing their ability to do so, using a descriptive survey based on the Theory of Planned Behavior (TPB).

Method

A sample of 97 registered nurses from two birthing units at a large, urban Canadian hospital participated in the study and provided data through self-administered questionnaires developed in an earlier pilot.

Theoretical Framework

"The TPB was selected to provide the framework for this study because it consists of well-defined constructs used to predict and understand factors that influence the intention to perform a behaviour (Ajzen, 1988). The TPB postulates that the central determinant of a person's behaviour is their intention to perform the behaviour. Intentions are influenced by three constructs: attitudes, subjective norms, and perceived behavioural control. Attitudes are defined as a person's beliefs about the consequences of a behaviour. Subjective norms refer to 'perceived social pressure to engage or not to engage in a behaviour' (Ajzen, 2008). Perceived behavioural control reflects an individual's perception of how difficult it is to perform a given behaviour (Ajzen, 1988; Francis et al., 2004)" (p. 407).

Key Findings

■ In these case scenarios, nurses had lower intention, subjective norm, and attitude scores to provide continuous labour support to women with EA compared to women without.

■ Nurses reported providing continuous labour support almost half as often to women with EA relative to women without EA.

■ The strongest predictor of nurses' intentions to provide continuous labour support was the expectations of others to perform this behaviour.

■ Nurses reported their top four organizational barriers as: (1) unit acuity, (2) methods of patient assignment, (3) need to cover other nurses for breaks, and (4) ratio of nurses to patients.

CRITICAL THINKING SUGGESTIONS

1. Answer questions 1 and 3 through 8 from Box 8.1 (p. 138) regarding this study.
2. Also consider the following targeted questions, which may assist you in further assessing aspects of the study:
   a. Is there another model or theory that was described in this chapter that could have been used to study nurse intentions? If yes, would this model have been a better choice for a framework than the TPB?
   b. Nurse researchers in several countries, including the United States, United Kingdom, and Australia, have tested the TPB for explaining nurse intentions and beliefs and have found support for the theory. What does this suggest about the cross-cultural utility of the TPB?
   c. Were the authors' findings consistent with the Theory of Planned Behavior?
3. If the results of this study are valid and reliable, what are some of the uses to which the findings might be put into clinical practice?

(Research Examples and Critical Thinking Activities continues on page 140)

Research Examples and Critical Thinking Activities (continued)

EXAMPLE 2 ■ Qualitative Research

Aspects of a qualitative nursing study, featuring terms and concepts discussed in this chapter, are presented below, followed by some questions to guide critical thinking.

Study

"The lived experience of suffering: A Parse research method study" (Pilkington & Kilpatrick, 2008)

Statement of Purpose

The purpose of the study was to enhance understanding about the lived experience of suffering from the perspective of older persons living in an institution.

Method

The study participants were 12 elderly persons residing in two long-term care facilities in Canada. Data collection and analysis were completed through "dialogical engagement, extraction-synthesis, heuristic interpretation, and artistic expression" (p. 230).

Theoretical Framework

Parse's Human Becoming Theory provided the theoretical perspective for the study and guided the descriptive exploratory methods used. The Human Becoming Theory has three principles that centre on the themes of meaning, rhythmicity, and transcendence. To explore how suffering shapes health and quality of life, the lived experience of suffering was viewed in light of these principles, "as a process of structuring meaning multidimensionally in light of the possibility of nonbeing, while cocreating reality in the paradoxical processes of human-universe relating and moving beyond the now moment" (p. 230).

Key Findings

The findings consisted of three core concepts that describe suffering from the participants' perspectives. The concepts were synthesized into the following structure: "Suffering is unbounded desolation emerging with resolute acquiescence with benevolent affiliations" (p. 235).

CRITICAL THINKING SUGGESTIONS

1. Answer questions 1 and 3 through 9 from Box 8.1 (p. 138) regarding this study.

2. Also consider the following targeted questions, which may assist you in further assessing aspects of the study:
   a. Was this study a test of Parse's theory?
   b. Did Pilkington and Kilpatrick operationalize Parse's concepts in this study?
   c. In what way was the use of theory different in this study than in the previous study by Payant et al.?

3. If the results of this study are trustworthy, what are some of the uses to which the findings might be put into clinical practice?

Summary Points

· ·

> ⇒ A **theory** is a broad characterization of phenomena. As classically defined, a theory is an abstract generalization that systematically explains the relationships among phenomena. **Descriptive theory** thoroughly describes a phenomenon.

> ⇒ The overall objective of theory is to make research findings meaningful, summarize existing knowledge into coherent systems, stimulate and provide direction to new research, and explain the nature of relationships among variables.

> ⇒ The basic components of a theory are concepts. Classically defined theories consist of a set of propositions about interrelationships among concepts, arranged in a logical system that permits new statements to be derived from them.

> ⇒ Concepts are also the basic elements of **conceptual models,** but the concepts are not linked to one another in a logically ordered, deductive system.

⇝ **Schematic models** (or **conceptual maps**) are symbolic representations of phenomena that depict a conceptual model through the use of symbols or diagrams.

⇝ **A framework** is the conceptual underpinnings of a study. In many studies, the framework is implicit and not fully explicated.

⇝ Several conceptual models of nursing have been developed and have been used in nursing research (e.g., Moyra Allen's McGill Model of Nursing). The concepts that are central to models of nursing are person, environment, health, and nursing.

⇝ Nonnursing theories used by nurse researchers (e.g., Lazarus and Folkman's Theory of Stress and Coping) are referred to as **borrowed theories;** when the appropriateness of borrowed theories for nursing inquiry is confirmed, the theories become **shared theories.**

⇝ In some qualitative research traditions (e.g., phenomenology), the researcher strives to suspend previously held substantive conceptualizations of the phenomena under study, but nevertheless there is a rich theoretical underpinning associated with the tradition itself.

⇝ Some qualitative researchers specifically seek to develop *grounded theories*, data-driven explanations to account for phenomena under study (**substantive theories**) through inductive processes.

⇝ In classical applications of theory, quantitative researchers test hypotheses deduced from a theory. A particularly fruitful approach involves testing two competing theories in one study.

⇝ In both qualitative and quantitative studies, researchers sometimes use a theory or model as an organizing framework or as an interpretive tool.

⇝ Researchers sometimes develop a problem, design a study, and *then* look for a conceptual framework; such an after-the-fact selection of a framework is less compelling than the systematic testing of a particular theory.

STUDIES CITED IN CHAPTER 8*

This reference list contains only those studies that were cited in this chapter. Citations pertaining to theoretical, methodologic, or nonempirical work are included together in a separate section at the end of the book (beginning on page 399).

Allen, F. M., & Warner, M. (2002). A developmental model of health and nursing. *Journal of Family Issues, 8*, 96–135.

Azjen, I., & Fishbein, M. (1980). *Understanding attitudes and predicting social behavior.* Englewood Cliffs, NJ: Prentice-Hall.

Azjen, I. (2005). *Attitudes, personality, and behavior* (2nd ed.). Milton Keynes, UK: Open University Press/McGraw-Hill.

Bakan, G., & Durmaz Akyol, A. (2007). Theory-guided interventions for adaptation to heart failure. *Journal of Advanced Nursing, 61*(6), 596–608.

Bandura, A. (1997). *Self-efficacy: The exercise of control.* New York: W. H. Freeman.

Barata, P. C., Mai, V., Howlett, R., Gagliardi, A. R., & Stewart, D. E. (2008). Discussions about self-obtained samples for HPV testing as an alternative for cervical cancer prevention. *Journal of Psychosomatic Obstetrics & Gynecology, 29*(4), 251–257.

Becker, M. H. (1974). *The health belief model and personal health behavior.* Thorofare, NJ: Slack.

Biggs, A. (2008). Orem's self-care deficit nursing theory: Update on the state of the art and science. *Nursing Science Quarterly, 21*(3), 200–206.

Black, C., & Ford-Gilboe, M. (2004). Adolescent mothers: resilience, family health work and health-promoting practices. *Journal of Advanced Nursing, 48*(4), 351–60.

Bluvol, A., & Ford-Gilboe, M. (2004). Hope, health work and quality of life in families of stroke survivors. *Journal of Advanced Nursing, 48*(4), 322–332.

Boudreau, F., & Godin, G. (2007). Using the theory of planned behaviour to predict exercise intention in obese adults. *Canadian Journal of Nursing Research, 39*(2), 112–125.

Boychuk Duchscher, J. E. (2007). *Professional Role Transition Into Acute-Care by Newly Graduated Baccalaureate Female Registered Nurses.* Unpublished doctoral dissertation, University of Alberta, Alberta, Canada.

Boychuk Duchscher, J. E. (2009). Transition shock: the initial stage of role adaptation for newly graduated registered nurses. *Journal of Advanced Nursing, 65*(5), 1103–13.

Doucet, T. J., & Bourner, D. A. (2007). Review of research related to Parse's theory of human becoming. *Nursing Science Quarterly, 20*(1), 16–32.

Fawcett, J. (1999). *The relationship between theory and research* (3rd ed.). Philadelphia: F. A. Davis.

Fawcett, J. (2004). Contemporary nursing knowledge: *Analysis and evaluation of conceptual models of nursing* (2nd ed.). Philadelphia: F. A. Davis.

Fetterman, D. M. (1998). *Ethnography: Step by step* (2nd ed.). Newbury Park, CA: Sage.

Fillion, L., Gagnon, P., Leblond, F., et al. (2008). A brief intervention for fatigue management in breast cancer survivors. *Cancer Nursing, 31*(2), 145–159.

Folkman, S. (1997). Positive psychological states and coping with severe stress. *Social Science and Medicine, 45*, 1207–1221.

Ford-Gilboe, M. (2002). Developing knowledge about family health promotion by testing the Developmental Health Model. *Journal of Family Nursing, 8*, 140–156.

Godin, G., Roy, E., Haley, N., Leclerc, P., & Boivin, J. F. (2008). Maintenance of a high intention of avoiding initiation into drug injection among street youths: A longitudinal study. *Addiction Research and Theory, 16*(4), 339–351.

Gottlieb, L. N., & Gottlieb, B. (2007). The developmental/health framework within the McGill model of nursing: "Laws of nature" guiding whole person care. *Advances in Nursing Science, 30*(1), E43–E57.

Laudenbach, L., & Ford-Gilboe, M. (2004). Psychometric evaluation of the Health Options Scale with adolescents. *Journal of Family Nursing, 10*(1), 121–138.

Lazarus, R. S., & Folkman, S. (1984). *Stress, appraisal, and coping.* New York: Springer.

Lowry, L., Beckman, S., Reed Gehrling, K., & Fawcett, J. (2007). Imagining nursing practice: The Neuman systems model in 2050. *Nursing Science Quarterly, 20*(3), 226–231.

McCormick, K. M., Naimark, B. J., & Tate, R. B. (2006). Uncertainty, symptom distress, anxiety, and functional status in patients awaiting coronary artery bypass surgery. *Heart and Lung, 35*(1), 34–45.

Morse, J. M. (2004). Constructing qualitative derived theory: Concept construction and concept typologies. *Qualitative Health Research, 14*, 1387–1395.

Neuman, B., & Reed, K. (2007). A Neuman systems model perspective on nursing in 2050. *Nursing Science Quarterly, 20*(2), 111–113.

O'Farrell, B., & Zou, G. Y. (2008). Implementation of the Canadian neurological scale on an acute care neuroscience unit: A program evaluation. *Journal of Neuroscience Nursing, 40*(4), 201–211.

Parse, R. R. (2007). The human becoming School of Thought in 2050. *Nursing Science Quarterly, 20*(4), 308–311.

Payant, L., Davies, B., Graham, I. D., Peterson, W. E., & Clinch, J. (2008). Nurses' intentions to provide continuous labor support to women. *Journal of Obstetric, Gynecologic, & Neonatal Nursing, 37*, 405–414.

Pearson, A. (2008). Dead poets, nursing theorists and contemporary nursing practice (3). *International Journal of Nursing Practice, 14*, 1–2.

Perrett, S. E. (2007). Review of Roy adaptation model-based qualitative research. *Nursing Science Quarterly, 20*(4), 349–356.

Pilkington, F. B., & Kilpatrick, D. (2008). The lived experience of suffering: A Parse research method study. *Nursing Science Quarterly, 21*(3), 228–237.

Porrett, T., & Cox, C. L. (2008). Coping mechanisms in women living with pelvic floor dysfunction. *Gastrointestinal Nursing, 6*(3), 30–39.

Racher, F. E., & Annis, R. C. (2008). Community health action model: Health promotion by the community. *Research and Theory for Nursing Practice: An International Journal, 22*(3), 182–191.

Rogers, M. E. (1986). Science of unitary human beings. In V. Malinski (Ed.), *Explorations on Martha Rogers' science of unitary human beings*. Norwalk, CT: Appleton-Century-Crofts.

Rosenstock, I., Stretcher, V., & Becker, M. (1988). Social learning theory and the Health Belief Model. *Health Education Quarterly, 15*, 175–183.

Sandelowski, M. (1993). Theory unmasked: The uses and guises of theory in qualitative research. *Research in Nursing & Health, 16*, 213–218.

Sampaio, F. A. A., Aquino, P. S., Leite de Araújo, T. L., & Galvao, M. T. G. (2007). Nursing care to an ostomy patient: Application of the Orem's theory. *Acta Paulista de Enfermagem, 21*(1), 94–100.

Sato, M. K., & Senesac, P. M. (2007). Imagining nursing practice: The Roy adaptation model in 2050. *Nursing Science Quarterly, 20*(1), 47–50.

Sgarbossa, D., & Ford-Gilboe, M. (2004). Mother's friendship quality, parental support, quality of life and family health work in families led by adolescent mothers of preschool children. *Journal of Family Nursing, 10*(2), 232–261.

Silva, M. C. (1986). Research testing nursing theory: State of the art. *Advances in Nursing Science, 9*, 1–11.

Sook Kim, T., Sook Park, J., & Ae Kim, M. (2008). The relation of meditation to power and well-being. *Nursing Science Quarterly, 21*(1), 49–58.

Spearman, S. A., Duldt, B. W., & Brown, S. (1993). Research testing theory: A selective review of Orem's self-care theory, 1986–1991. *Journal of Advanced Nursing, 18*(10), 1626–1631.

Todaro-Franceschi, V. (2007). Imagining nursing practice in the year 2050: Looking through a Rogerian looking glass. *Nursing Science Quarterly, 20*(3), 229–231.

Wright, B. W. (2007). The evolution of Roger's science of unitary human beings: 21st century reflections. *Nursing Science Quarterly, 20*(1), 64–67.

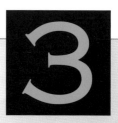

PART 3

Designs for Nursing Research

9 Scrutinizing Quantitative Research Design

On completing this chapter, you will be able to:

1. Discuss decisions that are embodied in a research design for a quantitative study

2. Describe and evaluate experimental, quasi-experimental, preexperimental, and nonexperimental designs

3. Distinguish between and evaluate cross-sectional and longitudinal designs

4. Identify and evaluate alternative methods of controlling extraneous variables

5. Understand various threats to the validity of quantitative studies

6. Evaluate a quantitative study in terms of its overall research design and method of controlling extraneous variables

7. Define new terms in the chapter

DIMENSIONS OF RESEARCH DESIGN IN QUANTITATIVE STUDIES

▶

The research design of a quantitative study incorporates key methodologic decisions about the fundamental form of a study and spells out the researcher's strategies for obtaining information that is accurate and interpretable. Thus, it is crucial for you to understand the implications of researchers' design decisions. Typically, developing a quantitative research design involves decisions with regard to the following aspects of the study:

➤ *Will there be an intervention?* In some studies, nurse researchers examine the effects of a new intervention (e.g., an innovative program to promote smoking cessation); in others, researchers gather information about existing phenomena. As noted in Chapter 2, this is a distinction between experimental and nonexperimental research. When there is an intervention, the research design specifies its features.

➤ *What types of comparison will be made?* Researchers usually design their studies to involve comparisons that enhance the interpretability of the results. Consider the example presented in Chapter 4 (Box 4.2), in which women who had an abortion were compared with women who delivered a baby in terms of emotional well-being. Without a comparison group, the researchers would not have known whether the abortion group members' emotional status was anomalous. Sometimes researchers use a before–after comparison (e.g., preoperative versus postoperative), and sometimes different groups are compared.

⇒ *How will extraneous variables be controlled?* The complexity of relationships among variables makes it difficult to test hypotheses unambiguously unless efforts are made to control confounding factors (i.e., to control *extraneous variables*). This chapter discusses techniques for achieving such control.

⇒ *When and how many times will data be collected?* In many studies, data are collected from participants at a single point in time, but some studies include multiple contacts with participants, for example, to determine how things have changed over time. The research design designates the frequency and timing of data collection.

⇒ *In what setting will the study take place?* Data for quantitative studies sometimes are collected in real-world settings, such as in clinics or people's homes. Other studies are conducted in highly controlled environments established for research purposes (e.g., laboratories).

There is no single typology of research designs because they vary along a number of dimensions. The dimensions involve whether researchers control the independent variable, what type of comparison is made, how many times data are collected, and whether researchers look forward or backward in time for the occurrence of the independent and dependent variables (Table 9.1). Each dimension is, with a few exceptions, independent of the others. For example, an experimental design can be a between-subjects or within-subjects design; experiments can be cross-sectional or longitudinal, and so forth (these terms are discussed later). The sections that follow describe different designs for quantitative nursing research. Qualitative research design is discussed in Chapter 10.

TABLE 9.1	DIMENSIONS OF QUANTITATIVE RESEARCH DESIGN	
DIMENSION	DESIGN	MAJOR FEATURES
Control over independent variable	Experimental	Manipulation of independent variable; control group; randomization
	Quasi-experimental	Manipulation of independent variable; no randomization and/or no comparison group; but efforts to compensate for this lack
	Preexperimental	Manipulation of independent variable; no randomization or no comparison group; limited control over extraneous variables
	Nonexperimental	No manipulation of independent variable
Type of group comparison	Between-subjects	Subjects in groups being compared are different people
	Within-subjects	Subjects in groups being compared are the same people at different times or in different conditions
Timeframes	Cross-sectional	Data are collected at a single point in time
	Longitudinal	Data are collected at two or more points in time over an extended period
Observance of independent and dependent variables	Retrospective	Study begins with dependent variable and looks backward for cause or influence
	Prospective	Study begins with independent variable and looks forward for the effect
Setting	Naturalistic setting	Data collected in real-world setting
	Laboratory	Data collected in contrived laboratory setting

EXPERIMENTAL, QUASI-EXPERIMENTAL, AND NONEXPERIMENTAL DESIGNS

This section describes designs that differ with regard to the amount of control the researcher has over the independent variable. We begin with research designs that offer the greatest amount of control: experimental designs.

Experiments

Experiments differ from nonexperimental studies in one key respect: researchers using an experimental design are active agents rather than passive observers. Early physical scientists found that, although observation of natural phenomena is valuable, the complexity of naturally occurring events often obscures relationships. This problem was addressed by isolating phenomena in laboratories and controlling the conditions under which they occurred. Procedures developed by physical scientists were adopted by biologists during the 19th century, resulting in many medical achievements. Researchers interested in human behaviour began using experimental methods in the 20th century.

Characteristics of Experiments

To qualify as an experiment, a research design must have three properties:

1. *Manipulation.* Experimenters do something to participants in the study.
2. *Control.* Experimenters introduce controls, including the use of a control group.
3. *Randomization.* Experimenters assign participants to control or experimental groups randomly.

Using **manipulation,** experimenters consciously vary the independent variable and then observe its effect on the dependent variable. Researchers manipulate the independent variable by administering an experimental *treatment* (or *intervention*) to some subjects while withholding it from others. To illustrate, suppose we were investigating the effect of physical exertion on mood in healthy adults. One experimental design for this research problem is a **pretest–posttest design** (or *before–after design*). This design involves the observation of the dependent variable (mood) at two points in time: before and after the treatment. Participants in the experimental group are subjected to a demanding exercise routine, whereas those in the control group undertake a sedentary activity. This design permits us to examine what changes in mood were *caused* by the exertion because only some people were subjected to it, providing an important comparison. In this example, we met the first criterion of a true experiment by manipulating physical exertion, the independent variable.

This example also meets the second requirement for experiments, the use of a control group. Campbell and Stanley (1963), in a classic monograph on research design, noted that scientific evidence requires at least one comparison. But not all comparisons provide equally persuasive evidence. Let us look at an example. If we were to supplement the diet of a sample of premature neonates with special nutrients for 2 weeks, the infants' weight at the end of the 2-week period would give us no information about the treatment's effectiveness. At a minimum, we would need to compare posttreatment weight with pretreatment weight to determine whether, at least, their weights had increased. But suppose we find an average weight gain of 400 g. Does this finding indicate that there is a causal relationship between the nutritional supplements (the independent variable) and weight gain (the dependent variable)? No, it does not. Infants normally gain weight as they mature. Without a control group—a group that does not receive the supplements—it is impossible to separate the effects of maturation from those of the treatment. The term **control group** refers to a group of participants whose performance on a dependent variable is used to evaluate the performance of the **experimental group** (the group receiving the intervention) on the same dependent variable.

Experimental designs also involve placing subjects in groups at random. Through **randomization** (or *random assignment*), each participant has an equal chance of being in any group. If people are randomly assigned, there is no systematic bias in the groups with respect to attributes that may affect the dependent variable. *Randomly assigned groups are expected to be comparable, on average, with respect to an infinite number of biological, psychological, and social traits at the outset of the study.* Group differences observed after random assignment can then be inferred as resulting from the treatment.

Random assignment can be accomplished by flipping a coin or pulling names from a hat. Researchers typically either use computers to perform the randomization or rely on a *table of random numbers*, a table displaying hundreds of digits arranged in a random order.

TIP

How can you tell if a study is experimental? Researchers usually indicate in their reports (in the method section) when they have used an experimental design, but they may also refer to the design as a *randomized design* or *clinical trial* (see Chapter 11). If such terms are missing, you can conclude that a study is experimental if the report says that a goal of the study was to "test," "evaluate," "assess," or "examine the effectiveness of" an "intervention," "treatment," or "innovation," *and* if individual participants were put into groups (or exposed to different conditions) at *random*.

Experimental Designs

Basic Designs. The most basic experimental design involves randomizing subjects to different groups and subsequently measuring the dependent variable. This design is a **posttest-only** (or *after-only*) **design.** A more widely used design, discussed previously, is the pretest–posttest design, which involves collecting **pretest data** (or **baseline data**) on the dependent variable before the intervention and **posttest data** (*outcome data*) after it.

Example of an after-only experimental design
Godin et al. (2008) used an after-only design to test the impact of completing a questionnaire about blood donation on subsequent blood donation behaviour in experienced blood donors: The two dependent variables measured were the number of registrations at each blood drive and number of successful blood donations. Measurements were made 6 months and 1 year after the questionnaire was completed.

Factorial Design. Researchers sometimes manipulate two or more variables simultaneously. Suppose we are interested in comparing two therapeutic strategies for premature infants: tactile stimulation versus auditory stimulation. We are also interested in learning whether the *amount* of stimulation affects infants' progress.

TYPE OF STIMULATION

		Auditory A1	Tactile A2
15 min.	B1	A1 B1	A2 B1
30 min.	B2	A1 B2	A2 B2
45 min.	B3	A1 B3	A2 B3

DAILY EXPOSURE

FIGURE 9.1   Schematic diagram of a factorial experiment.

Figure 9.1 illustrates the structure of this experiment. This **factorial design** allows us to address three questions: (1) Does auditory stimulation have a different effect on infant development than tactile stimulation? (2) Is the amount of stimulation (independent of modality) related to infant development? and (3) Is auditory stimulation most effective when linked to a certain dose and tactile stimulation most effective when coupled with a different dose?

The third question demonstrates a strength of factorial designs: they permit us to evaluate not only **main effects** (effects resulting from the manipulated variables, as in questions 1 and 2) but also **interaction effects** (effects resulting from combining the treatments). Our results may indicate, for example, that 15 minutes of tactile stimulation and 45 minutes of auditory stimulation are the most beneficial treatments. We could not have learned this by conducting two separate experiments that manipulated one independent variable at a time.

In factorial experiments, subjects are assigned at random to a combination of treatments. In our example, premature infants would be assigned randomly to one of the six cells. The term *cell* is used to refer to a treatment condition and is represented in a schematic diagram as a box. In a factorial design, the independent variables are referred to as *factors*. Type of stimulation is factor A, and amount of exposure is factor B. Each factor must have two or more *levels*. Level 1 of factor A is *auditory*, and level 2 of factor A is *tactile*. The research design in Figure 9.1 would be described as a 2 × 3 factorial design: two levels of factor A times three levels of factor B.

Example of a factorial design
Lespérance et al. (2007) used a 2 × 2 factorial design to test the effects of Citalopram and interpersonal psychotherapy (IPT) on depression in patients with coronary artery disease. Participants were randomly assigned to one of four treatment groups containing different combinations of IPT, Citalopram, and placebo control.

Crossover Design. Thus far, we have described experiments in which subjects who are randomly assigned to treatments are different people. For instance, the infants given 15 minutes of auditory stimulation in the factorial experiment are not the same infants as those exposed to other treatment conditions. This broad class of designs is called **between-subjects designs** because the comparisons are *between* different people. When the same subjects are compared, the designs are **within-subjects designs.**

A crossover design (sometimes called a *repeated measures design*) involves exposing participants to more than one treatment. Such studies are true experiments only if participants are randomly assigned to different treatment orders. For example, if a crossover design were used to compare the effects of auditory and tactile stimulation on infants, some subjects would be randomly assigned to receive auditory stimulation first followed by tactile stimulation, and others would receive tactile stimulation first. In such a study, the three conditions for an experiment have been met: there is manipulation, randomization, and control—with *subjects serving as their own control group.*

A crossover design has the advantage of ensuring the highest possible equivalence between subjects exposed to different conditions. Such designs are inappropriate for certain research questions, however, because of possible *carryover effects*. When subjects are exposed to two different treatments, they may be influenced in the second condition by their experience in the first. Drug studies rarely use a crossover design because drug B administered after drug A is not necessarily the same treatment as drug B before drug A.

TIP

Research reports do not always identify the specific experimental design that was used; this may have to be inferred from information about the data collection plan (in the case of after-only and before–after designs) or from such statements as "The subjects were used as their own controls" (in the case of a crossover design). Before–after and crossover designs are the most commonly used experimental designs in nursing research.

Example of a crossover design
Johnston et al. (2008) used a crossover design to determine the impact of Kangaroo mothercare (KMC) on pain from heel lance in preterm neonates. Infants were assigned to receive the experimental treatment and control condition in random sequence. In the experimental condition, the infant was held in KMC for 15 minutes prior to and for the duration of the heel lance procedure. In the control condition, the infant was in prone position swaddled in a blanket in an incubator.

Experimental and Control Conditions

In designing experiments, researchers make many decisions about what the experimental and control conditions entail, and these decisions can affect the results.

To give an experimental intervention a fair test, researchers need to carefully design one that is appropriate and of sufficient intensity and duration that effects on the dependent variable might reasonably be expected. Researchers delineate the full nature of the intervention in formal *protocols* that stipulate exactly what the treatment is for those in the experimental group; research protocols usually are summarized in research reports.

The control group condition used as a basis of comparison is sometimes called the *counterfactual*. Researchers have choices about what to use as the counterfactual, and the decision has implications for interpreting the findings. Among the possibilities for the counterfactual are the following:

⇒ No intervention—the control group gets no treatment at all

⇒ An alternative treatment (e.g., auditory versus tactile stimulation)

≈ A **placebo** or pseudo-intervention presumed to have no therapeutic value

≈ Standard methods of care—normal procedures used to treat patients

≈ A lower dose or intensity of treatment, or only parts of the treatment

≈ Delayed treatment (i.e., exposure to the experimental treatment at a later point)

Methodologically, the best possible test is between two conditions that are as different as possible, as when the experimental group gets a strong treatment and the control group gets no treatment. Ethically, however, the most appealing counterfactual is probably the delayed treatment approach, which may be difficult to do pragmatically. Testing two alternative interventions is also appealing ethically, but the risk is that the results will be inconclusive because it may be difficult to detect differential effects on the outcomes.

Ideally, participants should be *blinded* to which treatment group they are in, to avoid the risk that the outcomes would be affected by their *expectations* rather than by the actual intervention—although it is not always possible to mask the intervention.

Example of blinding

Scott and colleagues (2005) compared the efficacy of two diets before bowel cleansing in preparation for a colonoscopy. The standard liquid diet was compared to a liberalized diet that included a normal breakfast and a low-residue lunch, the day before the colonoscopy. Patients knew what group they were in, but the colonoscopists, who rated overall cleansing efficacy, did not. This is an example of a single-blind study.

Advantages and Disadvantages of Experiments

Experiments are the most powerful designs for testing hypotheses of cause-and-effect relationships. Because of its special controlling properties, an experiment offers greater corroboration than other research designs in that the independent variable (e.g., diet, drug dosage) affects the dependent variable (e.g., weight loss, blood pressure).

Lazarsfeld (1955) identified three criteria for causality. First, a cause must precede an effect in time. To test the hypothesis that saccharin causes bladder cancer, we would need to ensure that subjects had not developed cancer before exposure to saccharin. Second, there must be an empirical relationship between the presumed cause and the presumed effect. Thus, we would need to demonstrate an association between the ingestion of saccharin and the presence of cancer (i.e., that people who used saccharin experienced a higher incidence of cancer than those who did not). The final criterion for causality is that the relationship cannot be due to the influence of a third variable. Suppose that people who use saccharin tend also to drink more coffee than nonusers. Thus, a relationship between saccharin use and bladder cancer may reflect an underlying causal relationship between a substance in coffee and bladder cancer. It is particularly because of this third criterion that experimental designs are so strong. Through the controlling properties of manipulation, control groups, and randomization, alternative explanations to a causal interpretation can often be ruled out.

Experiments also have some limitations. First, not all variables of interest are amenable to manipulation. Many human characteristics, such as disease or health habits, cannot be randomly conferred on people. Second, there are many variables that could technically—but not ethically—be manipulated. For example, to date there have been no experiments to study the effect of cigarette smoking on lung cancer. Such an experiment would require us to assign people randomly to a smoking group (people forced to smoke) or a nonsmoking group (people prohibited from smoking).

In many health care settings, experimentation may not be feasible because it is impractical. It may, for instance, be impossible to secure the necessary cooperation from administrators or other key people to conduct an experiment.

Another potential problem is the **Hawthorne effect,** a term derived from a series of experiments conducted at the Hawthorne plant of the Western Electric Corporation in which various environmental conditions (e.g., light, working hours) were varied to determine their effect on worker productivity. Regardless of what change was introduced (i.e., whether the light was made better or worse), productivity increased. Thus, knowledge of being in a study may cause people to change their behaviour, thereby obscuring the effect of the research variables.

In health care settings, researchers sometimes contend with a double Hawthorne effect. For example, if an experiment investigating the effect of a new postoperative procedure were conducted, nurses as well as patients might be aware of participating in a study, and both groups could alter their actions accordingly. It is for this reason that **double-blind experiments,** in which neither the subjects nor those administering the treatment know who is in the experimental or control group, are so powerful. Unfortunately, the double-blind approach is not feasible in most nursing research because nursing interventions are often difficult to disguise.

In summary, experimental designs have some limitations that make them difficult to apply to real-world problems; nevertheless, experiments have a clearcut superiority to other designs for testing causal hypotheses.

Quasi-Experiments

Quasi-experiments look a lot like experiments because they also involve the manipulation of an independent variable (i.e., the institution of a treatment). Quasi-experiments, however, lack either the randomization or control-group features of true experiments—features whose absence weakens the ability to make causal inferences.

Quasi-Experimental Designs

There are several quasi-experimental designs, but only the two most commonly used by nurse researchers are discussed here.

Nonequivalent Control Group Design. The most frequently used quasi-experimental design is the **nonequivalent control-group before–after design,** which involves two or more groups of subjects observed before and after the implementation of an intervention. As an example, suppose we wanted to study the effect of primary nursing on nursing staff morale in an urban hospital. The new system of nursing care is being implemented throughout the hospital, so randomization of nurses is not possible. Therefore, we decide to collect comparison data from nurses in a similar hospital that is not instituting primary nursing. We gather data on staff morale in both hospitals before implementing the primary nursing system (the pretest) and again after its implementation (the posttest).

This quasi-experimental research design is identical to the before–after experimental design discussed in the previous section, *except* subjects were not randomly assigned to the groups. The quasi-experimental design is weaker because, without randomization, *it cannot be assumed that the experimental and comparison groups are equivalent at the outset.* The design is, nevertheless, strong because the collection of pretest data allows us to determine whether the groups had similar morale initially. If the comparison and experimental groups were similar at the pretest, we could be relatively confident that posttest differences in self-reported morale resulted from the intervention. (Note that in quasi-experiments, the term **comparison group** is generally used in lieu of *control group* to refer to the group against which experimental group outcomes are evaluated.)

Now suppose we had been unable to collect pretest data before primary nursing care was introduced (i.e., only posttest data were collected). This design has a serious flaw because we have no basis for judging the initial equivalence of the two nursing staffs. If we found higher postintervention morale in the experimental group, could we conclude that primary nursing caused an improvement in staff morale? There could be several alternative explanations for such differences. Campbell and Stanley (1963), in fact, called this *nonequivalent control group after-only design* a **preexperimental design** rather than quasi-experimental because we would be constrained from making the desired inferences. Thus, even though quasi-experiments lack some of the controlling properties of experiments, the hallmark of quasi-experiments is the effort to introduce some controls.

Example of a nonequivalent control group before–after design

Drummond et al. (2008) tested the effectiveness of teaching an early parenting approach in enhancing maternal and infant mutual responsiveness within a community-based support service for adolescent mothers. Participants were sequentially assigned to groups according to the order in which they were recruited into the study—The first participant was assigned to the experimental group and the second to the control, and so forth. Also, outcome data were collected before and after teaching was executed.

Time-Series Design. In the designs just described, a control group was used, but randomization was not. The next design has neither a control group nor randomization. Suppose that a hospital was adopting a requirement that all its nurses accrue a certain number of continuing education credits before being eligible for a promotion. Administrators want to assess the effect of this mandate on turnover rate and number of promotions awarded. Let us assume there is no other hospital that can serve as a reasonable comparison for this study, so the only kind of comparison that can be made is a before–after contrast. If the requirement were inaugurated in January, one could compare the turnover rate, for example, for the 3-month period before the new rule with the turnover rate for the subsequent 3-month period.

This one-group before–after design seems logical, but it has a number of problems. What if one of the 3-month periods is atypical, apart from the mandate? What about the effect of any other rules instituted during the same period? What about the effects of external factors, like changes in the local economy? The design in question, which is preexperimental, offers no way of controlling any of these factors—although the design can be beneficial in assessing the effectiveness of short-term educational interventions.

Example of a preexperimental before–after design

Atack and Luke (2008) used a one-group preexperimental design to measure the impact of an online course on infection control and prevention competencies. Seventy-six health care professionals completed three modules on infection control related to core competencies: hand hygiene, routine practices, and the chain of transmission. They also completed pretest and posttest measures of their perceptions of infection control competencies. There was no control group and inadvertently an absence of randomization.

The inability to obtain a control group does not eliminate the possibility of conducting research with integrity. The previous design could be modified so that at least some of the alternative explanations for change in nurses' turnover rate could be ruled out. One such design is the **time-series design,** which involves collecting data over an extended time period, and introducing the treatment during that period. Our study could be designed with four observations before the new continuing education rule and four observations after it. For example, the first observation could be the number of resignations between January and March in the year before the new rule, the second observation could be the number of resignations between April and June, and so forth. After the rule is implemented, data on turnover would be collected for four consecutive 3-month periods, giving us observations 5 through 8.

Although the time-series design does not eliminate all the problems of interpreting changes in turnover rate, the extended time perspective strengthens our ability to attribute change to the intervention. This is because the time-series design rules out the possibility that changes in resignations represent a random fluctuation of turnover measured at only two points.

Example of a time-series design
Mastel-Smith and colleagues (2006) used a time series design to evaluate the effectiveness of an intervention—therapeutic life review—to reduce depression in home-dwelling older women. Depression scores were obtained for the participants for 10 weeks before the intervention and during the 6-week intervention period.

Advantages and Disadvantages of Quasi-Experiments

Quasi-experiments are sometimes practical—it is not always feasible to conduct true experiments. In research in natural settings, it may be difficult to deliver an innovative treatment randomly to some people but not to others. Quasi-experimental designs introduce some research control when full experimental rigor is not possible.

The major disadvantage of quasi-experiments is that cause-and-effect inferences cannot be made as easily as with experiments. With quasi-experiments, there are alternative explanations for observed results. Suppose we wanted to evaluate the effect of a nursing intervention for infants of heroin-addicted mothers on infants' weight gain. If we use no comparison group or if we use a nonequivalent control group and then observe a weight gain, we must ask the following questions: Is it plausible that some other factor influenced the gain? Is it plausible that pretreatment group differences resulted in differential weight gains? Is it plausible that the changes would have occurred without an intervention? If the answer to any of these *rival hypotheses* is yes, inferences about treatment effectiveness are weakened. With quasi-experiments, there is almost always at least one plausible rival explanation.

TIP

How can you tell if a study is quasi-experimental? Researchers do not always identify their studies as quasi-experimental (or preexperimental). If a study involves an intervention (i.e., if the researcher has control over the independent variable) and if the report does not explicitly mention random assignment, it is probably safe to conclude that the design is quasi-experimental or preexperimental. Oddly, quite a few researchers *misidentify* true experimental designs as quasi-experimental. If individual subjects are randomized to groups or conditions, the design is *not* quasi-experimental.

Nonexperimental Studies

Many research problems cannot be addressed with an experimental or quasi-experimental design. For example, suppose we were interested in studying the effect of widowhood on physical health. Our independent variable here is widowhood versus nonwidowhood. Clearly, we cannot manipulate widowhood; people lose their spouses by a process that is neither random nor subject to control. Thus, we would have to proceed by taking the two groups (widows and nonwidows) as they naturally occur and comparing their physical well-being. There are various reasons for doing a **nonexperimental study** (sometimes referred to as an *observational study* by medical researchers because the study involves making observations rather than intervening). Sometimes the independent variable inherently cannot be manipulated, and in other cases, it is unethical to manipulate it. Also, an experimental design is not appropriate if the study purpose is description.

Types of Nonexperimental Studies

One class of nonexperimental research is **correlational** (or *ex post facto*) **research.** The literal translation of the Latin term *ex post facto* is "from after the fact," indicating that the research has been conducted after variation in the independent variable has occurred.

The basic purpose of correlational research is the same as that of experimental research: to study relationships among variables. However, it is difficult to infer causal relationships in correlational studies. In experiments, investigators make a prediction that a deliberate variation in X, the independent variable, will result in changes to Y, the dependent variable. In correlational research, on the other hand, investigators do not control the independent variable—the presumed causative factor—because it has already occurred. It is risky to draw cause-and-effect conclusions in such a situation. A famous research dictum is relevant: *correlation does not prove causation*. That is, the mere existence of a relationship between variables does not warrant the conclusion that one variable caused the other, even if the relationship is strong.

Correlational studies that explore causal relationships can be classified as either retrospective or prospective. In correlational studies with a **retrospective design,** a phenomenon observed in the present is linked to phenomena occurring in the past: the researcher focuses on a presently occurring outcome and then tries to ascertain antecedent factors that have caused it. For example, in retrospective lung cancer research, the investigator begins with a sample of people who have lung cancer and those who do not. The researcher then looks for differences between the groups in antecedent behaviours or conditions, such as smoking habits.

Correlational studies with a **prospective design,** by contrast, start with a presumed cause and then go forward to the presumed effect. For example, in prospective lung cancer studies, researchers start with a sample of smokers and non-smokers and later compare the two groups in terms of lung cancer incidence. Prospective studies are more costly than retrospective studies but are considerably stronger. For one thing, any ambiguity concerning the temporal sequence of phenomena is resolved in prospective research (i.e., the smoking is known to precede the lung cancer). In addition, samples are more likely to be representative of smokers and nonsmokers, and investigators may be in a position to rule out competing explanations for observed effects.

Example of a prospective nonexperimental study

Metcalfe and colleagues (2008) examined the predictors of contralateral prophylactic mastectomy among 927 women with a BRCA1 or BRCA2 mutation. The participants were followed for at least 1.5 years. Younger age was found, among other factors, to predict undertaking of a contralateral prophylactic mastectomy.

Researchers can sometimes strengthen a retrospective study, using a **case-control design.** This design involves comparing "cases" with a certain condition (e.g., breast cancer) with controls (women without breast cancer) who are selected to be similar to the cases with regard to background factors (e.g., family history of breast cancer) that could be linked to the condition. If researchers can demonstrate similarity between cases and controls with regard to extraneous traits, the inferences regarding the contribution of the independent variable (e.g., diet) to the disease are enhanced.

A second broad class of nonexperimental studies is **descriptive research.** The purpose of descriptive studies is to observe, describe, and document a phenomenon. For example, an investigator may wish to determine the percentage of teenaged mothers who receive adequate prenatal care. Sometimes, a report refers to the study design as **descriptive correlational,** meaning that researchers were interested in describing relationships among variables, without seeking to establish causal connections. For example, researchers might be interested in describing the relationship between fatigue and psychological distress in HIV patients. Because the intent in these situations is not specifically to explain or to understand the underlying causes of the variables of interest, a nonexperimental design is appropriate.

Advantages and Disadvantages of Nonexperimental Research

The major disadvantage of nonexperimental research is its inability to reveal causal relationships with assurance. Although this is not a problem when the aim is purely descriptive, correlational studies are often undertaken with an underlying desire to discover causes. Yet such studies are susceptible to faulty interpretation because researchers work with preexisting groups that have formed through **self-selection.** Kerlinger and Lee (2000) indicate that "self-selection occurs when the members of the groups being studied are in the groups, in part, because they differentially possess traits or characteristics extraneous to the research problem, characteristics that possibly influence or are otherwise related to the variables of the research problem" (p. 560). In other words, preexisting differences may be a plausible explanation for any observed group differences on the dependent variable.

As an example of such interpretive problems, suppose we studied differences in depression of patients with cancer who do or do not have adequate social support (i.e., emotional sustenance through a social network). The independent variable is social support, and the dependent variable is depression. Suppose we found that patients without social support were more depressed than patients with adequate support. We could interpret this to mean that people's emotional state is influenced by the adequacy of their social support, as diagrammed in Figure 9.2A. There are, however, other explanations for the findings. Perhaps a third variable influences *both* social support and depression, such as patients' family configuration. It may be that having family nearby affects how depressed cancer patients feel *and* the quality of their social support, as diagrammed in Figure 9.2B. A third possibility may be reversed causality, as shown in Figure 9.2C. Depressed cancer patients may find it more difficult to elicit social support than patients who are more cheerful. In this interpretation, it is the person's emotional state that causes the amount of received social support, and not the other way around. The point here is that correlational results should be interpreted cautiously, especially if the research has no theoretical basis.

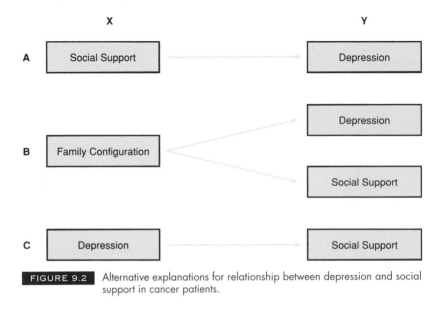

FIGURE 9.2   Alternative explanations for relationship between depression and social support in cancer patients.

TIP

Be prepared to think critically when a researcher claims to be studying the "effects" of an independent variable on a dependent variable in a nonexperimental study. For example, if a report is titled "The Effects of Dieting on Depression," the study is likely nonexperimental (i.e., subjects were not randomly assigned to dieting or not dieting). In such a situation, you might ask, Did dieting have an effect on depression—or did depression have an effect on dieting? or, Did a third variable (e.g., obesity) have an effect on both?

Despite interpretive problems, correlational studies are important in nursing because many interesting problems cannot be studied experimentally. Correlational research is often an efficient means of collecting a large amount of data about an area of interest. For example, it would be possible to collect extensive information about people's health problems and diet. Researchers could then study which health problems correlate with which nutritional patterns. By doing this, many relationships could be discovered in a short time. By contrast, an experimenter looks at only a few variables at a time. For example, one experiment might manipulate foods with different amounts of fat to observe the effects on physical outcomes, whereas another experiment might manipulate protein consumption, and so forth.

Quantitative Designs and Research Evidence

There is often a logical progression to knowledge expansion that begins with rich description, including description from qualitative research. Descriptive studies can be invaluable in documenting the prevalence, nature, and intensity of health-related conditions and behaviours and are critical in the conceptualization of effective interventions.

Correlational studies are often undertaken in the next phase of developing a knowledge base. Exploratory retrospective studies may pave the way for more rigorous case-control studies and prospective studies. As the evidence builds, conceptual models may be developed and tested using nonexperimental theory-testing strategies. These studies can provide hints about how to structure an intervention, who can most profit from it, and when it can best be instituted. Thus, the next important phase is to design interventions to improve health outcomes. Evidence regarding the effectiveness of interventions and health strategies is strongest when it comes from experiments. For this reason, experimental designs have earned the reputation among many of being the "gold standard" in an evidence-based practice environment. However, evidence for nursing practice depends on descriptive, correlational, and experimental research.

RESEARCH DESIGN AND THE TIME DIMENSION

The research design incorporates decisions about when and how often data will be collected in a study. In some studies, data are collected in a single time period, but others involve data collection on multiple occasions. Indeed, several designs involving multiple measurements have already been discussed, such as pretest–posttest designs, time-series designs, and prospective designs.

There are four situations in which it is appropriate to design a study with multiple points of data collection:

1. *Time-related processes.* Certain research problems involve phenomena that evolve over time. Examples include healing and recidivism.

2. *Time-sequenced phenomena.* It is sometimes important to ascertain the sequencing of phenomena. For example, if it is hypothesized that infertility contributes to depression, it would be important to determine that depression did not precede infertility.

3. *Comparative purposes.* Sometimes, multiple data points are used to compare phenomena over time. One example is a time-series study, in which the intent is to determine whether changes over time can be attributed to an intervention.

4. *Enhancement of research control.* Some designs collect data at multiple points to enhance interpretability of the results. For example, in nonequivalent control-group designs, the collection of preintervention data allows researchers to determine initial group differences.

Because of the importance of the time dimension in designing research, studies are sometimes categorized in terms of time. The major distinction is between cross-sectional and longitudinal designs—terms that are most often (although not always) used to describe nonexperimental studies.

Cross-Sectional Designs

Cross-sectional designs involve the collection of data at one point in time (or multiple times in a short time period, such as 2 hours and 4 hours postoperatively). All phenomena under study are captured during one data collection period. Cross-sectional designs are appropriate for describing the status of phenomena or relationships among phenomena at a fixed point. For example, a researcher might study whether children's behaviour is correlated contemporaneously with their diet. Retrospective studies are almost always cross-sectional. Data with regard to the independent and dependent variables are collected concurrently (e.g., the lung cancer status of respondents and their smoking habits), but the independent variable usually captures events or behaviours occurring in the past.

When cross-sectional designs are used to study time-related phenomena, the designs are weaker than longitudinal ones. Suppose, for example, we were studying changes in children's health promotion activities between ages 7 and 10 years. One way to investigate this would be to interview the same children at age 7 and then 3 years later at age 10—a longitudinal design. On the other hand, we could use a cross-sectional design by interviewing different children ages 7 and 10 at one point in time and then comparing their responses. If 10-year-olds engaged in more health-promoting activities than the 7-year-olds, it might be inferred that children became more conscious of making good health choices as they age. To make this kind of inference, we would have to assume that the older children would have responded as the younger ones did had they been questioned 3 years earlier, or, conversely, that 7-year-olds would report more health-promoting activities if they were questioned again 3 years later.

The main advantage of cross-sectional designs is that they are economical and easy to manage. There are, however, problems in inferring changes over time using a cross-sectional design. The amount of social and technological change that characterizes our society makes it questionable to assume that differences in the behaviours or characteristics of different age groups are the result of the passage through time rather than cohort or generational differences. In the previous example, 7- and 10-year-old children may have different attitudes toward health and health promotion independent of maturational factors. In cross-sectional studies, there are often competing explanations for observed differences.

Example of a cross-sectional study

Using a descriptive cross-sectional design, Ateah and Hamelin (2008) studied maternal bedsharing practices and experiences with their infants, and awareness of potential risks involved. Although a majority of mothers consented to risks involved in bedsharing such as rolling onto their infants, almost three quarters of them reported bedsharing on a regular or occasional basis.

Longitudinal Designs

Studies that collect data more than twice over an extended period use **longitudinal designs.** Longitudinal designs are useful for examining changes over time and for ascertaining the temporal sequencing of phenomena.

Three types of longitudinal studies deserve special mention: trend, panel, and follow-up studies. **Trend studies** are investigations in which samples from a population are studied over time with respect to some phenomenon. Different samples are selected from the same population at repeated intervals. In trend studies, researchers can examine patterns of change and make predictions about future directions.

Example of a trend study

Milke et al. (2008) conducted an evaluation of the effectiveness of a restraint-reduction initiative within a multisite, multimodel Canadian continuing care organization. Restraint data from four annual data collections between 2003 and 2006, involving approximately 1200 cases per year, were analysed to examine the trends in restraint use within the organization.

In **panel studies,** the same people provide data at two or more points in time. The term *panel* refers to the sample of people in the study. Panel studies typically yield more information than trend studies because researchers can identify individuals who did and did not change and then explore characteristics that differentiate the two groups. Panel studies are appealing as a method of studying change but are difficult and expensive to manage. The most serious challenge is the loss of participants over time—a problem known as **attrition.** Subject attrition is problematic because those who drop out of the study may differ in important respects from those who continue to participate, resulting in potential biases and concerns about the generalizability of the findings.

Example of a panel study

Benzies, Keown, and Magill-Evans (2009) followed a sample of 975 children drawn from the Candian National Longitudinal Survey of Children and Youth to study the immediate and sustained effects of parenting on physical aggression in Canadian children from birth to 6 years of age. Data on parenting style and parent-reported aggression in the children were collected at birth, 2, 4, and 6 years of age.

Follow-up studies are undertaken to determine the subsequent status of subjects with a specified condition or who received a specified intervention. For example, patients who have received a smoking intervention may be followed up to ascertain its long-term effect. To take a nonexperimental example, samples of premature infants may be followed up to assess their later perceptual and motor development.

Example of a follow-up study

Using a randomized controlled trial (RCT) design, Harrison et al. (2008) studied the effectiveness of nurse clinic versus home delivery of evidence-based community leg ulcer care. Data on wound healing were collected at baseline and patients were followed every 3 months until healing occurred. In addition, post wound healing follow-up data were collected 1 year after wound healing had occurred.

In longitudinal studies, the number of data collection points and the time intervals between them depend on the nature of the study. When change or development is rapid, numerous data collection points at relatively short intervals may be required to document the pattern. By convention, however, the term *longitudinal* implies multiple data collection points over an extended period of time.

TIP

Not all longitudinal studies are prospective because sometimes the independent variable occurred well before the initial wave of data collection. And not all prospective studies are longitudinal in the classic sense. For example, an experimental study that collects data 2, 4, and 6 hours after a treatment would be prospective but not longitudinal (i.e., the independent variable occurred first, but outcome data are not collected over a long time period).

TECHNIQUES OF RESEARCH CONTROL

A major purpose of research design in quantitative studies is to maximize researchers' control over extraneous variables. There are two basic types of extraneous variables that need to be controlled—those that are intrinsic to study participants and those that are external, stemming from the research situation.

Controlling External Factors

Various external factors, such as the research environment, can affect study outcomes. In carefully controlled quantitative research, steps are taken to minimize situational contaminants (i.e., to achieve **constancy of conditions** for the collection of data) so that researchers can be confident that the conditions are not affecting the data.

The environment has been found to influence people's emotions and behaviour, and so, in designing quantitative studies, researchers strive to control the environmental context. Control over the environment is most easily achieved in laboratory experiments, in which all subjects are brought into an environment structured by the experimenter. Researchers have less control over the environment in studies that occur in natural settings, but some opportunities exist. For example, in interview studies, researchers can restrict data collection to one type of setting (e.g., respondents' homes).

A second external factor that may need to be controlled is time. Depending on the research topic, the dependent variable may be influenced by the time of day or the time of year in which data are collected. In these cases, researchers should ensure that constancy of time is maintained. If an investigator were studying fatigue, for example, it would matter whether the data were gathered in the morning, afternoon, or evening, and so data from all subjects should be collected at the same time of day.

Another issue concerns constancy of communications to subjects. Formal scripts are often prepared to inform subjects about the study purpose, the use that will be made of the data, and so forth. In research involving an intervention, formal research protocols are developed. For example, in an experiment to test the effectiveness of a new medication, care would be needed to ensure that subjects in the experimental group received the same chemical substance and the same dosage, that the substance was administered in the same way, and so forth.

Example of controlling external factors

Markle-Reid et al. (2007) took care to ensure constancy of conditions in their RCT study, which tested the effectiveness of using a multifactorial and interdisciplinary health care (MIHC) team approach to reduce fall risk for frail older home-care clients over a 6-month period. The MIHC team received 1-day training sessions on an ongoing basis; were provided with a systematic, standardized, and evidence-based approach to their initial and ongoing assessments; and attended weekly conferences to discuss their assessment of client risk status and their progress toward their goals. In addition, the trained interviewers who assessed participants for fall risk status were blinded to the study purpose and participant treatment group assignment.

Controlling Intrinsic Factors

Control of study participants' extraneous characteristics is especially important. For example, suppose we were investigating the effects of an innovative physical training program on the cardiovascular functioning of nursing home residents. In this study, variables such as the subjects' age, gender, and smoking history would be extraneous variables; each is likely to be related to the outcome variable (cardiovascular functioning), independent of the physical training program. In other words, the effects that these variables have on the dependent variable are extraneous to the study. In this section, we review methods of controlling extraneous subject characteristics.

Methods of Controlling Subject Characteristics

Randomization. We have already discussed the most effective method of controlling subject characteristics: randomization. The primary function of randomization is to secure comparable groups, that is, to equalize groups with respect to extraneous variables. A distinct advantage of randomization is that it controls all possible sources of extraneous variation, without any conscious decision by researchers about which variables need to be controlled. In our example of the physical training intervention, random assignment of subjects to an experimental (intervention) group and control (no intervention) group would be an excellent control mechanism. Presumably, the two groups would be comparable in terms of age, gender, smoking history, and thousands of other preintervention characteristics. Randomization within a crossover design is especially powerful: participants serve as their own controls, thereby totally controlling all extraneous variables.

Example of randomization with crossover

Using a randomized crossover design, Johnston et al. (2009) compared the effects of maternal touch and talk versus an absence of maternal contact with infants and toddlers less than 3 years of age, on physiological stability and recovery during invasive procedures in the pediatric intensive care unity (PICU).

Homogeneity. When randomization is not feasible, other methods of controlling extraneous subject characteristics can be used. One alternative is **homogeneity,** in which only subjects who are homogeneous with respect to extraneous variables are included in the study. Extraneous variables, in this case, are not allowed to vary. In the physical training example, if gender were considered a confounding variable, we could recruit only men (or women) as participants. If we were concerned about the confounding effect of participants' age on physical fitness, participation could be limited to those within a specified age range. This strategy of using a homogeneous sample is easy, but its limitation is that the findings can be generalized only to the type of subjects who participated. If the physical training program were found to have beneficial effects on the cardiovascular functioning of men aged 65 to 75 years, its usefulness for improving the cardiovascular status of women in their 80s would need to be tested in a separate study.

Example of control through homogeneity

Zelkowitz et al. (2008) examined whether a brief psychoeducation intervention was effective in reducing maternal anxiety and developing sensitive interaction skills between mothers and their very low-birth-weight infants; to subsequently improve developmental outcomes in the infants at 6 months. Because maternal anxiety could be influenced by mother–infant interactions but also infant health status, the principle of homogeneity was used to restrict the sample. For example, infants could not be in a highly unstable medical condition that could lead to death, and they could not have a major congenital anomaly or sensory handicap.

Matching. A third method of dealing with extraneous variables is matching. **Matching** involves using information about subject characteristics to form comparison groups. For example, suppose we began with a sample of nursing home residents already set to participate in the physical training program. A comparison group of nonparticipating residents could be created by matching subjects, one by one, on the basis of important extraneous variables (e.g., age and gender). This procedure results in groups known to be comparable in terms of the extraneous variables of concern. Matching is the technique used to form comparable groups in case-control designs.

Matching has some drawbacks as a control method. To match effectively, researchers must know in advance what the relevant extraneous variables are. Also, after two or three variables, it becomes difficult to match. Suppose we wanted to control the age, gender, race, and length of nursing home stays of the participants. In this situation, if participant 1 in the physical training program were an African American woman, aged 80 years, whose length of stay was 5 years, we would have to seek another woman with these same or similar characteristics as a comparison group counterpart. With more than three variables, matching becomes cumbersome. Thus, matching as a control method is usually used only when more powerful procedures are not feasible.

Example of matching

Rush, McCracken, and Talley (2008) used a nonequivalent group design to assess the extent to which students participating in different clinical teaching models perceived themselves as insiders in the practice culture. Students participating in a 6-week intensive externship program offered by two hospitals were matched according to age, sex, race, educational background, and nursing experience, to a comparison group of students receiving traditional instructor led practicums.

Statistical Control. Another method of controlling extraneous variables is through statistical analysis. You may be unfamiliar at this point with basic statistical procedures, let alone sophisticated ones such as those referred to here. Therefore, a detailed description of powerful statistical control mechanisms, such as **analysis of covariance,** will not be attempted. You should recognize, however, that nurse researchers are increasingly using powerful statistical techniques to control extraneous variables. A brief description of methods of statistical control is presented in Chapter 15.

Example of statistical control
In a prospective cohort study, Markle-Reid et al. (2007) documented the association between the 6-month use of publicly funded home support services, and quality of life and use of health services among older people. The sample was divided into three groups based on average use of home support services over 6 months and differences in the baseline characteristics of participants between groups (such as depression, cognitive impairment, and efficacy of coping styles) were statistically controlled using repeated-measures analysis of covariance.

Evaluation of Control Methods

Overall, random assignment is the most effective approach to controlling extraneous variables because randomization tends to cancel out individual variation on all possible extraneous variables. Crossover designs are especially powerful, but they cannot be applied to all nursing problems because of the possibility of carryover effects. The three remaining alternatives described here have two disadvantages in common. First, researchers must know which variables to control in advance. To select homogeneous samples, match, or perform an analysis of covariance, researchers must decide which variables to control. Second, these three methods control only for identified characteristics, possibly leaving others uncontrolled.

Although randomization is the best mechanism for controlling extraneous subject characteristics, randomization is not always possible. If the independent variable cannot be manipulated, other techniques should be used. It is far better to use matching or analysis of covariance than simply to ignore the problem of extraneous variables.

CHARACTERISTICS OF GOOD DESIGN

In evaluating the merits of a quantitative study, one overarching question is whether the research design did the best possible job of providing valid and reliable evidence. Cook and Campbell (1979), in their classic book on research design, describe four important considerations for evaluating quantitative research design. The questions that researchers must address (and consumers must evaluate) regarding research design are as follows:

1. What is the strength of the evidence suggesting that a relationship exists between two variables?
2. If a relationship exists, what is the strength of the evidence that the independent variable of interest (e.g., an intervention), rather than extraneous factors, caused the outcome?
3. What is the strength of evidence suggesting that observed relationships are generalizable across people, settings, and time?
4. What are the theoretical constructs underlying the related variables, and are those constructs adequately captured?

These questions, respectively, correspond to four aspects of a study's validity: (1) statistical conclusion validity, (2) internal validity, (3) external validity, and (4) construct validity. In this section we discuss aspects of the first three types of validity; construct validity, which concerns the measurement of variables, is discussed in Chapter 14.

Statistical Conclusion Validity

As noted earlier, the first criterion for establishing causality is demonstrating that there is, in fact, an empirical relationship between the independent and dependent variables. Statistical methods are used to determine whether such a relationship exists. Design decisions can influence whether statistical tests will actually detect true relationships, and so researchers need to make decisions that protect against reaching false statistical conclusions. Although we cannot at this point in the text discuss all aspects of **statistical conclusion validity,** we can describe a few design issues that can be threats to making valid statistical inferences.

One issue that concerns **statistical power** is the ability of the design to detect true relationships among variables. Adequate statistical power can be achieved in various ways, the most straightforward of which is to use a sufficiently large sample. When small samples are used, statistical power tends to be low, and the analyses may fail to show that the independent and dependent variables are related— *even when they are*. Power and sample size are discussed in Chapter 12.

Another aspect of a powerful design concerns the construction or definition of the independent variable and the counterfactual. Both statistically and substantively, results are clearer when differences between the groups being compared are large. To enhance statistical conclusion validity, researchers should aim to maximize group differences on the independent variables so as to maximize differences on the dependent variable. If the groups or treatments are not very different, the statistical analysis might not be sufficiently sensitive to detect differences that actually exist.

A related issue is that the strength of an intervention (and hence statistical power) can be undermined if the intervention is not as powerful in reality as it is "on paper." An intervention can be weakened by a number of factors, such as lack of standardization, inadequate training, or premature withdrawal of subjects from the intervention. It is the researchers' responsibility to monitor the integrity of treatments in studies and to report deficiencies in achieving it.

Example of monitoring treatment integrity

Feeley et al. (2008) assessed the feasibility and acceptability of an intervention to reduce anxiety and enhance sensitivity among mothers of very low-birth-weight infants. Interveners kept standardized records of the details of each intervention session. The records were subsequently reviewed by the principal investigator to verify that the intervention had been delivered as planned and monitor any difficulties as encountered. In addition, interveners were supervised and monitored throughout the study through monthly meetings with the investigators.

Thus, if you are evaluating a study that indicates that groups being compared were not statistically different with respect to outcomes, one possibility is that the study had low statistical conclusion validity. The report might give clues about this possibility (e.g., too small a sample or substantial subject attrition) that should be taken into consideration when drawing conclusions about the study's evidence.

Internal Validity

Internal validity is the extent to which it is possible to make an inference that the independent variable is truly causing or influencing the dependent variable. Experiments possess a high degree of internal validity because randomization to different groups enables researchers to rule out competing explanations. With quasi-experiments and correlational studies, investigators must contend with rival hypotheses. There are various types of competing explanations, or *threats to internal validity*.

Threats to Internal Validity

History. The **history threat** is the occurrence of events concurrent with the independent variable that can affect the dependent variable. For example, suppose we were studying the effectiveness of an outreach program to encourage flu shots among community-dwelling elders using a time-series design. Now let us further suppose that, at about the same time the outreach program was initiated, there was a national public media campaign focusing on the flu. Our dependent variable in this case, number of flu shots administered, is subject to the influence of at least two forces, and it would be difficult for us to disentangle the two effects. In experiments, history is not typically an issue because external events are as likely to affect one group as another. The designs most likely to be affected by the history threat are one-group before–after designs and time-series designs.

Selection. The **selection threat** encompasses biases resulting from preexisting differences between groups. When people are not assigned randomly to groups, the groups being compared may not be equivalent. In such a situation, researchers contend with the possibility that any group difference in the dependent variable is due to extraneous factors rather than to the independent variable. Selection biases are the most problematic threats to the internal validity of studies not using an experimental design (e.g., nonequivalent control group designs, case-control designs) but can be partially addressed using the control mechanisms described in the previous section.

Maturation. The **maturation threat** arises from processes occurring as a result of time (e.g., growth, fatigue) rather than the independent variable. For example, if we wanted to test the effect of a special sensorimotor development program for developmentally delayed children, we would have to contend with the fact that progress would occur even without the intervention. Remember that the term *maturation* here does not refer to developmental changes exclusively but rather to any kind of change that occurs as a function of time. Phenomena such as wound healing and postoperative recovery can occur with little nursing intervention, and thus maturation may be a rival explanation for positive posttreatment outcomes. One-group before–after designs are especially vulnerable to this threat.

Mortality. The **mortality threat** stems from differential attrition from groups. The loss of subjects during the study may differ among groups because of initial differences in interest or motivation. For example, suppose we used a nonequivalent control-group design to assess nurses' morale in two hospitals, only one of which initiated primary nursing. Nursing morale is measured before and after the intervention. The comparison group, which may have no particular commitment to the study, may be reluctant to complete a posttest questionnaire. Those who do fill it out may be unrepresentative of the group as a whole; they may be highly critical of their work environment, for example. Thus, on the average, it may appear that the morale of nurses in the comparison hospital declined, but this might only be an artefact of the *mortality* of a select segment of this group.

Internal Validity and Research Design

Quasi-experimental, preexperimental, and correlational studies are especially susceptible to threats to internal validity. These threats represent alternative explanations (rival hypotheses) that compete with the independent variable as a cause of the dependent variable. *The aim of a good quantitative research design is to rule out these competing explanations.* The control mechanisms previously reviewed are strategies for improving the internal validity of studies—and thus for strengthening the quality of evidence they yield.

An experimental design normally eliminates competing explanations, but this is not always the case. For example, if constancy of conditions is not maintained for experimental and control groups, history might be a rival explanation for obtained results. Experimental mortality is, in particular, a salient threat: because the experimenter offers differential treatment to the experimental and control groups, members of the two groups may drop out of the study differentially. This is particularly likely to happen if the experimental treatment is stressful or time-consuming or if the control condition is boring or aggravating. When this happens, participants remaining in the study may differ from those who left, thereby nullifying the initial equivalence of the groups.

You should pay careful attention to the possibility of competing explanations for reported results, especially in studies that do not use an experimental design. When the investigator does not have control over critical extraneous variables, caution in interpreting results and drawing conclusions about the evidence is appropriate.

External Validity

External validity is the generalizability of research findings to other settings or samples, an issue of great importance for those interested in an evidence-based practice. Quantitative studies are rarely conducted with the intention of discovering relationships among variables for a single group of people. If a nursing intervention is found to be effective—and if the study results are internally valid—then others will want to adopt it. Therefore, an important question is whether an intervention will work in another setting or with different patients.

One aspect of a study's external validity concerns the adequacy of the sampling design. If the characteristics of the sample are representative of those of the population, the generalizability of the results to the population is enhanced. Sampling designs are described in Chapter 12.

Various aspects of a research situation also affect the study's external validity. For example, when a treatment is new (e.g., a new protocol for pain management), participants and researchers alike might alter their behaviour. People may be either enthusiastic or sceptical about new methods of doing things. Thus, the results may reflect reactions to the novelty rather than to the intrinsic qualities of the treatment. Results may also reflect study participants' awareness of being in a study (the Hawthorne effect) or their expectations about benefits of an intervention, independent of the actual intervention (a **placebo effect**). It is because of these risks that experimental blinding should be used whenever possible.

Example of a possible Hawthorne effect

Winterburn and Fraser (2000) used an experimental design to test the effect of long versus short postnatal stay on the decisions of first-time mothers to breastfeed. Length of hospital stay was unrelated to breastfeeding behaviours at 1 month, but in both groups, the breastfeeding rate was higher than citywide rates. The researchers speculated that this could reflect a Hawthorne effect.

Sometimes, the demands for internal and external validity conflict. If a researcher exercises tight control in a study to maximize internal validity, the setting may become too artificial to generalize to a more naturalistic environment. Therefore, a compromise must sometimes be reached. The importance of replicating studies in different settings with new study participants cannot be overemphasized.

CRITIQUING QUANTITATIVE RESEARCH DESIGNS

The overriding consideration in evaluating a research design is whether the design enables the researcher to answer the research question conclusively. This must be determined in terms of both substantive and methodologic considerations.

Substantively, the issue is whether the researcher selected a design that matches the aims of the research. If the research purpose is descriptive or exploratory, an experimental design is not appropriate. If the researcher is searching to understand the full nature of a phenomenon about which little is known, a

BOX 9.1   GUIDELINES FOR CRITIQUING RESEARCH DESIGNS IN QUANTITATIVE STUDIES

1. Does the study involve an intervention? If yes, was an experimental, quasi-experimental, or preexperimental design used—and was this the most appropriate design?
2. If the study was experimental or quasi-experimental, was "blinding" used? Who was blinded?
3. If the study was nonexperimental, why did not the researcher manipulate the independent variable? Was the decision regarding manipulation appropriate?
4. Was the study longitudinal or cross-sectional? Was the number of data collection points appropriate, given the research question?
5. What type of comparisons were called for in the research design (e.g., was the study design within-subjects or between-subjects)? Are the comparisons the most appropriate for illuminating the relationship between the independent and dependent variables?
6. What did the researcher do to control extraneous external factors and intrinsic subject characteristics? Were the procedures appropriate and adequate?
7. What steps did the researcher take in designing the study to enhance statistical conclusion validity? Were these steps adequate?
8. What steps did the researcher take to enhance the internal validity of the study? To what extent were those steps successful? What types of alternative explanations must be considered—what are the threats to internal validity? Does the design enable the researcher to draw causal inferences about the relationship between the independent and dependent variables?
9. To what extent is the study externally valid?
10. What are the major limitations of the design used? Are these limitations acknowledged by the researcher and taken into account in interpreting results?

structured design that allows little flexibility might block insights (flexible designs are discussed in Chapter 10). We have discussed research control as a mechanism for reducing bias, but sometimes too much control can introduce bias, for example, when the researcher tightly controls the ways in which the phenomena under study can be manifested and thereby obscures their true nature.

Methodologically, the main design issue in quantitative studies is whether the research design provides the most accurate, unbiased, interpretable, and replicable evidence possible. Indeed, there usually is no other aspect of a quantitative study that affects the quality of evidence as much as the research design. Box 9.1 provides questions to assist you in evaluating the methodologic aspects of quantitative research designs; these questions are key to a meaningful critique of a quantitative study.

RESEARCH EXAMPLES AND CRITICAL THINKING ACTIVITIES

EXAMPLE 1 ■ Experimental Design

Aspects of an experimental nursing study, featuring terms and concepts discussed in this chapter, are presented below, followed by some questions to guide critical thinking.

Study
"When the bough breaks: Provider-initiated comprehensive care is more effective and less expensive for sole-support parents on social assistance" (Browne, Byrne, Roberts, Gafni, & Whittaker, 2001)

Statement of Purpose
The purpose of the study was to examine the comparative effects and expense of proactively offering different mixes of provider-initiated health and social service packages to single parents and their children on social assistance (designated as sole-support families).

Treatment Groups

The study employed four treatment groups and one control group. All groups received basic social assistance: Group 1 received a full package of services that included health promotion, employment retraining, and the recreation/childcare/skills development program; Group 2 received health promotion; Group 3 received employment retraining; Group 4 received age-appropriate recreation/childcare/skills development programs; and Group 5 received no additional services (self-directed care).

Design and Method

A single blind five-armed randomized controlled trial was implemented over a 5-year period. A sample of 765 sole supporters were drawn from two study centres located in the Department of Social Assistance in the neighbouring regions of Hamilton-Wentworth and Halton in central Ontario, Canada. Study participants were equally randomized to each of the four treatment groups and the control group. Data were collected by interviewers who were blind to the study purpose, from all sole-support families (comprising the single parents sharing their home with at least one child) before random assignment and then at three follow-up points: at 1year, 2 years, and 4 years following enrolment into the study. Outcome data measured included parental mood disorders, adult social adjustment, child-hood behaviour disorders, child competence, social independence, and the dollar value of health and social services use. In addition, sociodemographic information describing the parent and engagement rate—a measure of dose of interventions, was obtained. All consent-ing participants were initially contacted by phone to schedule home visits, during which outcome data were collected. After the 2-year follow-up point, 404 families were lost to attrition; therefore, the results presented reflect data collected up to that point.

Key Findings

- The treatment and control groups did not differ significantly with respect to adult social adjustment scores from baseline to 2-year follow-up.

- There was no statistically significant decline in parental mood disorders and childhood behaviour disorders between the treatment and control groups at 2 years.

- A statistically significant proportion of parents in group I reported that they had not used any form of social assistance in the entire previous 12 months compared to the control group.

- At 2 years, all groups except groups III and V had at least a 50% reduction in per parent expenditures.

- Children with any behaviour disorder at baseline had higher competence rates if they received the recreation component compared to those who did not.
  1. Answer questions 1, 2, and 4 through 9 from Box 9.1 (p. 166) regarding this study.

  2. Also consider the following targeted questions, which may assist you in further assess-ing aspects of the study:
     a. What specific experimental design was used in this study? Was this appropriate?
     b. Could a crossover design have been used?
     c. Was randomization successful?

  3. If the results of this study are valid and reliable, what are some of the uses to which the findings might be put in clinical practice?

EXAMPLE 2 ■ Quasi-Experimental Design

Aspects of a quasi-experimental nursing study, featuring terms and concepts discussed in this chapter, are presented below, followed by some questions to guide critical thinking.

Study

"Effects of a two-generation Canadian preschool program on parenting stress, self-esteem, and life skills" (Benzies et al., 2009)

(Research Examples and Critical Thinking Activities continues on page 168)

Research Examples and Critical Thinking Activities (continued)

Statement of Purpose

The purpose of the study was to examine the effects on Canadian parents of a two-generation preschool program, which included centre-based early childhood education, parenting and life skills education, and family support.

Treatment Conditions

The intervention comprised a two-generation program comprising social, educational, and economic supports to parents and their children. Parent education involved a 6-week series of parenting and life skills training including group and one-on-one classes. In addition to education, a minimum of four home visits per year by a registered social worker was provided to families. For the children, centre-based preschool and kindergarten programming was offered for 4 days a week for 5 hours each day for 10 months. As an additional level of support, children who were assessed by developmental specialists to have a developmental delay were eligible for additional government funding to cover assessment and intervention costs.

Design and Method

Parents with low income as determined by their taxation documents and their children were eligible to attend the intervention program if they had additional risk factors such as housing instability, parental mental illness, or involvement with child welfare. Fifty-five caregivers of 76 children were recruited into the study and outcome data were collected using questionnaires, at intake into the program before the commencement of the 6-week education series (Time 1), and upon completion of the program (Time 2). Outcome measures included parenting stress, self-esteem and life skills at times 1 and 2. Participants were used as their own control and thus a different comparison group was not employed.

Key Findings

- Statistically significant increases in self-esteem and daily life management skills were found for parents at Time 2 compared to Time 1.
- Statistically significant decreases in certain aspects of parenting stress as measured by the Parenting Stress Index—Short Form Questionnaire were found, at Time 2 compared to Time 1.

CRITICAL THINKING SUGGESTIONS

1. Answer questions 1, 2, and 4 through 9 from Box 9.1 (p. 166) regarding this study.
2. Also consider the following targeted questions, which may assist you in further assessing aspects of the study:
   a. What specific design was used in this study? Was this appropriate?
   b. Comment on the researchers' decision to use the particular setting for their study.
3. If the results of this study are valid and reliable, what are some of the potential clinical uses?

EXAMPLE 3 ■ Nonexperimental Design

1. Read the method section from the study by Bryanton and collegues in Appendix A of this book, and then answer the relevant questions in Box 9.1 (p. 166).
2. Also consider the following targeted questions, which may further sharpen your critical thinking skills and assist you in assessing aspects of the study's merit:
   a. Was this study retrospective or prospective? Discuss the effect of the design on the researchers' ability to draw inferences about the direction of influence between the independent and dependent variables.
   b. In addition to the independent variables used in this study, can you think of other possible predictors of parenting self-efficacy? Can any of your suggested predictors be experimentally manipulated?

Summary Points

....

⇒ The **research design** is the researcher's overall plan for answering research questions. In quantitative studies, the design indicates whether there is an intervention, the nature of any comparisons, the methods used to control extraneous variables, and the timing and location of data collection.

⇒ **Experiments** involve **manipulation** (the researcher manipulates the independent variable by introducing a *treatment* or *intervention*), control (including the use of a **control group** that is compared to the **experimental group**), and **randomization** (wherein subjects are allocated to groups at random to make them comparable at the outset).

⇒ **Posttest-only** (or *after-only*) **designs** involve collecting data only once—after random assignment and the introduction of the treatment; in **pretest–posttest** (or *before–after*) **designs,** data are collected both before and after the experimental manipulation.

⇒ **Factorial designs,** in which two or more variables are manipulated simultaneously, allow researchers to test both **main effects** (effects from the experimentally manipulated variables) and **interaction effects** (effects resulting from combining the treatments).

⇒ **Between-subjects designs,** in which different sets of people are compared, contrast with **within-subjects designs,** which involve comparisons of the same subjects.

⇒ In a **crossover** (or *repeated-measures*) **design,** subjects are exposed to more than one experimental condition in random order and serve as their own controls.

⇒ **Quasi-experiments** involve manipulation but lack a comparison group or randomization. Quasi-experimental designs introduce controls to compensate for these missing components. By contrast, **preexperimental designs** have no such safeguards.

⇒ **The nonequivalent control-group before–after design** involves the use of a **comparison group** that was not created through random assignment and the collection of pretreatment data that permits an assessment of initial group equivalence.

⇒ In a **time-series design,** there is no comparison group; information on the dependent variable is collected over a period of time before and after the treatment.

⇒ **Nonexperimental research** includes **descriptive research**—studies that summarize the status of phenomena—and **correlational** (or *ex post facto)* **studies** that examine relationships among variables but involve no manipulation of the independent variable.

⇒ Researchers use **retrospective** and **prospective** correlational designs to infer causality, but the findings from such studies are generally open to several interpretations.

⇒ **Cross-sectional designs** involve the collection of data at one time period, whereas **longitudinal designs** involve data collection two or more times over an extended period. Three types of longitudinal studies, which are used to study changes or development over time, are **trend studies, panel studies,** and **follow-up studies.**

⇒ Quantitative researchers strive to control external factors that could affect the study outcomes (e.g., the environment) and extraneous subject characteristics.

⇒ Techniques for controlling subject characteristics include **homogeneity** (restricting the sample to eliminate variability on the extraneous variable); **matching** (matching subjects to make groups comparable); statistical procedures, such as

analysis of covariance; and **randomization**—the most effective control procedure because it controls all possible extraneous variables without researchers having to identify or measure them.

⇝ A well-designed study attends to statistical conclusion validity, internal validity, external validity, and construct validity.

⇝ **Statistical conclusion validity** concerns the strength of evidence that a relationship exists between two variables. Threats to statistical conclusion validity include low **statistical power** (the ability to detect true relationships) and a weak treatment.

⇝ **Internal validity** concerns the degree to which outcomes can be attributed to the independent variable. *Threats to internal validity* include **history, selection, maturation,** and **mortality** (caused by subject **attrition**).

⇝ **External validity** refers to the generalizability of study findings to other samples and situations.

STUDIES CITED IN CHAPTER 9*

This reference list contains only those studies that were cited in this chapter. Citations pertaining to theoretical, methodologic, or nonempirical work are included together in a separate section at the end of the book (beginning on page 399).

Atack, L., & Luke, R. (2008). Impact of online course on infection control and prevention competencies. *Journal of Advanced Nursing, 63*(2), 175–180.

Ateah, C. A., & Hamelin, K. J. (2008). Maternal bedsharing practices, experiences, and awareness of risks. *Journal of Obstetric, Gynecologic, and Neonatal Nursing, 37,* 274–281.

Benzies, K., Keown, L.-A., & Magill-Evans, J. (2009). Immediate and sustained effects of parenting on physical aggression in Canadian children to 6 years of age. *The Canadian Journal of Psychiatry, 54*(1), 55–64.

Benzies, K., Tough, S., Edwards, N., et al. (2009). Effects of a two-generation Canadian preschool program on parenting stress, self-esteem, and life skills. *Early Childhood Services: An Interdisciplinary Journal of Effectiveness, 3*(1), 19–32.

Browne, G., Byrne, C., Roberts, J., Gafni, A., & Whittaker, S. (2001). When the bough breaks: Provider-initiated comprehensive care is more effective and less expensive for sole-support parents on social assistance. *Social Science and Medicine, 53,* 1697–1710.

Campbell, D. T., & Stanley, J. C. (1963). *Experimental and quasi-experimental designs for research.* Chicago: Rand McNally.

Cook, T. D., & Campbell, D. T. (1979). *Quasi-experimental design and analysis issues for field settings.* Chicago: Rand McNally.

Drummond, J. E., Letourneau, N., Neufeld, S. M., Stewart, M., & Weir, A. (2008). Effectiveness of teaching an early parenting approach within a community-based support service for adolescent mothers. *Research in Nursing and Health, 31*(1), 12–22.

Feeley, N., Zelkowitz, P., Carbonneau, L., et al. (2008). Assessing the feasibility and acceptability of an intervention to reduce anxiety and enhance sensitivity among mothers of very low birthweight infants. *Advances in Neonatal Care, 8*(5), 276–284.

Godin, G., Sheeran, P., Conner, M., & Germain, M. (2008). Asking questions changes behaviour: Mere measurement effects on frequency of blood donation. *Health Psychology, 27*(2), 179–184.

Harrison, M. B., Graham, I. D., Lorimer, K., et al. (2008). Nurse clinic versus home delivery of evidence-based community leg ulcer care: A randomized health services trial. *BMC Health Services Research, 8,* 243.

Johnston, C. C., Filion, F., Campbell-Yeo, M., et al. (2008). Kangaroo mothercare diminishes pain from heel lance in very preterm neonates: A crossover trial. *BMC Pediatrics, 8*(13), 1–9.

Johnston, C. C., Rennick, J., Filion, F., et al. (2009). Maternal touch and talk for invasive procedures in infants and toddlers in the PICU. Manuscript under review.

Kerlinger, F. N., & Lee, H. B. (2000). *Foundations of behavioral research* (4th ed.). Orlando, FL: Harcourt College Publishers.

Lazarsfeld, P. (1955). Foreword. In H. Hyman (Ed.), *Survey design and analysis.* New York: The Free Press.

Lespérance, F., Frasure-Smith, N., Koszycki, D., et al. (2007). Effects of Citalopram and interpersonal psychotherapy on depression in patients with coronary artery disease: The Canadian cardiac randomized evaluation of antidepressant and psychotherapy efficacy (CREATE) trial. *JAMA, 297*(4), 367–379.

Markle-Reid, M., Henderson, S., Hecimovich, C., et al. (2007). Reducing fall risk for frail older home-care clients using a multifactorial and interdisciplinary team approach: Design of a randomized controlled trial. *Journal of Patient Safety, 3*(3), 149–157.

Mastel-Smith, B., Binder, B., Malecha, A., Hersch, G, Symes, L., & McFarlane, J. (2006). Testing therapeutic life review offered by home care workers to decrease depression among home-dwelling older women. *Issues in Mental Health Nursing, 27*(10), 1037–1049.

Menihan, C. A., Phipps, M., & Weitzen, S. (2006). Fetal heart rate patterns and sudden infant death syndrome. *Journal of Obstetric, Gynecologic, & Nenonatal Nursing, 35*(1), 116–122.

Metcalfe, K. A., Lubinski, J., Ghadirian, P., et al. (2008). Predictors of contralateral prophylactic mastectomy in women with a BRCA1 or BRCA2 mutation: The hereditary breast cancer clinical study group. *Journal of Clinical Oncology, 26*(7), 1093–1097.

Milke, D. L., Kendall, S., Neumann, I., Wark, C. F., & Knopp, A. (2008). A longitudinal evaluation of restraint reduction within a multi-site, multi-model Canadian continuing care organization. *Canadian Journal on Aging, 27*(1), 35–43.

Poochikian-Sarkissian, S., Wennberg, R. A., & Sidani, S. (2008). Examining the relationship between patient-centred care and outcomes on a neuroscience unit: A pilot project. *Canadian Journal of Neuroscience Nursing, 30*(2), 14–19.

Rush, K. L., McCracken, B., & Talley, C. (2008). Nursing students' self-perceptions as insiders in the practice culture. *Nurse Education in Practice*. Epub ahead of print.

Scott, S., Raymond, P., Thompson, W., & Galt, D. (2005). Efficacy and tolerance of sodium phosphates oral solution after diet liberalization. *Gastroenterology Nursing, 28*(2), 133–139.

Winterburn, S., & Fraser, R. (2000). Does the duration of postnatal stay influence breastfeeding rates at one month in women giving birth for the first time? A randomized control trial. *Journal of Advanced Nursing, 32*, 1152–1157.

Zelkowitz, P., Feeley, N., Shrier, I., et al. (2008). The Cues and Care Trial: A randomized controlled trial of an intervention to reduce maternal anxiety and improve developmental outcomes in very low birthweight infants. *BMC Pediatrics, 8*, 38.

10 Understanding Qualitative Research Design

On completing this chapter, you will be able to:

1. Discuss the rationale for emergent designs in qualitative research and describe qualitative design features

2. Identify the major research traditions for qualitative research and describe the domain of inquiry of each

3. Describe the main features of ethnographic, phenomenological, and grounded theory studies

4. Discuss the goals and methods of various types of research with an ideological perspective

5. Define new terms in the chapter

THE DESIGN OF QUALITATIVE STUDIES

Quantitative researchers specify a research design before collecting their data and adhere to that design once the study is underway; they *design* and then they *do*. In qualitative research, by contrast, the research design typically evolves during the study; qualitative researchers *design* as they *do*. Decisions about how best to obtain data and from whom to obtain data are made in the field, as the study unfolds. Qualitative research design is an **emergent design**—a design that emerges as researchers make ongoing decisions reflecting what has already been learned. As noted by Lincoln and Guba (1985), an emergent design in qualitative studies is not the result of researchers' sloppiness or laziness, but rather of their desire to base the inquiry on the realities and viewpoints of those under study—realities and viewpoints that are not known at the outset.

TIP

Design decisions for a qualitative study are usually summarized in the method section of a report (e.g., a decision to interview a subset of study participants a second time), but the decision-making process for design decisions is rarely described.

Characteristics of Qualitative Research Design

Qualitative inquiry has been guided by a number of different disciplines, and each has developed methods best suited to address questions of interest. However, some general characteristics of qualitative research design apply across disciplines. Qualitative design:

❧ is flexible and elastic, capable of adjusting to what is being learned during the course of data collection;

❧ requires researchers to become intensely involved, often remaining in the field for lengthy periods of time;

❧ requires ongoing analysis of the data to formulate subsequent strategies and to determine when fieldwork is done;

❧ tends to be holistic, striving for an understanding of the whole; and

❧ typically involves a merging together of various data collection strategies.

With regard to the last characteristic, qualitative researchers tend to put together a complex array of data from various sources. This tendency has been described as **bricolage,** and qualitative researchers have been referred to as bricoleurs, people who are "adept at performing a large number of diverse tasks, ranging from interviewing to observing, to interpreting personal and historical documents, to intensive reflection and introspection" (Denzin & Lincoln, 1994, p. 2).

Qualitative Design and Planning

Although design decisions are not made upfront, qualitative researchers typically do advance planning that supports their flexibility in developing an emergent design. In the absence of planning, design choices might actually be constrained. For example, a researcher initially might project a 6-month data collection period, but may need to be prepared to spend even longer in the field to pursue emerging opportunities. In other words, qualitative researchers plan for broad contingencies that may pose decision options in the field. Advance planning is usually important with regard to the following:

❧ Selection of the research tradition (described in the next section) that will guide certain design and analytic decisions

❧ Selection of a study site and identification of settings within the site that are likely to be especially fruitful for data collection

❧ Identification of the key *gatekeepers* who can provide (or deny) access to key data sources and can make arrangements for gaining entry

❧ Determination of the maximum time available for the study

❧ Identification of all needed equipment for the collection and analysis of data in the field (e.g., audio and video recording equipment)

Thus, qualitative researchers plan for a variety of circumstances, but decisions about how they will deal with them must be resolved when the social context of time, place, and human interactions is better understood.

One further task that qualitative researchers typically undertake before (and during) data collection is an analysis of their own biases and ideology. Qualitative researchers tend to accept that research is subjective and may be ideologically driven. Decisions about research design are not value free. Qualitative researchers, then, often take on as an early research challenge the identification of their own biases (discussed further in the section on *descriptive phenomenology*). Such an activity is particularly important in qualitative inquiry because of the intensely personal nature of the data collection and analysis experience.

Example regarding disclosure of possible bias
Hale, Treharne, and Kitas (2007) present an interesting discussion on embracing personal bias in qualitative research rather than "'bracketing' (Meadows & Morse, 2001), whereby the researcher attempts to suspend their own preconceived ideas and interpretations of an event or experience, so they do not re-interpret participants' words in the light of these personal experiences … an emotional detachment from the process, so that personal beliefs and values are not used in the analysis of data. However, complete objectivity can never be achieved in any research project, because we make value judgements throughout the design, execution and dissemination process" (p. 143).

QUALITATIVE RESEARCH TRADITIONS

Although qualitative research designs share some features, there is a wide variety of approaches. There is no readily agreed-on taxonomy, but one useful system is to describe qualitative research according to disciplinary traditions. As we have noted previously, these traditions vary in their view of what questions are important to ask in understanding human experiences. This section provides an overview of qualitative research traditions (some of which we have previously introduced), and subsequent sections describe ethnographies, phenomenological studies, and grounded theory studies in greater detail. In the discussion that follows, we describe *traditional* qualitative inquiry, but a later section examines qualitative studies that adopt a *critical* perspective.

Overview of Qualitative Research Traditions

The research traditions that have provided an underpinning for qualitative studies come primarily from anthropology, psychology, and sociology. As shown in Table 10.1, each discipline has tended to focus on one or two broad domains of inquiry.

TABLE 10.1 OVERVIEW OF QUALITATIVE RESEARCH TRADITIONS

DISCIPLINE	DOMAIN	RESEARCH TRADITION	AREA OF INQUIRY
Anthropology	Culture	Ethnography Ethnoscience (cognitive anthropology)	Holistic view of a culture Mapping of the cognitive world of a culture; a culture's shared meanings, semantic rules
Psychology/ philosophy	Lived experience	Phenomenology Hermeneutics	Experiences of individuals within their lifeworld Interpretations and meanings of individuals' experiences
Psychology	Behaviour and events	Ethology Ecologic psychology	Behaviour observed over time in natural context Behaviour as influenced by the environment
Sociology	Social settings	Grounded theory Ethnomethodology	Social structural processes within a social setting Manner by which shared agreement is achieved in social settings
Sociolinguistics	Human communication	Discourse analysis	Forms and rules of conversation
History	Past behaviour, events, and conditions	Historical analysis	Description and interpretation of historical events

The discipline of anthropology is concerned with human cultures. **Ethnography** is the primary research tradition within anthropology and provides a framework for studying the meanings, patterns, and experiences of a defined cultural group in a holistic fashion. **Ethnoscience** (or *cognitive anthropology*) focuses on the cognitive world of a culture, with particular emphasis on the semantic rules and the shared meanings that shape behaviour. Ethnoscientific studies may rely on quantitative as well as qualitative data.

Example of an ethnoscientific study

Neufeld, Harrison, Stewart, and Hughes (2008) used an ethnographic approach to explore advocacy as a proactive response to nonsupportive interactions with health and social service professionals among women caring for a relative with a chronic condition.

Phenomenology has its roots in both philosophy and psychology. As noted in Chapter 3, phenomenology is concerned with describing the lived experiences of humans. This research method attests that only those who have experienced the phenomenon can truly relate meaning from it for others. A closely related research tradition is **hermeneutics,** which uses the lived experiences of people as a tool to better understand the social, political, and historical context in which those experiences occur. Hermeneutic inquiry almost always focuses on meaning and interpretation—how socially and historically conditioned individuals interpret the world within their given context.

The discipline of psychology has several research traditions that focus on behaviour. Human **ethology,** which is sometimes described as the biology of human behaviour, studies behaviour as it evolves in its natural context. Human ethologists use observational methods to explore universal behavioural structures.

Example of an ethological study

Spiers (2006) used video ethology to examine the interactions and experiences expressing and responding to suffering and stoicism in home-care nurse–patient interactions. The analysis was based on 31 videotaped visits.

Ecological psychology focuses on the environment's influence on human behaviour and attempts to identify principles that explain the interdependence of humans and the environment. Viewed from an ecological context, people are affected by (and affect) a multilayered set of systems, including family, peer group, and neighbourhood, as well as the more indirect effects of health care and social services systems and the larger cultural belief and value systems of the society in which individuals live.

Example of an ecological study

Dwyer et al. (2008) explored the experiences and challenges faced by parents in Ontario, in supporting healthy eating and physical activity in their preschool children. Ecological analysis of data from focus group transcripts led to the categorization of themes according to intrapersonal and interpersonal levels, as well as the broader physical environment.

Sociologists study the social world and have developed several research traditions of importance to qualitative researchers. The grounded theory tradition (described earlier and elaborated on in a later section of this chapter) seeks to understand the key social psychological and structural processes that occur in a social setting.

Ethnomethodology seeks to discover how people make sense of everyday activities and interpret their social world so as to behave in socially acceptable ways. Within this tradition, researchers attempt to understand a social group's norms and assumptions that are so deeply ingrained that members no longer think about the underlying reasons for their behaviours.

Example of an ethnomethodologic study

Buus (2006) explored the exchange of knowledge at nursing shift handovers using one year's fieldwork data at two adjacent mental health hospital wards in Denmark. Ethnomethodology and conversation analysis revealed that "clinical knowledge was conventionalised knowledge because the production, negotiation, and distribution of knowledge were shaped by the local practices for handing over" (p. 1094).

The domain of inquiry for sociolinguists is human communication. The tradition called discourse analysis seeks to understand the rules, mechanisms, and structure of conversations, given the belief that language is never value-free. The data for **discourse analysis** typically are transcripts from naturally occurring conversations, such as those between nurses and their patients, but can also include images, magazine and newspaper articles, documents, and fieldnotes. There are various approaches to this tradition, including critical discourse analysis which has been used to explore the language different speakers bring to a debate over issues of interest (Smith, 2007).

Example of a discourse analysis

Chambers and Narayanasamy (2008) analysed interviews with 12 registered U.K. nurses using discourse analysis to explore nurses' personal constructions of health to show if this influences their health promotion practices with patients. The findings exposed two contradictory value systems (public and private accounts), which may lead to difficulty in fulfilling nurses' role obligations.

Finally, **historical research**—the systematic collection and critical evaluation of data relating to past occurrences—is also a tradition that relies primarily on qualitative data, as well as quantitative data. Similarly to other types of research, the goal of historical inquiry is to discover *new* knowledge. Generally, historical research is undertaken to answer questions about phenomena or issues relating to past events that may shed light on present behaviours or practices. Historical research can take many forms (e.g., bibliographical, social, intellectual, and technological histories) (Polit & Beck, 2008). It is important not to confuse historical research with a review of the literature about historical events.

Example of historical research

Bonifacio and Boschma (2008) examined the controversy surrounding family visitation in postanesthesia care units in North America. Using studies reported in the *Journal of Perianesthesia Nursing* during the period of 1984 to 2006 as the main data source, the authors explored the inconsistencies between current clinical practice (which tends to discourage visitors) and research (which supports the benefits of visitation for both patients and their families), proposing focused investigation of beliefs and workplace culture as a means of resolving remaining barriers.

It should be noted that some qualitative research reports do not identify a research tradition but simply say the study was qualitative. In some cases, a research tradition can be inferred from information about the types of questions that were asked or the methods used to collect and analyze data. However, not all qualitative research *has* a link to one of the traditions we have discussed. Some *descriptive qualitative studies* simply focus on describing a phenomenon in a holistic fashion.

Ethnography

Ethnographies are inquiries that involve the description and interpretation of cultural behaviour. Ethnographies are a blend of a process and a product: fieldwork and a written text. *Fieldwork* is the process by which ethnographers come to understand a culture; ethnographic texts are how that culture is communicated and portrayed. Because culture is, in itself, not visible or tangible, it must be constructed through ethnographic writing. Culture is inferred from the words, actions, and products of members of a group.

Ethnographic research is in some cases concerned with broadly defined cultures (e.g., a Haitian village culture) in a *macroethnography*. However, ethnographies sometimes focus on more narrowly defined cultures in a *microethnography*, which is an exhaustive, fine-grained study of a small unit within a group or culture (e.g., the culture of homeless shelters). An underlying assumption of ethnographers is that every human group eventually evolves a culture that guides the members' view of the world and the way they structure their experiences.

Example of a microethnography
Oudshoorn, Ward-Griffin, and McWilliam (2007) undertook a microethnographic exploration of the client–nurse relationship specific to home-based palliative care in Ontario. The researchers were interested in the sources and exercise of power under such circumstances.

Ethnographers seek to learn from (rather than to study) members of a cultural group. Ethnographers sometimes refer to emic and etic perspectives. An **emic perspective** is the way members of the culture envision their world—the insiders' view. The emic is the local concepts or means of expression used by the members of the group under study to characterize their experiences. The **etic perspective,** by contrast, is the outsiders' interpretation of the culture's experiences; it is the language used by those doing the research to refer to the same phenomena. Ethnographers strive to acquire an emic perspective of a culture. Moreover, they strive to reveal **tacit knowledge,** information about the culture that is so deeply embedded in cultural experiences that members do not talk about it or may not even be consciously aware of it.

Ethnographic research is a labour-intensive and time-consuming endeavour—months and even years of fieldwork may be required to learn about a cultural group. The study of a culture requires a certain level of intimacy with members of the cultural group, and such intimacy can only be developed over time and by working directly with those members as active participants. The concept of *researcher as instrument* is used by anthropologists to describe the significant role ethnographers play in analyzing and interpreting a culture.

Three broad types of information are usually sought by ethnographers: cultural behaviour (what members of the culture do), cultural artefacts (what members of the culture make and use), and cultural speech (what people say). This implies that ethnographers rely on various data sources, including observations, in-depth interviews, and other types of physical evidence (photographs, diaries, letters, and so forth). Ethnographers typically conduct in-depth interviews with about 25 to 50 informants. They also typically use a strategy known as **participant observation** in which they make observations of a community or group while participating in its activities (see Chapter 13).

The products of ethnographic research are rich, holistic descriptions of a culture. Ethnographers also make cultural interpretations, describing normative behavioural and social patterns. Among health care researchers, ethnography provides information about the health beliefs and health-related practices of a culture or subculture. Ethnographic inquiry can thus facilitate understanding of behaviours affecting health and illness.

Phenomenology

Phenomenology, rooted in a philosophical tradition developed by Germans, Husserl, and Heidegger, is an approach to thinking about people's life experiences. Phenomenological researchers ask: What is the *essence* of this phenomenon as experienced by these people at this point in time, and what does it *mean*? Phenomenologists assume there is an essence—an essential invariant structure—that can be understood, in much the same way that ethnographers assume that cultures exist. Phenomenologists investigate subjective phenomena in the belief that key *truths* about reality are grounded in people's lived experiences. The phenomenological approach is especially useful when a phenomenon has been poorly understood. The topics appropriate to phenomenology are ones that are fundamental to the life experiences of humans; for health researchers, these include such topics as the meaning of stress or the experience of bereavement.

Phenomenologists believe that lived experience gives meaning to each person's perception of a particular phenomenon. The goal of phenomenological inquiry is to understand fully lived experience and the perceptions to which it gives rise. Four aspects of lived experience that are of interest are *lived space*, or spatiality; *lived body*, or corporeality; *lived time*, or temporality; and *lived human relation*, or relationality.

Phenomenologists view human existence as meaningful and interesting because of people's consciousness of that existence. The phrase **being-in-the-world** (or *embodiment*) is a concept that acknowledges people's physical ties to their world—they think, see, hear, feel, and are conscious through their bodies' interaction with the world.

In phenomenological studies, the main data source is in-depth conversations with individuals who have experienced the phenomenon of interest, with researchers and informants as coparticipants. Through in-depth conversations, researchers strive to gain entrance into the informants' world, to have full access to their experiences as lived. Two or more separate interviews are sometimes needed. Typically, phenomenological studies involve a small number of study participants—often 10 or fewer—to explore the experience of each informant in sufficient depth. Using this method, the researcher continues sampling until **saturation** is reached (or no new data emerges). For some phenomenological researchers, the inquiry includes not only gathering information from informants but also efforts to experience the phenomenon in the same way, typically through participation, observation, and introspective reflection.

There are a number of variants and methodologic interpretations of phenomenology. The two main schools of thought are descriptive phenomenology and interpretive phenomenology (hermeneutics).

Example of a phenomenological study

Murphy (2007) examined nurses' perceptions of quality care, including the reported barriers and facilitators, for seniors in long-term care in Ireland. In-depth interviews were conducted with 20 nurses, revealing three major themes relevant to quality care: *it should be like home; striving for excellence,* and *making a difference.*

Descriptive Phenomenology

Descriptive phenomenology was developed first by Husserl (1962), who was interested in the question: What do we know as persons? His philosophy emphasized descriptions of human experience. Descriptive phenomenologists insist on the careful description of ordinary conscious experience of everyday life—a description of things as people experience them. These *things* include hearing, seeing, believing, feeling, remembering, deciding, evaluating, acting, and so forth.

Descriptive phenomenological studies often involve four steps: bracketing, intuiting, analyzing, and describing. **Bracketing** refers to the process of identifying and holding in abeyance preconceived beliefs about the phenomenon under study. Although bracketing can never be achieved totally, researchers strive to bracket out the world and any presuppositions in an effort to confront the data in pure form. Phenomenological researchers (as well as other qualitative researchers) often maintain a *reflexive journal* in their efforts to bracket.

Intuiting occurs when researchers remain open to the meanings attributed to the phenomenon by those who have experienced it. Phenomenological researchers then proceed to the analysis phase (i.e., extracting significant statements, categorizing, and making sense of the essential meanings of the phenomenon). Chapter 16 provides further information regarding data analysis in phenomenological studies. Finally, the descriptive phase occurs when researchers come to understand and define the phenomenon.

Example of a descriptive phenomenological study

Mansour and Porter (2008) did a phenomenolocial study designed to describe the experience of teaching nursing research to undergraduates. They elicited descriptions of the experience in e-mail interviews with 12 nurse educators, using three open-ended questions.

Interpretive Phenomenology

Heidegger, a student of Husserl, moved away from his professor's philosophy into **interpretive phenomenology,** or hermeneutics. To Heidegger (1962), the critical question is: What is Being? He stressed interpreting and understanding—not just describing—human experience. Heidegger argued that hermeneutics is a basic characteristic of human existence. Indeed, the term hermeneutics refers to the art and philosophy of interpreting the meaning of an object (such as a *text*, work of art, and so forth). The goals of interpretive phenomenological research are to enter another's world and to discover the practical wisdom, possibilities, and understandings found there.

It should be noted that an important distinction between descriptive and interpretive phenomenology is that in an interpretive phenomenological study, bracketing does not occur. For Heidegger, it was not possible to bracket one's being-in-the-world. Hermeneutics presupposes prior understanding of the phenomenon of interest on the part of the researcher.

Example of an interpretive phenomenological study

Gantert, McWilliam, Ward-Griffin, and Allen (2008) used interpretive phenomenology to explore seniors' perceptions on relationship building, including the barriers and facilitators encountered, with in-home providers within a home care program in Ontario.

Interpretive phenomenologists, like descriptive phenomenologists, rely primarily on in-depth interviews with individuals who have experienced the phenomenon of interest, but, as in the above example, they may go beyond a traditional approach to gathering and analyzing data. For example, interpretive phenomenologists sometimes augment their understandings of the phenomenon through an analysis of supplementary texts, such as novels, poetry, or other artistic expressions—or they use such materials in their conversations with study participants.

Example of a hermeneutic study using artistic expression
Pilkington and Kilpatrick (2008) studied the lived experience of suffering through dialogical engagement (or discussions) with elderly persons living in long-term care. The researchers chose a painting of an elderly man wrapped in a quilt covered in images of memories from his life to represent their new knowledge gleaned through the study.

Grounded Theory

Grounded theory has become an important method for the study of nursing problems and has contributed to the development of many middle-range theories of phenomena of relevance to nurses. Grounded theory began more as a systematic method of qualitative research than as a philosophy. It was developed in the 1960s by two sociologists, Glaser and Strauss (1967), whose theoretical roots were in *symbolic interactionism*, a perspective which focuses on the manner in which people make sense of social interactions and the interpretations they attach to social symbols (e.g., language).

TIP

How can you tell if a phenomenological study is descriptive or interpretive? Phenomenologists often use key terms in their report that can help you make a determination. In a descriptive phenomenological study, such terms may be bracketing, description, essence, Husserl, and phenomenological reduction. The names of Colaizzi, Van Kaam, and Giorgi may be found in the method section. In an interpretive phenomenological study, key terms can include being-in-the-world, shared interpretations, hermeneutics, understanding, and Heidegger. The names van Manen, Benner, and Diekelmann may appear in the method section. These names will be discussed in Chapter 16.

As noted in Chapter 3, grounded theory comprises methods for studying social processes and social structures. The focus of most grounded theory studies is on the discovery of a basic social psychological problem that a group of people experience and on the social psychological stages or phases that characterize the process used to cope with or resolve this basic problem. The primary purpose is to generate a theory that explains a pattern of behaviour that is problematic and relevant to study participants.

Grounded theory methods constitute an entire approach to the conduct of field research. For example, a study that truly follows Glaser and Strauss' precepts does not begin with the identification of a specific research problem. In grounded theory, both the research problem and the process used to resolve it are discovered during the study. A fundamental feature of grounded theory research is that data collection, data analysis, and sampling of participants occur simultaneously. The grounded theory process is recursive; researchers collect data, categorize them, describe the emerging central phenomenon, and then recycle earlier steps.

A procedure called **constant comparison** is used to identify the basic problem and to develop and refine theoretically relevant categories. The categories elicited from the data are constantly compared with data obtained earlier so that commonalities and variations can be determined, and categories can be condensed and collapsed. As data collection proceeds, the inquiry becomes focused on emerging theoretical concerns and core processes. Data analysis in grounded theory studies is described in Chapter 16.

Example of a grounded theory study

Turris and Johnson (2008) conducted a grounded theory study to understand women's experiences seeking treatment for the symptoms of potential cardiac illness—how they interpreted their symptoms, made decisions about seeking treatment, and understood experiences of care in the emergency department. Data were collected through researcher fieldnotes, 17 in-depth interviews with women, and 3 interviews with nurses.

In-depth interviews are the most common data source in grounded theory studies, but observation (including participant observation) and existing documents may also be used. Typically, a grounded theory study involves interviews with a sample of about 25 to 50 informants.

TIP

Grounded theory studies often use gerunds in their titles, which suggest action and change. A gerund is a part of speech ending in "ing." It is part verb (signifying action) and part noun. An example is the title *Living with Dying: The Evolution of Family Members' Experience of Mechanical Ventilation* by Sinuff et al. (2009).

Alternative Views of Grounded Theory

In 1990, Strauss and Corbin published what became a controversial book, *Basics of Qualitative Research: Grounded Theory Procedures and Techniques*. Strauss and Corbin stated that the purpose of the book was to provide beginning grounded theory students with a more concrete description of the procedures involved in building theory at the substantive level.

Glaser, however, disagreed with some of the procedures advocated by Strauss (his original coauthor) and Corbin (a nurse researcher). Glaser published a rebuttal in 1992, *Emergence Versus Forcing: Basics of Grounded Theory Analysis*. Glaser believed that Strauss and Corbin developed a method that is not grounded theory but rather what he calls "full conceptual description." According to Glaser, the purpose of grounded theory is to generate concepts and theories about their relationships that explain and interpret variation in behaviour in the substantive area under study. *Conceptual description*, in contrast, is aimed at describing the full range of behaviour of what is occurring in the substantive area, "irrespective of relevance and accounting for variation in behavior" (Glaser, 1992, p. 19).

Nurse researchers have conducted grounded theory studies using both the original Glaser and Strauss and the Strauss and Corbin approaches. We discuss aspects of the two approaches in more detail in the chapter on data analysis (see Chapter 16).

Formal Grounded Theory

Glaser and Strauss (1967) distinguished two types of grounded theory: substantive and formal. **Substantive theory** is grounded in data on a specific substantive area, such as postpartum depression. It can serve as a springboard for **formal grounded theory,** which involves developing a higher, more abstract level of theory from a compilation of substantive grounded theory studies regarding a particular phenomenon. Glaser and Strauss' (1971) theory of status passage is an example of a formal grounded theory.

Kearney (1998) used an interesting analogy to differentiate substantive theories (custom-tailored clothing) and formal theory (ready-to-wear clothing). Formal grounded theories were likened to clothing sold in department stores that can fit a wider variety of users. Formal grounded theory is not personally tailored like substantive theory, but rather provides a conceptualization that applies to a broader population experiencing a common phenomenon. Formal grounded theories are not situation specific. The best data for constructing formal grounded theories are substantive grounded theories.

Example of a formal grounded theory

Furlong and Wuest (2008) used a formal grounded theory approach to explore the self-care behaviours of nine spousal caregivers of persons with Alzheimer's disease in eastern Canada. The concept of *finding normalcy for self* was discovered, which provides much-needed direction for effective policy in the area.

TIP

Avoid jumping to conclusions about the research tradition of a study based on the report's title. For example, the study *The personal significance of home: Habitus and the experience of receiving long-term home care* (Angus, Kontos, Dyck, McKeever, & Poland, 2005) is not a phenomenological study but rather an ethnographic study of home care in 16 homes in Ontario—even though the word *experience* in the title might suggest otherwise. As another example, despite the title's suggestion of a focus on cultural issues, *Giving birth: The voices of orthodox Jewish women living in Canada* (Semenic, Callister, & Feldman, 2004) is a phenomenological study, not an ethnographic one.

RESEARCH WITH IDEOLOGICAL PERSPECTIVES

An emerging trend in nursing research is to conduct inquiries within ideological frameworks, typically to draw attention to certain social problems or the needs of certain groups. These approaches, which represent important investigative avenues, usually rely primarily on qualitative data and interpretive methods of analysis.

Critical Theory

Critical theory originated within a group of Marxist-oriented German scholars in the 1920s, collectively referred to as the Frankfurt School. Essentially, critical researchers are concerned with a critique of society and with envisioning new possibilities.

Critical research is typically action-oriented. Its broad aim is to integrate theory and practice so that people become aware of contradictions and disparities in their beliefs and social practices, and become inspired to change them. Critical researchers reject the idea of an objective, disinterested inquirer, and are oriented toward a transformation process. Critical theory calls for inquiries that foster enlightened self-knowledge and sociopolitical action. Moreover, critical theory involves a self-reflexive aspect. To prevent a critical theory of society from becoming yet another self-serving ideology, critical theorists must account for their own transformative effects.

The design of research within critical theory often begins with a thorough analysis of certain aspects of a problem. For example, critical researchers might analyze and critique taken-for-granted assumptions that underlie a problem, the

TABLE 10.2 ⊙	COMPARISON OF TRADITIONAL QUALITATIVE RESEARCH AND CRITICAL RESEARCH	
ISSUE	TRADITIONAL QUALITATIVE RESEARCH	CRITICAL RESEARCH
Research aims	Understanding; reconstruction of multiple constructions	Critique; transformation; consciousness raising; advocacy
View of knowledge	Transactional/subjective; knowledge is created in interaction between investigator and participants	Transactional/subjective; value mediated and value dependent; importance of historical insights
Method	Dialectic: truth arrived at logically through conversations	Dialectic and didactic: dialogue designed to transform naivety and misinformation
Evaluative criteria for inquiry quality	Authenticity; trustworthiness	Historical situatedness of the inquiry; erosion of ignorance; stimulus for change
Researcher's role	Facilitator of multivoice reconstruction	Transformative agent; advocate; activist

language used to depict the situation, and the biases of prior researchers investigating the problem. Critical researchers often triangulate multiple methodologies and emphasize multiple perspectives (e.g., alternative racial or social class perspectives) on problems. Critical researchers interact with study participants in ways that emphasize participants' expertise. Some of the features that distinguish more traditional qualitative research and critical research are summarized in Table 10.2.

Critical theory has played an especially important role in ethnography. *Critical ethnography* focuses on raising consciousness and aiding emancipatory goals in the hope of effecting social change. Critical ethnographers address the social, political, and economic dimensions of cultures and their value-laden agendas. An assumption in critical ethnographic research is that actions and thoughts are mediated by power relationships. Critical ethnographers attempt to increase the political dimensions of cultural research and undermine oppressive systems.

Example of a critical ethnography

Martin and Kipling (2006) undertook a critical ethnographic study to explore the undergraduate experience for Canadian Aboriginal nursing students, with the goal of uncovering best strategies for their recruitment and retention.

Feminist Research

Feminist research uses approaches that are similar to those of critical theory research, but it focuses sharply on gender domination and discrimination within patriarchal societies. Like critical researchers, feminist researchers seek to establish collaborative, nonexploitive relationships with their informants, to avoid objectification, and to conduct research that is transformative. Feminist researchers stress *intersubjectivity* between researchers and participants and the mutual creation of knowledge.

Gender is the organizing principle in feminist research, and investigators seek to understand how gender and a gendered social order have shaped women's lives. The aim is to alter the "invisibility and distortion of female experience in ways relevant to ending women's unequal social position" (Lather, 1991, p. 71). The purpose of feminist research is to provide information *for* women, not just *about* women.

The scope of feminist research ranges from studies of the particular and subjective views of individual women, to studies of social movements and broad policies that affect (and often exclude) women. Olesen (1994), a sociologist who studied nurses' career patterns and definitions of success, has noted that some of the best feminist research on women's subjective experiences has been done in the area of women's health.

Feminist research methods generally include in-depth, collaborative individual interviews or group interviews that offer the possibility of reciprocally educational encounters. Feminists generally seek to negotiate the meanings of the results with those participating in the study, and to be self-reflexive about what they themselves are experiencing and learning. In feminist research, the researcher's history, assumptions, interests, motives, and interpretations are explicitly scrutinized in the process of the study.

Feminist research, like other research with an ideological perspective, has raised the bar for the conduct of ethical research. With the emphasis on trust, empathy, and nonexploitive relationship, proponents of these newer modes of inquiry view any type of deception or manipulation as abhorrent. As Punch (1994) has noted in speaking about ethics and feminist research, "you do not rip off your sisters" (p. 89).

Example of feminist research
Peters, Jackson, and Rudge (2007) conducted a feminist study to explore the differences between perceptions of *success* portrayed by assisted reproductive technology (ART) services in Australia and New Zealand, and experienced by participant couples who have accessed these services. By examining textual data from formal reports and ART websites, as well as interviews with participant couples, the researchers found that the perceptions portrayed by ART services "are disparate to those held by participant couples, and as statistics are manipulated to promote further patronage of ART services, the likelihood of 'success' is overstated" (p. 130).

Participatory Action Research

Participatory action research (PAR) is closely allied to both critical research and feminist research. PAR, one of several types of *action research* that originated in the 1940s with social psychologist Kurt Lewin, is based on a recognition that the use and production of knowledge can be political and can be used to exert power. PAR researchers typically work with groups or communities that are vulnerable to the control or oppression of a dominant group or culture.

PAR is, as the name implies, participatory. There is collaboration between researchers and study participants in the definition of the problem, the selection of an approach and research methods, the analysis of the data, and the use to which findings are put. The aim of PAR is to produce not only knowledge but also action and consciousness-raising. Researchers specifically seek to empower people through the process of constructing knowledge. The PAR tradition has as its starting point a concern for the powerlessness of the group under study. Thus, a key objective is to produce action that is directly used to make improvements through education and sociopolitical action.

In PAR, the research methods take second place to emergent processes of collaboration and dialogue that can motivate, increase self-esteem, and generate solidarity. Thus, data-gathering strategies are not only the traditional methods of interview and observation (including both qualitative and quantitative approaches) but also may include storytelling, sociodrama, drawing and painting, and other activities designed to encourage people to find creative ways to explore their lives and recognize their own strengths.

Example of participatory action research

Etowa, Wiens, Bernard, and Clow (2007) used PAR to study the experiences of African-Canadian women living in rural and remote communities in Nova Scotia, with regards to their health status, health care delivery and health services utilization. The *On the Margins* project collected a range of data, including 237 in-depth one-on-one interviews and 12 focus groups with this marginalized population.

CRITIQUING QUALITATIVE DESIGNS

Evaluating a qualitative design is often difficult. Qualitative researchers do not always document design decisions and are even less likely to describe the process by which such decisions were made. Researchers often do, however, indicate whether the study was conducted within a specific qualitative tradition. This information can be used to come to some conclusions about the study design. For example, if a report indicated that the researcher conducted 1 month of fieldwork for an ethnographic study, there would be reason to suspect that insufficient time had been spent in the field to obtain a true emic perspective of the culture under study. Ethnographic studies may also be critiqued if their only source of information was from interviews, rather than from a broader range of data sources including observations.

In a grounded theory study, you might also be concerned if the researcher relied exclusively on data from interviews; a stronger design might have been obtained by including participant observations. Also, look for evidence about when the data were collected and analyzed. If the researcher collected all the data before analyzing any of it, you might question whether the constant comparative method was used correctly.

In critiquing a phenomenological study, you should first determine whether the study is descriptive or interpretive. This will help you to assess how closely the researcher kept to the basic tenets of that qualitative research tradition. For example, in a descriptive phenomenological study, did the researcher bracket?

No matter what qualitative design is identified in a study, look to see if the researchers stayed true to a single qualitative tradition throughout the study or if they mixed qualitative traditions, possibly weakening the rigour of the study. For example, did the researcher state that a grounded theory design was used, but then present results that described *themes* instead of generating a substantive theory?

The guidelines in Box 10.1 are intended to assist you in critiquing the designs of qualitative studies.

BOX 10.1 GUIDELINES FOR CRITIQUING QUALITATIVE DESIGNS

1. Is the research tradition for the qualitative study identified? If none was identified, can one be inferred? If more than one was identified, is this justifiable or does it suggest method *slurring*?

2. Is the research question congruent with a qualitative approach and with the specific research tradition (i.e., is the domain of inquiry for the study congruent with the domain encompassed by the tradition)? Are the data sources, research methods, and analytic approach congruent with the research tradition?

3. How well is the research design described? Are design decisions explained and justified? Does it appear that the researcher made all design decisions up-front, or did the design emerge during data collection, allowing researchers to capitalize on early information?

4. Is the design appropriate, given the research question? Does the design lend itself to a thorough, in-depth, intensive examination of the phenomenon of interest? What design elements might have strengthened the study (e.g., a longitudinal perspective rather than a cross-sectional one)?

5. Was there appropriate evidence of reflexivity in the design?

6. Was the study undertaken with an ideological perspective? If so, is there evidence that ideological methods and goals were achieved? (e.g., Was there evidence of full collaboration between researchers and participants? Did the research have the power to be transformative, or is there evidence that a transformative process occurred?)

TIP

In this age of the Internet, students and researchers have access to information on qualitative design at their fingertips. Two important websites are:

www.phenomenologyonline.com
www.groundedtheory.com

RESEARCH EXAMPLES AND CRITICAL THINKING ACTIVITIES

EXAMPLE 1 ■ Discourse Analysis

Aspects of a nursing study applying discourse analysis, featuring terms and concepts discussed in this chapter, are presented here, followed by some questions to guide critical thinking.

Study

"A discourse and Foucauldian analysis of nurses health beliefs: Implications for nurse education" (Chambers & Narayanasamy, 2008)

Aim

The aim of the study was to investigate nurses' personal constructions of health to establish what influence these have on their health promotion practices.

Method

The study used discourse analysis of hierarchial focused interviews with 12 registered nurses in the United Kingdom. The analysis consisted of reading and re-reading the interview transcripts; examining in detail "the regularity and variability of patterns, use of rhetoric, adoption of subject positions, resistance and acceptance of dominant discourses"; labelling the identified domains; "interpreting the nature of the variability and the prevalence of any patterns in the variability"; and finally, consultation with validators (or colleagues uninvolved in the research) to ensure the validity of findings (p. 158).

Key Findings

- Two opposing values emerged—a holistic view and an individualistic or victim blaming view. Nurses need to be critically reflective of such contradictory views.

- These contradicting values imply that although nurses enact their expected role in terms of providing care, "… the nurse is also capable of displaying converse attitudes to those relatives and patients whose values are contradictory to his or her own" (p. 161).

CRITICAL THINKING SUGGESTIONS

1. Answer questions 1 through 6 from Box 10.1 (p. 185) regarding this study.
2. Also consider the following targeted questions, which may assist you in further assessing aspects of the study:
   a. What are hierarchical focused interviews? Why was this type of interviewing suited to this study?
   b. Why was discourse analysis chosen?
   c. Could this study have been conducted as a phenomenological study? As a grounded theory study? Why or why not?
3. If the results of this study are trustworthy, what are some of the uses to which the findings might be put into clinical practice?

EXAMPLE 2 ■ Grounded Theory Study

Aspects of a grounded theory study, featuring terms and concepts discussed in this chapter, are presented below, followed by some questions to guide critical thinking.

Study

"Maintaining integrity: Women and treatment seeking for the symptoms of potential cardiac illness" (Turris & Johnson, 2008)

Statement of Purpose

The purpose of this grounded theory study was to understand how women seeking treatment for the symptoms of potential cardiac illness interpreted their symptoms, made decisions about seeking treatment, and understood experiences of care in the emergency department.

Context

The researchers acknowledged the gender debate concerning cardiac illness and its treatment, presentation of symptoms, and delay in seeking treatment.

Method

The researchers chose a grounded theory approach because, "In the complicated world of health care, a sense of 'what is going on here?'—with a focus on overall meaning, rather than discrete events—is invaluable for creating theory. The focus of grounded theory is on understanding the basic social and/or psychological process that is taking place" (p. 1464). Data were collected through researcher fieldnotes, 17 in-depth interviews with women, and 3 interviews with nurses, over a year long period at two emergency departments in a Canadian city. Open, selective and theoretical coding processes were utilized.

Key Findings

The basic social psychological process of maintaining integrity . . . . the process the women used to keep intact their sense of self and to keep going in the context of their daily lives, despite the threat . . . " (p. 1466) emerged across personal, social and physical dimensions. The women were also seen to go through three phases: (1) "resisting disruption (pre-hospital)"; (2) "suspending agency" (in-hospital); and (3) "integrating new knowledge and experience" (after discharge) (p. 1466).

CRITICAL THINKING SUGGESTIONS

1. Answer questions 1 through 6 from Box 10.1 (p. 185) regarding this study.
2. Also consider the following targeted questions, which may assist you in further assessing aspects of the study:
   a. Did the researchers develop a substantive theory or a formal theory?
   b. Was this study longitudinal or cross-sectional?
   c. Could this study have been conducted as a phenomenological study? As an ethnographic study? Why or why not?
3. If the results of this study are trustworthy, what are some of the uses to which the findings might be put into clinical practice?

Summary Points

- ➤ Qualitative research typically involves an **emergent design**—a design that emerges as the study unfolds.
- ➤ As **bricoleurs,** qualitative researchers are creative and intuitive, putting together data drawn from many sources to arrive at a holistic understanding of a phenomenon.
- ➤ Although qualitative design is flexible, qualitative researchers nevertheless plan for broad contingencies that are expected to pose decision opportunities for design decisions in the field.

⇝ A naturalistic inquiry typically progresses through three broad phases in the field: an orientation phase to determine what it is about the key phenomenon that is salient, a focused exploration phase that closely examines important aspects of the phenomenon, and a confirmation and closure phase to confirm findings.

⇝ Qualitative research traditions have their roots in anthropology (e.g., *ethnography* and **ethnoscience**), philosophy (*phenomenology* and **hermeneutics**), psychology (**ethology, ecological psychology**), sociology (*grounded theory, ethnomethodology*), sociolinguistics (**discourse analysis**), and history (**historical research**).

⇝ Some *descriptive qualitative* studies are not linked to any research tradition and are designed to describe some phenomenon in an in-depth, holistic fashion.

⇝ Ethnography focuses on the culture of a group of people and relies on extensive fieldwork. The ethnographer strives to acquire an **emic,** or insider's, **perspective** of the culture under study and to discover deeply embedded **tacit knowledge;** the outsider's perspective is known as **etic.**

⇝ Phenomenology seeks to determine the essence and meaning of a phenomenon as it is experienced by people.

⇝ In **descriptive phenomenology,** researchers describe lived experiences by **bracketing out** any preconceived views and **intuiting** the essence of the phenomenon by remaining open to the meanings attributed to it by those who have experienced it.

⇝ Bracketing is not a feature of **interpretive phenomenology** (hermeneutics), which focuses on interpreting the meaning of experiences.

⇝ *Grounded theory* is an approach to generating a theory to explain a pattern of behaviour that is problematic and relevant to participants. This approach uses **constant comparison** – categories elicited from the data are constantly compared with data obtained earlier so that shared patterns and variations can be determined.

⇝ There are two types of grounded theory: **substantive theory,** which is grounded in data on a specific substantive area, and **formal grounded theory** (often using data from substantive theory studies) that is at a higher level of abstraction.

⇝ Research is sometimes conducted within an ideological perspective, and such research tends to rely primarily on qualitative research.

⇝ **Critical theory** is concerned with a critique of existing social structures; critical researchers conduct inquiries that involve collaboration with participants and foster enlightened transformation. *Critical ethnography* uses the principles of critical theory in the study of cultures.

⇝ **Feminist research,** like critical research, is designed to be transformative, but the focus is sharply on how gender domination and discrimination shape women's lives.

⇝ **Participatory action research** (PAR) produces knowledge through close collaboration with groups or communities that are vulnerable to control or oppression by a dominant culture. In PAR, research methods take second place to emergent processes that can motivate people and generate community solidarity.

STUDIES CITED IN CHAPTER 10*

This reference list contains only those studies that were cited in this chapter. Citations pertaining to theoretical, methodologic, or nonempirical work are included together in a separate section at the end of the book (beginning on page 399).

Angus, J., Kontos, P., Dyck, I., McKeever, P., & Poland, B. (2005). The personal significance of home: Habitus and the experience of receiving long-term home care. *Sociology of Health & Illness, 27*(2), 161–187.

Bonifacio, N. C., & Boschma, G. (2008). Family visitation in the PACU, 1984–2006. *Journal of Perianesthesia Nursing, 23*(2), 94–101.

Buus, N. (2006). Conventionalized knowledge: Mental health nurses producing clinical knowledge at intershift handovers. *Issues in Mental Health Nursing, 27*(10), 1079–1096.

Chambers, D., & Narayanasamy, A. (2008). A discourse and Foucauldian analysis of nurses health beliefs: Implications for nurse education. *Nurse Education Today, 28*(2), 155–162.

Denzin, N. K., & Lincoln, Y. S. (Eds.). (1994). *Handbook of Qualitative Research*, Thousand Oaks, CA: Sage.

Etowa, J., Wiens, J., Bernard, W. T., & Clow, B. (2007). Determinants of black women's health in rural and remote communities. *Canadian Journal of Nursing Research, 39*(3), 56–76.

Furlong, K. E., & Wuest, J. (2008). Self-care behaviours of spouses caring for significant others with Alzheimer's disease: The emergence of self-care worthiness as a salient condition. *Qualitative Health Research, 18*(12), 1662–1672.

Gantert, T. W., McWilliam, C. L., Ward-Griffin, C., & Allen, N. J. (2008). The key to me: Seniors' perceptions of relationship-building with in-home service providers. *Canadian Journal on Aging, 27*(1), 23–34.

Hale, E. D., Treharne, G. J., & Kitas, G. D. (2007). Qualitative methodologies 1: Asking research questions with reflexive insight. *Musculoskeletal Care, 5*(3), 139–147.

Mansour, T., & Porter, E. J. (2008). Educators' experience of teaching nursing research to undergraduates. *Western Journal of Nursing Research, 30*(7), 888–904.

Martin, D. E., & Kipling, A. (2006). Factors shaping Aboriginal nursing students' experiences. *Nurse Education Today, 26*(8), 688–696.

Murphy, K. (2007). A qualitative study explaining nurses' perceptions of quality care for older people in long-term care settings in Ireland. *Journal of Clinical Nursing, 16*(3), 477–485.

Neufeld, A., Harrison, M. J., Stewart, M., & Hughes, K. (2008). Advocacy of women family caregivers: Response to nonsupportive interactions with professionals. *Qualitative Health Research, 18*(3), 301–310.

Oudshoorn, A., Ward-Griffin, C., & McWilliam, C. (2007). Client-nurse relationships in home-based palliative care: A critical analysis of power relations. *Journal of Clinical Nursing, 16*(8), 1435–1443.

Peters, K., Jackson, D., & Rudge, T. (2007). Failures of reproduction: Problematising "success" in assisted reproductive technology. *Nursing Inquiry, 14*(2), 125–131.

Pilkington, F. B., & Kilpatrick, D. (2008). The lived experience of suffering: A Parse research method study. *Nursing Science Quarterly, 21*(3), 228–337.

Semenic, S. E., Callister, L. C., & Feldman, P. (2004). Giving birth: The voices of orthodox Jewish women living in Canada. *Journal of Obstetric, Gynecologic, and Neonatal Nursing, 33*(1), 80–87.

Sinuff, T., Giacomini, M., Shaw, R., Swinton, M., & Cook, D. J. (2009). Living with dying: the evolution of family members' experience of mechanical ventilation. *Critical Care Medicine, 37*(1), 154–8.

Spiers, J. (2006). Expressing and responding to pain and stoicism in home-care nurse-patient interactions. *Scandinavian Journal of Caring Sciences, 20*(3), 293–301.

Turris, S. A., & Johnson, J. L. (2008). Maintaining integrity: Women and treatment seeking for the symptoms of potential cardiac illness. *Qualitative Health Research, 18*(11), 1461–1476.

11 Examining Specific Types of Research

On completing this chapter, you will be able to:

1. Identify the purposes and some of the distinguishing features of specific types of research (e.g., clinical trials, surveys)

2. Determine whether researchers' primary approach (qualitative versus quantitative) and design were appropriate for the type of research

3. Identify several advantages of mixed method research and describe specific applications

4. Define new terms in the chapter

All quantitative studies can be categorized as either experimental, quasi-experimental/pre-experimental, or nonexperimental, as discussed in Chapter 9. And, most qualitative studies lie within one of the research traditions described in Chapter 10. This chapter describes types of qualitative and quantitative research that vary according to study purpose rather than according to research design or tradition. The chapter also describes mixed method research that combines qualitative and quantitative approaches in a single project.

STUDIES THAT ARE TYPICALLY QUANTITATIVE

The research described in this section usually uses quantitative approaches, but it is important to note that for certain types of research (e.g., evaluation research), qualitative methods may also be added as a component in a mixed method strategy.

Clinical Trials

Clinical trials are studies designed to assess the effectiveness of clinical interventions. Methods associated with clinical trials have been developed for medical and epidemiological research, but nurse researchers are increasingly adopting these methods to test nursing interventions.

Clinical trials undertaken to test innovative therapies often are designed in a series of phases.

➤ *Phase I* of the trial occurs after the initial development of the drug or therapy and is designed primarily to determine things like drug dose (or strength of the therapy), safety, and patient tolerance. This phase typically uses pre-experimental designs (e.g., before–after designs without a control group). The focus is not on efficacy, but on developing the best possible treatment.

⮞ *Phase II* of the trial involves seeking preliminary evidence of the effectiveness of the treatment as it has been designed in Phase I. This is typically done by using a pre-experimental or quasi-experimental design or sometimes an experimental design with a small sample. During this phase, researchers assess the feasibility of launching a larger, more rigorous test, seek evidence that the treatment holds promise, and look for possible side effects. This phase is considered a *pilot test* of the treatment. There have been clinical trials of drug therapies that have shown such powerful effects during this phase that further phases were considered unnecessary and even unethical, but this would rarely be true in nursing studies.

Example of a Phase II clinical trial
Keefe and colleagues (2006) developed REST interventions (reassurance, empathy, support, and time-out) for parents of irritable infants, based on a theory of infant colic that Keefe herself had previously developed. The trial to test the efficacy of REST involved randomly assigning infants to two sites, either treatment or control group.

⮞ *Phase III* is a full experimental test of the treatment, involving random assignment to groups or to orderings of treatment conditions. The objective of this phase is to determine the efficacy of the innovation compared with the standard treatment or an alternative counterfactual. When the term *clinical trial* is used in the nursing literature, it usually is referring to a Phase III trial, which may also be called a **randomized clinical trial** (RCT). Phase III clinical trials usually involve the use of a large and heterogeneous sample of subjects, frequently selected from multiple, geographically dispersed sites to ensure that findings are not unique to a single setting.

⮞ *Phase IV* of a trial occurs after the decision to adopt an innovation has been made. In this phase, researchers monitor the long-term consequences of the intervention as it is used in actual practice, including both benefits and side effects. This phase might use a nonexperimental, pre-experimental, or quasi-experimental design.

Example of a multisite randomized clinical trial
Brown-Etris et al. (2008) conducted a 19-month prospective, randomized, multisite clinical evaluation of a transparent absorbent acrylic dressing (TAAD) and a hydrocolloid dressing (HD) in the management of stage II and shallow stage III pressure ulcers. A total of 72 patients who were evenly randomly assigned to either the TAAD or HD treatments were enrolled across five study sites, four of which were in the United States and one in Canada. In addition, patients were recruited from a variety of health care settings, including extended care facilities, outpatient wound care clinics, and home-care agencies.

Evaluations

Evaluations are used to find out how well a program, treatment, or policy works. Clinical nurses, nurse administrators, and nursing educators often need to pose such questions as the following: How are current practices working? Should a new practice be adopted? Which approach is most effective? In this era of accountability, evaluations of the effectiveness of nursing actions are common. Evaluations can employ experimental, quasi-experimental, or nonexperimental designs and can be either cross-sectional or longitudinal. Although most evaluations are quantitative, certain aspects of programs are often evaluated using qualitative methods.

Clinical trials are sometimes evaluations. As an example, Steel-O'Connor et al. (2003) evaluated the effectiveness of two public health nurse follow-up programs (home visits and telephone follow-up) in terms of infant health problems, breast-feeding rates, and use of postpartum health services. Their program evaluation involved a multisite clinical trial in Ontario. Generally, the term *evaluation research* is used when researchers are trying to determine the effectiveness of a rather complex program, rather than when they are testing a specific entity (e.g., alternative drugs or sterilizing solutions). Thus, not all clinical trials would be called evaluations, and not all evaluations use methods associated with clinical trials. Moreover, evaluations often try to answer broader questions than simply whether an intervention is more effective clinically than care as usual. Evaluations may involve determining how the intervention was actually put into place, for example.

There are various types of evaluations. A **process analysis** (or an **implementation analysis**) obtains descriptive information about the process of implementing a new program or procedure and about its functioning in actual operation. Process evaluations, which often rely on both qualitative and quantitative data, are designed to address such questions as the following: What are the strongest and weakest aspects of the program? What exactly *is* the treatment, and how does it differ from traditional practices? What were the barriers to implementing the program successfully?

Example of a process analysis

Baumbusch et al. (2008) described the process of developing a collaborative participatory approach to knowledge translation during an ongoing program of research concerning equitable care for diverse populations. Documented were the complexities of translating knowledge within the political landscape of health care delivery, the need to negotiate researchers and practitioners' agendas in a collaborative approach, and resources needed to support the process.

An **outcome analysis** documents the extent to which the goals of a program are attained, to obtain preliminary evidence about program success (e.g., the extent to which positive outcomes are in line with the original intent). Outcome analyses are descriptive and do not use experimental designs; before–after designs without a comparison group are common.

Example of an outcome analysis

As part of a larger study to evaluate the contribution of nurse practitioners to acute care settings, Sidani (2008) examined patients' perceptions of the extent to which acute care nurse practitioners provided patient-centred care (PCC), and the effects of PCC on patient outcomes such as functional status, self care ability, and satisfaction with care.

An **impact analysis** attempts to identify the *impacts* or *net effects* of an intervention (i.e., the effects over and above what would have occurred in its absence). Impact analyses use an experimental or quasi-experimental design because their goal is to attribute a causal connection between outcomes and the intervention. Many nursing evaluations are impact analyses, although they are not necessarily labelled as such.

Example of an impact analysis

Using a quasi-experimental design, Marchand et al. (2008) studied the impact of clinical implementation of a scrub less chlorhexidine/ethanol preoperative surgical hand rub on the incidence of surgical site infection rates, reported skin irritations, and health care personnel acceptance in a 160-bed university affiliated heart institute. Retrospective data analysis was used to compare outcome measures collected during the first year of implementation of the new method, to the last full year of the standard surgical scrub preparation.

Finally, evaluations sometimes include a **cost–benefit analysis** to determine whether the monetary benefits of a program outweigh the costs. Administrators make decisions about resource allocations for health services not only on the basis of whether something "works" but also on the basis of whether it is economically viable. Cost–benefit analyses are typically done in connection with impact analyses and Phase III clinical trials, that is, when researchers establish solid evidence regarding program effectiveness.

Example of a cost analysis

Guerriere et al. (2008) assessed the costs and determinants of privately financed home-based health care in Ontario. Five hundred and fourteen clients were interviewed by telephone and asked to provide information about time and monetary costs of care. The mean total cost of care for a 4-week period was $7,670.67 (CAN) and 75% of these costs were associated with private expenditures. Higher age, activities of daily living impairment, being female and having four or more chronic conditions predicted higher private expenditures.

Outcomes Research

Outcomes research, designed to document the effectiveness of health care services, is gaining momentum in nursing and health care fields. Although outcomes research overlaps with evaluation research, evaluations typically appraise a specific new intervention, whereas outcomes research is a more global assessment of health care services. The impetus for outcomes research comes from the quality assessment and quality assurance functions that grew out of the professional standards review organizations (PSROs) in the 1970s. Outcomes research represents a response to the increasing demand from policy makers, insurers, and the public to justify care practices in terms of improved patient outcomes and costs.

Although many nursing studies are concerned with examining patient outcomes and patient satisfaction, specific efforts to appraise and document the quality of nursing care—as distinct from the care provided by the overall health care system—are not numerous. A major obstacle is attribution—that is, linking patient outcomes to specific nursing actions, distinct from the actions of other members of the health care team. It is also difficult in some cases to determine a causal connection between outcomes and health care interventions because factors outside the health care system (e.g., patient characteristics) affect outcomes in complex ways.

Nevertheless, outcomes research continues to expand. There is increasing interest, for example, in describing the work that nurses do in terms of established classification, and there is also interest in maintaining complete and accurate records of nursing actions in computerized data sets (referred to as *nursing minimal data sets* or *NMDS*). A number of research-based classification systems of nursing interventions are being developed, refined, and tested, including the Nursing Diagnoses Taxonomy of the North American Nursing Diagnosis Association (NANDA) and the Nursing Intervention Classification (NIC) developed at the University of Iowa. Studies with these classification systems have thus far focused on descriptions of patient problems and nursing interventions, and assessments of the utility of these systems.

Example of a study using the NIC system

Lunney (2006) examined the effects of implementing NANDA diagnoses, interventions from NIC, and outcomes from the NOC on nurses' power and children's health outcomes, using nurses' reports of health visits with children in six schools.

Just as there have been efforts to develop classifications of nursing interventions, work has been undertaken to develop outcome classification systems. Of particular note is the Nursing Outcomes Classification (NOC) developed by nurses at the University of Iowa College of Nursing to complement the NIC (Johnson & Maas, 1998). The NOC system was designed to measure patient outcomes that are sensitive to nursing care and to help standardize these outcomes. The NOC includes 260 patient outcomes categorized into seven domains: functional health, physiologic health, psychosocial health, health knowledge and behaviour, perceived health, family health, and community health.

Sidani, Doran, and Mitchell (2004) recently advocated a theory-driven approach to evaluating the quality of nursing care. Their approach focuses on the identification of patient, professional, and setting characteristics that affect processes of health care that, in turn, affect patient outcomes.

Example of outcomes research
Kyung and Chin (2008) studied the outcomes of a 4-week pulmonary rehabilitation program for older patients with chronic obstructive pulmonary disease (COPD). The program was associated with significant improvement in exercise performance and reduced dyspnea.

Surveys

A **survey** obtains information regarding the prevalence, distribution, and interrelationships of variables within a population (e.g., political opinion polls). Surveys collect information on people's actions, knowledge, intentions, opinions, and attitudes.

Survey data are based on **self-reports**—respondents answer questions posed by researchers. Survey data can be collected in a number of ways, but the most respected method is through **personal interviews** (or *face-to-face interviews*), in which interviewers meet with respondents to ask them questions. Personal interviews are usually costly because they tend to involve a lot of personnel time. Nevertheless, personal interviews are considered the best means of collecting survey data because the quality of data they yield is higher than other methods and because relatively few people refuse to be interviewed in person. **Telephone interviews** are a less costly, but often less effective, method of gathering survey data. When the interviewer is unknown, respondents may be uncooperative on the telephone. Telephoning can, however, be a convenient method of collecting information if the interview is short and not too personal. Telephone interviews may be difficult for certain groups of respondents, including low-income people (who do not always have a telephone) and the elderly (who may have hearing problems).

Survey researchers can also distribute **questionnaires,** which are self-administered. Because respondents differ in their reading levels and in their ability to communicate in writing, questionnaires are *not* merely a printed form of an interview. Self-administered questionnaires are economical but are not appropriate for surveying certain populations (e.g., the elderly, children). Survey questionnaires are generally distributed through the mail but may also be distributed in other ways (e.g., through the Internet).

Survey research is highly flexible: it can be applied to many populations, and it can focus on a wide range of topics. Survey data tend, however, to be relatively superficial. Survey research is better suited to extensive rather than intensive analysis. Although surveys can be done within the context of experiments, they are usually nonexperimental.

Example of a survey
Kulig et al. (2008) conducted a survey of Canadian nurses practicing in rural and remote regions to learn about their experiences and perceptions. Questionnaires were mailed to more than 5700 nurses, using postal codes from RN registration data, to locate nurses in all provinces and northern territories.

STUDIES THAT CAN BE QUALITATIVE OR QUANTITATIVE

The studies described in the previous section are typically conducted with formal instruments designed to yield quantitative data. The types of studies described in this section can be either qualitative or quantitative.

Case Studies

Case studies are in-depth investigations of a single entity or a small number of entities. The entity may be an individual, family, group, community, or other social unit. In a case study, researchers obtain a wealth of descriptive information and may examine relationships among different phenomena. Case study researchers attempt to analyze and understand issues that are important to the history, development, or circumstances of the person or entity under study.

One way to think of a case study is to consider what is centre stage. In most studies, whether qualitative or quantitative, a certain phenomenon or variable (or set of variables) is the core of the inquiry. In a case study, the *case* itself is central. As befits an intensive analysis, the focus of case studies is typically on determining the dynamics of *why* an individual thinks, behaves, or develops in a particular manner rather than on *what* his or her status or actions are. It is not unusual for probing research of this type to require detailed study over a considerable period. Data are often collected that relate not only to the person's present state but also to past experiences and situational factors relevant to the problem being examined.

The greatest strength of case studies is the depth that is possible when a limited number of individuals or groups are being investigated. On the other hand, this same strength is a potential weakness because researchers' familiarity with the person or group may make objectivity more difficult. The biggest criticism of case studies concerns generalizability: if researchers discover important relationships, it is difficult to know whether the same relationships would occur with others. However, case studies can often play a critical role in challenging generalizations based on other types of research.

It is important to recognize that case study research is not simply anecdotal descriptions of a particular incident or patient. Case study research is a disciplined process and typically requires an extended period of systematic data collection.

Example of a qualitative case study
Using in-depth interviews, Macdonald et al. (2008) conducted a case study of a bereaved mother. Nine months following the death of her daughter from a traumatic brain injury, the researchers sought to better understand the moral and medical complexities involved in clinician–family interactions around brain death, organ donation, and issues involving life and death.

Secondary Analysis

Secondary analysis involves the use of data gathered in a previous study to test new hypotheses or explore new phenomena. In a typical study, researchers collect far more data than can be analyzed. Secondary analysis of existing data is efficient because data collection is typically the most time-consuming and expensive part of a study. Nurse researchers have done secondary analyses with both large national data sets and smaller, localized sets, and with both qualitative and quantitative data.

A number of avenues are available for making use of an existing set of quantitative data. For example, variables and relationships among variables that were previously unanalyzed can be examined (e.g., a dependent variable in the original study could become the independent variable in the secondary analysis). Or, the secondary analysis can focus on a particular subgroup rather than on the full original sample (e.g., survey data about health habits from a national sample could be analyzed by studying smoking among urban teenagers). As another example, the unit of analysis can be changed. A **unit of analysis** is the basic unit that yields data for an analysis; in nursing studies, each individual subject is typically the unit of analysis. However, data are sometimes aggregated to yield information about larger units (e.g., a study of individual nurses from 25 hospitals could be converted to aggregated data about the hospitals). In qualitative studies, wider theories can be generated by using data from several different data sets. Or, a qualitative researcher could scrutinize an existing data set for particular themes or content coverage that was previously unexplored.

The use of available data makes it possible to bypass time-consuming steps in a study, but there are some noteworthy disadvantages in working with existing data. In particular, if researchers do not play a role in collecting the data, the chances are pretty high that the data set will be deficient in one or more ways, such as in the sample used, the variables measured, and so forth. Researchers may continuously face "if only" problems: if only they had asked questions on a certain topic or had measured a particular variable differently. Nevertheless, existing data sets present exciting opportunities for exploring phenomena of importance to nurses.

Example of a secondary analysis of quantitative data
Loiselle and Dubois (2009) used data from Loiselle's initial study on the impact of multimedia patient education tools on psychosocial adjustment to cancer to further document the impact of the educational intervention on health service utilization among women with breast cancer and men with prostate cancer.

Example of a secondary analysis of qualitative data
Molzahn, Bruce, and Sheilds (2008) used narratives from a book containing 100 stories reported by patients living with a chronic kidney disease (CKD) to explore how people with CKD describe experiences of liminality (i.e., a situation or threshold which can lead to new perspectives) associated with the disease and its treatment.

Methodologic Research

Methodologic research examines methods of obtaining and analyzing research data and addresses the development, validation, and evaluation of instruments or methods. Nurse researchers have become increasingly interested in methodologic research; this is not surprising in light of growing demands for sound and reliable outcome measures and for sophisticated procedures for obtaining and analyzing qualitative and quantitative data.

Quantitative methodologic studies often focus on instrument development and testing. For example, suppose we developed and evaluated an instrument to measure patients' satisfaction with nursing care. In such a study, we would not examine levels of patient satisfaction, nor how satisfaction relates to characteristics of nurses or patients. Our goal would be to develop an effective, trustworthy instrument that could be used by others.

Most methodologic studies are descriptive and nonexperimental, but occasionally quantitative researchers use an experimental or quasi-experimental design to test competing methodologic strategies. For example, a researcher might test whether a financial incentive increases the number of volunteers willing to participate in a study. Potential participants could be randomly assigned to an incentive or no-incentive condition. The dependent variable in this case is whether people agree to participate.

In qualitative research, methodologic issues often arise within the context of a substantive study, as the study is not a purely methodologic endeavour. In such instances, however, the researcher typically performs separate analyses designed to highlight a methodologic issue and to generate strategies for solving a methodologic problem.

Methodologic research may appear less provocative than substantive research, but it is virtually impossible to produce high-quality research evidence on a substantive topic with inadequate research methods.

Example of a quantitative methodologic study
Kelly et al. (2007) sough to ascertain the cost implications and predictors of success of gathering follow-up data from a cohort of high-risk adolescent girls who took part in a reproductive health promotion intervention. The study also examined which approaches were particularly effective through follow-up interviews.

Example of a qualitative methodologic study
Hansen-Ketchum and Myrick (2008) examined how perspectives of realism and relativism may shape epistemological understandings and influence type and use of photo methods in qualitative research. The authors sought to uncover the range of researchers' assumptions that guide the use of photo methods in qualitative research and how knowledge generated as such is perceived.

MIXED METHOD STUDIES

An emerging trend, and one that we believe will gain momentum, is the planned integration of qualitative and quantitative data within single studies or coordinated clusters of studies. This section discusses the rationale for such **mixed method** (or **multimethod**) studies and presents several applications.

Rationale for Mixed Method Studies

The dichotomy between quantitative and qualitative data represents a key methodologic distinction in the social, behavioural, and health sciences. Some argue that the paradigms that underpin qualitative and quantitative research are fundamentally incompatible. Others, however, believe that many areas of inquiry can be enriched and the evidence base enhanced through the judicious blending of qualitative and quantitative data. The advantages of such a triangulated design include the following:

⇒ *Complementarity.* Qualitative and quantitative data represent words and numbers, the two fundamental languages of human communication. The strengths and weaknesses of these two types of data and associated methods are complementary. By using multiple methods, researchers can allow each method to do what it does best, possibly avoiding the limitations of a single approach.

⇒ *Incrementality.* Progress on a topic tends to be incremental, relying on multiple feedback loops. Qualitative findings can generate hypotheses to be tested, and quantitative findings can be clarified through in-depth probing. It can be productive to build such a loop into the design of a single study.

⇒ *Enhanced validity.* When a hypothesis or model is supported by multiple and complementary types of data, researchers can be more confident about the validity of their results.

⇒ *Creating new frontiers.* Sometimes qualitative and quantitative findings are inconsistent with each other. This lack of congruity—when it happens in a single study—can lead to insights that can further develop a line of inquiry. Inconsistencies in separate studies may reflect differences in study participants and circumstances rather than theoretically meaningful distinctions. In a single study, discrepancies can be used as a springboard for further exploration.

TIP

Mixed method studies rarely combine qualitative and quantitative findings in a single report. Typically, the quantitative findings are reported in one journal article, and the qualitative findings appear in a separate article in a different journal. This sometimes makes it difficult for readers to grasp the contributions of all the components.

Applications of Mixed Method Research

The integration of qualitative and quantitative data can be used to address various research goals.

1. *Instrumentation.* Researchers sometimes collect qualitative data for the development and validation of formal instruments used in research or clinical settings. The questions for such an instrument are sometimes derived from clinical experience or prior research, but when a construct is new, these sources may be inadequate to capture its full complexity. Qualitative data can be used to generate questions for instruments that are subsequently subjected to rigorous testing in methodologic studies.

Example of instrumentation
Loiselle and Lambert (2009) developed a scale to measure individuals' profiles of preferences for cancer information. In-depth interviews with individuals with cancer revealed five patterns of preferences for cancer information. These patterns formed the basis for developing the scale. The scale is currently being pilot tested to assess its psychometric properties.

2. *Hypothesis generation and testing.* In-depth qualitative studies consist of insights about constructs or relationships among them. These insights then can be tested and confirmed in quantitative studies, and the generalizability of the insights can be assessed. This most often happens in the context of discrete investigations. One problem, however, is that it usually takes years to conduct a study and publish the results, which means that considerable time may elapse between qualitative insights and formal quantitative testing of hypotheses based on those insights. A research team interested in a phenomenon might wish to collaborate in a research program that has both hypothesis generation and testing as an explicit goal.

Example of hypothesis generation
Judith Wuest's grounded theory research on women's caregiving gave rise to a *theory of precarious ordering* (i.e., the multiple competing and changing demands on women). On the basis of this grounded theory, Wuest and colleagues (2007) developed hypotheses about how the nature and quality of the relationship between the caregiver and a care recipient predict health consequences for women caregivers. The hypotheses received support in a qualitative study among 236 women caregivers of adult family members.

3. *Illustration.* Qualitative data are sometimes used to illustrate the meaning of quantitative descriptions or relationships. Such illustrations help to clarify

important concepts, to corroborate the findings from the statistical analysis, and to guide the interpretation of results. Qualitative materials can be used to illustrate specific statistical findings and to provide more global and dynamic views of the phenomena under study, sometimes in the form of illustrative case studies.

4. *Understanding relationships and causal processes.* Quantitative methods can demonstrate that variables are systematically related but may fail to provide insights about *why* they are related. Interpretations are often speculative, representing hypotheses that could be tested in future studies. When a study integrates qualitative and quantitative data, however, the researcher may be in a stronger position to derive meaning directly from the statistical findings.

Example of illustrating with qualitative data
As a follow-up to a quantitative study revealing that large proportions of lung cancer patients, despite having a high level of distress associated with unmet needs, do not desire assistance with these needs, Steele and Fitch (2008) conducted a qualitative study to explore reasons for the phenomenon. Identified reasons for not asking for help included, believing staff were too busy, the problem would go away with time, an unawareness of possible help options, not wanting help from professionals, and having access to outside community resources.

Example of illuminating with qualitative data
Dubois and Loiselle (in press) studied the impact of patient education interventions on health service utilization using a mixed method approach. First, in a quasi-experimental longitudinal study, Loiselle and Dubois (2009) documented how cancer informational support intervention guided service use among 250 individuals newly diagnosed with cancer. A qualitative follow-up study of a new sample of 20 individuals, also newly diagnosed with cancer, further delineated in more depth, how cancer informational support guided (or not) subsequent health care service use.

5. *Theory building, testing, and refinement.* The most ambitious application of mixed method research is in the area of theory development. A theory gains acceptance as it escapes disconfirmation, and the use of multiple methods provides great opportunity for potential disconfirmation of a theory. If the theory can survive these assaults, it can provide a stronger context for the organization of clinical and intellectual work.

Example of theory building
Bourgault et al. (2008a, 2008b) conducted a mixed methods study to examine the help-seeking process in women with irritable bowel syndrome. Qualitatively, a grounded theory approach was used because it allows for the understanding of behaviours and actions and theory construction. Quantitative data on abdominal pain and psychological distress were collected concurrently to describe these variables in the study sample. A concurrent triangulation approach, which allows for analysis and integration of qualitative and quantitative data, was subsequently used for building a theoretical model.

Mixed Method Strategies

The ways in which researchers can design studies to integrate qualitative and quantitative methods are almost limitless. The three following scenarios are especially common:

1. *Adding qualitative methods to a survey.* Once researchers have gained the cooperation of survey respondents, they may be in a good position to collect more

in-depth data from them. If in-depth interviews can be postponed until after the analysis of quantitative data, researchers can further investigate the reasons for any obtained results. The second-stage respondents, in other words, can be used as informants to help researchers interpret outcomes.

2. *Embedding quantitative measures into an ethnography.* Although qualitative data prevail in ethnographic field studies, ethnographers can often profit from the collection of structured information, either from the study participants or from a larger or more representative sample. Having already gained entrée into the community and the cooperation of its members, ethnographers may be in an ideal position to conduct a survey or a record-extraction activity. For example, if a researcher's in-depth fieldwork focused on family violence, community-wide police and hospital records could be used to gather systematic data amenable to statistical analysis.

3. *Embedding qualitative approaches into experimental research.* Qualitative data can often enrich clinical trials and evaluations that rely on experimental designs. Through in-depth approaches, researchers can, for example, better understand qualitative differences between groups, including differences in the experiences and processes underlying experimental effects. Qualitative data may be especially useful when researchers are evaluating complex interventions. When an experimental treatment is straightforward (e.g., a new drug), it might be easy to interpret the results. However, many nursing interventions are more complicated; they may involve new ways of interacting with patients or new approaches to organizing the delivery of care. At the end of the experiment, even when hypothesized results are obtained, people may ask, What was it that really caused the group differences? In-depth qualitative data may help researchers to address the **black box** question—understanding what it is about the intervention that is driving observed effects. Also, mixed method approaches are sometimes useful in the early stages of an experiment or clinical trial. For example, through in-depth questioning, researchers can gather information about the feasibility and acceptability of an intervention, or about how best to promote it.

Example of qualitative data collection in a clinical trial
Within a larger clinical trial to test the effectiveness of a support group intervention, Clarke, Butler and Esplen (2008) examined the experiences of BRCA1/2 carriers in communicating genetic risk information to their biological offspring, using verbatim transcriptions of dialogue during videotaped support group therapy sessions.

CRITIQUING STUDIES DESCRIBED IN THIS CHAPTER

It is somewhat difficult to provide guidance on critiquing the types of studies described in this chapter because they are so diverse and many of the fundamental methodologic issues that would be critiqued concern the overall design. Table 11.1 provides a very crude guide to the types of quantitative research designs that are usually considered appropriate for the various types of studies described in this chapter. Note that qualitative approaches could be integrated as an adjunct in *any* of these types in a mixed method study, and in some cases (e.g., a process analysis), qualitative data could be collected exclusively in lieu of quantitative data. Despite the limitations of the table, you can see, for example, that an impact analysis or Phase III clinical trial using a preexperimental design would be problematic.

TABLE 11.1 GUIDE TO STUDY TYPES AND QUANTITATIVE RESEARCH DESIGNS

TYPE OF STUDY	USUAL TYPE OF QUANTITATIVE DESIGN
Clinical trial	
Phase I	Preexperimental, nonexperimental*
Phase II	Small-scale experimental, quasi-experimental
Phase III	Experimental
Phase IV	Nonexperimental, preexperimental, quasi-experimental
Evaluation	
Process analysis	Nonexperimental*
Outcome analysis	Preexperimental
Impact analysis	Experimental, quasi-experimental
Cost–benefit analysis	Experimental, quasi-experimental
Outcomes research	Nonexperimental,* preexperimental, quasi-experimental, experimental
Survey	Nonexperimental
Case study	Nonexperimental*
Secondary analysis	Nonexperimental*
Methodologic	Nonexperimental, pre-experimental, quasi-experimental, experimental*

*Information collected could be qualitative data rather than quantitative data. In deliberately mixed method studies, both qualitative and quantitative data could be gathered for *any* of these types of study.

You should also consider whether researchers took appropriate advantage of the possibilities of a mixed method design. Collecting both qualitative and quantitative data is not always necessary or practical, however, you can consider whether the study would have been strengthened by triangulating different types of data. In studies in which mixed methods were used, you should carefully consider whether the inclusion of both types of data was justified and whether the researcher really made use of both types of data to enhance knowledge on the research topic.

Box 11.1 offers a few specific questions for critiquing the types of studies included in this chapter.

BOX 11.1 GUIDELINES FOR CRITIQUING STUDIES DESCRIBED IN THIS CHAPTER

1. Does the study purpose match the study design? Was the best possible design (or research tradition) used to address the study purpose?
2. Is the study exclusively qualitative or exclusively quantitative? If so, could the study have been strengthened by including both types of data?
3. If both qualitative and quantitative data were collected, was the use of both types justified? How (if at all) did the inclusion of both types of data strengthen the study and further the aims of the research?

▶ RESEARCH EXAMPLES AND CRITICAL THINKING ACTIVITIES

EXAMPLE 1 ■ Mixed Method Research—Survey and Qualitative Inquiry

Aspects of a coordinated series of studies on ovarian cancer using qualitative and quantitative approaches are presented below, followed by some questions to guide critical thinking.

Study

"Using mixed methods for evaluating an integrative approach to cancer care: A case study" (Brazier, Cooke, & Moravan, 2008)

Statement of Purpose

The purpose of the study was to evaluate the impact of participating in an integrative cancer care program on patients' lifestyle, quality of life, and overall well-being.

Method

A mixed methods observation case study using a pretest/posttest design with no control group was implemented at the Centre For Integrated Healing in Vancouver, British Columbia. All new patients starting at the Centre between May and September 2004 were invited to participate in study with 46 of 77 new patients consenting to take part in the study. Quantitative outcome measures on quality of life, social support, anxiety and depression, locus of control, and hope were assessed at baseline (preprogram start), at 6 weeks and 5 months from the start of the program. In addition, qualitative data, through focus groups and one-on-one interviews were collected midway through the follow-up period to further explore the program's impacts.

Key Findings

A few highlights of the findings are presented.

- No statistically significant improvements or declines were noted on the quantitative outcome measures between baseline and the 5-month follow-up.
- Qualitative findings revealed that patients' active engagement in their cancer care involved empowered decision making and personal change.
- Facilitators of active engagement qualitatively identified included healing, partnerships with practitioners, information and resources, managing the integration of complementary and conventional therapies, emotional support, and a sense of hope.

CRITICAL THINKING SUGGESTIONS

1. Answer the questions from Box 11.1 (p. 201) regarding this study.
2. Also consider the following targeted questions, which may assist you in further assessing aspects of the study:
   a. Comment on the researchers' decision to collect self-report data.
   b. Comment on the sequencing of the survey and the in-depth interviews.
3. If the results of this study are valid and trustworthy, what are some of the potential clinical uses?

EXAMPLE 2 ■ Mixed Method Study: Quantitative Measures and In-Depth Interviews

Aspects of a mixed method nursing study, featuring terms and concepts discussed in this chapter, are presented below, followed by some questions to guide critical thinking.

Study

"Younger women's perceptions of coping with breast cancer" (Manuel et al., 2007)

Statement of Purpose

The purpose of the study was to explore young women's perceptions of coping with breast cancer and to examine the coping strategies employed.

Method

A cross-sectional mixed method approach was used to address the study objectives. Quantitative and qualitative methods were employed to examine coping strategies used by 201 women who were aged 50 years or younger at diagnosis and were 6 months to 3.5 years postdiagnosis. A questionnaire called the Ways of Coping Scale—Cancer version, which is used to identify different coping strategies used by cancer patients, was used as the primary quantitative outcome measure. In conjunction, one-on-one interviews using open-ended questions were used to collect qualitative data on the participants' perceptions of coping with breast cancer.

Key Findings

- The quantitative portion revealed that the most frequently used coping strategies were wishful thinking, making changes, and cognitive restructuring.

- Qualitative data revealed several additional strategies used by the participants such as being physically active, seeking information, resting, and using medication, complementary and alternative therapies—elements not included in the Ways of Coping Scale.

- Qualitative data also suggested that the young women found different coping strategies particularly useful depending on the specific stressor.

CRITICAL THINKING SUGGESTIONS

1. Answer the questions from Box 11.1 (p. 201) regarding this study.

2. Also consider the following targeted questions, which may assist you in further assessing aspects of the study:
   a. Would you consider this study an evaluation? Why or why not?
   b. The results of the qualitative and quantitative portions of the study are somewhat different. Why do you think that might be the case?

3. If the results of this study are valid and trustworthy, what are some of the clinical implications?

Summary Points

- Quantitative and qualitative studies vary according to purpose as well as design and tradition. Several specific types of study are described in this chapter.

- **Clinical trials**—studies designed to assess the effectiveness of clinical interventions—are often designed in a series of phases. *Phase I* is designed to finalize the features of the intervention; *Phase II* involves seeking preliminary evidence of treatment effectiveness; *Phase III* is a full experimental test of the treatment, often called a **randomized clinical trial** (RCT); and *Phase IV* monitors generalizability and long-term consequences.

- **Evaluations,** which assess the effectiveness of a program, policy, or procedure, can answer a variety of questions. **Process** or **implementation analyses** describe the process by which a program gets implemented and how it functions in practice. **Outcome analyses** describe the status of some condition after the introduction of an intervention. **Impact analyses** test whether an intervention caused any *net effects* relative to a counterfactual. **Cost–benefit analyses** examine whether the monetary costs of a program are outweighed by benefits.

- **Outcomes research** is undertaken to document the quality and effectiveness of health care and nursing services. Classification systems that help to standardize descriptions of nursing actions and outcomes sensitive to nursing care can contribute to outcomes research.

✎ **Surveys** examine people's characteristics, attitudes, and intentions by asking them questions. The preferred survey method is through **personal interviews,** in which interviewers meet respondents face-to-face and question them. **Telephone interviews** are more economical, but are not suitable for lengthy surveys or for ones with sensitive questions. **Questionnaires** are self-administered; that is, questions are read by respondents, who then give written responses.

✎ **Case studies** are intensive investigations of a single entity or small number of entities (e.g., people, organizations). Such studies, which can be qualitative or quantitative, typically involve data collection over an extended period.

✎ **Secondary analysis** refers to studies in which researchers analyze previously collected data—either qualitative or quantitative. Secondary analysts may examine unanalyzed concepts, focus on a particular subsample, or change the **unit of analysis.**

✎ In **methodologic research,** investigators are concerned with the development and assessment of methodologic tools or strategies.

✎ **Mixed method (or multimethod) research,** the blending of qualitative and quantitative data in a single project, can be advantageous in developing an evidence base for nursing practice. Qualitative and quantitative methods have complementary strengths and weaknesses, and an integrated approach can lead to theoretical and substantive insights.

✎ In nursing, one of the most frequent uses of multimethod research has been in the area of instrument development and refinement. Qualitative data are also used to illustrate, clarify, or amplify the meaning of quantified descriptions or relationships. Multimethod studies can help to interpret relationships and can also be used to generate and test hypotheses.

✎ Researchers can implement a multimethod study in a variety of ways, including the use of qualitative data as an adjunct in clinical trials, experimental evaluations, and surveys. The collection of quantitative data within the context of a primarily qualitative study is somewhat less common, but is most likely to happen in ethnographies.

STUDIES CITED IN CHAPTER 11*

This reference list contains only those studies that were cited in this chapter. Citations pertaining to theoretical, methodologic, or nonempirical work are included together in a separate section at the end of the book (beginning on page 399).

Baumbusch, J. L., Kirkham, S. R., Khan, K. B., et al. (2008). Pursuing common agendas: A collaborative model for knowledge translation between research and practice in clinical settings. *Research in Nursing and Health, 31*(2), 130–140.

Bourgault, P., Devroede, G., St-Cyr-Tribble, D., Marchand, S., & de Souza, J. (2008a). Help seeking process in women with irritable bowel syndrome. Part 1: Study results. *Gastrointestinal Nursing, 6*(9), 24–31.

Bourgault, P., Devroede, G., St-Cyr-Tribble, D., Marchand, S., & de Souza, J. (2008b). Help seeking process in women with irritable bowel syndrome. Part 2: Discussion. *Gastrointestinal Nursing, 6*(10), 28–32.

Brazier, A., Cooke, K., & Moravan, V. (2008). Using mixed methods for evaluating an integrative approach to cancer care: A case study. *Integrative Cancer Therapies, 7*(1), 5–17.

Brown-Etris, M., Milne, C., Orsted, H., et al. (2008). A prospective, randomized, multisite clinical evaluation of a transparent absorbent acrylic dressing and a hydrocolloid dressing in the management of stage II and shallow stage III pressure ulcers. *Skin & Wound Care, 21*(4), 169–174.

Clarke, S., Butler, K., & Esplen, M. J. (2008). The phases of disclosing BRCA1/2 genetic information to offspring. *Psychooncology, 17*(8), 797–803.

Dubois, S., & Loiselle, C. G. (2009). Cancer informational support and health care service use among individuals newly diagnosed: A mixed methods approach. *Journal of Evaluation in Clinical Practice, 15,* 346–359.

Guerriere, D. N., Wong, A. Y. M., Croxford, R., Leong, V. W., McKeever, P., & Coyte, P. C. (2008). Costs and determinants of privately financed home-based health care in Ontario, Canada. *Health and Social Care in the Community, 16*(2), 126–136.

Hansen-Ketchum, P., & Myrick, F. (2008). Photo methods for qualitative research in nursing: An ontological and epistemological perspective. *Nursing Philosophy*, *9*(3), 205–213.

Johnson, M., & Maas, M. (1998). The nursing outcomes classification. *Journal of Nursing Care Quality*, *12*, 9–20.

Keefe, M. R., Karlsen, K. A., Lobo, M. L., Kotzer, A. M., & Dudley, W. N. (2006). Reducing parenting stress in families with irritable infants. *Nursing Research*, *55*(3), 198–205.

Kelly, P., Ahmed, A., Martinez, E., & Peralez-Dieckmann, E. (2007). Cost analysis of obtaining postintervention results in a cohort of high-risk adolescents. *Nursing Research*, *56*(4), 269–274.

Kulig, J. C., Andrews, M. E., Stewart, N. L., et al. (2008). How do registered nurses define rurality? *Australian Journal of Rural Health*, *16*(1), 28–32.

Kyung, K., & Chin, P. (2008). The effect of a pulmonary rehabilitation programme on older patients with chronic pulmonary disease. *Journal of Clinical Nursing*, *17*(1), 118–125.

Loiselle, C. G., & Dubois, S. (2009). The impact of a multimedia cancer informational intervention as opposed to usual care on health care service use among individuals newly diagnosed with breast or prostate cancer. *Cancer Nursing*, *32*(1), 37–44.

Loiselle, C. G., & Lambert, S. D. (2009). The development of the profile of preferences for cancer information (PPCI) scale. *Submitted to Supportive Care in Cancer*.

Lunney, M. (2006). NANDA diagnoses, NIC interventions, and NOC outcomes used in an electronic health record with elementary school children. *Journal of School Nursing*, *22*(2), 94–101.

Macdonald, M. E., Liben, S., Carnevale, F. A., & Cohen, S. R. (2008). Signs of life and signs of death: Brain death and other mixed messages at the end of life. *Journal of Child Health Care*, *12*(2), 92–105.

Manuel, J., Burwell, S., Crawford, S., et al. (2007). Younger women's perceptions of coping with breast cancer. *Cancer Nursing*, *30*(2), 85–94.

Marchand, R., Theoret, S., Dion, D., & Pellerin, M. (2008). Clinical implementation of a scrubless chlorhexidine/ethanol pre-operative surgical hand rub. *Canadian Operating Room Nursing Journal*, *26*(2), 21–31.

Molzahn, A. E., Bruce, A., & Sheilds, L. (2008). Learning from stories of people with chronic kidney disease. *Nephrology Nursing Journal*, *35*(1), 13–20.

Sidani, S. (2008). Effects of patient-centered care on patient outcomes: An evaluation. *Research and Theory for Nursing Practice*, *22*(1), 24–37.

Sidani, S., Doran, D. M., & Mitchell, P. H. (2004). A theory-driven approach to evaluating quality of nursing care. *Journal of Nursing Scholarship*, *36*, 60–65.

Steele, R., & Fitch, M. I. (2008). Why patients with lung cancer do not want help with some needs. *Supportive Care in Cancer*, *16*(3), 251–259.

Steele-O'Connor, K. O., Mowat, D. L., Scott, H. M., et al. (2003). A Randomized trial of two public health nurse follow-up programs after early obstetrical discharge. *Canadian Journal of Public Health*, *94*, 98–103.

Wuest, J., Hodgins, M., Malcolm, J., Merritt-Gray, M., & Seamon, P. (2007). The effects of past relationship and obligation on health and health promotion in women caregivers of adult family members. *Advances in Nursing Science*, *30*(3), 206–220.

12 Examining Sampling Plans

On completing this chapter, you will be able to:

1. Describe the rationale for sampling in research

2. Identify differences in the logic and evaluation criteria used in sampling for quantitative versus qualitative studies

3. Distinguish between nonprobability and probability samples and compare their advantages and disadvantages

4. Identify several types of sampling in qualitative and quantitative studies and describe their main characteristics

5. Evaluate the appropriateness of the sampling method and sample size used in a study

6. Define new terms in the chapter

Sampling is a process familiar to all of us—we gather information, make decisions, and formulate predictions about phenomena based on contact with a limited portion of them. Researchers, too, draw conclusions from samples. In testing the efficacy of a nursing intervention for patients with cancer, nurse researchers reach conclusions without testing the intervention with every victim of the disease. However, researchers cannot afford to draw conclusions about nursing interventions and health-related phenomena based on flawed samples. The consequences of faulty inferences are more far-reaching in professional decisions than in private ones.

BASIC SAMPLING CONCEPTS
▶

Sampling is an important step in the research process. In quantitative studies in particular, the findings can be seriously compromised by sampling inadequacies. Let us first consider some terms associated with sampling—terms that are used primarily (but not exclusively) in connection with quantitative studies.

Populations

A **population** is the entire aggregation of cases that meet specified criteria. For instance, if a researcher was studying Canadian nurses with doctoral degrees, the population could be defined as all Canadian citizens who are RNs and who have acquired a DNSc, PhD, or other doctoral-level degree. Other possible populations might be all cardiac patients hospitalized at the University of Alberta Hospital in 2009; all individuals under the age of 30 diagnosed with schizophrenia in Calgary; or all children in New Brunswick with leukemia. Thus, a population may be broadly defined, involving thousands of individuals, or narrowly specified to include a few hundred.

Populations are not restricted to human subjects. A population might consist of all the shift reports from the Shriners Hospital from 2004 to 2008, or all Canadian high schools with clinics that dispense contraceptives. Whatever the basic unit, the population comprises the aggregate of entities in which a researcher is interested.

Researchers (especially quantitative researchers) specify the characteristics that delimit the study population through the **eligibility criteria** (or *inclusion criteria*). For example, consider the population of Canadian nursing students. Would this population include part-time students? Would RNs returning to school for a bachelor's degree be included? Researchers establish these criteria to determine whether a person qualifies as a member of the population—although a population is sometimes defined in terms of traits that people must *not* possess through *exclusion criteria* (e.g., excluding people who do not speak English).

Example of eligibility criteria in a quantitative study

Semenic, Loiselle, and Gottlieb (2008) studied potential influences on the length of exclusive breastfeeding among Canadian primiparous mothers recruited from three large teaching hospitals in Montreal: "Eligible women were all first-time mothers (to control for previous breastfeeding experience) who planned to breastfeed exclusively for at least 6 weeks (as is commonly advised to ensure adequate milk production). Additional inclusion criteria were: minimum of 18 years of age; birth of a single, healthy, full-term baby; able to speak and read English; and, living with a spouse/partner who could read English. Exclusion criteria included any maternal or infant illness or abnormality that potentially could interfere with the initiation of breastfeeding" (pp. 429–430).

Example of eligibility criteria in a qualitative study

Neufeld et al. (2008) conducted an ethnographic study of women caregivers' proactive responses to negative interactions with health professionals. The eligibility criteria for the study included: (1) caregivers' relationship to the family member and type of condition being cared for (i.e., they could be mothers of premature infants or mothers of children with juvenile diabetes or asthma or women caring for an adult family member with cancer or dementia); (2) caregivers both residing and not residing with care recipient; (3) English speaking; and (4) living within 100 km of the city in which the study was completed.

Quantitative researchers sample from an accessible population in the hope of generalizing to a target population. The **target population** is the entire population in which a researcher is interested. The **accessible population** comprises cases from the target population that are accessible to the researcher as a pool of subjects. For example, the researcher's target population might consist of all patients with diabetes in Canada, but, in reality, the population that is accessible to him or her might consist of patients with diabetes who receive health care at a particular clinic.

TIP

Evidence-based practice is dependent on good information about the population about whom research has been conducted. Many quantitative researchers fail to identify their target populations, or to discuss the issue of generalizability of their findings. Researchers should clearly identify their populations so that users will know whether the findings have external validity and are relevant to groups with whom they work.

Samples and Sampling

Sampling is the process of selecting a portion of the population to represent the entire population. A **sample,** then, is a subset of the population. The entities that make up the samples and populations are *elements*. In nursing research, the elements are usually humans.

Researchers work with samples rather than with populations because it is more practical to do so. Researchers have neither the time nor the resources to study all members of a population. Furthermore, it is unnecessary to study everyone because it is usually possible to obtain reasonably good information from a sample.

Still, information from samples can lead to erroneous conclusions. In quantitative studies, *the overriding criterion of adequacy is a sample's representativeness—* the extent to which the sample is similar to the population. Unfortunately, there is no method for ensuring that a sample is representative. Certain sampling plans are less likely to result in biased samples than others, but there is never a guarantee of a representative sample. Researchers operate under conditions in which error is possible, but quantitative researchers strive to minimize or control those errors. Consumers must assess their success in having done so; their success in minimizing sampling bias.

Sampling bias is the systematic overrepresentation or underrepresentation of some segment of the population in terms of a characteristic relevant to the research question. Sampling bias is affected by many things, including the homogeneity of the population. If the elements in a population were all identical on the critical attribute, any sample would be as good as any other. Indeed, if the population exhibited no variability at all, a single element would be a sufficient sample for drawing conclusions about the population. For many physical or physiologic attributes, it may be safe to assume a reasonable degree of homogeneity. For example, the blood in a person's veins is relatively homogeneous; hence, a single blood sample chosen haphazardly from a patient is adequate for clinical purposes. Most human attributes, however, are not homogeneous. Variables, after all, derive their name from the fact that traits vary from one person to the next. Age, blood pressure, and stress level, for example, are all attributes that reflect human heterogeneity.

Strata

Populations consist of subpopulations or **strata.** Strata are mutually exclusive segments of a population based on a specific trait. For instance, a population consisting of all RNs in Ontario could be divided into two strata based on gender. Strata are used in the sample selection process in quantitative studies to enhance the sample's representativeness.

TIP

The sampling plan is usually discussed in a report's Method section, sometimes in a subsection called "Sample," "Subjects," or "Participants." A description of sample characteristics, however, may be reported in the Results section. If researchers have undertaken analyses to detect sample biases, these may be described in either the Method or Results section (e.g., researchers might compare the characteristics of patients who were invited to participate in the study but who declined to do so with those of patients who actually became subjects).

SAMPLING DESIGNS IN QUANTITATIVE STUDIES

Quantitative and qualitative researchers have different approaches to sampling. Quantitative researchers develop a sampling plan before data collection begins, with the goals of achieving statistical conclusion validity and generalizing their results to a population. Qualitative researchers, by contrast, focus on achieving an in-depth, holistic understanding of the phenomenon of interest. They allow sampling decisions to emerge during the course of data collection based on informational needs. This section provides information about sampling strategies used by quantitative researchers, and the next section focuses on sampling in qualitative investigations.

The two main sampling design issues in quantitative studies are how the sample is selected and how many elements are included. There are two broad types of sampling designs in quantitative research: nonprobability and probability sampling.

Nonprobability Sampling

In **nonprobability sampling,** researchers select elements by nonrandom methods. There is no way to estimate the probability of including each element in a nonprobability sample, and every element does *not* have a chance for inclusion. Three methods of nonprobability sampling used in quantitative studies are convenience, quota, and purposive sampling.

Convenience and Snowball Sampling

Convenience sampling (or *accidental sampling*) entails using the most conveniently available people as participants. A nurse who distributes questionnaires about vitamin use to the first 100 available community-dwelling elders is using a convenience sample. The problem with convenience sampling is that available subjects might be atypical of the population; therefore, the price of convenience is the risk of bias.

Another type of convenience sampling is **snowball sampling** (or *network sampling* or *chain sampling*). With this approach, early sample members are asked to refer others who meet the eligibility criteria. This method of sampling is often used when the population consists of people with specific traits who might be difficult to identify by ordinary means (e.g., people who are afraid of hospitals).

Convenience sampling is the weakest but most widely used form of sampling for quantitative studies. In heterogeneous populations, there is no other sampling method in which the risk of bias is greater—and there is no way to evaluate the biases. Caution is needed in interpreting findings and generalizing results from quantitative studies based on convenience samples. However, it is important to note that convenience samples are useful as a starting point when little evidence exists on a particular issue, or when other sampling methods conflict with overriding research ethics.

Example of a convenience sample
Spagrud et al. (2008) studied the impact of type of venous access and adult–child interaction on the pain and distress experienced by children during routine blood sampling at two major Canadian cancer centres. Their study was undertaken with a convenience sample of 55 pediatric oncology patients aged between 3 and 18 years, who were enrolled into the study arms according to the central venous device already in place.

Quota Sampling

In **quota sampling,** researchers identify strata of the population and then determine how many participants are needed from each stratum to meet a quota. By using information about population characteristics, researchers can ensure that diverse segments are represented.

As an example, suppose we were interested in studying the attitudes of undergraduate nursing students toward working on an AIDS unit. The accessible population is a nursing school with an enrolment of 500 undergraduates; a sample size of 100 students is desired. With a convenience sample, we could distribute

TABLE 12.1	NUMBERS AND PERCENTAGES OF STUDENTS IN STRATA OF A POPULATION, CONVENIENCE SAMPLE, AND QUOTA SAMPLE		
STRATA	POPULATION	CONVENIENCE SAMPLE	QUOTA SAMPLE
Male	100 (20%)	5 (5%)	20 (20%)
Female	400 (80%)	95 (95%)	80 (80%)
Total	500 (100%)	100 (100%)	100 (100%)

questionnaires to 100 students as they entered the nursing school library. Suppose, however, that we suspect that male and female students have different attitudes toward working with AIDS victims. A convenience sample might result in too many men, or too few. Table 12.1 presents some fictitious data showing the gender distribution for the population and for a convenience sample (second and third columns). In this example, the convenience sample seriously overrepresents women and underrepresents men. In a quota sample, researchers can guide the selection of subjects so that the sample includes an appropriate number of cases from both strata. The far-right panel of Table 12.1 shows the number of men and women required for a quota sample for this example.

If we pursue this example a bit further, you may better appreciate the dangers of a biased sample. Suppose a key question in this study was: Would you be willing to work on a unit that cared exclusively for patients with AIDS? The percentage of students in the population who would respond "yes" to this question is shown in the first column of Table 12.2. Of course, these values would not be known; they are displayed to illustrate a point. Within the population, males are more likely than females to express willingness to work on an AIDS unit, yet men were underrepresented in the convenience sample. As a result, there is a notable discrepancy between the population and sample values; nearly twice as many students in the population are favourable toward working with AIDS victims (20%) than in the convenience sample (11%). The quota sample, on the other hand, does a reasonably good job of reflecting the population's views.

Except for identifying key strata, quota sampling is similar to convenience sampling; subjects are a convenience sample from each population stratum. Because of this fact, quota sampling shares many of the weaknesses of convenience

TABLE 12.2	STUDENTS WILLING TO WORK ON AIDS UNIT: POPULATION, CONVENIENCE SAMPLE, AND QUOTA SAMPLE		
	NUMBER IN POPULATION	NUMBER IN CONVENIENCE SAMPLE	NUMBER IN QUOTA SAMPLE
Willing males	28 (out of 100)	2 (out of 5)	6 (out of 20)
Willing females	72 (out of 400)	9 (out of 95)	13 (out of 80)
Total number of willing students	100 (out of 500)	11 (out of 100)	19 (out of 100)
Percentage willing	20%	11%	19%

sampling. For instance, if we were required by the quota sampling plan to interview 20 male nursing students, a trip to the dormitories might be a convenient method of recruiting those subjects. Yet this approach would fail to give any representation to male students living off campus, who may have distinctive views about working with patients with AIDS. Despite its problems, however, quota sampling is an important improvement over convenience sampling. Quota sampling is a relatively easy way to enhance the representativeness of a nonprobability sample, and does not require sophisticated skills. Surprisingly, few researchers use this strategy.

Example of a quota sample

Wilson et al. (2008) conducted a study to examine generational differences in job satisfaction among Ontario registered nurses. The sample of 6541 who returned questionnaires were stratified according to nurses' birth dates into "Baby Boomer," "Generation X," or "Generation Y."

Purposive Sampling

Purposive sampling (or *judgmental sampling*) is based on the belief that researchers' knowledge about the population can be used to hand pick the cases (or types of cases) to be included in the sample. Researchers might decide purposely to select the widest possible variety of respondents or might choose subjects who are judged to be typical of the population in question or knowledgeable about the issues under study. Sampling in this subjective manner, however, provides no external, objective method for assessing the typicality of the selected subjects. Nevertheless, this method can be used to advantage in certain instances. For example, sometimes researchers want to ask questions to a group of experts. Also, as discussed in a later section, purposive sampling is often used productively by qualitative researchers.

Example of a purposive sample

Lugg and Ahmed (2008) conducted a study to explore U.K. nurses' knowledge, perceptions, and self-reported practices regarding meticillin-resistant *Staphylococcus aureus* (MRSA)—a concern for hospitals internationally. The study utilized a self-administered questionnaire with a purposive sample of 45 adult and 50 pediatric nurses.

Evaluation of Nonprobability Sampling

Nonprobability samples are rarely representative of the target population—some segment of the population is likely to be systematically underrepresented. And, when there is sampling bias, there is a good chance that the results will be misleading. Why, then, are nonprobability samples used at all in quantitative research? Clearly, the advantage of these designs lies in their convenience and economy. Probability sampling requires resources and time. There may be no option but to use a nonprobability sampling plan. Researchers using a nonprobability sample out of necessity should be cautious about their conclusions, and you as a reader should be alert to the possibility of sampling bias.

TIP

How can you tell what type of sampling design was used in a quantitative study? Researchers who have made explicit efforts to achieve a representative sample usually indicate the type of sampling design used. If the sampling design is not specified, it is probably safe to assume that a sample of convenience was used.

Probability Sampling

Probability sampling involves the random selection of elements from the population. *Random selection* should not be confused with *random assignment*, which was described in Chapter 9. Random assignment is the process of allocating subjects to different treatments on a random basis in experimental designs. Random assignment has no bearing on how subjects in the experiment were selected in the first place. A **random selection** process is one in which each element in the population has an equal, independent chance of being selected. Because probability samples involve selecting units at random, some confidence can be placed in their representativeness. The four most commonly used probability sampling designs are simple random, stratified random, cluster, and systematic sampling.

Simple Random Sampling

Simple random sampling is the most basic probability sampling design. Because more complex probability sampling designs incorporate features of simple random sampling, the procedures are briefly described so that you can understand what is involved.

After defining the population, researchers establish a *sampling frame*, the technical name for the actual list of population elements. If nursing students at McGill University were the accessible population, then a student roster would be the sampling frame. If the population of interest were 300-bed or larger hospitals in Ontario, then a list of all those hospitals would be the sampling frame. Populations are sometimes defined in terms of an existing sampling frame. For example, a researcher might use a telephone directory as a sampling frame. In such a case, the population would be defined as the residents of a certain community who have listed telephone numbers. After a list of population elements has been developed, the elements are numbered consecutively. A table of random numbers or a computer program is then used to draw, at random, a sample of the desired size.

Samples selected randomly in such a fashion are not subject to researcher biases. There is no *guarantee* that the sample will be representative of the population, but random selection does guarantee that differences between the sample and the population are purely a function of chance. The probability of selecting a deviant sample through random sampling is low, and this probability decreases as the sample size increases.

Simple random sampling is a laborious process. The development of the sampling frame, enumeration of the elements, and selection of the sample are time-consuming steps, particularly with a large population. Moreover, it is rarely possible to get a complete listing of population elements; hence, other methods are often used.

Example of a random sample
Loughrey (2008) explored the issue of gender roles with male nurses in the Republic of Ireland. A validated measure (short-form Bem sex role inventory) was mailed to a random sample of 250 male registered nurses with the Irish Nursing Board.

Stratified Random Sampling

In **stratified random sampling,** the population is divided into homogeneous subsets from which elements are selected at random. As in quota sampling, the aim of stratified sampling is to enhance the sample's representativeness. The most common procedure for drawing a stratified random sample is to group together those elements that belong to a stratum and to randomly select the desired number of elements.

Researchers may sample either proportionately (in relation to the size of the stratum) or disproportionately. If a population of students in a nursing school in Canada consisted of 10% Asian, 5% Aboriginals, and 85% Caucasians, a **proportionate sample** of 100 students, stratified on race/ethnicity, would consist of 10, 5, and 85 students from the respective strata. Researchers often use a **disproportionate sample** whenever comparisons between strata of unequal size are desired. In our example, the researcher might select 20 Asian, 20 Aboriginal, and 60 Caucasians to ensure a more adequate representation of the viewpoints of the two racial minorities. (When disproportionate sampling is used, however, it is necessary to make a mathematic adjustment—**weighting**—to arrive at the best estimate of overall population values.)

By using stratified random sampling, researchers can sharpen the representativeness of their samples. Stratified sampling may, however, be impossible if information on the stratifying variables is unavailable (e.g., a student roster might not include information on race and ethnicity). Furthermore, a stratified sample requires even more labour than simple random sampling because the sample must be drawn from multiple enumerated listings.

Example of a stratified random sample

Curtis (2008) conducted a survey of nurses to examine the impact of biographical factors (i.e., gender, age, nursing education, current position at work, and length of time in current workplace) on job satisfaction. A stratified random sample according to these factors was drawn from eligible registrants with the Irish Nursing Board.

Cluster Sampling

For many populations, it is impossible to obtain a listing of all elements. For example, there is no listing of all full-time nursing students in Canada. Large-scale studies rarely use simple or stratified random sampling. The most common procedure for national surveys is cluster sampling.

In **cluster sampling,** there is a successive random sampling of units. The first unit to be sampled is large groupings or clusters. For example, in drawing a sample of nursing students, researchers might first draw a random sample of nursing schools and then sample students from the selected schools. The usual procedure for selecting samples from a general population is to sample such administrative units as provinces, cities, census tracts, and then households, successively. Because of the successive stages of sampling, this approach is sometimes referred to as *multistage sampling*.

For a specified number of cases, cluster sampling tends to contain more sampling error than simple or stratified random sampling. Nevertheless, cluster sampling is more economical and practical when the population is large and widely dispersed.

Example of a cluster/multistage sample

Vlack et al. (2007) obtained survey estimates of immunization coverage for indigenous Australian children aged 2 years in the state of Queensland, and compared this with those from the national Immunization Register for the same age group. To select a survey sample, they first stratified 153 geographical areas in Queensland according to their accessibility creating four strata (from "highly accessible" to "very remote"), and then randomly selected 30 of them for a total target sample of 210 children—seven eligible children from each area. This represented 6% of the estimated population.

Systematic Sampling

Systematic sampling involves the selection of every kth case from a list or group, such as every 10th person on a patient list. Systematic sampling can be applied in such a way that an essentially random sample is drawn. First, the size of the population is divided by the size of the desired sample to obtain the sampling interval width. The *sampling interval* is the standard distance between the selected elements. For instance, if we wanted a sample of 50 from a population of 5000, our sampling interval would be 100 (5000/50 = 100). In other words, every 100th case would be sampled. Next, the first case would be selected randomly (e.g., by using a table of random numbers). If the random number chosen were 73, the people corresponding to numbers 73, 173, 273, and so forth would be included in the sample. Systematic sampling conducted this way is essentially identical to simple random sampling and is often preferable because of its convenience.

Example of a systematic random sample
Douglas, Wollin, and Windsor (2008) surveyed chronic pain among people with multiple sclerosis in an Australian community. Approximately 1200 people from the MS Society of Queensland membership database met the study inclusion criteria, with systematic random sampling selecting every third person, to a total of 500 participants.

Evaluation of Probability Sampling

Probability sampling is the only reliable method of obtaining representativeness because it avoids the risk of conscious or unconscious biases. If all the elements in the population have an equal probability of being selected, there is a high likelihood that the sample will represent the population adequately. Probability sampling also allows researchers to estimate the magnitude of sampling error. **Sampling error** is the difference between population values (e.g., the average heart rate of the population) and sample values (e.g., the average heart rate of the sample). It is rare that a sample is perfectly representative of a population and contains no sampling error; however, probability sampling permits estimates of the degree of expected error. On the other hand, probability sampling is expensive and demanding. Unless the population is narrowly defined, it is beyond the scope of most researchers to draw a probability sample.

> **TIP**
>
> The quality of the sampling plan is of particular importance in survey research because the purpose of surveys is to obtain descriptive information about the prevalence or average values for a population. All national surveys, such as the National Population Health Survey in Canada, use probability samples (usually multistage samples). Probability samples are rarely used in experimental and quasi-experimental studies, in part because the main focus of such inquiries is on between-group differences rather than absolute values for a population.

Sample Size in Quantitative Studies

Sample size, the number of subjects in a sample, is a major issue in quantitative research. No simple equation can determine how large a sample is needed, but quantitative researchers are generally advised to use the largest sample possible. The larger the sample, the more representative it is likely to be. Every time researchers calculate a percentage or an average based on sample data, the purpose is to estimate a population value. The larger the sample, the smaller the sampling error.

Let us illustrate this with an example of estimating monthly aspirin consumption in a nursing home. The population is 15 nursing home residents whose aspirin consumption averages 16 per month. Two simple random sam-

TABLE 12.3	COMPARISON OF POPULATION AND SAMPLE VALUES AND AVERAGES IN NURSING HOME ASPIRIN CONSUMPTION EXAMPLE		
NUMBER IN GROUP	GROUP	VALUES (MONTHLY NUMBER OF ASPIRINS CONSUMED)	AVERAGE
15	Population	2, 4, 6, 8, 10, 12, 14, 16, 18, 20, 22, 24 26, 28, 30	16.0
2	Sample 1A	6, 14	10.0
2	Sample 1B	20, 28	24.0
3	Sample 2A	16, 18, 8	14.0
3	Sample 2B	20, 14, 26	20.0
5	Sample 3A	26, 14, 18, 2, 28	17.6
5	Sample 3B	30, 2, 26, 10, 4	14.4
10	Sample 4A	18, 16, 24, 22, 8, 14, 28, 20, 2, 6	15.8
10	Sample 4B	14, 18, 12, 20, 6, 14, 28, 12, 24, 16	16.4

ples with sample sizes of 2, 3, 5, and 10 were drawn from this population (Table 12.3). Each sample average on the right represents an estimate of the population average, which we know is 16. (Under ordinary circumstances, the population value would be unknown, and we would draw only one sample.) With a sample size of 2, our estimate might have been wrong by as many as eight aspirins (sample 1B). As the sample size increases, the average gets closer to the population value, *and* differences in the estimates between samples A and B get smaller. As the sample size increases, the probability of getting a deviant sample diminishes because large samples provide the opportunity to counterbalance atypical values.

Sophisticated researchers estimate how large their samples should be to test their research hypotheses adequately through **power analysis** (Cohen, 1988). A simple example can illustrate basic principles of power analysis. Suppose we were testing an intervention to help people quit smoking; we assign smokers randomly to either an experimental or a control group. How many subjects should we use in this study? When using power analysis, researchers estimate how big group differences will be on the outcomes (e.g., the difference in the average number of cigarettes smoked a week after the intervention). The estimate might be based on previous research, on our personal experience, or on other factors. When expected differences are large, it does not take a large sample to ensure that the differences will be revealed in a statistical analysis; but when small differences are predicted, large samples are needed. Cohen (1988) claimed that, for new areas of research, group differences are likely to be small. In our example, if we expected a small group difference in postintervention smoking, the sample size needed to test the effectiveness of the new program, assuming standard statistical criteria, would be about 800 smokers (400 per group). If a medium-sized difference were expected, the total sample size would still need to be several hundred smokers.

When samples are too small, researchers run the risk of gathering data that will not support their hypotheses—even when those hypotheses are correct. This poses a potential threat to the study's statistical conclusion validity. Large samples are no assurance of accuracy. However, with nonprobability sampling even a large sample can harbour extensive bias. The famous example from the United States illustrating this point is the 1936 U.S. presidential poll conducted by the magazine *Literary Digest*, which predicted that Alfred M. Landon would defeat Franklin D. Roosevelt by a landslide. An extremely large sample—about 2.5 million people—participated in this poll, but biases arose because the sample was drawn from telephone directories and automobile registrations during a Depression year when only the well-to-do (who favoured Landon) had a car or telephone.

A large sample cannot correct for a faulty sampling design; nevertheless, a large nonprobability sample is preferable to a small one. When critiquing quantitative studies, you must assess both the sample size and the sample selection method to judge how representative the sample likely was. Although nurse researchers conduct increasingly more pilot work, there is currently limited guidance from the research community to calculate adequate sample size for these studies. Hertzog (2008) provides some recommendations by study aim for those seeking to justify their approach, but still advises that interpretation of pilot data should remain cautionary.

TIP

The sampling plan is often one of the weakest aspects of quantitative research. Most nursing studies use samples of convenience, and many are based on samples that are too small to provide an adequate test of the hypotheses. Most quantitative studies are based on samples of fewer than 200 participants, and a great many studies have fewer than 100 participants. Power analysis is not used by many nurse researchers, and research reports typically offer no justification for the size of the study sample. Small samples run a high risk of leading researchers to erroneously reject their research hypotheses. Therefore, you should be especially prepared to critique the sampling plan of studies that fail to support research hypotheses.

SAMPLING IN QUALITATIVE RESEARCH

Qualitative studies typically use small, nonrandom samples. This does not mean that qualitative researchers are unconcerned with the quality of their samples, but rather that they use different criteria for selecting participants. This section examines sampling considerations in qualitative studies.

The Logic of Qualitative Sampling

Quantitative research is concerned with measuring attributes and relationships in a population, and therefore a representative sample is needed to ensure that the measurements accurately reflect and can be generalized to the population. The aim of most qualitative studies is to discover meaning and to uncover multiple realities; therefore, generalizability, as quantitative researchers use this term, is not a guiding criterion.

Qualitative researchers ask such sampling questions as: Who would be an information-rich data source for my study? Whom should I talk to, or what should I observe to maximize my understanding of the phenomenon? A critical first step in qualitative sampling is selecting settings with high potential for "information richness."

As the study progresses, new sampling questions emerge, such as the following: Whom can I talk to or observe to confirm my understandings? To challenge, modify, or enrich my understandings? Thus, as with the overall design in qualitative studies, sampling design is an emergent one that capitalizes on early learning to guide subsequent direction.

Types of Qualitative Sampling

Qualitative researchers usually eschew probability samples. A random sample is not the best method of selecting people who will make good informants (i.e., people who are knowledgeable, articulate, reflective, and willing to talk at length with a researcher).

Convenience and Snowball Sampling

Qualitative researchers sometimes begin with a convenience sample, which can be referred to as a **volunteer sample.** Volunteer samples are especially useful when researchers need participants to come forward to identify themselves (e.g., by placing notices in newspapers for people with certain experiences) or when they need to rely on referrals from others.

Sampling by convenience is efficient, but it is not usually a preferred sampling approach, even in qualitative studies. The key aim in qualitative studies is to extract the greatest possible information from the small number of informants in the sample, and a convenience sample may not provide the most information-rich sources. Convenience sampling is frequently used as a way to begin the sampling process.

Qualitative researchers also use snowball sampling (or *nominated sampling*), asking early informants to make referrals for other study participants. Researchers may use this method to gain access to people who are difficult to identify. A weakness of this approach is that the eventual sample might be restricted to a rather small network of acquaintances. Moreover, the quality of the referrals may be affected by whether the referring sample member trusted the researcher and truly wanted to cooperate.

Example of a snowball sample
Profetto-McGrath et al. (2007) conducted a pilot study exploring evidence use by clinical nurse specialists in a health region in Western Canada. The researchers recruited an initial group of clinical nurse specialists, who then in turn referred others as possible participants.

Purposive Sampling

Qualitative sampling may begin with volunteer informants and may be supplemented with new participants through snowballing, but many qualitative studies eventually evolve to a purposive (or *purposeful*) sampling strategy—a strategy in which researchers hand pick the cases or types of cases that will best contribute to the information needs of the study. Qualitative researchers often strive to select sample members purposefully based on the information needs emerging from the early findings: whom to sample next depends on who has been sampled already.

Example of a purposive sample
Gantert et al. (2008) explored seniors' experiences in Ontario relating to in-home service providers. Their purposive sample was derived from a list generated by case managers of potential participants who were willing to be contacted for the purposes of the study. The final sample of 15 seniors were chosen to give "maximal variation" in terms of gender, age, diagnosis, duration of relationships with providers, and type of in-home service received.

Within purposive sampling, several strategies have been identified (Patton, 2002), only some of which are mentioned here. Note that researchers themselves do not necessarily refer to their sampling plans with Patton's labels. His classification shows the kind of diverse strategies qualitative researchers have adopted to meet the conceptual needs of their research:

⇝ **Maximum variation sampling** involves purposefully selecting cases with a range of variation on dimensions of interest

⇝ **Homogeneous sampling** involves a deliberate reduction of variation to permit a more focused inquiry

⇝ **Extreme/deviant case sampling** provides opportunities for learning from the most unusual and extreme informants (e.g., outstanding successes and notable failures)

⇝ **Typical case sampling** involves selecting participants who will illustrate or highlight what is typical or average

⇝ **Criterion sampling** involves studying cases that meet a predetermined criterion of importance

Example of maximum variation sampling

In a multiphased research study, Williamson et al. (2006) studied the use of health-related services by low-income Canadians in two large urban cities. Individual interviews were conducted with 99 low-income individuals in Edmonton and 100 in Toronto, using purposive sampling to select those with incomes equal to or below the Statistics Canada low-income definition. The authors stated that: "The sample size was determined by our desire that participants represent a variety of socio-demographic characteristics and low-income situations (e.g., working poor, social assistance recipients, unemployed) . . . [which] led to a larger sample size than is usual in many qualitative studies" (p. 110).

Maximum variation sampling is often the sampling mode of choice in qualitative research because it is useful in documenting the scope of a phenomenon and in identifying important patterns that cut across variations. Other strategies can also be used advantageously, however, depending on the nature of the research question.

TIP

A qualitative research report will not necessarily use such terms as "maximum variation sampling" but may describe the researcher's selection of a diverse sample of participants.

A strategy of sampling confirming and disconfirming cases is another purposive strategy that is used toward the end of data collection in qualitative studies. As researchers note trends and patterns in the data, emerging conceptualizations may need to be checked. **Confirming cases** are additional cases that fit researchers' conceptualizations and offer enhanced credibility. **Disconfirming cases** are new cases that do not fit and serve to challenge researchers' interpretations. These "negative" cases may offer new insights about how the original conceptualization needs to be revised or expanded.

TIP

Some qualitative researchers appear to call their sample purposive simply because they "purposely" selected people who experienced the phenomenon of interest. However, experience with the phenomenon is actually an eligibility criterion—the population of interest comprises people with that experience. If the researcher then recruits *any* person with that experience, the sample is selected by convenience, not purposively. Purposive sampling implies an intent to carefully choose *particular* exemplars or *types* of people who can best enhance the researcher's understanding of the phenomenon.

Theoretical Sampling

Theoretical sampling is a method of sampling used in grounded theory studies. Glaser (1978) defined this sampling approach as "the process of data collection for generating theory whereby the analyst jointly collects, codes, and analyzes his data and decides what data to collect next and where to find them, in order to develop his theory as it emerges" (p. 36). This complex sampling technique requires researchers to be involved with multiple lines and directions as they go back and forth between data and categories as the theory emerges.

Theoretical sampling is not the same as purposeful sampling. The purpose of theoretical sampling is to discover categories and their properties and to offer interrelationships that occur in the substantive theory. Glaser noted that the basic question in theoretical sampling is: what groups or subgroups should the researcher turn to next? The groups are chosen as they are needed for their theoretical relevance in furthering the emerging conceptualization.

Example of a theoretical sample

Mills, Francis, and Bonner (2007) used theoretical sampling in their grounded theory study of Australian rural nurses' experiences of mentoring. Nine participants were interviewed, with data collection and analysis undertaken concurrently. "Theoretical sampling occurred on the basis of this ongoing analysis and interview aide memoirs were amended to reflect current constructions and questions that remained unanswered" (p. 585).

Sample Size in Qualitative Studies

There are no rules for sample size in qualitative research. Sample size is largely a function of the purpose of the inquiry, the quality of the informants, and the type of sampling strategy used. For example, a larger sample is likely to be needed with maximum variation sampling than with typical case sampling. Patton argues that purposive sample sizes should "be judged on the basis of the purpose and rationale of each study... The sample, like all other aspects of qualitative inquiry, must be judged in context..." (2002, p. 245).

A guiding principle in qualitative sampling is **data saturation** (i.e., sampling to the point at which no new information is obtained). Information redundancy can typically be achieved with a fairly small number of cases, if the information from each is of sufficient depth. Morse (2000) noted that the number of participants needed to reach saturation depends on a number of factors. For example, the broader the scope of the research question, the more participants will likely be needed. Data quality can also affect sample size. If participants are good informants who are able to reflect on their experiences and communicate effectively, saturation can be achieved with relatively few informants. Also, if longitudinal data are collected, fewer participants may be needed because each will provide a greater amount of information. As discussed in the next section, sample size is also partly a function of the type of qualitative inquiry that is undertaken.

TIP

The sample size adequacy for quantitative studies can be estimated by consumers after the fact through power analysis. However, sample size adequacy in a qualitative study is more difficult to critique because redundancy of information is difficult for consumers to judge. Some qualitative reports explicitly state that data saturation was achieved.

Sampling in the Three Main Qualitative Traditions

There are similarities among the various qualitative traditions with regard to sampling: samples are generally small, probability sampling is almost never used, and final sampling decisions generally take place during data collection. However, there are some differences as well.

Sampling in Ethnographic Studies

Ethnographers often begin by adopting a "big net" approach—that is, mingling with and having conversations with as many members of the culture under study as possible. Starting with this wide-angle lens of the culture provides ethnographers with the "lay of the land."

Although they may converse with many people (usually 25 to 50), ethnographers often rely on a smaller number of **key informants,** who are highly knowledgeable about the culture and who develop special, ongoing relationships with them. These key informants are ethnographers' main link to the "inside."

Key informants usually are chosen purposively, guided by ethnographers' informed judgments (although sampling may become more theoretical as the study progresses). Developing a pool of potential key informants often depends on ethnographers' prior knowledge to construct a relevant framework. For example, an ethnographer might make decisions about different types of key informants to seek out based on roles (e.g., physicians, nurse practitioners) or on some other theoretically meaningful distinction. Once a pool of potential key informants is developed, the main considerations for final selection are their level of knowledge about the culture and how willing they are to collaborate with the ethnographer in revealing and interpreting the culture. Ethnographers typically attempt to develop relationships with as diverse a group of informants as possible.

Sampling in ethnography typically involves more than selecting informants because observation and other data sources play a big role in helping researchers understand a culture. Ethnographers have to decide not only *whom* to sample but also *what* to sample. For example, ethnographers have to make decisions about observing *events* and *activities*, about examining *records* and *artefacts*, and about exploring *places* that provide clues about the culture. Key informants can help ethnographers decide what to sample.

Example of an ethnographic sample

Scott and Pollock (2008) conducted an ethnological study to examine the influence of organizational culture on nurses' research utilization. Fieldwork was undertaken on a pediatric critical care unit in a Canadian children's hospital, as there is evidence to suggest that research utilization may increase in specialized health care environments. The first author collected over 120 hours of observations at all shifts and days of the week, as well as 29 individual interviews with nurses, managers, or other health professionals on the unit. The authors state that: "A maximum variation sampling strategy (Patton, 2002) was used to sample events where research utilization was expected to occur (e.g., rounds and reports)" (p. 300).

Sampling in Phenomenological Studies

Phenomenologists tend to rely on very small samples of participants—typically 10 or fewer. There is one guiding principle in selecting the sample for a phenomenological study: all participants must have experienced the phenomenon under study and must be able to articulate what it is like to have lived that experience. Although phenomenological researchers seek participants who have had the targeted experiences, they also want to explore diversity of individual experiences. Thus, as described by Porter (1999), they may specifically look for people with demographic or other differences who have shared a common experience. To study a phenomenon of interest in depth, phenomenologists may also sample experiences of place and of events in time because a person's experience of the phenomenon under study is situated in a specific place and time.

Example of a sample in a phenomenological study

Gantert et al. (2008) conducted a Canadian phenomenological study of the experience of being a senior receiving in-home care, in terms of developing the client–care provider relationship.

Interpretive phenomenologists may, in addition to sampling people, sample artistic or literary sources. Experiential descriptions of the phenomenon may be selected from a wide array of literature, such as poetry, novels, biographies, diaries, and journals. These sources can help increase phenomenologists' insights into the phenomena under study. Art—including paintings, film, photographs, and music—is viewed as another source of lived experience by interpretive phenomenologists. Each artistic medium is viewed as having its own specific language or way of expressing the experience of the phenomenon.

Sampling in Grounded Theory Studies

Grounded theory research is typically done with samples of about 20 to 30 people, using theoretical sampling. The goal in a grounded theory study is to select informants who can best contribute to the evolving theory. Sampling, data collection, data analysis, and theory construction occur concurrently, and so study participants are selected serially and contingently—that is, contingent on the emerging conceptualization. Theoretical sampling is used to develop and refine categories. As grounded theorists identify gaps or holes in their emerging theory, they go back to the field and sample data to fill in thin areas. At this point in their research, grounded theorists become very selective in their sampling: participants are sampled only in regard to specific issues. Theoretical sampling is used not to increase the sample size but to refine the developing theory and to gain more insight into the properties of the categories. Sampling might evolve as follows:

1. The researcher begins with a general notion of where and with whom to start. The first few cases may be solicited purposively, by convenience, or through snowballing.

2. In the early part of the study, a strategy such as maximum variation sampling might be used to gain insights into the range and complexity of the phenomenon under study.

3. The sample is adjusted in an ongoing fashion. Emerging conceptualizations help to focus the sampling process to maximize understanding of the categories.

4. Sampling continues until saturation is achieved.

5. Final sampling often includes a search for confirming and disconfirming cases to test, refine, and strengthen the theory.

Example of a sample in a grounded theory study

In their grounded study of women's experiences seeking treatment for potential symptoms of cardiac illness, Turris and Johnson (2008) recruited participants from two emergency departments in a large Canadian city. Although initial sampling was by convenience, emerging themes provided direction for theoretical sampling. For example, younger participants were sought to better understand the possible influence of age on treatment seeking decisions. From an initial group of 10 participants, the final study sample totalled 16.

CRITIQUING THE SAMPLING PLAN

The sampling plan of a study—particularly a quantitative study—merits particular scrutiny because, if the sample is seriously biased or too small, the findings may be misleading or just plain wrong. In critiquing a sampling plan, you should consider two issues. The first is whether the researcher has adequately described the sampling strategy. Ideally, research reports should include a description of the following aspects of the sample:

☞ The type of sampling approach used (e.g., convenience, snowball, purposive, simple random)

☞ The population under study and the eligibility criteria for sample selection in quantitative studies; the nature of the setting and study group in qualitative ones (qualitative studies may also articulate eligibility criteria)

☞ The number of participants in the study and a rationale for the sample size

☞ A description of the main characteristics of participants (e.g., age, gender, medical condition, race/ethnicity, and so forth) and, in a quantitative study, of the population

☞ In quantitative studies, the number and characteristics of potential subjects who declined to participate in the study

If the description of the sample is inadequate, you may not be in a position to deal with the second and principal issue, which is whether the researcher made good sampling decisions.

Critiquing Quantitative Sampling Plans

We have stressed that the main criterion for assessing a sampling plan in quantitative research is whether the sample is representative of the population. You will never be able to know for sure, of course, but if the sampling strategy is weak or if the sample size is small, there is reason to suspect some bias. When researchers have adopted a sampling plan in which the risk for bias is high, they should take steps to estimate the direction and degree of this bias so that readers can draw some informed conclusions.

Even with a rigorous sampling strategy, the sample may contain some bias if not all people invited to participate in a study agree to do so. If certain segments of the population refuse to participate, then a biased sample can result, even when probability sampling is used. The research report ideally should provide information about **response rates** (i.e., the number of people participating in a study relative to the number of people sampled) and about possible **nonresponse bias**—differences between participants and those who declined to participate (also sometimes referred to as *response bias*).

In developing the sampling plan, quantitative researchers make decisions about the specification of the population as well as the selection of the sample. If the target population is defined broadly, researchers may have missed opportunities to control extraneous variables, and the gap between the accessible and the target population may be too great. Your job as reviewer is to come to conclusions about the reasonableness of generalizing the findings from the researcher's sample to the accessible population and from the accessible population to a broader target population. If the sampling plan is seriously flawed, it may be risky to generalize the findings at all.

Box 12.1 presents some guiding questions for critiquing the sampling plan of a quantitative research report.

BOX 12.1 GUIDELINES FOR CRITIQUING QUANTITATIVE SAMPLING DESIGNS

1. Is the population under study identified and described? Are eligibility criteria specified? Are the sample selection procedures clearly delineated?
2. What type of sampling plan was used? Would an alternative sampling plan have been preferable? Was the sampling plan one that could be expected to yield a representative sample?
3. How were participants recruited into the sample? Does the method suggest potential biases?
4. Did some factor other than the sampling plan (e.g., a low response rate) affect the representativeness of the sample?
5. Are possible sample biases or weaknesses identified?
6. Are key characteristics of the sample described (e.g., mean age, percent female)?
7. Is the sample size sufficiently large? Was the sample size justified on the basis of a power analysis or other rationale?
8. To whom can the study results reasonably be generalized?

Evaluating Qualitative Sampling Plans

In a qualitative study, sampling can be evaluated in terms of adequacy and appropriateness (Morse, 1991). *Adequacy* refers to the sufficiency and quality of the data the sample yielded. An adequate sample provides data without any "thin" spots. When the researcher has truly obtained saturation with a sample, informational adequacy has been achieved, and the resulting description or theory is richly textured and complete.

Appropriateness concerns the methods used to select a sample. An appropriate sample is one resulting from the identification and use of study participants who can best supply information according to the conceptual requirements of the study. Researchers must use a strategy that will yield the fullest possible understanding of the phenomenon of interest. A sampling approach that excludes negative cases or that fails to include participants with unusual experiences may not meet the information needs of the study.

Another important issue concerns the potential for transferability of the findings. The degree of transferability of study findings is a function of the similarity between the study sample and the people at another site to which the findings might be applied. **Fittingness** is the degree of congruence between these two groups. Thus, in critiquing a report, you should see whether the researcher provided an adequately thick description of the sample, setting, and context so that someone interested in transferring the findings could make an informed decision.

Further guidance to critiquing sampling in a qualitative study is presented in Box 12.2.

BOX 12.2 GUIDELINES FOR CRITIQUING QUALITATIVE SAMPLING DESIGNS

1. Is the setting or context adequately described? Is the setting appropriate for the research question?
2. Are the sample selection procedures clearly delineated? What type of sampling strategy was used?
3. Were the eligibility criteria for the study specified? How were participants recruited into the study? Did the recruitment strategy yield information-rich participants?
4. Given the information needs of the study—and, if applicable, its qualitative tradition—was the sampling approach appropriate? Are dimensions of the phenomenon under study adequately represented?
5. Is the sample size adequate and appropriate for the qualitative tradition of the study? Did the researcher indicate that information redundancy had been achieved? Do the findings suggest a richly textured and comprehensive set of data without any apparent "holes" or thin areas?
6. Are key characteristics of the sample described (e.g., age, gender)? Is a rich description of participants provided, allowing for an assessment of the transferability of the findings?

▶ **RESEARCH EXAMPLES AND CRITICAL THINKING ACTIVITIES**

EXAMPLE 1 ■ Quantitative Research

Aspects of a quantitative nursing study, featuring terms and concepts discussed in this chapter, are presented below, followed by some questions to guide critical thinking.

Study

"A survey of oncology advanced practice nurses in Ontario: Profile and predictors of job satisfaction" (Bryant-Lukosius et al., 2007)

Purpose

The purpose of this study was to examine professional role structures and processes, and determine their influence on job satisfaction among oncology advance practice nurses (APN) in Ontario.

Design

The researchers conducted a cross-sectional, mailed, self-report survey that identified participant demographics; perceptions of role preparedness, confidence and competence; educational needs; role characteristics; role processes (according to the domains of direct patient care, education, research, organizational leadership, and scholarly/professional development); and included a validated measure of nurse practitioner job satisfaction.

Sampling Plan

The sample included all nurses working for at least 6 months in a defined APN role with direct oncology patient care. As there was no current provincial system in place to draw this sample, a snowball sampling method was used over a 5-month period to identify potential participants. "First, the research team generated a list of potential participants known to them through regional, provincial and national oncology nursing initiatives. This list was circulated to a provincial network . . . [who] reviewed the list with local and regional colleagues to identify additional APNs. Other participants were identified from Ontario members listed on the Canadian Association of Nurses in Oncology (CANO) website and through recruitment efforts at two conferences held by CANO and the Canadian Association of APNs. The research team and provincial network reviewed each updated list. The process concluded on a fifth review when no new participants were identified and all feasible strategies to identify APNs were exhausted" (p. 53).

Key Findings

- Although the sample reported significant nursing experience (average of 21.5 years), there was a large representation of novice APNs (average length of time in the role at 3.62 years) with many in their first APN role (49.3%).

- APNs were minimally satisfied with their roles, with role confidence and number of overtime hours positive and negative predictors of job satisfaction, respectively.

- APNs are not fully implementing the five domains of role processes, with the sample reporting the least amount of time in research-related activities.

CRITICAL THINKING SUGGESTIONS

1. Answer questions 1 through 5, 7, and 8 from Box 12.1 (p. 223) regarding this study.

2. Also consider the following targeted questions, which may assist you in further assessing aspects of the study:
   a. What are some of the potential biases that may arise from the type of sampling method used?
   b. Are the results of this sample generalizable?

3. If the results of this study are valid and reliable, what are some of the uses to which the findings might be put into clinical practice?

EXAMPLE 2 ■ Qualitative Research

Aspects of a qualitative nursing study, featuring terms and concepts discussed in this chapter, are presented below, followed by some questions to guide critical thinking.

Study

"The role of nursing unit culture in shaping research utilization behaviors" (Scott & Pollock, 2008)

Research Purpose

Scott and Pollock undertook an ethnographic study to examine the influence of organizational culture on nurses' general research utilization behaviours.

Method

The researchers conducted an ethnographical study of one pediatric critical care unit over a period of 7 months. The first author collected over 120 hours of unit observations, as well as 29 individual interviews with nurses, managers, or other health care professionals on the unit. All interviews were recorded and transcribed for analysis. Concurrent data collection and analysis continued until data saturation on the phenomenon of interest was reached. An audit trail was conducted to optimise the validity of study findings.

Sampling Plan

The researchers applied a maximum variation sampling strategy to gain a comprehensive view of unit culture. The first author observed nursing rounds, report times, breaks, communication patterns, and unit routines across all shifts and days of the week. A broad sampling of interviewees was employed to prevent "elite bias." (p. 300)

Key Findings

The study revealed empirical data to support hypothesized, as well as unanticipated cultural influences, namely *the hierarchical structure of authority*, *nature of nurses' work*, *workplace ethos*, and *valued knowledge forms*. The researchers surmised that "Nurses learned the culture of the unit and it was a culture in which they were told what to do, and in which they had little scope for independent decision-making or, indeed, little input into decision-making. Within such a culture, they were unwilling and unable to use research to inform their practice" (p. 306).

CRITICAL THINKING SUGGESTIONS

1. Answer questions 1 through 6 from Box 12.2 (p. 223) regarding this study.

2. Also consider the following targeted questions, which may assist you in further assessing aspects of the study:
   a. Comment on the researchers' decision to include other health care professionals as interviewees in a study of nursing unit culture.
   b. What conclusions can be drawn from this research, given that the study describes the culture on a specific unit?

3. If the results of this study are trustworthy, what are some of the uses to which the findings might be put into clinical practice?

EXAMPLE 3 ■ Quantitative Research

1. Read the Method section from the study by Bryanton and colleagues found in Appendix A of this book and then answer the relevant questions in Box 12.1 (p. 223).

2. Also consider the following targeted questions, which may further sharpen your critical thinking skills and assist you in assessing aspects of the study:
   a. What modifications to the sampling plan may have improved the representativeness of the sample?
   b. The report indicates that participants and nonparticipants (those declining to participate in the study) differed in some respects. Discuss the nature of the differences and what effect this may have had on the study findings.

(Research Examples and Critical Thinking Activities continues on page 226)

Research Examples and Critical Thinking Activities (continued)

EXAMPLE 4 ■ **Qualitative Research**

1. Read the Method section from the study by Woodgate, Ateah, and Secco found in Appendix B of this book and then answer the relevant questions in Box 12.2 (p. 223).
2. Also consider the following targeted questions, which may further sharpen your critical thinking skills and assist you in assessing aspects of the study.
   a. Comment on the lack of single parents in the sample and the effect it may have had on the study findings.
   b. Comment on the limited number of fathers in the sample and the fact that none participated in individual interviews.

Summary Points

⇝ **Sampling** is the process of selecting a portion of the **population,** which is an entire aggregate of cases.

⇝ An *element* (the basic unit about which information is collected) must meet the **eligibility criteria** to be included in the sample.

⇝ The main consideration in assessing a sample in a quantitative study is its *representativeness*—the extent to which the sample is similar to the population and avoids bias. **Sampling bias** refers to the systematic overrepresentation or underrepresentation of some segment of the population.

⇝ Quantitative researchers usually sample from an **accessible population** but typically want to generalize to a larger **target population.**

⇝ **Nonprobability sampling** (wherein elements are selected by nonrandom methods) includes convenience, quota, and purposive sampling. Nonprobability sampling designs are convenient and economical; a major disadvantage is their potential for bias.

⇝ **Convenience sampling** (or *accidental sampling*) uses the most readily available or most convenient group of people for the sample. **Snowball sampling** is a type of convenience sampling in which referrals for potential participants are made by those already in the sample.

⇝ **Quota sampling** divides the population into homogeneous **strata** (subgroups) to ensure representation of those subgroups in the sample; within each stratum, researchers select participants by convenience sampling.

⇝ In **purposive** (or *judgmental*) **sampling,** participants or types of participants are hand picked based on the researcher's knowledge about the population.

⇝ **Probability sampling** designs, which involve the **random selection** of elements from the population, yield more representative samples than nonprobability designs and permit estimates of the magnitude of **sampling error.** Probability samples, however, are expensive and demanding.

⇝ **Simple random sampling** involves the selection of elements on a random basis from a *sampling frame* that enumerates all the elements.

⇝ **Stratified random sampling** divides the population into homogeneous subgroups from which elements are selected at random.

⇝ **Cluster sampling** (or *multistage sampling*) involves the successive selection of random samples from larger to smaller units by either simple random or stratified random methods.

⪼ **Systematic sampling** is the selection of every kth case from a list. By dividing the population size by the desired sample size, the researcher establishes the *sampling interval*, which is the standard distance between the selected elements.

⪼ In addition to representativeness, **sample size** is another important concern in quantitative studies, especially with regard to a study's statistical conclusion validity.

⪼ Advanced researchers use **power analysis** to estimate sample size needs. Large samples are preferable to small ones in quantitative studies because larger samples tend to be more representative, but even large samples do not guarantee representativeness.

⪼ Qualitative researchers use the theoretical demands of the study to select articulate and reflective informants with certain types of experience in an emergent way, capitalizing on early learning to guide subsequent sampling decisions.

⪼ Qualitative researchers most often use purposive or, in grounded theory studies, **theoretical sampling** to guide them in selecting data sources that maximize information richness.

⪼ Various purposive sampling strategies have been used by qualitative researchers. One strategy is **maximum variation sampling,** which entails purposely selecting cases with a wide range of variation. Other strategies include **homogeneous sampling** (deliberately reducing variation), **extreme case sampling** (selecting the most unusual or extreme cases), and **criterion sampling** (studying cases that meet a predetermined criterion of importance).

⪼ Another strategy in qualitative research is **sampling confirming and disconfirming cases,** that is, selecting cases that enrich and challenge the researchers' conceptualizations.

⪼ Samples in qualitative studies are typically small and based on information needs. A guiding principle is **data saturation,** which involves sampling to the point at which no new information is obtained and redundancy is achieved.

⪼ Ethnographers make numerous sampling decisions, including not only *whom* to sample but also *what* to sample (e.g., activities, events, documents, artefacts); these decisions are often aided by **key informants** who serve as guides and interpreters of the culture.

⪼ Phenomenologists typically work with a small sample of people (10 or fewer) who meet the criterion of having lived the experience under study.

⪼ Grounded theory researchers typically use theoretical sampling and work with samples of about 20 to 30 people.

⪼ Criteria for evaluating qualitative sampling are informational adequacy and appropriateness; potential for transferability is another issue of concern.

STUDIES CITED IN CHAPTER 12*

This reference list contains only those studies that were cited in this chapter. Citations pertaining to theoretical, methodologic, or nonempirical work are included together in a separate section at the end of the book (beginning on page 399).

Bryant-Lukosius, D., Green, E., Fitch, M., et al. (2007). A survey of oncology advanced practice nurses in Ontario: Profile and predictors of job satisfaction. *Nursing Leadership, 20*(2), 50–68.

Cohen, J. (1988). *Statistical power analysis for the behavioral sciences* (2nd ed.). Mahwah, NJ: Erlbaum.

Curtis, E. A. (2008). The effects of biographical variables on job satisfaction among nurses.*British Journal of Nursing, 17*(3), 174–180.

Douglas, C., Wollin, J. A., & Windsor, C. (2008). Illness and demographic correlates of chronic pain among a community-based sample of people with multiple sclerosis. *Archives of Physical Medicine and Rehabilitation, 89*(10), 1923–1932.

Gantert, T. W., McWilliam, C. L., Ward-Griffin, C., & Allen, N. J. (2008). The key to me: Seniors' perceptions of relationship-building with in-home service providers. *Canadian Journal on Aging, 27*(1), 23–34.

Glaser, B. G. (1978). *Theoretical sensitivity: Advances in the methodology of grounded theory.* Mill Valley, CA: Sociology Press.

Hertzog, M. A. (2008). Considerations in determining sample size for pilot studies. *Research in Nursing & Health, 31,* 180–191.

Loughrey, M. (2008). Just how male are male nurses? *Journal of Clinical Nursing, 17*(10), 1327–1334.

Lugg, G. R., & Ahmed, H. A. (2008). Nurses' perceptions of meticillin-resistant *Staphylococcus aureus*: Impacts on practice. *British Journal of Infection Control, 9*(1), 8–14.

Mills, J., Francis, K., & Bonner, A. (2007). Live my work: Rural nurses and their multiple perspectives of self. *Journal of Advanced Nursing, 59*(6), 583–590.

Morse, J. M. (1991). Strategies for sampling. In J. M. Morse (Ed.), *Qualitative nursing research: A contemporary dialogue.* Newbury Park, CA: Sage.

Morse, J. M. (2000). Determining sample size. *Qualitative Health Research, 10,* 3–5.

Neufeld, A., Harrison, M. J., Stewart, M., & Hughes, K. (2008). Advocacy of women family caregivers: Response to nonsupportive interactions with professionals. *Qualitative Health Research, 18*(3), 301–310.

Patton, M. Q. (2002). *Qualitative evaluation and research methods* (3rd ed.). Newbury Park, CA: Sage.

Porter, E. J. (1999). Defining the eligible, accessible population for a phenomenological study. *Western Journal of Nursing Research, 21,* 796–804.

Profetto-McGrath, J., Smith, K. B., Hugo, K., Taylor, M., & El-Hajj, H. (2007). Clinical nurse specialists' use of evidence in practice: A pilot study. *Worldviews on Evidence-Based Nursing, 4*(2), 86–96.

Scott, S. D., & Pollock, C. (2008). The role of nursing unit culture in shaping research utilization behaviors. *Research in Nursing & Health, 31*(4), 298–309.

Semenic, S., Loiselle, C., & Gottlieb, L. (2008). Predictors of the duration of exclusive breastfeeding among first-time mothers. *Research in Nursing & Health, 31*(5), 428–441.

Spagrud, L. J., von Baeyer, C. L., Kaiser, A., et al. (2008). Pain, distress, and adult-child interaction during venipuncture in pediatric oncology: An examination of three types of venous access. *Journal of Pain and Symptom Management, 36*(2), 173–184.

Turris, S. A., & Johnson, J. L. (2008). Maintaining integrity: Women and treatment seeking for the symptoms of potential cardiac illness. *Qualitative Health Research, 18*(11), 1461–1476.

Vlack, S., Foster, R., Menzies, R., Williams, G., Shannon, C., & Riley, I. (2007). Immunisation coverage of Queensland indigenous two-year-old children by cluster sampling and by register. *Australian & New Zealand Journal of Public Health, 31*(1), 67–72.

Williamson, D. L., Stewart, M. J., Hayward, K., et al. (2006). Low-income Canadians' experiences with health-related services: Implications for health care reform. *Health Policy, 76*(1), 106–121.

Wilson, B., Squires, M., Widger, K., Cranley, L., & Tourangeau, A. (2008). Job satisfaction among a multigenerational nursing workforce. *Journal of Nursing Management, 16*(6), 716–723.

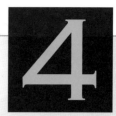

Data
Collection

13 Scrutinizing Data Collection Methods

On completing this chapter, you will be able to:

1. Identify phenomena that lend themselves to self-reports, observation, and physiologic measurement

2. Distinguish between and evaluate structured and unstructured self-reports; open-ended and closed-ended questions; and interviews and questionnaires

3. Distinguish between and evaluate structured and unstructured observations and describe various methods of collecting, sampling, and recording observational data

4. Describe the major features of biophysiologic measures

5. Critique a researcher's decisions regarding the data collection plan (degree of structure, general method, mode of administration) and its implementation

6. Define new terms in the chapter

The concepts in which researchers are interested must be measured, observed, or recorded. The task of selecting or developing methods for gathering data is among the most challenging in the research process.

OVERVIEW OF DATA COLLECTION AND DATA SOURCES

There are many alternative approaches to data collection, and these approaches vary along several dimensions. This section provides an overview of some important dimensions.

Existing Data Versus New Data

One of the first data decisions that a researcher makes concerns the use of existing data versus new data gathered specifically for the study. While most of this chapter is devoted to the latter, better data archiving (or storage) techniques have allowed researchers to increasingly take advantage of existing information, which conserves time and resources. However, it is important to note that use of existing data must adhere to the ethical guidelines under which it was originally collected—for example, participants' consents specify the limits imposed on data access and use.

We have already discussed several types of studies that rely on existing data. Meta-analyses and meta-syntheses (see Chapter 7) are examples of studies that involve analyses of available data—that is, data from research reports. Historical research (see Chapter 10) typically relies on available data in the form of written, narrative records of the past: diaries, letters, newspapers, minutes of meetings, and so forth. As we discussed in Chapter 11, researchers sometimes perform a secondary analysis, which is the use of data gathered in a previous study to test new hypotheses or address new research questions.

An important existing data source for nurse researchers is **records.** Hospital records, nursing charts, physicians' order sheets, and care plan statements all constitute rich data sources. Records are an economical and convenient source of information. Because the researchers were not responsible for collecting and recording information, however, they may be unaware of the records' limitations, biases, or incompleteness. If the records available for use are not the entire set of all possible records, investigators must consider the records' representativeness. Existing records have been used in both qualitative and quantitative nursing studies.

Example of a study using records
Avis et al. (2007) used the medical records of 10,287 2-year-olds to determine the rates of childhood immunization in each residential neighbourhood in Saskatoon to identify factors that could influence low adherence.

TIP

Researchers describe their data collection plan in the "Methods" section of a research report. In a report for a quantitative study, the specific data collection methods are often described in a subsection labelled "Measures" or "Instruments." The actual steps taken to collect the data are sometimes described in a separate subsection with the heading "Procedures."

Major Types of Data for Nursing Studies

If existing data are unavailable or unsuitable for a research question, researchers must collect new data. In developing their data collection plan, researchers make many decisions, including the basic type of data to gather. Three types have been used most frequently by nurse researchers: self-reports, observations, and biophysiologic measures. **Self-reports** are participants' responses to questions posed by the researcher, as in an interview. Direct **observation** of people's behaviours or characteristics is an alternative to self-reports for certain research questions. Nurses also use **biophysiologic measures** to assess important clinical variables. Sections of this chapter are devoted to these three major types of data collection.

In quantitative studies, researchers decide up front how to operationalize their variables and how best to gather their data. Their data collection plans are almost always "cast in stone" before a single piece of data is collected. Self-reports are the most common data collection approach in quantitative nursing studies.

Qualitative researchers typically go into the field knowing the most likely sources of data, but they do not rule out other possible data sources that might come to light as data collection progresses. As in quantitative studies, the primary method of collecting qualitative data is through self-report, that is, through interviews with study participants. Observation is often a part of many qualitative studies as well. Physiologic data are rarely collected in a naturalistic inquiry.

Table 13.1 compares the types of data used by researchers in the three main qualitative traditions, as well as other aspects of the data collection process for each tradition. Ethnographers almost always triangulate data from various

TABLE 13.1 ▶ **DATA COLLECTION IN THE THREE MAIN QUALITATIVE TRADITIONS**

ISSUE	ETHNOGRAPHY	PHENOMENOLOGY	GROUNDED THEORY
Type of data	Primarily participant observation and interviews, plus documents, artefacts, maps, photographs, social network diagrams, genealogies	Primarily in-depth interviews, sometimes diaries, artwork, or other materials	Primarily individual interviews, sometimes group interviews, participant observations, journals
Unit of data collection	Cultural systems	Individuals	Individuals
Period of data collection	Extended period, many months or years	Typically moderate	Typically moderate
Salient field issues	Gaining entrée, determining a role, learning how to participate, encouraging candor, identification with group, premature exit	Bracketing one's views, building rapport, encouraging candor, listening intently while preparing next question, keeping "on track," handling personal emotions	Building rapport, encouraging candor, keeping "on track," listening intently while preparing next question, handling personal emotions

sources, with observation and interviews being the most important methods. Ethnographers also gather or examine products of the culture under study, such as documents, records, artefacts, photographs, and so forth. Phenomenologists and grounded theory researchers rely primarily on in-depth interviews with individual participants, although observation also plays a role in some grounded theory studies.

Key Dimensions of Data Collection Methods

Data collection methods vary along several important dimensions, regardless of the type of data collected in a study:

❧ *Structure.* Research data can be collected in a highly structured manner: the same information is gathered from all participants in a comparable, prespecified way. Sometimes, however, it is more appropriate to be flexible and to allow participants to reveal relevant information in a naturalistic way.

❧ *Quantifiability.* Data that will be analyzed statistically must be gathered in such a way that they can be quantified. On the other hand, data that are to be analyzed qualitatively are collected in narrative form. Structured data collection approaches tend to yield data that are more easily quantified.

❧ *Obtrusiveness.* Data collection methods differ in terms of the degree to which people are aware of their status as study participants. If participants are fully aware of their role in a study, their behaviour and responses might not be normal. When data are collected unobtrusively, however, ethical problems may emerge.

❧ *Objectivity.* Some data collection approaches require more subjective judgment than others. Quantitative researchers generally strive for methods that are as objective as possible. In qualitative research, however, the researcher's subjective judgment is considered a valuable tool.

Research questions may dictate where on these four dimensions the data collection method will lie. For example, questions that are best suited for a phenomenological study tend to use methods that are low on structure, quantifiability, and objectivity, whereas research questions appropriate for a survey tend to require methods that are high on all four dimensions. However, researchers often have latitude in selecting or designing appropriate data collection plans.

TIP

Most data that are analyzed quantitatively actually begin as qualitative data. If a researcher asked respondents if they have been severely depressed, moderately depressed, somewhat depressed, or not at all depressed in the past week, they answer in words, not numbers. The words are transformed, through a coding process, into quantitative categories.

SELF-REPORT METHODS

A good deal of information can be gathered by directly questioning people. If, for example, we were interested in learning about patients' perceptions of hospital care, their preoperative fears, or their health-promoting activities, we would likely talk to them and ask them questions. For some research variables, alternatives to direct questioning exist, but the unique ability of humans to communicate verbally on a sophisticated level ensures that self-reports will always be a fundamental tool in nurse researchers' repertoire of data collection techniques.

Self-report techniques can vary in structure—from loosely organized methods that do not involve a formal set of questions, to tightly structured methods involving the use of forms such as questionnaires. Some characteristics of different self-report approaches are discussed next.

Qualitative Self-Report Techniques

Self-report methods used in qualitative studies offer flexibility. When these unstructured methods are used, researchers do not have a set of questions that must be asked in a specific order and worded in a given way. Instead, they start with some general questions and allow respondents to tell their stories in a naturalistic, narrative fashion. In other words, unstructured or semistructured interviews are conversational in nature.

Unstructured interviews, which are used by researchers in all qualitative research traditions, encourage respondents to define the important dimensions of a phenomenon and to elaborate on what is relevant to them, rather than being guided by investigators' *a priori* notions of relevance. Unstructured interviews are the mode of choice when researchers lack a precise understanding of what it is they do not know.

Types of Qualitative Self-Reports

There are several approaches to collecting qualitative self-report data. **Completely unstructured interviews** are used when researchers have no preconceived view of the content or flow of information to be gathered. Their aim is to elucidate respondents' perceptions of the world without imposing the researchers' views. Typically, researchers begin by asking a broad **grand tour question** such as "What happened when you first learned that you had AIDS?" Subsequent questions usually are more focused and are guided by initial responses. Ethnographic and phenomenological studies sometimes use completely unstructured interviews.

Semistructured (or *focused*) **interviews,** which are used more frequently than totally unstructured interviews, rely on a list of topics or broad questions that must be addressed in an interview. Interviewers use a written **topic guide** (or *interview guide*) to ensure that all question areas are covered. The interviewer's function is to encourage participants to talk freely about all the topics on the guide, and probe for greater detail when necessary.

Focus group interviews are interviews with groups of about 5 to 10 people whose opinions and experiences are solicited simultaneously. The interviewer (or *moderator*) guides the discussion according to a topic guide or set of questions. Another researcher will often sit in as a silent observer to note any nonverbal cues that may enrich the data and to validate, in discussion with the moderator, a general description of the session. The advantages of a group format are that it is efficient and can generate a lot of dialogue. Some people, however, are uncomfortable expressing their views or describing their experiences in front of a group. It is an important skill in moderating therefore to encourage the quieter individuals, while politely limiting the more dominant ones. Focus groups have been used by researchers in many qualitative research traditions and can play a particularly important role in feminist, critical theory, and participatory action research.

Example of semistructured interviews

Fairbairn et al. (2008) explored the effect of Vancouver's supervised injection facility on violence and related risk during the injection process, with 25 female injection drug users through semistructured interviews employing a topic guide.

Example of focus group interviews

Brazier, Cooke, and Moravan (2008) evaluated an integrative cancer care program in Vancouver using a mixed-method approach. While the small sample size ($n = 46$) limited the quantitative results in terms of statistical significance, the focus group data collected midway through the follow-up period revealed a rich description of active patient engagement in their cancer care. Four focus groups were held, each approximately 2.5 hours in duration, which followed a series of guiding questions such as "Can you please describe any ways that your experience at the Centre may have affected your healing and/or recovery from cancer?" (p. 8)

Life histories are narrative self-disclosures about individual life experiences. With this approach, researchers ask respondents to describe, often in chronologic sequence, their experiences regarding a specified theme, either orally or in writing. Some researchers have used this approach to obtain a total life health history.

The **think aloud method** is a qualitative method that has been used to collect data about cognitive processes, such as thinking, problem solving, and decision making. This method involves having people use audio-recording devices to talk about decisions as they are being made or while problems are being solved, over an extended period (e.g., throughout a shift). The method produces an inventory of decisions and underlying processes as they occur in a naturalistic context.

Example of the think aloud method

Atack, Luke, and Chien (2008) tested the usability of an online patient education system developed to tailor best health evidence to the needs of individual patients. One part of the testing involved each participant sitting with a researcher at the computer and going through a number of predetermined online education packages, while thinking aloud. The 75-minute session was audio-taped, observed by an unseen second researcher, and the mouse movements tracked to highlight any difficulties encountered.

Personal **diaries** have long been used as a source of data in historical research. It is also possible to generate new data for a nonhistorical study by asking participants to maintain a diary or journal over a specified period. Diaries can be useful in providing an intimate description of a person's everyday life. The diaries may be completely unstructured; for example, individuals who have undergone organ transplantation could be asked simply to spend 10 to 15 minutes a day jotting down their thoughts and feelings. Frequently, however, participants are requested to make entries into a diary regarding some specific aspect of their experience (e.g., about fatigue).

The **critical incidents technique** is a method of gathering information about people's behaviours by examining specific incidents relating to the behaviour under study. The technique focuses on a factual *incident*—an integral episode of human behaviour; *critical* means that the incident must have had a discernible impact on some outcome. The technique differs from other self-report approaches in that it focuses on something specific about which respondents can be expected to testify as expert witnesses.

Example of the critical incident technique

Meijers and Gustafsson (2008) used critical incidents technique in their study of patients' self-determination in two separate intensive care units in Sweden. They asked participating intensive care nurses to elaborate on a specific successful incident where they believed their actions strengthened their patient's self-determination, as well as a negative incident that had the reverse effect.

Gathering Qualitative Self-Report Data

Researchers gather narrative self-report data to develop a construction of a phenomenon that is consistent with that of participants. This goal requires researchers to take steps to overcome communication barriers and to enhance the flow of meaning. For example, researchers should strive to learn if a group under study uses any special terms or jargon.

Although qualitative interviews are conversational, this does not mean that researchers engage in them casually. Conversations are purposeful and require advance thought and preparation. For example, the wording of questions should make sense to respondents and reflect their worldview. In addition to being good questioners, researchers must be good listeners. Only by attending carefully to what respondents are saying can in-depth interviewers develop appropriate follow-up questions.

Unstructured interviews are typically long—sometimes lasting several hours. The issue of how best to record such abundant information is a difficult one. Some researchers take sketchy notes as the interview progresses, filling in the details after the interview is completed—but this method is risky in terms of data accuracy. Most prefer tape recording the interviews for later transcription. Although some respondents are self-conscious when their conversation is recorded, they typically forget about the presence of recording equipment after a few minutes. It is always necessary first to seek permission from the interviewee before taping; refusal may ultimately result in exclusion from the study.

Quantitative Self-Report Techniques

Structured approaches to collecting self-report data are appropriate when researchers know in advance exactly what they need to know and can, therefore, frame appropriate questions to obtain the needed information. Structured self-report data are usually collected by means of a formal, written document—an **instrument.** The instrument is an **interview schedule** when the questions are asked orally in either a face-to-face or telephone format and is a **questionnaire** when respondents complete the instrument themselves.

Question Form

In a structured instrument, respondents are asked to respond to the same questions in the same order, and they are given the same set of response options. **Closed-ended questions** (also called **fixed-alternative questions**) are ones in which the **response alternatives** are prespecified by the researcher. The alternatives may range from a simple yes or no to complex expressions of opinion. The purpose of using questions with fixed alternatives is to ensure comparability of responses and to facilitate analysis.

Many structured instruments also include some **open-ended questions,** which allow participants to respond to questions in their own words. In questionnaires, respondents must write out their responses to open-ended questions. In interviews, the interviewer writes down responses verbatim. Some examples of open-ended and closed-ended questions are presented in Box 13.1.

Both open-ended and closed-ended questions have strengths and weaknesses. Closed-ended questions are more difficult to construct than open-ended ones but easier to administer and, especially, to analyze. Closed-ended questions are more efficient: people can complete more closed-ended questions than open-ended ones in a given amount of time. Also, respondents may be unwilling to compose lengthy written responses to open-ended questions in questionnaires.

The major drawback of closed-ended questions is that researchers might overlook some potentially important responses. Another concern is that closed-ended questions can be superficial; open-ended questions allow for richer and fuller information if the respondents are verbally expressive and cooperative. Finally, some respondents object to choosing from alternatives that do not reflect their opinions precisely.

Instrument Construction

In drafting questions for a structured instrument, researchers must carefully monitor the wording of each question for clarity, sensitivity to respondents' psychological state, absence of bias, and (in questionnaires) reading level. Questions must be sequenced in a psychologically meaningful order that encourages cooperation and candour.

Draft instruments are usually critically reviewed by colleagues and then pretested with a small sample of respondents. A *pretest* is a trial run to determine whether the instrument is useful in generating desired information. In large studies, the development and pretesting of self-report instruments may take many months to refine the instrument and gather adequate psychometrics.

Interviews Versus Questionnaires

Researchers using structured self-reports must decide whether to use interviews or questionnaires. You should be aware of the limitations and strengths of these alternatives because the decision may affect the findings and the quality of the evidence. Questionnaires, relative to interviews, have the following advantages:

⮞ Questionnaires are less costly and require less time and effort to administer; this is a particular advantage if the sample is geographically dispersed. Web-based questionnaires are especially economical.

⮞ Questionnaires offer the possibility of complete anonymity, which may be crucial in obtaining information about illegal or deviant behaviours or about embarrassing traits.

Example of mailed questionnaires
Pinelli et al. (2008) sought patterns of change in family functioning, resources, coping, and parental depression in parents of sick newborns over the year after birth. Baseline questionnaires were administered by a research assistant within the first 4 days of admission to the NICU, and then mailed to participants at 3, 6, and 12 months postdischarge to identify any changes over time.

BOX 13.1 EXAMPLES OF QUESTION TYPES

Open-Ended

■ What led to your decision to stop smoking?

■ What did you do when you discovered you had AIDS?

Closed-Ended

1. ***Dichotomous Question***
   Have you ever been hospitalized?
   ❏ 1. Yes
   ❏ 2. No

2. ***Multiple-Choice Question***
   How important is it to you to avoid a pregnancy at this time?
   ❏ 1. Extremely important
   ❏ 2. Very important
   ❏ 3. Somewhat important
   ❏ 4. Not at all important

3. ***"Cafeteria" Question***
   People have different opinions about the use of hormone-replacement therapy for women in menopause. Which of the following statements best represents your point of view?
   ❏ 1. Hormone replacement is dangerous and should be totally banned.
   ❏ 2. Hormone replacement may have some undesirable side effects that suggest the need for caution in its use.
   ❏ 3. I am undecided about my views on hormone-replacement therapy.
   ❏ 4. Hormone replacement has many beneficial effects that merit its promotion.
   ❏ 5. Hormone replacement is a wonder cure that should be administered widely to menopausal women.

4. ***Rank-Order Question***
   People value different things about life. Below is a list of principles or ideals that are often cited when people are asked to name things they value most. Please indicate the order of importance of these values to you by placing a 1 beside the most important, 2 beside the next most important, and so forth.
   ❏ Career achievement/work
   ❏ Family relationships
   ❏ Friendships and social interaction
   ❏ Health
   ❏ Money
   ❏ Religion

5. ***Forced-Choice Question***
   Which statement most closely represents your point of view?
   ❏ 1. What happens to me is my own doing.
   ❏ 2. Sometimes I feel I don't have enough control over my life.

6. ***Rating Question***
   On a scale from 0 to 10, where 0 means extremely dissatisfied and 10 means extremely satisfied, how satisfied are you with the nursing care you received during your hospitalization?

   Extremely dissatisfied   Extremely satisfied
   0   1   2   3   4   5   6   7   8   9   10

The strengths of interviews far outweigh those of questionnaires. These strengths include the following:

⇝ Response rates tend to be high in face-to-face interviews. Respondents are less likely to refuse to talk to an interviewer than to ignore a questionnaire, especially a mailed questionnaire. Low response rates can lead to bias because respondents are rarely a random subset of those sampled. Longitudinal studies pose even more challenge for researchers as participants are asked to complete questionnaires at various timepoints. In the mailed questionnaire study described earlier (Pinelli et al., 2008), 20% of families dropped out over the course of the study. Researchers, therefore, must allow for attrition in their original sample size calculations.

⇒ Many people simply cannot fill out a questionnaire; examples include young children, the blind, and the very elderly. Interviews are feasible with most people.

⇒ Interviewers can produce additional information through observation of respondents' living situation, level of understanding, degree of cooperativeness, and so forth—all of which can be useful in interpreting responses.

Most advantages of face-to-face interviews also apply to telephone interviews. Complicated or detailed instruments are not well suited to telephone interviewing, but for relatively brief instruments, the telephone interview combines relatively low costs with high response rates.

Example of in-person interviews

Maheu and Thorne (2008) explored the experiences of 21 Canadian women who received inconclusive BRCA1/2 genetic testing after a diagnosis of breast or ovarian cancer. In-depth, open-ended interviews were conducted with participants within a range of 3 to 18 months after receiving their test results, with recruitment continuing until the data revealed consistent themes.

Scales and Other Special Forms of Structured Self-Reports

Several special types of structured self-reports are used by nurse researchers. These include composite social–psychological scales, vignettes, and Q sorts.

Scales

Social–psychological scales are often incorporated into a questionnaire or interview schedule. A **scale** is a device designed to assign a numeric score to people to place them on a continuum with respect to attributes being measured, like a scale for measuring weight. Social–psychological scales quantitatively discriminate among people with different attitudes, motives, perceptions, and needs.

The most common scaling technique is the **Likert scale,** which consists of several declarative statements (or *items*) that express a viewpoint on a topic. Respondents are asked to indicate how much they agree or disagree with the statement. Table 13.2 presents an illustrative, five-point Likert scale for measuring attitudes toward condom use. In this example, agreement with positively worded statements and disagreement with negatively worded statements are assigned higher scores. The first statement is positively phrased; agreement indicates a favourable attitude toward condom use. Because the item has five response alternatives, a score of 5 would be given to someone strongly agreeing, 4 to someone agreeing, and so forth. The responses of two hypothetical respondents are shown by a check or an X, and their item scores are shown in the right-hand columns. Person 1, who agreed with the first statement, has a score of 4, whereas person 2, who strongly disagreed, has a score of 1. The second statement is negatively worded, and so the scoring is reversed—a 1 is assigned to those who strongly agree and so forth. This reversal is necessary so that a high score consistently reflects positive attitudes toward condom use. A person's total score is determined by summing item scores; hence, these scales are sometimes called **summated rating scales.** The total scores of the two respondents reflect a considerably more positive attitude toward condoms on the part of person 1 (score = 26) than person 2

TABLE 13.2 ⓘ	EXAMPLE OF A LIKERT SCALE TO MEASURE ATTITUDES TOWARD CONDOMS							

DIRECTION OF SCORING*	ITEM	RESPONSES†					SCORE	
		SA	A	?	D	SD	Person 1 (✓)	Person 2 (X)
+	1. Using a condom shows you care about your partner.		✓			X	4	1
−	2. My partner would be angry if I talked about using condoms.			X		✓	5	3
−	3. I wouldn't enjoy sex as much if my partner and I used condoms.			X	✓		4	2
+	4. Condoms are a good protection against AIDS and other sexually transmitted diseases.				✓	X	3	2
+	5. My partner would respect me if I insisted on using condoms.	✓				X	5	1
−	6. I would be too embarrassed to ask my partner about using a condom.			X		✓	5	2
	Total score						26	11

*Researchers would not indicate the direction of scoring on a Likert scale administered to subjects. The scoring direction is indicated in this table for illustrative purposes only.

†SA, strongly agree; A, agree; ?, uncertain; D, disagree; SD, strongly disagree.

(score = 11). Summing item scores makes it possible to make fine discriminations among people with different points of view. A six-item scale, such as the one in Table 13.2, could yield a range of possible scores, from a minimum of 6 (6 × 1) to a maximum of 30 (6 × 5).

Example of a Likert scale

Muller-Staub et al. (2008) studied the effect of guided clinical reasoning on nursing diagnoses, related interventions, and patient outcomes in a cluster-randomized trial. Nurses across three Swiss hospital wards received the guided clinical reasoning intervention while a further three wards acted as the control, receiving standard educational practice only. An instrument containing an 18-item Likert-type five-point (0 to 4) scale was used to evaluate the intervention at baseline and 3 to 7 months postintervention.

Another technique for measuring attitudes is the **semantic differential** (SD). With the SD, respondents rate concepts (e.g., primary nursing, team nursing) on a series of *bipolar adjectives*, such as good/bad, strong/weak, important/unimportant. Respondents are asked to place a check at the appropriate point on a seven-point scale that extends from one extreme of the dimension to the other. An example of an SD format is shown in Figure 13.1. The SD method is flexible and easy to construct. The concept being rated can be virtually anything—a person, concept, issue, and so forth. Scoring is similar to that for Likert scales. Scores from 1 to 7 are assigned to each bipolar scale response, and responses are then summed across the scales to yield a total score.

Nurse practitioners

Competent	7*	6	5	4	3	2	1		Incompetent
Worthless	1	2	3	4	5	6	7		Valuable
Important									Unimportant
Pleasant									Unpleasant
Bad									Good
Cold									Warm
Responsible									Irresponsible
Successful									Unsuccessful

*The score values would not be printed on the form administered to actual subjects. The numbers are presented here solely for the purpose of illustrating how semantic differentials are scored.

FIGURE 13.1   Example of a semantic differential.

Another type of psychosocial measure is the **visual analog scale** (VAS), which can be used to measure subjective experiences, such as pain, fatigue, and dyspnoea. The VAS is a straight line, the end anchors of which are labelled as the extreme limits of a sensation. Participants mark a point on the line corresponding to the amount of sensation experienced. Traditionally, a VAS line is 100 mm in length, which makes it easy to derive a score from 0 to 100 by simply measuring the distance from one end of the scale to the mark on the line. An example of a VAS is presented in Figure 13.2.

Scales permit researchers to efficiently quantify subtle gradations in the strength or intensity of individual characteristics. Scales can be administered either verbally or in writing and thus are suitable for use with most people. Scales are susceptible to several common problems, however, the most troublesome of which are referred to as **response set biases.** The most important biases include the following:

Example of a visual analog scale
Sawyer et al. (2008) conducted a pain prevalence study at a large Canadian teaching hospital using two self-administered pain measurements instruments, one of which included a visual analog scale (i.e., the short form McGill Pain Questionnaire).

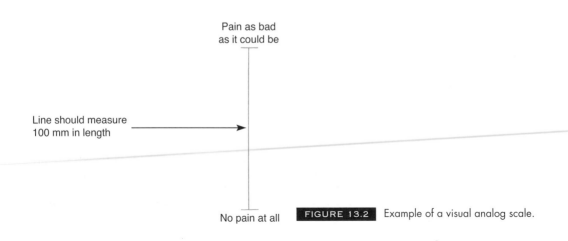

Pain as bad
as it could be

Line should measure
100 mm in length

No pain at all   **FIGURE 13.2**   Example of a visual analog scale.

❧ *Social desirability response set bias*—a tendency to misrepresent attitudes or traits by giving answers that are consistent with prevailing social views.

❧ *Extreme response set bias*—a tendency to consistently express attitudes or feelings in extreme responses (e.g., strongly agree), leading to distortions because extreme responses may not necessarily signify the greatest intensity of the trait being measured.

❧ *Acquiescence response set bias*—a tendency to agree with statements regardless of their content by people who are referred to as *yea-sayers*. Other people (*nay-sayers*) disagree with statements independently of the question content.

These biases can be reduced through such strategies as *counterbalancing* positively and negatively worded statements, developing sensitively worded questions, creating a nonjudgmental atmosphere, and guaranteeing the confidentiality of responses.

TIP

Most studies that collect self-report data involve one or more social–psychological scale. Typically, the scales are ones that were developed previously by other researchers as these will already have psychometric evidence to support validation.

Vignettes

Vignettes are brief descriptions of situations to which respondents are asked to react. The descriptions are structured to elicit information about respondents' perceptions, opinions, or knowledge about a phenomenon. Questions about the vignettes can be open ended (e.g., How would you recommend handling this situation?) or closed ended (e.g., On the seven-point scale below, rate how well you think the nurse handled the situation?).

Vignettes are an economical means of eliciting information about how people might behave in situations that would be difficult to observe in daily life. For example, we might want to assess how patients would react to or feel about nurses with different cultural backgrounds. The principal problem with vignettes concerns response validity. If respondents describe how they would react in a situation portrayed in the vignette, how accurate is that description of their actual behaviour? Thus, although the use of vignettes can be profitable, the possibility of response biases should be recognized.

Example of vignettes
Thompson et al. (2008) studied the effects of clinical experience and time pressure on nurses' decision making, using samples drawn from four countries—Australia, United Kingdom, Canada, and the Netherlands. Experienced acute care nurses (n = 241) were given 50 vignettes based on real clinical risk assessments and were asked whether or not to intervene. Just over half of the vignettes were administered with a 10-second response limit to test nurses' decision making under time pressure.

Q Sorts

In a **Q sort,** participants are presented with a set of cards on which statements or phrases are written. Participants are asked to sort the cards along a specified bipolar dimension, such as agree/disagree. Typically, there are between 60 and 100 cards to be sorted into 9 or 11 piles, with the number of cards to be placed in each pile predetermined by the researcher.

The sorting instructions in a Q sort can vary. For example, personality can be studied by writing descriptions of personality traits on the cards; participants can then be asked to sort items on a continuum from "exactly like me" to "not at all like me." Or, patients could be asked to rate various aspects of their treatment on a most distressing to least distressing continuum.

Q sorts can be useful, but they also have drawbacks. On the positive side, Q sorts are versatile and can be applied to a wide variety of problems. Requiring people to place a predetermined number of cards in each pile eliminates many response biases. On the other hand, it is time-consuming to administer Q sorts to a large sample of people. Some critics argue that the forced distribution of cards according to researchers' specifications is artificial and excludes information about how participants would ordinarily distribute their responses.

Example of a Q sort

Cragg, Marsden, and Wall (2008) used Q sort as an approach to studying the role of clinical directors in the U.K. health care system, from the perspective of colleagues. A sample of 30 staff drawn from various stakeholder groups was asked to rank a set of 80 statements according to a nine-point scale (strongly agree to strongly disagree). The statements were derived from previous stakeholder interviews and literature review.

Evaluation of Self-Report Methods

Self-report techniques—the most common method of data collection in nursing studies—are strong with respect to their directness. If researchers want to know how people feel or what they believe, the most direct approach is to ask them. Moreover, self-reports frequently yield information that would be impossible to gather by other means. Behaviours can be directly *observed*, but only if people are willing to engage in them publicly. It is usually impossible for researchers to observe such behaviours as contraceptive practices or drug use. Furthermore, observers can only observe behaviours occurring at the time of the study; self-report instruments can gather retrospective data about activities that occurred in the past or about behaviours in which participants plan to engage in the future. Information about feelings, values, opinions, and motives can sometimes be inferred through observation, but people's actions do not always indicate their state of mind. Self-report instruments can be used to measure psychological characteristics through direct communication with participants.

Despite these advantages, self-report methods have some weaknesses. The most serious issue concerns the validity and accuracy of self-reports: How can we be sure that respondents feel or act the way they say they do? How can we trust the information that respondents provide, particularly if the questions ask them to admit to potentially undesirable traits? Investigators often have no alternative but to assume that most respondents have been frank. Yet, we all have a tendency to present ourselves in the best light, and this may conflict with the truth. When reading research reports, you should be alert to potential biases in self-reported data, particularly with respect to behaviours or feelings that society judges to be controversial or wrong.

You should also be familiar with the merits of unstructured and structured self-reports. In general, unstructured (qualitative) interviews are of greatest utility when a new area of research is being explored. A qualitative approach allows researchers to ascertain what the basic issues are, how individuals conceptualize and talk about a phenomenon, and what the range is of opinions or behaviours that are relevant to the topic. Qualitative methods may also help elucidate the underlying meaning of a pattern or relationship repeatedly observed in quantitative research.

Qualitative methods, however, are extremely time-consuming and demanding and are not appropriate for capturing the measurable aspects of a phenomenon, such as incidence (e.g., the percentage of women who experience postpartum depression, or PPD), frequency (how often symptoms of PPD are experienced),

---

BOX 13.2 GUIDELINES FOR CRITIQUING SELF-REPORTS

1. Does the research question lend itself to a self-report method of data collection? Would an alternative method have been more appropriate?
2. Is the degree of structure consistent with the nature of the research question?
3. Given the research question and respondent characteristics, did the researcher use the best possible mode for collecting the data (i.e., personal interviews, telephone interviews, or self-administered questionnaires)?
4. Do the questions included in the instrument or topic guide adequately cover the complexities of the problem under investigation?
5. If a composite scale was used, does its use seem appropriate? Does the scale adequately capture the target research variable?
6. If a vignette or Q sort was used, does its use seem appropriate?

---

duration (e.g., average time period during which PPD is present), or magnitude (e.g., degree of severity of PPD). Structured self-reports are also appropriate when researchers want to test hypotheses concerning relationships.

Critiquing Self-Reports

One of the first questions you should ask is whether the researcher made the right decision in obtaining the data by self-report rather than by an alternative method. Attention then should be paid to the adequacy of the actual methods used. Box 13.2 presents some guiding questions for critiquing self-reports.

It may be difficult to perform a thorough critique of self-report methods in studies reported in journals because researchers seldom include detailed descriptions of the data collection methods. What you can expect is information about the following aspects of the self-report data collection:

⤳ The degree of the structure used in the questioning

⤳ Whether interviews or questionnaires (or variants such as a Q sort) were used

⤳ How the instruments were administered (e.g., by telephone, in person, by mail, over the Internet)

⤳ Where the interviews (if relevant) took place

Degree of structure is especially important in your assessment of a data collection plan. The decision about an instrument's structure should be based on considerations that you can often evaluate. For example, respondents who are not very articulate are more receptive to instruments with many closed-ended questions than to questioning that forces them to compose lengthy answers. Other considerations include the amount of time available (structured instruments are more efficient); the expected sample size (open-ended questions and qualitative interviews are difficult to analyze with large samples); the status of existing information on the topic (in a new area of inquiry, a quantitative approach may not be warranted); and, most important, the nature of the research question.

TIP

In research reports, descriptions of data collection instruments are often quite brief. For example, if a study involved the use of a depression scale (e.g., the Center for Epidemiological Studies Depression Scale, or CES-D), the research report most likely would not describe individual items on this scale—although the report should provide an appropriate reference. Moreover, there is typically insufficient space in journals for detailed rationales (e.g., a rationale for choosing the CES-D instead of the Beck Depression Scale). As such, it may be hard for you to undertake a thorough critique of the data collection plan. It is acceptable to e-mail the author for further details, if necessary.

OBSERVATIONAL METHODS

For some research questions, direct observation of people's behaviour is an alternative to self-reports. Within nursing research, observational methods have broad applicability, particularly for clinical inquiries. Nurses are in an advantageous position to observe, relatively unobtrusively, the behaviours and activities of patients, their families, and health care staff. Observational methods can be used to gather such information as the characteristics and conditions of individuals (e.g., patients' sleep–wake state), verbal communication (e.g., exchange of information at change-of-shift), nonverbal communication (e.g., body language), activities (e.g., patients' self-grooming activities), and environmental conditions (e.g., noise levels in nursing homes).

In observational studies, researchers have flexibility with regard to several issues:

⇒ *The focus of the observation.* The focus can be broadly defined events (e.g., patient mood swings) or small, specific behaviours (e.g., facial expressions).

⇒ *Concealment.* As discussed in Chapter 5, awareness of being observed may cause people to behave abnormally, thereby jeopardizing the validity of the observations. The problem of behavioural distortions due to the known presence of an observer is called **reactivity.**

⇒ *Duration of observation.* Some observations can be made in a short period of time, but others, particularly those in ethnographic and other field studies, may require months or years in the field.

⇒ *Method of recording observations.* Observations can be made through the human senses and then recorded by paper-and-pencil methods, but they can also be done with sophisticated technical equipment (e.g., video, audio-recording equipment).

In summary, observational techniques can be used to measure a broad range of phenomena and are versatile. Like self-report techniques, an important dimension for observational methods is degree of structure—that is, whether the observational data are amenable to qualitative or quantitative analysis.

Qualitative Observational Methods

Qualitative researchers collect observational data with a minimum of structure and researcher-imposed constraints. Skilful unstructured observation permits researchers to see the world as the study participants see it, to develop a rich understanding and appreciation of key phenomena, to extract meaning from events and situations, and to grasp the subtleties of cultural variation.

Naturalistic observations often are made in field settings through a technique called **participant observation.** A participant observer participates in the functioning of the group or institution under study and strives to observe and record information within the contexts, experiences, and symbols that are relevant to the participants. By assuming a participating role, observers may have insights that would have eluded more passive observers. Of course, not all qualitative observational studies use *participant* observation; some unstructured observations involve watching and recording unfolding behaviours without the observers' participation in activities. The great majority of qualitative observations, however, do involve some participation, particularly in ethnographic and grounded theory research.

Example of qualitative nonparticipant observation
Miller et al. (2008) conducted a study exploring nursing emotion work (or "the management of the emotions of self and others in order to improve patient care") and how it applies to interprofessional collaboration in general internal medicine wards across three urban Canadian hospitals. Data collection methods included nonparticipant observation, shadowing, and semistructured interviews.

The Observer-Participant Role in Participant Observation

In participant observation, the role observers play in the social group under study is important because their social position determines what they are likely to see. That is, the behaviours that are likely to be available for observation depend on the observers' position in a network of relations.

The extent of the observers' actual participation in a group is best thought of as a continuum. At one extreme of the continuum is complete immersion in the setting, with researchers assuming full participant status; at the other extreme is complete separation, with researchers assuming an onlooker status. Researchers may in some cases assume a fixed position on this continuum throughout the study.

On the other hand, researchers' role as participants may evolve over the course of the fieldwork. A researcher may begin primarily as a bystander, with participation in group activities increasing over time. In other cases, it might be profitable to become immersed in a social setting quickly, with participation diminishing to allow more time for pure observation.

TIP

It is not unusual to find research reports that state that participant observation was used when in fact the description of the method suggests that observation, but not participation, was involved. Some researchers appear to use the term "participant observation" to refer generally to unstructured observations conducted in the field.

Observers must overcome at least two major hurdles in assuming a satisfactory role vis-à-vis participants. The first is to gain entrée into the social group under study; the second is to establish rapport and develop trust within that group. Without gaining entrée, the study cannot proceed; but without the trust of the group, the researcher will typically be restricted to "front stage" knowledge—that is, information distorted by the group's protective facades (Leininger, 1985). The goal of participant observers is to "get back stage"—to learn about the true realities of the group's experiences and behaviours. On the other hand, being a fully participating member does not *necessarily* offer the best perspective for studying a phenomenon—just as being an actor in a play does not offer the most advantageous view of the performance.

Example of participant observation

O'Brien, Mill, and Wilson (2009) conducted an ethnographic study of cervical screening in Canadian First Nation Cree women, using participant observation and interviews. One of the authors is, herself, First Nations and spent time prior to data collection working as a health care provider in the sample community—" . . . she was a participant observer of community life and in an unique position to observe women's responses to both screening and illness" (p. 84).

Gathering Participant Observation Data

Participant observers typically place few restrictions on the nature of the data collected, in keeping with the goal of minimizing observer-imposed meanings and structure. Nevertheless, participant observers often do have a broad plan for the types of information to be gathered. Among the aspects of an observed activity likely to be considered relevant are the following:

1. *The physical setting—"where" questions.* Where is the activity happening? What are the main features of the physical setting?

2. *The participants—"who" questions.* Who is present? What are their characteristics and roles? Who is given free access to the setting—who "belongs?"

3. *Activities—"what" questions.* What is going on? What are participants doing? How do participants interact with one another?

4. *Frequency and duration—"when" questions.* When did the activity begin and end? How regularly does the activity recur?

5. *Process—"how" questions.* How is the activity organized? How does the event unfold?

6. *Outcomes—"why" questions.* Why is the activity happening, or why is it happening in this manner? What did *not* happen—and why?

The next decision is to identify a way to sample observations and to select observational locations. Researchers generally use a combination of positioning approaches. *Single positioning* means staying in a single location for a period to observe transactions. *Multiple positioning* involves moving around the site to observe behaviours from different locations. *Mobile positioning* involves following a person throughout a given activity or period.

Because participant observers cannot spend a lifetime in one site and cannot be in more than one place at a time, observation is usually supplemented with information from unstructured interviews or conversations. For example, informants may be asked to describe what went on in a meeting the observer was unable to attend, or to describe an event that occurred before the observer entered the field. In such cases, the informant functions as the observer's observer.

Recording Observations

The most common forms of record keeping in participant observation studies are logs and field notes, but photographs and videotapes may also be used. A **log** (or *field diary*) is a daily record of events and conversations. **Field notes** are broader, more analytic, and more interpretive. Field notes represent the observer's efforts to record information, synthesize, and understand the data.

Field notes can be descriptive or reflective. *Descriptive notes* (or *observational notes*) are objective, *thick* descriptions of events and conversations. Descriptions of what has transpired must include contextual information about time, place, and actors to fully portray the situation. *Reflective notes* document researchers' personal experiences and reflections while in the field. Reflective notes can serve various purposes. *Theoretical notes* are interpretive attempts to attach meaning to observations. *Methodologic notes* are instructions or reminders about how subsequent observations will be made. *Personal notes* are comments about the researcher's own feelings during the research process. Box 13.3 presents examples of various types of field notes from Beck's (2002) study of mothering twins.

The success of any participant observation study depends on the quality of the logs and field notes. Observers must develop the skill of making detailed mental notes that can later be written or tape-recorded. The use of laptop computers can greatly facilitate the recording and organization of notes in the field.

Quantitative Observational Methods

Structured observation differs from unstructured techniques in the specificity of what will be observed and in the advance preparation of forms. The creativity of structured observation lies not in the observation itself but rather in the development of a system for accurately categorizing, recording, and encoding the observations and sampling the phenomena of interest.

Categories and Checklists

The most common approach to making structured observations is to use a category system for classifying observed phenomena. A **category system** represents a

BOX 13.3   **EXAMPLE OF FIELD NOTES: MOTHERING MULTIPLES GROUNDED THEORY STUDY**
▶

Observational Notes: O.L. attended the Mothers of Multiples Support Group again this month but she looked worn out today. She wasn't as bubbly as she had been at the March meeting. She explained why she wasn't doing as well this month. She and her husband had just found out that their house has lead-based paint in it. Both twins do have increased lead levels. She and her husband are in the process of buying a new home.

Theoretical Notes: So far all the mothers have stressed the need for routine in order to survive the first year of caring for twins. Mothers, however, have varying definitions of routine. I.R. had the firmest routine with her twins. B.L. is more flexible with her routine, i.e., the twins are always fed at the same time but aren't put down for naps or bed at night at the same time. Whenever one of the twins wants to go to sleep is fine with her. B.L. does have a daily routine in regards to housework. For example, when the twins are down in the morning for a nap, she makes their bottles up for the day (14 bottles total).

Methodologic Notes: The first sign-up sheet I passed around at the Mothers of Multiples Support Group for women to sign up to participate in interviews for my grounded theory study consisted of only two columns: one for the mother's name and one for her telephone number. I need to revise this sign-up sheet to include extra columns for the age of the multiples, the town where the mother lives, and older siblings and their ages. My plan is to start interviewing mothers with multiples around 1 year of age so that the moms can reflect back over the process of mothering their infants for the first 12 months of their lives.

Right now I have no idea of the ages of the infants of the mothers who signed up to be interviewed. I will need to call the nurse in charge of this support group to find out the ages.

Personal Notes: Today was an especially challenging interview. The mom had picked the early afternoon for me to come to her home to interview her because that is the time her 2-year-old son would be napping. When I arrived at her house her 2-year-old ran up to me and said hi. The mom explained that he had taken an earlier nap that day and that he would be up during the interview. So in the living room with us during our interview were her two twin daughters (3 months old) swinging in the swings and her 2-year-old son. One of the twins was quite cranky for the first half hour of the interview. During the interview the 2-year-old sat on my lap and looked at the two books I had brought as a little present. If I didn't keep him occupied with the books, he would keep trying to reach for the microphone of the tape recorder.

From Beck, C. T. (2002). Releasing the pause button: Mothering twins during the first year of life. *Qualitative Health Research,* *12,* 593–608.

method of recording in a systematic fashion the behaviours and events of interest that transpire in a setting.

Some category systems are constructed so that *all* observed behaviours within in a specified domain (e.g., all body positions and movements) can be classified into one and only one category. A contrasting technique is to develop a system in which only particular types of behaviour (which may or may not be manifested) are categorized. For example, if we were studying autistic children's aggressive behaviour, we might develop such categories as "strikes another child" or "throws objects around the room." In this category system, many behaviours—all that are nonaggressive—would not be classified, and some children may exhibit *no* aggressive actions. Nonexhaustive systems are adequate for many purposes, but one risk is that resulting data might be difficult to interpret. When a large number of behaviours are not categorized, the investigator may have difficulty placing categorized behaviour into perspective.

Example of a nonexhaustive observational checklist
Benzies et al. (2008) examined interactions between first-time fathers and their 5- or 6-month-old infants. The researchers used an instrument called the Nursing Child Assessment Teaching Scale (NCATS), an observational checklist that taps 50 parent and 23 infant behaviours during a teaching task (i.e., introducing a new toy to their infant) using a yes/no scale. In this study, the parent–infant interactions were assessed at baseline and postintervention when the infants were approximately 8 months old.

One of the most important requirements of a category system is the careful and explicit operational definition of the behaviours and characteristics to be observed. Each category must be carefully explained, giving observers clearcut criteria for assessing the occurrence of the phenomenon. Even with detailed definitions of categories, observers often are faced with making numerous on-the-spot inferences. Virtually all category systems require observer inference, to a greater or lesser degree.

After a category system has been developed, researchers typically construct a **checklist,** which is the instrument used to record observations. The checklist is generally formatted with the list of behaviours from the category system on the left and space for tallying their frequency or duration on the right. The task of the observer using an exhaustive category system is to place *all* observed behaviours in one category for each integral unit of behaviour (e.g., a sentence in a conversation, a time interval). Checklists based on exhaustive category systems tend to be demanding because the recording task is continuous. With nonexhaustive category systems, categories of behaviours that may or may not be manifested by participants are listed. The observer's tasks are to watch for instances of these behaviours and to record their occurrence.

Example of low observer inference

Wells et al. (2008) evaluated a nurse-led clinic for patients undergoing radiotherapy to the head and neck in the United Kingdom. The study compared three groups—the traditional medical on-treatment review, nurse-led clinic, and an historical control group. A mixed-methods approach to data collection included the use of an observational clinic checklist to assess the nature of the consultations, which would be checked only if items occurred.

Rating Scales

Another approach to structured observations is to use a **rating scale,** which requires observers to rate some phenomena along a descriptive continuum. Observers may be required to make ratings of behaviour at intervals throughout the observation or to summarize an entire event or transaction after observation is completed.

Rating scales can be used as an extension of checklists, in which the observer records not only the occurrence of some behaviour but also some qualitative aspect of it, such as its magnitude or intensity. When rating scales are coupled with a category scheme in this fashion, considerably more information about the phenomena under study can be obtained, but this approach places an immense burden on observers.

Example of observational ratings

Bettazzoni et al. (2008) studied the intrusiveness of schizophrenia on life activities and interests, as well as subjective well-being, in 78 Canadian persons living with the illness. In addition to the data collected from the patients themselves, a clinician and a relative/friend were nominated by each participant to provide independent ratings. While a variety of measures were used to collect data in this study, the Barnes Rating Scale for Drug-Induced Akathisia (or patients' inner restlessness) is an example of rating scale used by an observer to measure the severity of the condition.

Observational Sampling

Researchers must decide when structured observational systems will be applied. Observational sampling methods provide a mechanism for obtaining representative examples of the behaviours being observed. One system is **time sampling,** which involves the selection of time periods during which observations will occur. Time frames may be systematically selected (e.g., every 30 seconds at 2-minute intervals) or selected at random.

Event sampling selects integral behaviours or events for observation. Event sampling requires researchers to either have knowledge about the occurrence of events or be in a position to wait for or precipitate their occurrence. Examples of integral events that may be suitable for event sampling include shift changes of nurses in a hospital or cast removals of pediatric patients. This sampling approach is preferable to time sampling when the events of interest are infrequent and may be missed if time sampling is used. When behaviours and events are relatively frequent, however, time sampling enhances the representativeness of the observed behaviours.

Evaluation of Observational Methods

The field of nursing is particularly well suited to observational research. Nurses are often in a position to watch people's behaviours and may, by training, be especially sensitive observers. Moreover, certain research questions are better suited to observation than to self-reports, such as when people cannot adequately describe their own behaviours. This may be the case when people are unaware of their own behaviour (e.g., stress-induced behaviour), when people are embarrassed to report their activities (e.g., aggressive actions), when behaviours are emotionally laden (e.g., grieving behaviour), or when people are not capable of articulating their actions (e.g., young children or the mentally ill). Observational methods have an intrinsic appeal for directly capturing behaviours and events. Furthermore, observational methods can provide information of great depth and variety. With this approach, humans—the observers—are used as measuring instruments and provide a uniquely sensitive (if fallible) tool.

Several of the shortcomings of the observational approach have already been mentioned. These include possible ethical difficulties and reactivity of the observed when the observer is conspicuous. However, one of the most pervasive problems is the vulnerability of observations to bias. A number of factors interfere with objective observations, including the following:

➢ Emotions, prejudices, and values of the observer may result in faulty inference.

➢ Personal interest and commitment may colour what is seen in the direction of what the observer wants to see.

➢ Anticipation of what is to be observed may affect what is perceived.

➢ Hasty decisions may result in erroneous conclusions or classifications.

Observational biases probably cannot be eliminated, but they can be minimized through careful observer training.

Both unstructured and structured observational methods have pros and cons. Qualitative observational methods potentially yield a richer understanding of human behaviours and social situations than is possible with structured procedures. Skilful participant observers can "get inside" a situation and lead to a solid understanding of its complexities. Furthermore, qualitative observational approaches are flexible and give observers freedom to reconceptualize the problem after becoming familiar with the situation. On the other hand, observer bias may pose a threat: once researchers begin to participate in a group's activities, the possibility of emotional involvement becomes a salient issue. Participant observers may develop a myopic

---

BOX 13.4 GUIDELINES FOR CRITIQUING OBSERVATIONAL METHODS

1. Does the research question lend itself to an observational approach? Would an alternative method have been more appropriate?
2. Is the degree of structure consistent with the nature of the research question?
3. To what degree were observers concealed during data collection? If there was no concealment, what effect might the observers' presence have had on the behaviours being observed?
4. To what degree did the observer participate in activities with those being observed, and was this appropriate?
5. Where did the observations take place? To what extent did the setting influence the naturalness of the behaviours observed?
6. How were data actually recorded (e.g., on field notes, checklists)? Did the recording procedure appear appropriate?
7. What was the plan by which events or behaviours were sampled? Did this plan appear appropriate?
8. What steps were taken to minimize observer biases?

---

view on issues of importance to the group. Another issue is that qualitative observational methods are highly dependent on the observational and interpersonal skills of the observer.

Researchers generally choose an approach that matches the research problem—and their paradigmatic orientation. Qualitative observational methods are especially profitable for in-depth research in which the investigator wishes to establish an adequate conceptualization of the important issues in a social setting or to develop hypotheses. Structured observation is better suited to formal hypothesis testing regarding measurable human behaviours.

Critiquing Observational Methods

As in the case of self-reports, the first question you should ask when critiquing an observational study is whether the data should have been collected by some other approach. The advantages and disadvantages of observational methods, discussed previously, should be helpful in considering the appropriateness of using observation.

Some additional guidelines for critiquing observational studies are presented in Box 13.4. A research report should usually document the following aspects of the observational plan:

⇝ The degree of structure in the observations
⇝ The focus of the observations
⇝ The degree to which the observer was concealed
⇝ For qualitative studies, how entry into the observed group was gained, the relationship between the observer and those observed, the time period over which data were collected, and the method of recording data
⇝ For quantitative studies, a description of the category system or rating scales and the settings in which observations took place
⇝ The plan for sampling events and behaviours to observe

BIOPHYSIOLOGIC MEASURES

One result of the trend toward clinical, patient-centred studies is greater use of biophysiologic and physical variables. Clinical nursing studies involve biophysiologic instruments both for creating independent variables (e.g., an intervention using biofeedback equipment) and for measuring dependent variables. For the most part, our discussion focuses on the use of biophysiologic measures as dependent (outcome) variables.

Nurse researchers have used biophysiologic measures in a variety of ways. Some have studied basic biophysiologic processes that have relevance for nursing care, using healthy participants or an animal species. Some have evaluated specific nursing interventions or products to enhance patient health or comfort. Yet others have examined the correlates of physiologic functioning in patients with health problems. Studies have also been undertaken to evaluate the measurement of biophysiologic information gathered by nurses, with an eye toward improving clinical measurements.

Example of evaluating clinical measurements

Moore et al. (2009) conducted a Canadian multisite randomized, controlled trial to determine whether catheter washouts with either saline or Contisol prevent or reduce blockage in long-term indwelling catheters. While the primary outcome measure was mean time to first catheter change, secondary outcome measures included urinary pH and incidence of microscopic hematuria and leukocytes.

Types of Biophysiologic Measures

Biophysiologic measures include both *in vivo* and *in vitro* measures. *In vivo* measures are performed directly within or on living organisms. Examples of *in vivo* measures include blood pressure and vital capacity measurement. The previously mentioned study by Johnston et al. (2009) involving enhanced kangaroo care in premature neonates is an example of this kind of research. *In vivo* instruments are available to measure all bodily functions, and technologic advances continue to improve the ability to measure biophysiologic phenomena more accurately and conveniently.

With *in vitro* measures, data are gathered from participants by extracting some biophysiologic material from them and subjecting it to laboratory analysis. The analysis is normally done by specialized laboratory technicians. *In vitro* measures include chemical measures (e.g., the measurement of hormone, sugar, or potassium levels), microbiologic measures (e.g., bacterial counts and identification), and cytologic or histologic measures (e.g., tissue biopsies). The previously mentioned study by Moore et al. (2009) involving catheter washouts is an example of this kind of research.

Evaluation of Biophysiologic Measures

Biophysiologic measures offer a number of advantages to nurse researchers. First, biophysiologic measures are relatively accurate and precise, especially when compared with psychological measures, such as self-report measures of anxiety, pain, and so forth. Biophysiologic measures are also objective. Two nurses reading from the same spirometer output are likely to record identical tidal volume measurements, and two different spirometers are likely to produce the same readouts. Patients cannot easily distort measurements of biophysiologic functioning deliberately. Finally, biophysiologic instrumentation provides valid measures of the targeted variables: thermometers can be depended on to measure temperature and not blood volume, and so forth. For nonbiophysiologic measures, there are typically concerns about whether an instrument is really measuring the target concept.

In short, biophysiologic measures are plentiful, tend to be accurate and valid, and are extremely useful in clinical nursing studies. However, care must be exercised in using them with regard to practical, ethical, medical, and technical considerations. For example, Canadian Aboriginal people regard these measures as particularly invasive, as biological samples are linked to their sense of spirituality.

Critiquing Biophysiologic Measures

As always, the most important consideration in evaluating a data collection strategy is the appropriateness of the measures for the research question. The objectivity, accuracy, and availability of biophysiologic measures are of little significance if an alternative method would have resulted in a better measurement of the key concepts. Stress, for example, could be measured in various ways: through self-report (e.g., through the use of a scale such as the State-Trait Anxiety Inventory); through direct observation of participants' behaviour during exposure to stressful stimuli; or by measuring heart rate, blood pressure, or levels of adrenocorticotropic hormone in urine samples. The choice of which measure to use must be linked to the way that stress is conceptualized in the research problem.

Additional criteria for assessing the use of biophysiologic measures are presented in Box 13.5. The general questions to consider are these: Did the researcher select the correct biophysiologic measure? Was care taken in the collection of the data? Did the researcher competently interpret the data?

TIP

Many nursing studies—especially qualitative ones—integrate a variety of data collection approaches. Qualitative studies are especially likely to combine unstructured observations and self-reports. If multiple approaches are used in a quantitative study, structured self-reports combined with biophysiologic measures are most common.

IMPLEMENTING THE DATA COLLECTION PLAN

In addition to selecting methods for collecting data, researchers must develop and implement a plan for gathering their data. This involves decisions that could affect the quality of the data being collected.

One important decision concerns who will collect the data. Researchers often hire assistants to collect data rather than doing it personally. This is especially true in large-scale quantitative studies. In other studies, nurses or other health care staff are asked to assist in the collection of data. From your perspective as a consumer, the critical issue is whether the people collecting data were able to produce valid and accurate data. In any research endeavour, adequate training of data collectors is essential.

Another issue concerns the circumstances under which data were gathered. For example, it may be essential to ensure total privacy to participants. In most cases, it is important for researchers to create a nonjudgmental atmosphere in which participants are encouraged to be candid or behave naturally. Again, you as a consumer must ask whether there is anything about the way in which the data were collected that could have created bias or otherwise affected data quality.

BOX 13.6 GUIDELINES FOR CRITIQUING DATA COLLECTION PROCEDURES

1. Who collected the research data? Were the data collectors qualified for their role, or is there something about them (e.g., their professional role, their relationship with study participants) that could undermine the collection of unbiased, high-quality data?

2. How were data collectors trained? Does the training appear adequate?

3. Where and under what circumstances were the data gathered? Were other people present during that data collection? Could the presence of others have created any distortions?

4. Did the collection of data place any undue burdens (in terms of time or stress) on participants? How might this have affected data quality?

In evaluating the data collection plan of a study, then, you should critically appraise not only the actual methods chosen but also the procedures used to collect the data. Box 13.6 provides some specific guidelines for critiquing the procedures used to collect research data.

RESEARCH EXAMPLES AND CRITICAL THINKING ACTIVITIES

EXAMPLE 1 ■ Unstructured Observation and Interviews

Aspects of a qualitative study, featuring terms and concepts discussed in this chapter, are presented below, followed by some questions to guide critical thinking.

Study
"Cervical screening in Canadian First Nation Cree women" (O'Brien et al., 2009)

Statement of Purpose
The purpose of this study was to determine attitudes toward cervical cancer and screening in First Nations Cree women, with the aim to increase utilization of these services by developing culturally sensitive approaches.

Method
The authors conducted a focused ethnography involving participant observation, researcher journaling, and interview. A sample of eight Cree women participated in the study after the appropriate ethics approvals from both the community and university were secured. The researchers did not approach potential study recruits; instead the First Nations Community Health Representative acted as a liaison. The third author conducted the interviews, as she had spent time in the community prior to and during the data collection, which "enabled her to record the context in which events that shaped attitudes occurred" (p. 84). Interviews ranged between 60 and 90 minutes and explored the attitudes and cultural beliefs of these women, who had all experienced cervical screening and/or cancer. Additional data collection approaches, such as journaling and participant observation, strengthened the findings.

Key Findings
■ While the women understood that screening was important, they feared the procedure as well as the possibility of a cancer diagnosis—regarded as "a death sentence." For some individuals, the fear motivated them to seek testing; yet for others it was the reverse.

■ Cree women prefer female health care providers as their traditional beliefs advocate modesty—believing that their partner was the only male who could see them naked.

■ Tension exists between the contradicting beliefs of the biomedical and traditional health care systems—an important finding that must be considered when developing culturally appropriate intervention.

(Research Examples and Critical Thinking Activities continues on page 254)

Research Examples and Critical Thinking Activities (continued)

CRITICAL THINKING SUGGESTIONS

1. Answer the following questions, many of which are adapted from the critiquing guidelines presented in this chapter:
   a. How much structure did the researchers use in their data collection? Is the degree of structure used appropriate for the study purpose?
   b. Some of the researchers' data were gathered through observation; does the research question lend itself to an observational approach? If the researchers had not done observations, would the findings likely be affected?
   c. The report indicated that *participant* observation was used, even prior to the study beginning. Describe why this approach was taken.
   d. Much of the data for this study were gathered through self-report; does the research question lend itself to a self-report approach? If the researchers had not gathered self-report data, would their findings likely have been affected?
   e. Comment on the fact that the interviews were not conducted in the Cree language.

2. If the results of this study are trustworthy, what are some of the uses to which the findings might be put into clinical practice?

EXAMPLE 2 ■ Physiologic and Observational Measures

Aspects of a quantitative nursing study, featuring terms and concepts discussed in this chapter, are presented below, followed by some questions to guide critical thinking.

Study

"Enhanced kangaroo mother care for heel lance in preterm neonates: A crossover trial" (Johnston et al., 2009)

Statement of Purpose

The Canadian study was designed to compare the effects of enhanced (i.e., rocking, singing, and sucking) versus traditional kangaroo care in preterm neonates.

Method

In a single-blind crossover design involving 90 neonates born between 32 and 36 weeks' gestational age, each mother spent 30 minutes with her baby in either regular (i.e., skin-to-skin contact only) or enhanced (i.e., rocking, singing, and sucking) kangaroo care. Baseline data were then collected on each neonate for 1 minute, before 1-minute heel warming and then lancing, at which point data were collected in 30-second intervals until the baby's heart rate returned to baseline. Measures taken included the Premature Infant Pain Profile (PIPP), which relies on heart rate, transcutaneous oxygen saturation, as well as facial action indicators, and the Neonatal Acute Physiology Version II (SNAP-II), which utilizes patients' medical record physiology data.

Key Findings

■ No significant difference was found between the pain responses of neonates exposed to enhanced versus regular kangaroo mother care. Therefore, nurses do not need to encourage or discourage mothers engaged in kangaroo care who wish to rock, sing, or let their baby suck.

CRITICAL THINKING SUGGESTIONS

1. Answer the following questions, many of which are adapted from the critiquing guidelines presented in this chapter:
   a. How much structure did the researchers use in their data collection? Is the degree of structure appropriate for the research question?
   b. Does the research question lend itself to an observational approach? If the researchers had not undertaken observational work, would the findings likely be affected?

    c. While not directly related to the primary outcome, which was decreasing procedural pain in neonates, would this study have benefited from mothers' self-report? What might the secondary outcome be if such measures were undertaken?

2. If the results of this study are valid and reliable, what are some of the uses to which the findings might be put into clinical practice?

EXAMPLE 3 ■ Structured Self-Reports and Physiologic Measures

1. Read the "Method" section from the study by Bryanton and colleagues in Appendix A of this book, and then answer questions 1 through 4 in Box 13.2 (p. 243).

2. Also consider the following targeted questions, which may further sharpen your critical thinking skills and assist you in assessing aspects of the study's merit:
    a. Comment on the researchers' decision to use self-report during a critical life event (within 12 to 48 hours of childbirth). Was this the best method to use?
    b. What justification do the researchers provide for their choice of measures?
    c. Comment on the fact that 46% of eligible women refused participation. How might this have been improved?

EXAMPLE 4 ■ Unstructured Self-Reports

1. Read the "Procedure" section from the study by Woodgate and colleagues in Appendix B of this book, and then answer questions 1 through 3 in Box 13.2. (p. 243)

2. Also consider the following targeted questions, which may further sharpen your critical thinking skills and assist you in assessing aspects of the study:
    a. Comment on the value of open-ended interview in this phenomenological study.
    b. Comment on the value of discussing preliminary interpretations with participants as the data collection proceeded?

Summary Points

- Some researchers use existing data in their studies—for example, those doing historical research, meta-analyses, secondary analyses, or analyses of available **records.**

- Data collection methods vary along four dimensions: structure, quantifiability, researcher obtrusiveness, and objectivity.

- The three principal data collection methods for nurse researchers are self-reports, observations, and biophysiologic measures.

- Self-reports are the most widely used method of collecting data for nursing studies. Qualitative studies—especially ethnographies—are more likely than quantitative studies to triangulate data from different sources.

- **Self-report** data are collected by means of an oral interview or written questionnaire. Self-report methods are an indispensable means of collecting data but are susceptible to errors of reporting.

- Unstructured self-reports, used in qualitative studies, include **completely unstructured interviews,** which are conversational discussions on the topic of interest; **semistructured** (or *focused*) **interviews,** using a broad **topic guide; focus group interviews,** which involve discussions with small groups; **life histories,** which encourage respondents to narrate their life experiences about a theme; the **think aloud method,** which involves having people talk about decisions as they are making them; **diaries,** in which respondents are asked to maintain daily records about some aspects of their lives; and the **critical incidents technique,** which involves probes about the circumstances surrounding an incident that is critical to an outcome of interest.

➤ Structured self-reports used in quantitative studies employ a formal **instrument**—a **questionnaire or interview schedule**—that may contain a combination of **open-ended questions** (which permit respondents to respond in their own words) and **closed-ended questions** (which offer respondents fixed alternatives from which to choose).

➤ Questionnaires are less costly than interviews, offer the possibility of anonymity, and run no risk of interviewer bias; however, interviews yield higher response rates, are suitable for a wider variety of people, and provide richer data than questionnaires.

➤ Social-psychological **scales** are self-report tools for quantitatively measuring the intensity of such characteristics as attitudes, needs, and perceptions.

➤ **Likert scales** (or **summated rating scales**) present respondents with a series of *items* worded favourably or unfavourably toward some phenomenon; responses indicating level of agreement or disagreement with each statement are scored and summed into a composite score.

➤ The **semantic differential** (SD) technique consists of a series of scales with bipolar adjectives (e.g., good/bad) along which respondents rate their reactions toward phenomena.

➤ A **visual analog scale** (VAS) is used to measure subjective experiences (e.g., pain, fatigue) along a line designating a bipolar continuum.

➤ Scales are versatile and powerful but are susceptible to **response set biases**—the tendency of some people to respond to items in characteristic ways, independently of item content.

➤ **Vignettes** are brief descriptions of some person or situation to which respondents are asked to react.

➤ With a **Q sort,** respondents sort a set of statements into piles according to specified criteria.

➤ Direct **observation** of phenomena, which includes both structured and unstructured procedures, is a technique for gathering data about behaviours and events.

➤ One type of unstructured observation is **participant observation,** in which the researcher gains entrée into the social group of interest and participates to varying degrees in its functioning while making in-depth observations of activities and events. **Logs** of daily events and **field notes** of the observer's experiences and interpretations constitute the major data collection instruments in unstructured observation.

➤ Structured observations, which dictate what the observer should observe, often involve **checklists**—tools based on **category systems** for recording the appearance, frequency, or duration of prespecified behaviours or events. Alternatively, the observer may use **rating scales** to rate phenomena along a dimension of interest (e.g., energetic/lethargic).

➤ Structured observations often use a sampling plan (such as **time sampling** or **event sampling**) for selecting the behaviours or events to be observed.

➤ Observational techniques are a versatile and important alternative to self-reports, but observational biases can pose a threat to the validity and accuracy of observational data.

➤ Data may also be derived from **biophysiologic measures,** which can be classified as either *in vivo* measurements (those performed within or on living organisms) or *in vitro* measurements (those performed outside the organism's body, such as blood tests). Biophysiologic measures have the advantage of being objective, accurate, and precise.

⇒ In developing a data collection plan, the researcher must decide who will collect the data, how the data collectors will be trained, and what the circumstances for data collection will be.

STUDIES CITED IN CHAPTER 13*

This reference list contains only those studies that were cited in this chapter. Citations pertaining to theoretical, methodologic, or nonempirical work are included together in a separate section at the end of the book (beginning on page 399).

Atack, L., Luke, R., & Chien, E. (2008). Evaluation of patient satisfaction with tailored online patient education information. *CIN: Computers, Informatics, Nursing, 26*(5), 258–264.

Avis, K., Tan, L., Anderson, C., Tan, B., & Muhajarine, N. (2007). Taking a closer look: An examination of measles, mumps, and rubella immunization uptake in Saskatoon. *Canadian Journal of Public Health, 98*(5), 417–421.

Beck, C. T. (2002). Releasing the pause button: Mothering twins during the first year of life. *Qualitative Health Research, 12*, 593–608.

Benzies, K., Magill-Evans, J., Harrison, M. J., MacPhail, S., & Kimak, C. (2008). Strengthening new fathers' skills in interaction with their 5-month-old infants: Who benefits from a brief intervention? *Public Health Nursing, 25*(5), 431–439.

Bettazzoni, M., Zipursky, R. B., Friedland, J., & Devins, G. M. (2008). Illness intrusiveness and subjective well-being in schizophrenia. *The Journal of Nervous & Mental Disease, 196*(11), 798–805.

Brazier, A., Cooke, K., & Moravan, V. (2008). Using mixed methods for evaluating an integrative approach to cancer care: A case study. *Integrative Cancer Therapies, 7*(1), 5–17.

Cragg, R., Marsden, N., & Wall, D. (2008). Perceptions of the clinical director role. *British Journal of Healthcare Management, 14*(2), 58–65.

Fairbairn, N., Small, W., Shannon, K., Wood, E., & Kerr, T. (2008). Seeking refuge from violence in street-based drug scenes: Women's experiences in North America's first supervised injection facility. *Social Science & Medicine, 67*(5), 817–823.

Johnston, C. C., Filion, F., Campbell-Yeo, M., et al. (2009). Enhanced kangaroo mother care for heel lance in preterm neonates: A crossover trial. *Journal of Perinatology, 29*(1), 51–56.

Leininger, M. M. (Ed.). 1985. *Qualitative research methods in nursing*. New York: Grune & Stratton.

Maheu, C., & Thorne, S. (2008). Receiving inconclusive genetic test results: An interpretive description of the BRCA1/2 experience. *Research in Nursing & Health, 31*(6), 553–562.

Meijers, K. E., & Gustafsson, B. (2008). Patient's self-determination in intensive care—From an action—and confirmation theoretical perspective. The intensive care nurse view. *Intensive & Critical Care Nursing, 24*(4), 222–232.

Miller, K. L., Reeves, S., Zwarenstein, M., Beales, J. D., Kenaszchuk, C., & Conn, L. G. (2008). Nursing emotion work and interprofessional collaboration in general internal medicine wards: A qualitative study. *Journal of Advanced Nursing, 64*(4), 332–343.

Moore, K. N., Hunter, K. F., McGinnis, R., et al. (2009). Do catheter washouts extend patency time in long-term indwelling urethral catheters? *Journal of Wound, Ostomy & Continence Nursing, 36*(1), 82–90.

Muller-Staub, M., Needham, I., Odenbreit, M., Lavin, M. A., & Van Achterberg, T. (2008). Implementing nursing diagnostics effectively: Cluster randomized trial. *Journal of Advanced Nursing, 63*(3), 291–301.

O'Brien, B. A., Mill, J., & Wilson, T. (2009). Cervical screening in Canadian First Nation Cree women. *Journal of Transcultural Nursing, 20*(1), 83–92.

Pinelli, J., Saigal, S., Wu, Y. W. B., et al. (2008). Patterns of change in family functioning, resources, coping and parental depression in mothers and fathers of sick newborns over the first year of life. *Journal of Neonatal Nursing, 14*, 156–165.

Sawyer, J., Haslam, L., Robinson, S., Daines, P., & Stilos, K. (2008). Pain prevalence study in a large Canadian teaching hospital. *Pain Management Nursing, 9*(3), 104–112.

Thompson, C., Dalgleish, L., Bucknall, T., et al. (2008). The effects of time pressure and experience on nurses' risk assessment decisions: A signal detection analysis. *Nursing Research, 57*(5), 302–311.

Wells, M., Donnan, P. T., Sharp, L., Ackland, C., Fletcher, J., & Dewar, J. A. (2008). A study to evaluate nurse-led on-treatment review for patients undergoing radiotherapy for head and neck cancer. *Journal of Clinical Nursing, 17*(11), 1428–1439.

14 Evaluating Measurements and Data Quality

On completing this chapter, you will be able to:

1. Describe the major characteristics of measurement and identify major sources of measurement error

2. Describe aspects of reliability and validity, and specify how each aspect can be assessed

3. Interpret the meaning of reliability and validity coefficients

4. Describe the four dimensions used in establishing the trustworthiness of qualitative data and identify methods of enhancing data quality in qualitative studies

5. Evaluate the overall quality of a measuring tool or data collection approach used in a study

6. Define new terms in the chapter

An ideal data collection procedure is one that captures a phenomenon or concept in a way that is relevant, accurate, truthful, and sensitive. For most concepts of interest to nurse researchers, few, if any, data collection procedures match this ideal. In this chapter, we discuss criteria for evaluating the quality of data obtained in both quantitative and qualitative studies.

MEASUREMENT AND THE ASSESSMENT OF QUANTITATIVE DATA

Quantitative studies derive data through the measurement of variables. Before discussing the assessment of quantitative measures, we briefly discuss the concept of measurement.

Measurement

Measurement involves rules for assigning numeric values to *qualities* of objects to designate the *quantity* of the attribute. No attribute inherently has a numeric value; human beings invent rules to measure concepts. An often-quoted statement by an American psychologist, L.L. Thurstone, summarizes a position assumed by many quantitative researchers: "Whatever exists, exists in some amount and can be measured." The notion here is that attributes are not constant: they vary from day to day or from one person to another. This variability is capable of a numeric expression that signifies *how much* of an attribute is present. Quantification is used to communicate that amount. The purpose of assigning numbers is to differentiate among people who possess varying degrees of the critical attribute.

Measurement requires numbers to be assigned to objects according to rules rather than haphazardly. The rules for measuring temperature, weight, and other physical attributes are widely known and accepted. Rules for measuring many variables, however, have to be invented. What are the rules for measuring patient satisfaction? Pain? Depression? Whether the data are collected through observation, self-report, or some other method, researchers must specify how numeric values are to be assigned.

Advantages of Measurement

A major strength of measurement is that it removes guesswork when gathering information. Consider how handicapped nurses and doctors would be in the absence of measures of body temperature, blood pressure, and so forth. Because measurement is based on explicit rules, the information tends to be objective: two people measuring a person's weight using the same scale would likely get identical results. Two people scoring responses to a self-report stress scale would likely arrive at identical scores. Not all quantitative measures are completely objective, but most incorporate rules for minimizing subjectivity.

Measurement also makes it possible to obtain reasonably precise information. Instead of describing Nathan as "rather tall," for example, we can depict him as a man who is 1.9 m tall. If it were necessary, we could obtain even more precise height measurements. Such precision allows researchers to differentiate among people who possess different amounts of an attribute.

Finally, measurement is a language of communication. Numbers are less vague than words and can thus communicate information broadly. If a researcher reported that the average oral temperature of a sample of patients was "somewhat high," different readers might develop different ideas about the sample's physiologic state. If the researcher reported an average temperature of 37.6°C, however, there is no ambiguity.

Errors of Measurement

Researchers work with fallible measures. Values and scores from even the best instruments have a certain amount of error. We can think of every piece of quantitative data as consisting of two parts: a true component and an error component. This can be written as an equation, as follows:

Obtained score = True score ± Error

The **obtained** (or observed) **score** could be, for example, a patient's heart rate or score on an anxiety scale. The **true score** is the true value that would be obtained if it were possible to have an infallible measure of the target attribute. The true score is hypothetical; it can never be known because measures are not infallible. The **error of measurement**—the difference between true and obtained scores—reflects extraneous factors that affect the measurement and distort the results. Many factors contribute to errors of measurement. Among the most common are the following:

⮞ *Situational contaminants.* Measurements can be affected by the conditions under which they are produced (e.g., people's awareness of an observer can affect their behaviour; environmental factors such as temperature or time of day can be sources of measurement error).

≫ *Response set biases.* A number of relatively enduring characteristics of respondents can interfere with accurate measures of an attribute (see Chapter 13).

≫ *Transitory personal factors.* Temporary personal factors (e.g., fatigue) can influence people's motivation or ability to cooperate, act naturally, or do their best.

≫ *Administration variations.* Alterations in the methods of collecting data from one person to the next can affect obtained scores (e.g., if some biophysiologic measures are taken before a feeding and others are taken postprandially).

≫ *Item sampling.* Errors can be introduced as a result of the sampling of items used to measure an attribute. For example, a student's score on a 100-item research methods test will be influenced to a certain extent by *which* 100 questions are included.

This list is not exhaustive, but it illustrates that data are susceptible to measurement error from a variety of sources.

Reliability

The reliability of a quantitative measure is a major criterion for assessing its quality. **Reliability** is the consistency with which an instrument measures the attribute. If a spring scale gave a reading of 50 kg for a person's weight one minute and a reading of 60 kg the next minute, we would naturally be wary of using such an unreliable scale. The less variation an instrument produces in repeated measurements, the higher is its reliability.

Another way to define reliability is in terms of accuracy. An instrument is reliable if its measures accurately reflect true scores. A reliable measure is one that maximizes the true score component and minimizes the error component of an obtained score.

Three aspects of reliability are of interest to quantitative researchers: stability, internal consistency, and equivalence.

Stability

The *stability* of a measure is the extent to which the same scores are obtained when the instrument is used with the same people on separate occasions. Assessments of stability are derived through **test–retest reliability** procedures. The researcher administers the same measure to a sample of people on two occasions, and then compares the scores.

TIP

Many psychosocial scales contain two or more *subscales,* each of which tap distinct, but related, concepts (e.g., a measure of independent functioning might include subscales for motor activities, communication, and socializing). The reliability of each subscale is typically assessed and, if subscale scores are summed for an overall score, the scale's overall reliability would also be assessed.

Suppose, for example, we were interested in the stability of a self-report scale that measured self-esteem in adolescents. Because self-esteem is a fairly stable attribute that would not change markedly from one day to the next, we would expect a reliable self-esteem measure to yield consistent scores on two separate tests. As a check on the instrument's stability, we arrange to administer the scale 3 weeks apart to a sample of teenagers. Fictitious data for this example are presented in Table 14.1. On the whole, differences on the two tests are not large. Researchers compute a **reliability coefficient,** a numeric index of a measure's reliability, to objectively determine exactly how small the differences are.

TABLE 14.1	FICTITIOUS DATA FOR TEST–RETEST RELIABILITY OF SELF-ESTEEM SCALE	
PARTICIPANT NUMBER	TIME 1	TIME 2
1	55	57
2	49	46
3	78	74
4	37	35
5	44	46
6	50	56
7	58	55
8	62	66
9	48	50
10	67	63

$r = .95$.

Reliability coefficients (designated as r) range from .00 to 1.00.* The higher the value, the more reliable (stable) is the measuring instrument. In the example shown in Table 14.1, the reliability coefficient is .95, which is quite high.

TIP

For most purposes, reliability coefficients higher than .70 are satisfactory, but coefficients in the .85 to .95 range are far preferable.

The test–retest approach to estimating reliability has certain disadvantages. The major problem is that many traits do change over time, independently of the instrument's stability. Attitudes, knowledge, and so forth can be modified by experiences between two measurements. Thus, stability indexes are most appropriate for relatively enduring characteristics, such as personality and abilities. Even with such traits, test–retest reliability tends to decline as the interval between the two administrations increases.

Example of test–retest reliability
Fillion et al. (2003) evaluated the French Canadian adaptation of the Multidimensional Fatigue Inventory among patients with cancer. Some study participants completed the scale twice—at weeks 2 and 4 of radiation treatment. The test–retest reliability for the total scale was .83, whereas that for subscales ranged from .51 (mental fatigue) to .78 (physical fatigue).

---

*Computation procedures for reliability coefficients are not presented in this textbook, but formulas can be found in the references cited at the end of this chapter. Although reliability coefficients can technically be less than .00 (i.e., a negative value), they are almost invariably a number between .00 and 1.00).

Internal Consistency

Scales that involve summing items usually are evaluated for their internal consistency. Ideally, scales are composed of items that all measure the same critical attribute and nothing else. On a scale to measure nurses' empathy, it would be inappropriate to include an item that is a better measure of spirituality than empathy. An instrument has **internal consistency** reliability to the extent that all its subparts measure the same characteristic. This approach to reliability assesses an important source of measurement error in multi-item measures: the sampling of items.

One of the oldest methods for assessing internal consistency is the *split-half technique*. In this approach, the items comprising a scale are split into two groups (usually, odd versus even items) and scored, and then scores on the two half-tests are used to compute a reliability coefficient. If the two half-tests are really measuring the same attribute, the correlation between the two and reliability coefficient will be high. Additional methods of estimating internal consistency include **Cronbach alpha** (or **coefficient alpha**). This method gives an estimate of split-half correlations for all possible ways of dividing the measure into two halves, not just odd versus even items. As with test–retest reliability coefficients, indexes of internal consistency range between .00 and 1.00. The higher the reliability coefficient, the more internally consistent the measure.

Example of internal consistency reliability

Watson, Oberle, and Deutscher (in press) conducted psychometric testing of the 36-item Nurses' Attitudes Toward Obesity and Obese Patients Scale (NATOOPS) with 598 nurses. Using the Statistical Package for Social Sciences (SPSS) computer program, a Cronbach alpha value of .81 was obtained for internal consistency.

Equivalence

The *equivalence* approach to estimating reliability—used primarily with observational instruments—determines the consistency or equivalence of the instrument by different observers or raters. As noted in Chapter 13, a potential weakness of direct observation is the risk for observer error. The degree of error can be assessed through **interrater** (or **interobserver**) **reliability,** which is estimated by having two or more trained observers make simultaneous, independent observations. The resulting data can then be used to calculate an index of equivalence or agreement. That is, a reliability coefficient can be computed to demonstrate the strength of the relationship between the observers' ratings. When two independent observers score some phenomenon congruently, the scores are likely to be accurate and reliable.

Example of interrater reliability

Using a crossover observational design, Gélinas and Johnston (2007) sought to validate the English version of the Critical-Care Pain Observation Tool (CPOT). Raters administered the instrument to 55 critically ill ventilated adults in the intensive care unit. Across the six data collection points, high interrater reliability ranging from .80 to .93 was obtained between raters.

Interpretation of Reliability Coefficients

Reliability coefficients are an important indicator of an instrument's quality. A measure with low reliability prevents an adequate testing of research hypotheses. If data fail to confirm a hypothesis, one possibility is that the measuring tool was unreliable—not necessarily that the expected relationships do not exist. Knowledge about an instrument's reliability thus is critical in interpreting research results, especially if research hypotheses are not supported.

Reliability estimates vary according to the procedure used to obtain them. Estimates of reliability computed by different procedures for the same instrument are not identical.

Example of different forms of reliability
Rossen and Gruber (2007) developed a scale to measure older adults' self-efficacy in relocating to independent living communities. Their 32-item scale had a test–retest reliability of .70 over a 2-week period. Cronbach alpha for the total scale was high, .97.

In addition, reliability of an instrument is related to sample heterogeneity. The more homogeneous the sample (i.e., the more similar the scores), the lower the reliability coefficient will be. This is because instruments are designed to measure differences, and if sample members are similar to one another, it is more difficult for the instrument to discriminate reliably among those who possess varying degrees of the attribute. Finally, longer instruments (i.e., those with more items) tend to have higher reliability than shorter ones.

> **TIP**
>
> If a research report provides information on the reliability of a quantitative scale without specifying the type of reliability measure used, it is probably safe to assume that internal consistency reliability was assessed by the Cronbach alpha method.

Validity

The second important criterion for evaluating a quantitative instrument is its validity. **Validity** is the degree to which an instrument measures what it is supposed to be measuring. If a researcher develops an instrument to measure patients' stress, he or she should take steps to ensure that the resulting scores validly reflect this variable and not some other concept.

The reliability and validity of an instrument are not totally independent. A measuring device that is not reliable cannot be valid. An instrument cannot validly be measuring the attribute of interest if it is erratic or inaccurate. An instrument can be reliable, however, without being valid. Suppose we had the idea to measure patients' anxiety by measuring the circumference of their wrists. We could obtain highly accurate, consistent, and precise measurements of wrist circumferences, but they would not be valid indicators of anxiety. Thus, the high reliability of an instrument provides no evidence of its validity; the low reliability of a measure *is* evidence of low validity.

>
>
> **TIP**
>
> Some methodologic studies are designed to determine the quality of instruments used by clinicians or researchers. In these *psychometric assessments,* information about the instrument's reliability and validity is carefully documented.

Like reliability, validity has a number of aspects and assessment approaches. One aspect is known as face validity. **Face validity** refers to whether the instrument *looks* as though it is measuring the appropriate construct. Although it is often useful for an instrument to have face validity, three other types of validity are of greater importance in assessing an instrument: content validity, criterion-related validity, and construct validity.

Content Validity

Content validity is concerned with adequate coverage of the content area being measured. Content validity is crucial for tests of knowledge. In such a context, the validity question is: How representative are the questions on this test of the universe of all questions that might be asked on this topic?

Content validity is also relevant in measures of complex psychosocial traits. A person who wanted to create a new instrument would begin by developing a thorough conceptualization of the construct of interest so that the measure would adequately capture the whole domain. Such a conceptualization might come from first-hand knowledge but is more likely to come from qualitative studies or from a literature review.

The content validity of an instrument is necessarily based on judgment. There are no totally objective methods for ensuring the adequate content coverage of an instrument. Experts in the content area are often called on to analyze the items' adequacy in representing the hypothetical content universe in the correct proportions. It is also possible to calculate a **content validity index** (CVI) that indicates the extent of expert agreement, but ultimately the experts' subjective judgments must be relied on.

Example of content validity

Rennick et al. (2008) developed the Children's Critical Illness Impact Scale as a measure of posthospitalization distress in children aged 6 to 12 years. To determine the content validity of the scale, individual interviews and focus groups were conducted with health professionals across three Canadian pediatric teaching hospitals, for their evaluation of the item relevance of the measure. A high content validity index of .87 was established.

Criterion-Related Validity

In **criterion-related validity** assessments, researchers seek to establish a relationship between scores on an instrument and some external criterion. The instrument, whatever attribute it is measuring, is said to be valid if its scores correspond strongly with scores on some criterion. (One difficulty of criterion-related validation, however, is finding a criterion that is, in itself, reliable and valid.) After a criterion is established, validity can be estimated easily. A **validity coefficient** is computed by using a mathematic formula that correlates scores on the instrument with scores on the criterion variable. The magnitude of the coefficient indicates how valid the instrument is. These coefficients (r) range between .00 and 1.00, with higher values indicating greater criterion-related validity. Coefficients of .70 or higher are desirable.

Sometimes, a distinction is made between two types of criterion-related validity. **Predictive validity** is an instrument's ability to differentiate between people's performances or behaviours on some future criterion. When a school of nursing correlates students' incoming high school grades with their subsequent grade-point averages, the predictive validity of the high school grades for nursing school performance is being evaluated. **Concurrent validity** refers to an instrument's ability to distinguish among people who differ in their present status on some criterion. For example, a psychological test to differentiate between patients in a mental institution who could and could not be released could be correlated with current ratings by nurses. The difference between predictive and concurrent validity, then, is the difference in the timing of obtaining measurements on a criterion.

Example of predictive validity

Perraud et al. (2006) developed The Depression Coping Self-Efficacy Scale—to measure depressed individuals' confidence in their ability to follow treatment recommendations. Scale scores at discharge from a psychiatric hospital were found to be predictive of rehospitalization 6 to 8 weeks later.

Construct Validity

Validating an instrument in terms of **construct validity** is challenging. Construct validity is concerned with the following question: What construct is the instrument actually measuring? The more abstract the concept, the more difficult it is to establish the construct validity of the measure; at the same time, the more abstract the concept, the less suitable it is to use a criterion-related validation approach. What objective criterion is there for concepts such as empathy and separation anxiety? Construct validation is addressed in several ways, but there is always an emphasis on testing relationships predicted on the basis of theoretical considerations. Researchers make predictions about the manner in which the construct will function in relation to other constructs.

One approach to construct validation is the **known-groups technique**. In this procedure, groups that are expected to differ on the critical attribute are administered the instrument, and group scores are compared. For instance, in validating a measure of fear of the labour experience, the scores of primiparas and multiparas could be contrasted. Women who had never given birth would likely experience more anxiety than women who had already had children; one might question the validity of the instrument if such differences did not emerge.

Another method of construct validation involves an examination of relationships based on theoretical predictions. Researchers might reason as follows: According to theory, construct X is related to construct Y; instrument A is a measure of construct X, and instrument B is a measure of construct Y; scores on A and B are related to each other, as predicted by the theory; therefore, it is inferred that A and B are valid measures of X and Y. This logical analysis is fallible, but it does offer supporting evidence.

Another approach to construct validation employs a statistical procedure known as **factor analysis,** which is a method for identifying clusters of related items on a scale. The procedure is used to identify and group together different measures of some underlying attribute and to distinguish them from measures of different attributes.

In summary, construct validation employs both logical and empirical procedures. Like content validity, construct validity requires a judgment pertaining to what the instrument is measuring. Construct validity and criterion-related validity share an empirical component, but, in the latter case, there is a pragmatic, objective criterion with which to compare a measure rather than a second measure of an abstract theoretical construct.

Interpretation of Validity

Like reliability, validity is not an all-or-nothing characteristic of an instrument. An instrument cannot really be said to possess or lack validity; it is a question of degree. The testing of an instrument's validity is not proved but rather is supported by an accumulation of evidence.

Example of construct validity

Cossette et al. (2008) conducted a methodologic study involving 531 nursing students to evaluate the construct validity of the Caring Nurse–Patient Interaction Short Scale. An exploratory factor analysis was used to assess the construct validity of the 23-item scale that reflects four caring domains: humanistic, relational, clinical, and comforting care.

Strictly speaking, researchers do not validate an instrument *per se* but rather some application of the instrument. A measure of anxiety may be valid for presurgical patients but may not be valid for nursing students before a final examination. Validation is a never-ending process: the more evidence that can be gathered that an instrument is measuring what it is supposed to be measuring, the greater the confidence researchers have in its validity.

In quantitative studies involving self-report or observational instruments, the research report usually provides validity and reliability information from an earlier study—often a study conducted by the person who developed the instrument. If the sample characteristics in the original study and the new study are similar, the citation provides valuable information about data quality in the new study. Ideally, researchers should also compute new reliability coefficients for the actual research sample.

Sensitivity and Specificity

Reliability and validity are the two most important criteria for evaluating quantitative instruments, but researchers sometimes need to consider other qualities. In particular, for screening and diagnostic instruments, sensitivity and specificity need to be evaluated.

Sensitivity is the ability of an instrument to correctly identify a "case," that is, to correctly screen in or diagnose a condition. An instrument's sensitivity is its rate of yielding "true positives." **Specificity** is the instrument's ability to correctly identify noncases, that is, to correctly screen *out* those without the condition. Specificity is an instrument's rate of yielding "true negatives." To determine an instrument's sensitivity and specificity, researchers need a reliable and valid criterion of "caseness" against which scores on the instrument can be assessed.

There is, unfortunately, a tradeoff between the sensitivity and specificity of an instrument. When sensitivity is increased to include more true positives, the number of true negatives declines. Therefore, a critical task is to develop the appropriate *cut-off point*, that is, the score value used to distinguish cases and noncases. Instrument developers use sophisticated procedures to make such a determination.

THE ASSESSMENT OF QUALITATIVE DATA

The assessment procedures described thus far cannot be meaningfully applied to such qualitative materials as narrative responses in interviews or participant observers' field notes. This does not imply, however, that qualitative researchers are unconcerned with data quality. The central question underlying the concepts of validity and reliability is: Do the data reflect the truth? Certainly, qualitative researchers are as eager as quantitative researchers to have data reflecting the true state of human experience.

Nevertheless, there has been considerable controversy about the criteria to use for assessing the "truth value" of qualitative research. Whittemore, Chase, and Mandle (2001), who listed different criteria recommended by 10 influential authorities, noted that the difficulty in achieving universally accepted criteria (or even universally accepted labels for those criteria) stems in part from various tensions, such as the tension between the desire for rigour and the desire for creativity.

The criteria currently thought of as the "gold standard" for qualitative researchers are those outlined by Lincoln and Guba (1985). As noted in Chapter 2, these researchers have suggested four criteria for establishing the **trustworthiness** of qualitative data: credibility, dependability, confirmability, and transferability. It should be noted that these criteria go beyond an assessment of qualitative *data* alone, but rather are concerned with evaluations of interpretations and conclusions as well. These standards are often used by researchers in all major qualitative research traditions.

TIP
Qualitative research reports are uneven in the amount of information they provide about data quality. Some do not address data quality issues at all, whereas others elaborate on the steps taken to assess trust-worthiness. The absence of information undermines consumers' ability to draw conclusions about the believability of qualitative findings.

Credibility

Careful qualitative researchers take steps to improve and evaluate data **credibility,** which refers to confidence in the truth of the data and interpretations of them. Lincoln and Guba note that the credibility of an inquiry involves two aspects: first, carrying out the investigation in a way that believability is enhanced; and second, taking steps to *demonstrate* credibility. Lincoln and Guba suggest various techniques for improving and documenting the credibility of qualitative data. A few that are especially relevant to the evaluation of qualitative studies are mentioned here.

Prolonged Engagement and Persistent Observation

Lincoln and Guba recommend activities that increase the likelihood of producing credible data and interpretations. A first and very important step is **prolonged engagement**—the investment of sufficient time in data collection activities to have an in-depth understanding of the culture, language, or views of the group under study and to test for misinformation. Prolonged engagement may also be essential for building trust and rapport with informants.

Credible data collection also involves **persistent observation,** which refers to the researcher's focus on the aspects of a situation that are relevant to the phenomena being studied. As Lincoln and Guba note, "If prolonged engagement provides scope, persistent observation provides depth" (1985, p. 304).

Example of prolonged engagement and persistent observation
Pauly (2008) employed an ethnographic design in the study of the underlying value tensions that impact nursing practice and affect equity in access to health care among substance use and homeless individuals. To ensure dependability of findings, data collection involved 203 hours of participant observation involving multiple observers and formal interviews with participants over a period of 10 months.

Triangulation

Triangulation can also enhance credibility. As previously noted, triangulation refers to the use of multiple referents to draw truthful conclusions. The aim of triangulation is to "overcome the intrinsic bias that comes from single-method, single-observer, and single-theory studies" (Denzin, 1989, p. 313). It has also been argued that triangulation helps to capture a more complete and contextualized portrait of the phenomenon under study—a goal shared by researchers in all qualitative traditions. Denzin (1989) identified four types of triangulation:

1. *Data source triangulation*: using multiple data sources in a study (e.g., interviewing diverse key informants such as nurses and patients about the same topic)

2. *Investigator triangulation*: using more than one person to collect, analyze, or interpret a set of data

3. *Theory triangulation:* using multiple perspectives to interpret a set of data

4. *Method triangulation*: using multiple methods to address a research problem (e.g., observations plus interviews)

Triangulation provides a basis for convergence on the truth. By using multiple methods and perspectives, researchers strive to distinguish true information from information with errors.

Example of investigator triangulation

Lobchuk, Udod, and Loiselle (2009) explored oncology nurses' perceptions of their relationships with family members within a Western Canadian ambulatory cancer care setting. All three researchers coded the interviews separately and then reviewed their findings together.

External Checks: Peer Debriefing and Member Checks

Two other techniques for establishing credibility involve external checks on the inquiry. **Peer debriefing** is a session held with objective peers to review and explore various aspects of the inquiry. Peer debriefing exposes investigators to the searching questions of others who are experienced in either qualitative research or in the phenomenon being studied, or both. Peer review can also be useful to researchers interested in testing some working hypotheses or in exploring new interpretive avenues.

Member checks involve soliciting study participants' reactions to preliminary findings and interpretations. Member checking can be carried out both informally in an ongoing way as data are being collected and more formally after data have been collected and analyzed. Lincoln and Guba (1985) consider member checking the most important technique for establishing the credibility of qualitative data. However, not all qualitative researchers use member checking to ensure credibility. For example, member checking is not a component of Giorgi's method of descriptive phenomenology. Giorgi (1989) argued that asking participants to evaluate the researchers' interpretation of their own descriptions exceeds the role of participants.

Example of peer debriefing and member checking

Brathwaite and Williams (2004) studied the childbirth experiences of professional Chinese Canadian women. Their qualitative study was based on in-depth interviews with six women. The researchers asked study participants to review their findings and confirm or refute them. They also validated emerging themes by consulting with three colleagues who were members of the Chinese Canadian community.

Searching for Disconfirming Evidence

Data credibility can be enhanced by researchers' systematic search for data that challenge an emerging conceptualization or descriptive theory. The search for **disconfirming evidence** occurs through purposive sampling but is facilitated through other processes already described, such as prolonged engagement and peer debriefings. The sampling of individuals who can offer conflicting viewpoints can greatly strengthen a comprehensive description of a phenomenon.

Lincoln and Guba (1985) refer to a similar activity of **negative case analysis**—a process by which researchers revise their hypotheses through the inclusion of cases that appear to disconfirm earlier hypotheses. The goal of this procedure is to refine a hypothesis or a theory continuously until it accounts for all cases.

Researcher Credibility

Another aspect of credibility discussed by Patton (2002) is **researcher credibility,** the faith that can be put in the researcher. In qualitative studies, researchers *are* the data collecting instruments—as well as creators of the analytic process—and, therefore, the researchers' training, qualifications, and experience are important in establishing confidence in the data.

Research reports ideally should contain information about the researchers, including information about credentials and about any personal connections the researchers had to the people, topic, or community under study. For example, it is relevant for a reader of a report on AIDS patients' coping mechanisms to know that the researcher is HIV positive. Patton argues that the researcher should report "any personal and professional information that may have affected data collection, analysis and interpretation—negatively or positively . . . " (2002, p. 566).

Dependability

The **dependability** of qualitative data refers to data stability over time and over conditions. It might be said that credibility (in qualitative studies) is to validity (in quantitative studies) what dependability is to reliability. Like the reliability–validity relationship in quantitative research, there can be no credibility in the absence of dependability.

One approach to assessing data dependability is to undertake a **stepwise replication.** This approach, which is conceptually similar to a split-half technique, involves having several researchers who can be divided into two teams. These teams deal with data sources separately and conduct, essentially, two independent inquiries through which data and conclusions can be compared.

Another technique relating to dependability is the **inquiry audit.** An inquiry audit involves a scrutiny of the data and relevant supporting documents by an external reviewer, an approach that also has a bearing on data confirmability, as we discuss next.

Example of dependability

Using individual interviews, Tse and Hall (2008) conducted an exploratory qualitative study to describe parents' perceptions of a behavioural sleep intervention. Interview transcripts and field notes were reviewed independently by the two researchers to determine themes around the research topic. Subsequently, comparisons were made between the researchers to identify congruence and to rectify incongruence between their respective analyses.

Confirmability

Confirmability refers to the objectivity or neutrality of the data, that is, the potential for congruence between two or more independent people about the data's accuracy, relevance, or meaning. Bracketing (in phenomenological studies) and maintaining a reflexive journal are methods that can enhance confirmability, although these strategies do not actually document that it has been achieved.

Inquiry audits can be used to establish both the dependability and confirmability of the data. In an inquiry audit, the investigator develops an **audit trail,** which is a systematic collection of documentation that allows an independent auditor to come to conclusions about the data. After the audit trail materials are assembled, the inquiry auditor proceeds to audit, in a fashion analogous to a financial audit, the trustworthiness of the data and the meanings attached to them. Examples of the classes of records that are important in creating an adequate audit trail include the raw data (e.g., field notes, interview transcripts), analytic products (e.g., documentation on working hypotheses, notes from member check sessions), and materials relating to intentions and dispositions (e.g., reflective notes).

Researchers can also enhance the **auditability** of their inquiry (i.e., the degree to which an outside person can follow the researchers' methods, decisions, and conclusions) by maintaining an adequate **decision trail.** A decision trail articulates the researchers' decision rules for categorizing data and making inferences in the analysis. When researchers share decision trail information in their research report, readers are in a better position to evaluate the soundness of the decisions and to draw conclusions about the trustworthiness of the study.

Transferability

In Lincoln and Guba's (1985) framework, **transferability** refers to the extent to which the findings from the data can be transferred to other settings and is thus similar to the concept of generalizability. This is, to some extent, an issue relating to sampling and design rather than to the soundness of the data *per se.* As Lincoln and Guba note, however, a researcher's responsibility is to provide sufficient descriptive data in the research report for consumers to evaluate the applicability of the data to other contexts: "Thus the naturalist cannot specify the external validity of an inquiry; he or she can provide only the thick description necessary to enable someone interested in making a transfer to reach a conclusion about whether transfer can be contemplated as a possibility" (1985, p. 316). **Thick description** refers to a rich, thorough description of the research setting and of the transactions and processes observed during the inquiry. Thus, if there is to be transferability, the burden rests with researchers to provide sufficient information to permit judgments about contextual similarity and dissimilarity.

> **TIP**
>
> Because the process of assessing data quality in qualitative studies may be inextricably linked to data analysis, discussions of data quality are sometimes included in the "Results" section rather than the "Method" section of the report. In some cases, the text will not explicitly point out that data quality issues are being discussed. Readers may have to be alert to evidence of triangulation or other verification techniques in such statements as "Informants' reports of experiences of serious illness were supported by discussions with three public health nurses."

CRITIQUING DATA QUALITY

If data are seriously flawed, the study cannot contribute useful evidence. Therefore, it is important for you as a consumer to consider whether researchers have taken appropriate steps to collect data that are accurate. In both qualitative and quantitative studies, you have the right—indeed, the obligation—to ask: Can I trust the data? Do the data accurately reflect the true state of the phenomenon under study?

In quantitative studies, you should expect some discussion of the reliability and validity of the measures—preferably, information collected directly with the sample under study (rather than evidence from other studies). You should be wary about the results of quantitative studies when the report provides no information about data quality or when it suggests unfavourable reliability or validity. Also, data quality deserves special scrutiny when the research hypotheses are not confirmed. There may be many reasons that hypotheses are not supported by data (e.g., too small a sample or a faulty theory), but the quality of the measures is an important area of concern. When hypotheses are not supported, one possibility is that the instruments were not good measures of the research constructs. Box 14.1 provides some guidelines for critiquing data quality in quantitative studies.

Information about data quality is equally important in qualitative studies. You should be particularly alert to information on data quality when a single researcher

BOX 14.1   GUIDELINES FOR EVALUATING DATA QUALITY IN QUANTITATIVE STUDIES

1. Is there congruence between the research variables as conceptualized (i.e., as discussed in the "Introduction" of the report) and as operationalized (i.e., as described in the "Method" section)?

2. If operational definitions (or scoring procedures) are specified, do they clearly indicate the rules of measurement? Do the rules seem sensible? Were data collected in such a way that measurement errors were minimized?

3. Does the report offer evidence of the reliability of measures? Does the evidence come from the research sample itself, or is it based on other studies? If the latter, is it reasonable to conclude that data quality would be similar for the research sample as for the reliability sample (e.g., are sample characteristics similar)?

4. If reliability is reported, which estimation method was used? Was this method appropriate? Should an alternative or additional method of reliability appraisal have been used? Is the reliability sufficiently high?

5. Does the report offer evidence of the validity of the measures? Does the evidence come from the research sample itself, or is it based on other studies? If the latter, is it reasonable to believe that data quality would be similar for the research sample as for the validity sample (e.g., are the sample characteristics similar)?

6. If validity information is reported, which validity approach was used? Was this method appropriate? Does the validity of the instrument appear to be adequate?

7. If there is no reliability or validity information, what conclusion can you reach about the quality of the data in the study?

8. If a diagnostic or screening tool was used, is information provided about its sensitivity and specificity, and were these qualities adequate?

9. Were the research hypotheses supported? If not, might data quality play a role in the failure to confirm the hypotheses?

has been responsible for collecting, analyzing, and interpreting all the data, as is frequently the case. Some guidelines for critiquing the trustworthiness of data in qualitative studies are presented in Box 14.2.

TIP

The amount of detail about data quality in a research report varies considerably. Some articles have virtually no information. Sometimes such information is not needed (e.g., when biophysiologic instrumentation with a proven and widely known record for accuracy is used). Most research reports, however, should provide some evidence that data quality was sufficiently high to answer the research questions. Normally, information about data quality is presented in the "Method" section of the report.

BOX 14.2   GUIDELINES FOR EVALUATING DATA QUALITY IN QUALITATIVE STUDIES

1. Does the report discuss efforts to enhance or evaluate the trustworthiness of the data? If so, is the description sufficiently detailed and clear? If not, is there other information that allows you to conclude that data are of high quality?

2. Which techniques (if any) did the researcher use to enhance and appraise the credibility of the data? Was the investigator in the field for an adequate amount of time? Was triangulation used, and if so, of what type? Did the researcher search for disconfirming evidence? Were there peer debriefings and/or member checks? Do the researcher's qualifications enhance the credibility of the data?

3. Which techniques (if any) did the researcher use to enhance and appraise the dependability, confirmability, and transferability of the data?

4. Given the efforts to enhance data quality, what can you conclude about the trustworthiness of the data? In light of this assessment, how much faith can be placed in the results of the study?

RESEARCH EXAMPLES AND CRITICAL THINKING ACTIVITIES

EXAMPLE 1 ■ Quantitative Research

Aspects of the quantitative study presented in Appendix A are presented below, followed by some questions to guide critical thinking.

Study

"Predictors of early parenting self-efficacy: Results of a prospective cohort study" (Bryanton, Gagnon, Hatem, & Johnston, 2008)

Statement of Purpose

The purpose of the study was to determine factors that are predictive of maternal parenting self-efficacy at 12 to 48 hours following childbirth and at 1-month postpartum.

Measure

To address the research question, parenting self-efficacy was measured using the Parent Expectations Survey (PES). This 25-item Likert-type scale was developed by Reece in 1992 and was later revised in 1998 by Reece and Harkless, with the addition of five items related to affective tasks of parenting. The PES includes items about a mother's self-efficacy in her abilities to feed and soothe her infant, meet other nonfeeding needs, and manage her lifestyle. For each item, women respond with a number from 0 (cannot do) to 10 (certain can do) that most closely represents how they feel about themselves as a new parent. Psychometric testing, including content validity, criterion-related validity, and internal consistency reliability, has been established for the scale.

Content Validity

Content validity was established by seven doctorally prepared nurses who rated each item on the scale as appropriate or inappropriate. After analyzing their responses, nurses were found to have a 92% agreement for the overall items. In addition, the questionnaire was reviewed by Bandura, the author of Self-Efficacy Theory, and four pediatric and family nurse practitioners.

CRITICAL THINKING SUGGESTIONS

1. Answer questions 3 through 6 and 8 from Box 14.1 (p. 271) regarding this study.
2. Also consider the following targeted questions, which may assist you in further assessing aspects of the study:
   a. After reviewing the psychometric properties of the scale, do you think the researchers made a good decision by including the PES?
   b. Each item on the PES is scored on an 11-point scale from 0 to 10. What is the range of possible scores on the scale?
3. What are the various ways that the PES might be used within clinical practice?

EXAMPLE 2 ■ Qualitative Research

Aspects of a qualitative nursing study, featuring terms and concepts discussed in this chapter, are presented below, followed by some questions to guide critical thinking.

Study

"Living in a world of our own: The experience of parents who have a child with autism" (Woodgate, Ateah, & Secco, 2008)

Statement of Purpose

The purpose of the study was to describe the lived experience of parents who have a child with autism.

Method

A hermeneutic phenomenological study involving the concurrent collection and analysis of data was used to address the study purpose. This approach allows the uncovering of the structure and internal meaning of the lived experience. Using in-depth interviews, data were collected from 21 parents of a total of 16 families of children with autism, over a period of 16 months. During the interviews, parents were asked to describe what life was like for them before, during, and after their child was diagnosed with autism. Parents were either interviewed individually or with their spouse and all interviews were audio taped. Data were subsequently transcribed from the audio recordings and reviewed in depth, in an attempt to find structure and meaning to the reported experiences, as well as emerging themes. Data collection continued until saturation—when there is replication of data concerning the emerging essential themes.

Credibility

The researchers enhanced credibility through prolonged engagement with participants and data: the researchers were in contact with the participants over a period of 16 months. Also, member checks were done by reviewing preliminary data interpretations with the participants during and following interviews. In addition, careful line-by-line analysis of transcripts and detailed memo writing were employed.

Dependability and Confirmability

The researchers maintained an audit trail, consisting of a written record of their methodological and theoretical decisions during data collection and data analysis.

Transferability

The research report contains information about the demographic characteristics of the participants, their family size, the severity of disability of the children with respect to communication, social relations, and repetitive or stereotyped behaviour; and their involvement with ancillary treatment services. Such information could be used to determine potential transferability.

Key Findings

Parents described a sense of isolation in caring for their children with autism and this sense was attributed to four main sources: society's lack of understanding of the nature of autism and what is involved in caring for an autistic child, missing a "normal" way of life due to the impact of autism on their lives, feeling disconnected from the rest of the family, and inadequate support received from child-related agencies and institutions. In addition to the identified sense of isolation, the researchers identified three themes that speak to how the parents struggled to remove the isolation they and their children were experiencing. These included vigilant parenting, sustaining the self and family, and fighting all the way.

CRITICAL THINKING SUGGESTIONS

1. Answer the questions from Box 14.2 (p. 271) regarding this study.
2. Also consider the following targeted questions, which may assist you in further assessing aspects of the study:
   a. Can you think of other types of confirmability of data that the researchers could have used?
   b. How did audiotaping and transcription enhance the trustworthiness of the data?
3. If the results of this study are trustworthy, what are some of the uses to which the findings might be put in clinical practice?

EXAMPLE 3 ■ Quantitative Research

1. Read the "Method" section from the quantitative study by Bryanton and colleagues (2008) in Appendix A and then answer questions 1 through 6 and 9 in Box 14.1 (p. 271).

EXAMPLE 4 ■ Qualitative Research

1. Read the "Method" section from the qualitative study by Woodgate and colleagues (2008) in Appendix B of this book, and then answer the relevant questions in Box 14.2 (p. 271).

Summary Points

· ·

- ➤ **Measurement** involves a set of rules according to which numeric values are assigned to objects to represent varying degrees of an attribute.

- ➤ Few quantitative measuring instruments are infallible. Sources of measurement error include situational contaminants, response biases, and transitory personal factors (e.g., fatigue).

- ➤ **Obtained scores** from an instrument consist of a **true score** component—the value that would be obtained if it were possible to have a perfect measure of the attribute—and an error component, or **error of measurement,** that represents measurement inaccuracies.

- ➤ **Reliability** is the degree of consistency or accuracy with which an instrument measures an attribute. The higher the reliability of an instrument, the lower the amount of error in the obtained scores.

- ➤ There are different methods for assessing reliability and computing a **reliability coefficient.** The *stability* aspect, which concerns the extent to which an instrument yields the same results on repeated administrations, is evaluated by **test–retest procedures.**

- ➤ The **internal consistency** aspect of reliability, which refers to the extent to which all the instrument's items are measuring the same attribute, is assessed using either the *split-half reliability technique* or, more likely, the **Cronbach alpha method.**

- ➤ When the focus of a reliability assessment is on establishing *equivalence* between observers in rating or coding behaviours, estimates of **interrater** (or **interobserver**) **reliability** are obtained.

- ➤ **Validity** is the degree to which an instrument measures what it is supposed to be measuring.

- ➤ **Face validity** refers to whether an instrument appears, on the face of it, to be measuring the appropriate construct.

- ➤ **Content validity** is concerned with the sampling adequacy of the content of a measure.

- ➤ **Criterion-related validity** focuses on the correlation between the instrument and an outside criterion.

- ➤ **Construct validity** refers to the adequacy of an instrument in measuring the construct of interest. One construct validation method is the **known-groups technique,** which contrasts the scores of groups that are presumed to differ on the attribute; another is **factor analysis,** a statistical procedure for identifying unitary clusters of items or measures.

- ➤ Sensitivity and specificity are criteria for evaluating screening or diagnostic instruments. **Sensitivity** is the instrument's ability to correctly identify a case, that is, its rate of true positives. **Specificity** is the instrument's ability to correctly identify a noncase, that is, its rate of true negatives.

- ➤ Qualitative researchers evaluate the **trustworthiness** of their data using the criteria of credibility, dependability, confirmability, and transferability.

- ➤ **Credibility,** roughly analogous to validity in a quantitative study, refers to the believability of the data. Techniques to improve the credibility of qualitative data include **prolonged engagement,** which strives for adequate scope of data, and **persistent observation,** which is aimed at achieving adequate depth.

- ➤ **Triangulation** is the process of using multiple referents to draw conclusions about what constitutes the truth. The four major forms are *data source triangulation, investigator triangulation, theoretical triangulation*, and *method triangulation.*

❧ Two important tools for establishing credibility are **peer debriefings,** wherein the researcher obtains feedback about data quality and interpretation from peers, and **member checks,** wherein informants are asked to comment on the researcher's conclusions and interpretations.

❧ **Dependability** of qualitative data refers to the stability of data over time and over conditions and is somewhat analogous to the concept of reliability in quantitative studies.

❧ **Confirmability** refers to the objectivity or neutrality of the data. Independent **inquiry audits** by external auditors can be used to assess and document dependability and confirmability.

❧ The **auditability** of a study is enhanced when researchers maintain and share portions of an **audit trail** and **decision trail** in their reports.

❧ **Transferability** is the extent to which findings from the data can be transferred to other settings or groups. Transferability can be enhanced through **thick descriptions** of the context of the data collection.

STUDIES CITED IN CHAPTER 14*

*This reference list contains only those studies that were cited in this chapter. Citations pertaining to theoretical, methodologic, or nonempirical work are included together in a separate section at the end of the book (beginning on page 399).

Brathwaite, A. C., & Williams, C. C. (2004). Childbirth experiences of professional Chinese Canadian women. *Journal of Obstetric, Gynecologic, and Neonatal Nursing, 33*(6), 748–755.

Bryanton, J., Gagnon, A. J., Hatem, M., & Johnston, C. (2008). Predictors of early parenting self-efficacy: Results of a prospective cohort study. *Nursing Research, 57*(4), 252–259.

Cossette, S., Pepin, J., Côté, J., & de Courval, F. P. (2008). The multidimensionality of caring: A confirmatory factor analysis of the Caring Nurse-Patient Interaction Short Scale. *Journal of Advanced Nursing, 61*(6), 699–710.

Fillion, L., Gélinas, S., Simard, S., Savard, J., & Gagnon, P. (2003). Validation evidence for the French Canadian adaptation of the Multidimensional Fatigue Inventory as a measure of cancer-related fatigue. *Cancer Nursing, 26*(2), 143–154.

Gélinas, C., & Johnston, C. (2007). Pain assessment in the critically ill ventilated adult: Validation of the Critical-Care Pain Observation Tool and physiologic indicators. *Clinical Journal of Pain, 23*(6), 497–505.

Lobchuk, M., Udod, S., & Loiselle, C. G. (2009). *A study of oncology nurses' perceptions of their relations with family members within a cancer care setting.* Research grant funded by the Canadian Association of Nurses in Oncology (CANO).

Pauly, B. B. (2008). Shifting moral values to enhance access to health care: Harm reduction as a context for ethical nursing practice. *International Journal of Drug Policy, 19*(3), 195–204.

Perraud, S., Fogg, L., Kopytko, E., & Gross, D. (2006). Predictive validity of the Depression Coping Self-Efficacy Scale (DCSES). *Research in Nursing & Health, 29*(2), 147–160.

Rennick, J. E., McHarg, L. F., Dell'Api, M., Johnston, C. C., & Stevens, B. (2008). Developing the Children's Critical Illness Impact Scale: Capturing stories from children, parents, and staff. *Pediatric Critical Care Medicine, 9*(3), 252–260.

Rossen, E., & Gruber, K. (2007). Development and psychometric testing of the relocation self-efficacy scale. *Nursing Research, 56*(4), 244–251.

Tse, L., & Hall, W. (2008). A qualitative study of parents' perceptions of a behavioural sleep intervention. *Child: Care, Health and Development, 34*(2), 162–172.

Watson, L., Oberle, K., & Deutscher, D. (2008). Development and psychometric testing of the nurses' attitudes toward obesity and obese patients (NATOOPS) scale. *Research in Nursing and Health, 31*(16), 586–593.

Whittemore, R., Chase, S. K., & Mandle, C. L. (2001). Validity in qualitative research. *Qualitative Health Research, 11*(4), 522–537.

Woodgate, R. L., Ateah, C., & Secco, L. (2008). Living in a world of our own: The experience of parents who have a child with autism. *Qualitative Health research, 18*(8), 1075–1083.

PART 5

Data Analysis

15 Analyzing Quantitative Data

On completing this chapter, you will be able to:

1. Identify the four levels of measurement and compare their characteristics

2. Identify and interpret various descriptive statistics

3. Describe the logic and purpose of tests of statistical significance and describe hypothesis testing procedures

4. Specify the appropriate applications for *t* tests, analysis of variance, chi-squared tests, correlation coefficients, multiple regression, and analysis of covariance

5. Understand the results of simple statistical procedures described in a research report

6. Define new terms in the chapter

The data collected in a study do not by themselves answer research questions or test hypotheses. Data need to be systematically analyzed so that patterns can be detected. This chapter describes procedures for analyzing quantitative data, and Chapter 16 discusses the analysis of qualitative data.

LEVELS OF MEASUREMENT

A quantitative measure can be classified according to its **level of measurement.** This classification is important because the analyses that can be performed on data depend on their measurement level. Of note, there is still debate about the merits of these classifications, particularly when it comes to measures in the behavioral sciences as opposed to basic or physical sciences. Traditionally, four levels of measurement are proposed:

1. **Nominal measurement,** the lowest level, involves using numbers simply to categorize attributes. Examples of variables that are nominally measured include gender and blood type. The numbers assigned in nominal measurement do not have quantitative meaning. If we code males as 1 and females as 2, the number 2 does not mean "more than" 1. Nominal measurement provides information only about categorical equivalence and nonequivalence; the numbers cannot be treated mathematically. It is nonsensical, for example, to compute the sample's average gender by adding the values of the codes and dividing by the number of subjects.

2. **Ordinal measurement** ranks objects based on their relative standing on an attribute. If a researcher rank-orders people from heaviest to lightest, this is ordinal measurement. As another example, consider this ordinal coding scheme for measuring ability to perform activities of daily living: 1 = completely dependent; 2 = needs another person's assistance; 3 = needs mechanical assistance; and 4 = completely independent. The numbers signify incremental ability to perform activities of daily living independently. Ordinal measurement does not, however, tell us how much greater one level is than another. For example, we do not know if being completely independent is twice as good as needing mechanical assistance. As with nominal measures, the mathematic operations permissible with ordinal-level data are restricted.

3. **Interval measurement** occurs when researchers can specify the ranking of objects on an attribute *and* the distance between those objects. Most psychological tests are based on interval scales. For example, the Stanford-Binet Intelligence Scale—a standardized intelligence quotient (IQ) test used in many countries—is an interval measure. A score of 140 on the Stanford-Binet is higher than a score of 120, which, in turn, is higher than 100. Moreover, the difference between 140 and 120 is presumed to be equivalent to the difference between 120 and 100. Interval scales expand analytic possibilities: interval-level data can be averaged meaningfully, for example. Many statistical procedures require interval measurements.

4. **Ratio measurement** is the highest level of measurement. Ratio scales, unlike interval scales, have a meaningful zero and therefore provide information about the absolute magnitude of the attribute. The Centigrade scale for measuring temperature (interval measurement) has an arbitrary zero point. Zero on the thermometer does not signify the absence of heat; it would not be appropriate to say that 30°C is twice as hot as 15°C. Many physical measures, however, are ratio measures with a real zero. A person's weight, for example, is a ratio measure. It is acceptable to say that someone who weighs 120 kg is twice as heavy as

someone who weighs 60 kg. Statistical procedures suitable for interval-level data are also appropriate for ratio-level data.

Example of ratio measurement
≫ Loiselle and Dubois (2009) conducted a quasi-experimental study comparing the impact of a multimedia patient education tool versus usual care on several outcome variables including reliance on health care services by individuals newly diagnosed with cancer. Several variables included ratio-level measurement, such as number of health care services used within the past 2 months and number of minutes spent with various health care providers.

Researchers usually strive to use the highest levels of measurement possible—especially for their dependent variables—because higher levels yield more information and are amenable to more powerful analysis than lower levels.

> **TIP**
>
> How can you tell the measurement level of a variable? A variable is *nominal* if the values could be interchanged (e.g., 1 = male, 2 = female, OR 1 = female, 2 = male—the codes are arbitrary). A variable is usually *ordinal* if there is a quantitative ordering of values AND if there are only a small number of values (e.g., very important, important, not too important, unimportant). A variable is usually considered *interval* if it is measured with a composite scale or psychological test. A variable is *ratio* level if it makes sense to say that one value is twice as much as another (e.g., 100 mg is twice as much as 50 mg).

DESCRIPTIVE STATISTICS

Statistical procedures enable researchers to organize, interpret, and communicate numeric information. Statistics are either descriptive or inferential. **Descriptive** statistics, such as averages and percentages, are used to synthesize and describe data. When such indexes are calculated on data from a population, they are called **parameters.** A descriptive index from a sample is a **statistic.** Most scientific questions are about parameters; researchers calculate statistics to estimate them.

Frequency Distributions

Data that are not analyzed or organized are overwhelming. It is not even possible to discern general trends without some structure. Consider the 60 numbers in Table 15.1. Let us assume that these numbers are the scores of 60 preoperative

TABLE 15.1		PATIENTS' ANXIETY SCORES							
22	27	25	19	24	25	23	29	24	20
26	16	20	26	17	22	24	18	26	28
15	24	23	22	21	24	20	25	18	27
24	23	16	25	30	29	27	21	23	24
26	18	30	21	17	25	22	24	29	28
20	25	26	24	23	19	27	28	25	26

TABLE 15.2	FREQUENCY DISTRIBUTION OF PATIENTS' ANXIETY SCORES	
SCORE	FREQUENCY	PERCENTAGE
15	1	1.7
16	2	3.3
17	2	3.3
18	3	5.0
19	2	3.3
20	4	6.7
21	3	5.0
22	4	6.7
23	5	8.3
24	9	15.0
25	7	11.7
26	6	10.0
27	4	6.7
28	3	5.0
29	3	5.0
30	2	3.3
	$N = 60$	100.0

patients on a six-item measure of anxiety—scores that we will consider to be on an interval scale. Visual inspection of the numbers in this table provides little insight on patients' anxiety levels.

Frequency distributions are a method of imposing order on numeric data. A **frequency distribution** is a systematic arrangement of numeric values from lowest to highest, together with a count (or percentage) of the number of times each value was obtained. The 60 anxiety scores are presented as a frequency distribution in Table 15.2. This arrangement makes it convenient to see at a glance the highest and lowest scores, the most common scores, and how many patients were in the sample (total sample size is typically designated as N in research reports). None of this was easily discernible before the data were organized.

Some researchers display frequency data graphically in a *frequency polygon* (Figure 15.1). In such graphs, scores are on the horizontal line, with the lowest value on the left, and frequency counts or percentages are on the vertical line. Distributions can be described by their shapes. **Symmetric distribution** occurs if, when folded over, the two halves of a frequency polygon would be superimposed

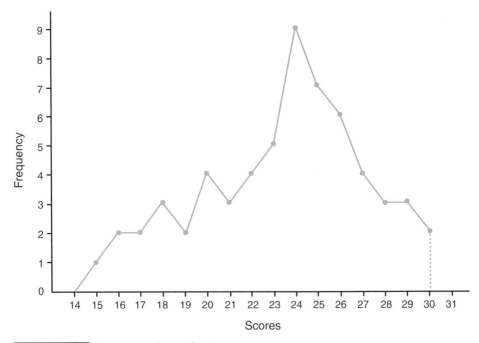

FIGURE 15.1 Frequency polygon of patients' anxiety scores.

(Figure 15.2). In an asymmetric or **skewed distribution,** the peak is off centre and one tail is longer than the other. When the longer tail is pointed toward the right, the distribution has a **positive skew,** as in the first graph of Figure 15.3. Personal income is an example of a positively skewed attribute. Most people have moderate incomes, with few high-income people at the right end of the distribution. If the longer tail points to the left, the distribution has a **negative skew,** as in the second graph in Figure 15.3. Age at death is an example: here, the bulk of people are at the far right end of the distribution, with relatively few people dying at an early age.

Another aspect of a distribution's shape concerns how many peaks or high points it has. A *unimodal distribution* has one peak (graph A, Figure 15.2), whereas a *multimodal distribution* has two or more peaks—that is, two or more values of high frequency. A multimodal distribution with two peaks is a *bimodal distribution*, illustrated in graph B of Figure 15.2.

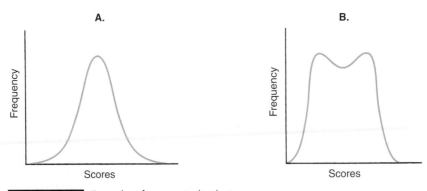

FIGURE 15.2 Examples of symmetric distributions.

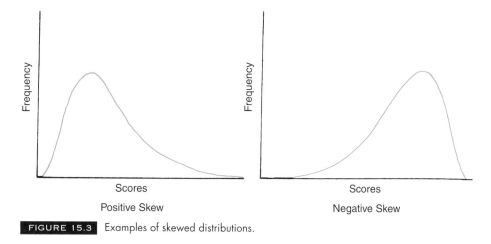

FIGURE 15.3 Examples of skewed distributions.

A distribution of particular interest is the **normal distribution** (sometimes called *a bell-shaped curve*). A normal distribution is symmetric, unimodal, and not very peaked, as illustrated in graph A of Figure 15.2. Many human attributes (e.g., height, intelligence) approximate a normal distribution.

Frequency distributions can be constructed with data for variables measured on any of the four measurement scales.

Example of frequency information

⇒ Table 15.3 presents distribution information on sample characteristics from a study of clients of adult day programs in Alberta (Ross-Kerr, Warren, Schalm, Smith, & Godkin, 2003). This table shows, for selected background characteristics, both the frequency and the percentage of participants in various categories. For example, 179 of the 477 clients (37.5%) were men and 298 (62.5%) were women. Most subjects were either married (41.5%) or widowed (46.1%).

Central Tendency

For variables on an interval or ratio scale, a distribution of values is usually of less interest than an overall summary. Researchers ask such questions as: What was the patients' average blood pressure? How depressed was the typical mother postpartum? These questions seek a single number that best represents the whole distribution. Such indexes are measures of **central tendency.** To lay people, the term *average* is normally used to designate central tendency. There are three commonly used kinds of averages, or measures of central tendency: the mode, the median, and the mean.

⇒ **Mode:** The mode is the number that occurs most frequently in a distribution. In the following distribution, the mode is 53:

150 51 51 52 53 53 53 53 54 55 56

The value of 53 occurred four times, a higher frequency than for other numbers. The mode of the patients' anxiety scores in Table 15.2 is 24. The mode, in other words, identifies the most popular value. The mode is used most often to describe typical or high-frequency values for nominal measures. For example, in the study by Ross-Kerr and co-researchers (see Table 15.3), we could make the following statement: The typical (modal) client was a widowed female.

TABLE 15.3 ⓘ	EXAMPLE OF TABLE WITH FREQUENCY INFORMATION: SELECTED CHARACTERISTICS OF CLIENTS ATTENDING ADULT DAY PROGRAMS	
CLIENT CHARACTERISTIC	NUMBER (N = 477)	PERCENTAGE
Type of program		
Adult day support program	234	49.1
Adult day hospital program	243	50.9
Gender		
Male	179	37.5
Female	298	62.5
Marital status		
Widowed	220	46.1
Married	198	41.5
Separated/divorced	30	6.3
Never married	29	6.1

Adapted from Rose-Kerr, J. C., Warren, S., Schalm, C., Smith, D., & Godkin, M. D. (2003). Adult day programs: Are they needed? *Journal of Gerontological Nursing, 29*(12), 1–7.

⇒ **Median:** The median is the point in a distribution that divides scores in half. Consider the following set of values:

2 2 3 3 4 5 6 7 8 9

The value that divides the cases in half is midway between 4 and 5, and thus 4.5 is the median. For the patient anxiety scores, the median is 24, the same as the mode. An important characteristic of the median is that it does not take into account individual values and is thus insensitive to extremes. In the above set of numbers, if the value of 9 were changed to 99, the median would remain 4.5. Because of this property, the median is the preferred index of central tendency to describe a highly skewed distribution. The median may be abbreviated as *Md* or *Mdn*.

⇒ **Mean:** The mean equals the sum of all values divided by the number of participants—commonly referred to as the average. The mean of the patients' anxiety scores is 23.4 (1405/60). As another example, here are the weights of eight people:

50 55 61 66 72 78 86 92

In this example, the mean is 70. Unlike the median, the mean is affected by every score. If we were to exchange the 92-kg person for one weighing 132 kg, the mean weight would increase from 70 to 75 kg. A substitution of this kind would leave the median unchanged. The mean is often symbolized as M or $\bar{X}$ (e.g., $\bar{X} = 145$).

For interval-level or ratio-level measurements, the mean, rather than the median or mode, is usually the statistic reported. The mean is the most stable of these indexes: if repeated samples were drawn from a population, the means would fluctuate less than the modes or medians. Because of its stability, the mean usually is the best estimate of a population central tendency. When a distribution is highly skewed, however, the mean does not characterize the centre of the distribution; in such situations, the median is preferred. For example, the median is a better central tendency measure of family income than the mean because income is positively skewed.

Variability

Two sets of data with identical means could be quite different with respect to **variability,** that is, how different people are from one another. Consider the distributions in Figure 15.4, which represent hypothetical scores of students from two schools on the Stanford-Binet IQ test. Both distributions have an average score of 100, but the two groups are very different. In school A, there is a wide range of scores—from scores below 70 to above 130. In school B, by contrast, there are few low scorers but also few outstanding performers. School A is more heterogeneous (i.e., more variable) than school B; school B is more homogeneous than school A.

Researchers compute an index of variability to summarize the extent to which scores in a distribution differ from one another. Several such indexes have been developed, the most important of which are the range and the standard deviation.

☞ **Range:** The range is the highest score minus the lowest score in a distribution. In the example of the patients' anxiety scores, the range is 15 (30 − 15). In the distributions in Figure 15.4, the range for school A is about 80 (140 − 60), whereas the range for school B is about 50 (125 − 75). The chief virtue of the range is ease of computation. Because it is based on only two scores, however, the range is unstable: from sample to sample drawn from the same population, the range tends to fluctuate widely. Moreover, the range ignores variations between the two extremes. In school B of Figure 15.4, if a single student obtained a score of 60 and another obtained a score of 140, the range of both schools would then be 80—despite clear differences in heterogeneity. For these reasons, the range is used largely as a gross descriptive index.

☞ **Standard deviation:** The most widely used variability index is the standard deviation. Like the mean, the standard deviation is calculated based on every value in a distribution. The standard deviation summarizes the *average* amount of deviation of values from the mean. In the anxiety scale example, the

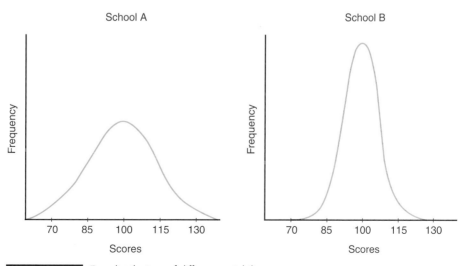

FIGURE 15.4   Two distributions of different variability.

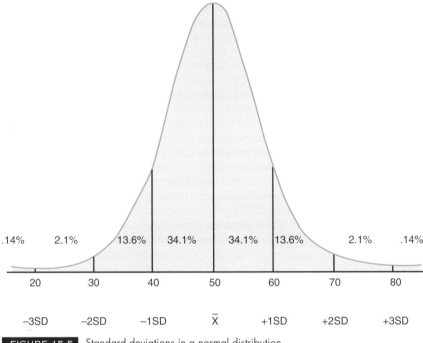

.14%   2.1%   13.6%   34.1%   34.1%   13.6%   2.1%   .14%

20   30   40   50   60   70   80

−3SD   −2SD   −1SD   X̄   +1SD   +2SD   +3SD

FIGURE 15.5 Standard deviations in a normal distribution.

standard deviation is 3.725.* In research reports, the standard deviation is often abbreviated as *s* or *SD*. Occasionally, the standard deviation is simply shown in relation to the mean without a formal label, such as M = 4.0 (1.5) or M = 4.0 ± 1.5, where 4.0 is the mean and 1.5 is the standard deviation.†

A standard deviation is more difficult to interpret than the range. With regard to the SD of the anxiety scores, you might ask, 3.725 *what*? What does the number mean? We can answer these questions from several angles. First, as discussed, the SD is an index of how variable scores in a distribution are. If male and female nursing students had means of 23 on the anxiety scale, but females had an SD of 7 and males had an SD of 3, we would immediately know that the males were more homogeneous (i.e., their scores were more similar to one another).

The SD represents the *average* of deviations from the mean. The mean tells us the single best point for summarizing an entire distribution, and an SD tells us how much, on average, the scores deviate from that mean. In the anxiety scale example, they deviated by an average of just under 4 points. A standard deviation might thus be interpreted as an indication of our degree of error when we use a mean to describe an entire sample.

In normal and near-normal distributions, there are roughly 3 SDs above and below the mean. Suppose we had a normal distribution with a mean of 50 and an SD of 10 (Figure 15.5). In such a distribution, a fixed percentage of cases fall within certain distances from the mean. Sixty-eight percent of all cases fall within 1 SD above and below the mean. Thus, in this example, nearly 7 of 10 scores are between 40 and 60. In a normal distribution, 95% of the scores fall within 2 SDs

---

*Formulas for computing the standard deviation, as well as other statistics discussed in this chapter, are not shown in this textbook. The emphasis here is on helping you to understand statistical applications. References at the end of the chapter can be consulted for computation formulas.

†Research reports occasionally refer to an index of variability known as the **variance.** The variance is simply the value of the standard deviation squared. In the example of the patients' anxiety scores, the variance is 3.725^2 or 13.88.

TABLE 15.4	EXAMPLE OF TABLE WITH DESCRIPTIVE STATISTICS: CHARACTERISTICS OF WOMEN IN TWO RESEARCH GROUPS			
	HOME VISIT GROUP (n = 117)		TELEPHONE TRIAGE GROUP (n = 120)	
CHARACTERISTIC	Mean	SD	Mean	SD
Age	31.3	4.7	30.4	5.6
Prepregnancy weight (kg)	60.7	11.3	60.7	11.8
Weight gain during pregnancy (kg)	15.0	15.9	14.0	15.7
Gestational age at delivery (week)	39.5	1.42	39.5	2.9

Adapted from Janssen, P. A., Iker, C. E., & Carty, E. A. (2003). Early labour assessment and support at home: A randomized controlled trial. *Journal of Obstetrics and Gynaecology Canada, 25*(9), 734–741.

from the mean. Only a handful of cases—about 2% at each extreme—lie more than 2 SDs from the mean. Using this figure, we can see that a person with a score of 70 had a higher score than about 98% of the sample.

Example of means and SDs

≈ Table 15.4 presents descriptive statistics from a clinical trial designed to assess the effect of alternative modes of early labour support for pregnant women (Janssen, Iker, & Carty, 2003). The table shows the means and SDs of selected background characteristics for the two research groups (women getting support through a home visit or through telephone triage). According to these data, the two groups had similar means with regard to age, weight, weight gain, and gestational age at delivery. The telephone triage group, however, tended to be slightly more heterogeneous. For example, the SD for gestational age was much larger in the telephone triage group than in the home visit group, even though the means were identical.

Bivariate Descriptive Statistics

So far, our discussion has focused on *univariate* (one-variable) *descriptive statistics*. The mean, mode, standard deviation, and so forth are used to describe one variable at a time. *Bivariate* (two-variable) *descriptive statistics* describe relationships between two variables.

Contingency Tables

A **contingency table** is a two-dimensional frequency distribution in which the frequencies of two variables are **cross-tabulated.** Suppose we had data on patients' gender and whether they were nonsmokers, light smokers (<1 pack of cigarettes a day), or heavy smokers (≥1 pack a day). The question is whether there is a tendency for the men to smoke more heavily than the women or *vice versa*. Some fictitious data on these two variables are shown in a contingency in Table 15.5. Six cells are created by using one variable (gender) for columns and the other variable (smoking status) for rows. After all subjects are allocated to the appropriate cells, percentages can be computed. This simple procedure allows us to see at a glance that, in this sample, women were more likely than men to be nonsmokers (45.4% versus 27.3%) and less likely to be heavy smokers (18.2% versus 36.4%). Contingency tables usually are used with nominal data or ordinal data that have few levels or ranks. In the present example, gender is a nominal measure and smoking status is an ordinal measure.

TABLE 15.5　CONTINGENCY TABLE FOR GENDER AND SMOKING STATUS RELATIONSHIP

| | GENDER | | | | | |
| | Female | | Male | | Total | |
SMOKING STATUS	n	%	n	%	n	%
Nonsmoker	10	45.4	6	27.3	16	36.4
Light smoker	8	36.4	8	36.4	16	36.4
Heavy smoker	4	18.2	8	36.4	12	27.3
Total	22	50.0	22	50.0	44	100.0

Example of a contingency table

❖ Table 15.6 presents a contingency table from a study by King, Parry, Southern, Faris, and Tsuyuki (2008) that examined, among other things, predictors of long-term pain and discomfort following sternotomy. Incision and breast pain data were collected using numeric rating scales at 5 days, 12 weeks, and 12 months following sternotomy. An abridged version of the contingency table presented examines the relationship between patients' report of pain at 12 weeks postoperatively and 12 months later. Overall, symptom presence at 12 months was related to symptom presence at 12 weeks; 79.7% of patients who reported any pain at 12 months had reported pain at 12 weeks.

A comparison between Tables 15.5 and 15.6 illustrates that cross-tabulated data can be presented in two ways: within each cell, percentages can be computed based on either row totals or column totals. In Table 15.5, the number 10 in the first cell (female nonsmokers) was divided by the column total (i.e., by the total number of females—22) to arrive at the percentage (45%) of females who were nonsmokers. The table could have shown 63% in this cell (10/16)—the percentage of nonsmokers who were female. In Table 15.6, the number 47 in the first cell was divided by the column total of 59 (i.e., the total number of patients who reported pain at 12 months postop irrespective of pain at 12 weeks postop) to yield 79.7%—the percentage of those who reported pain at 12 months, who also reported pain at 12 weeks. Computed the other way, the researchers would have gotten 25.5% (47/184)—the percentage of patients who reported pain at 12 weeks postop, who also reported pain at 12 months

TABLE 15.6　EXAMPLE OF A CONTINGENCY TABLE: USING PAIN REPORTED AT 12 WEEKS POSTOPERATIVELY (POST-OP) AS A PREDICTOR FOR PAIN AT 12 MONTHS POST-OP

| | PAIN AT 12 MONTHS? | | | | | |
| | Yes | | No | | Total | |
PAIN AT 12 WEEKS?	n	%	n	%	n	%
Yes	47	79.7	137	51	184	56.4
No	12	20.3	130	49	142	43.6
Total	59	18	267	82	326	100.0

Calculations and adaptations from King, K. M., Parry, M., Southern, D., Faris, P., & Tsuyuki, R. T. (2008). Women's recovery from Sternotomy-Extension (WREST-E) study: Examining long-term pain and discomfort following sternotomy and their predictors. Heart, 94, 493–497.

postop. Either approach is acceptable, although the former is often preferred because then the percentages in a column add up to 100%.

TIP

You may need to spend extra time inspecting contingency tables to determine which total—row or column—was used as the basis for calculating percentages.

Correlation

Relationships between two variables are usually described through **correlation** procedures. The correlation question is: To what extent are two variables related to each other? For example, to what degree are anxiety scores and blood pressure measures related? This question can be answered quantitatively by calculating a **correlation coefficient,** which describes the *intensity* and *direction* of a relationship.

Two variables that are related are height and weight: tall people tend to weigh more than short people. The relationship between height and weight would be a *perfect relationship* if the tallest person in a population was the heaviest, the second tallest person was the second heaviest, and so forth. The correlation coefficient summarizes how "perfect" a relationship is. The possible values for a correlation coefficient range from −1.00 through .00 to +1.00. If height and weight were perfectly correlated, the correlation coefficient expressing this would be 1.00 (the actual correlation coefficient is in the vicinity of .50 to .60 for a general population). Height and weight have a **positive relationship** because greater height tends to be associated with greater weight.

When two variables are unrelated, the correlation coefficient is zero. One might expect that women's shoe size is unrelated to their intelligence. Women with large feet are as likely to perform well on IQ tests as those with small feet. The correlation coefficient summarizing such a relationship would presumably be near .00.

Correlation coefficients running between .00 and −1.00 express a **negative,** or *inverse*, **relationship.** When two variables are inversely related, increments in one variable are associated with decrements in the second. For example, there is a negative correlation between depression and self-esteem: on average, people with *high* self-esteem tend to be *low* on depression. If the relationship were perfect (i.e., if the person with the highest self-esteem score had the lowest depression score, and so forth), then the correlation coefficient would be −1.00. In actuality, the relationship between depression and self-esteem is moderate—usually in the vicinity of −.40 or −.50. Note that the higher the *absolute value* of the coefficient (i.e., the value disregarding the sign), the stronger the relationship. A correlation of −.80, for instance, is much stronger than a correlation of +.20.

The most commonly used correlation index is the **product–moment correlation coefficient** (also called **Pearson's r**), which is computed with interval or ratio measures. One correlation index for ordinal measures is **Spearman's rank-order correlation** (r_s), sometimes referred to as **Spearman's rho.**

It is difficult to offer guidelines on what should be interpreted as strong or weak relationships because it depends on the nature of the variables. If we were to measure patients' body temperature both orally and rectally, a correlation (r) of .70 between the two measurements would be low. For most psychosocial variables (e.g., stress and severity of illness), however, an r of .70 would be rather high. Perfect correlations (+1.00 and −1.00) are extremely rare.

Correlation coefficients are often reported in tables displaying a two-dimensional **correlation matrix,** in which variables are displayed in both rows and columns. To read a correlation matrix, one finds the row for one variable and reads across until the row intersects with the column for another variable, and the intersection gives the corresponding value for r.

TABLE 15.7	EXAMPLE OF A CORRELATION MATRIX: PSYCHOSOCIAL CORRELATES OF CARDIOVASCULAR REACTIVITY TO ANTICIPATION OF AN EXERCISE STRESS TEST BEFORE ATTENDING CARDIAC REHABILITATION				
	1	2	3	4	5
1. Anxiety	1.00				
2. Self-efficacy	−.57	1.00			
3. Heart rate change	.47	−.61	1.00		
4. Systolic blood pressure change	.40	−.24	.34	1.00	
5. Diastolic blood pressure change	.10	−.04	.03	.61	1.00

Adapted from Fraser, S. N., Rodgers, W., & Daub, B. (2008). Psychosocial correlates of cardiovascular reactivity to anticipation of an exercise stress test prior to attending cardiac rehabilitation: A preliminary test. *Journal of Applied Biobehavioral Research, 13*(1), 20–41.

Example of a correlation matrix

⮞ Table 15.7 presents an abridged correlation matrix from a study by Fraser et al. (2008) that examined psychosocial factors associated with cardiovascular reactivity to anticipation of an exercise stress test, before attending cardiac rehabilitation (Fraser, Rodgers, & Daub, 2008). Study participants included both men and women; however, the table presented includes data on women exclusively. The table lists, on the left, two possible psychosocial factors (anxiety and self-efficacy) that are associated with cardiovascular reactivity (indicated by heart-rate change and systolic and diastolic blood pressure change). The numbers in the top row, from 1 to 5, correspond to the five variables: 1 is anxiety, 2 is self-efficacy, and so forth. At the intersection of row 1 and column 1, we find the value 1.00, which indicates that the variable "anxiety" is perfectly correlated with itself. The next entry at the intersection of row 3 and column 2 represents the correlation between self-efficacy and heart rate change. The value of −.61 indicates a negative correlation between the variables. As such, women with higher self-efficacy tended to report less changes in heart rate and vice versa.

INTRODUCTION TO INFERENTIAL STATISTICS

Descriptive statistics are useful for summarizing data, but researchers usually do more than simply describe. **Inferential statistics,** which are based on the *laws of probability*, provide a means for drawing conclusions about a population, given data from a sample.

Sampling Distributions

When using a sample to estimate population characteristics, it is important to obtain a sample that is representative of the population. Random sampling is the best means of securing such samples. Inferential statistics are based on the assumption of random sampling from populations—although this assumption is widely violated.

Even with random sampling, however, sample characteristics are seldom identical to those of the population. Suppose we had a population of 30,000 nursing school applicants whose mean score on a standardized entrance exam was 500 with a standard deviation of 100. Suppose that we do not know these parameters but that we must estimate them based on scores from a random sample of 25 applicants. Should we expect a sample mean of exactly 500 and a standard

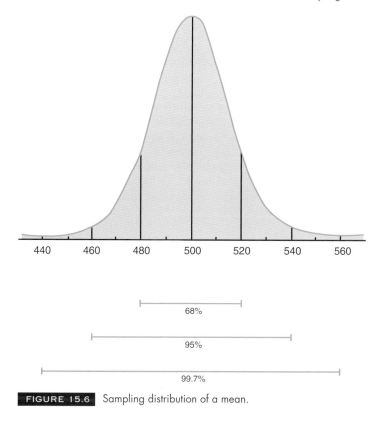

440   460   480   500   520   540   560

68%

95%

99.7%

FIGURE 15.6 Sampling distribution of a mean.

deviation of 100? It would be improbable to obtain identical values. Suppose that the sample mean was 505. If a completely new random sample of 25 students were drawn, the mean might be 497. Sample statistics fluctuate and are unequal to the population parameter because of sampling error. Researchers need a way to determine whether sample statistics are good estimates of population parameters.

To understand the logic of inferential statistics, we must perform a mental exercise. Consider drawing a sample of 25 students from the population of all applicants, calculating a mean test score, replacing the students, and drawing a new sample. Each mean is considered one datum. If we drew 10,000 samples of 25 applicants, we would have 10,000 means (data points) that could be used to construct a frequency polygon (Figure 15.6). This distribution is called a **sampling distribution of the mean,** which is a theoretical distribution rather than an actual distribution because in practice no one draws consecutive samples from a population and plots their means. Statisticians have demonstrated that (1) sampling distributions of means follow a normal distribution and (2) the mean of a sampling distribution for an infinite number of sample means equals the population mean. In our example, the mean of the sampling distribution is 500, the same as the population mean.

Remember that when scores are normally distributed, 68% of the cases fall between +1 SD and −1 SD from the mean. Because a sampling distribution of means is normally distributed, the probability is 68 out of 100 that any randomly drawn sample mean lies between +1 SD and −1 SD of the population mean. The problem is to determine the standard deviation of the sampling distribution—which is called the **standard error of the mean** (or SEM). The word *error* signifies that the sample means contain some error as estimates of the population mean. The smaller the standard error (i.e., the less variable the sample means), the more accurate are the means as estimates of the population value.

Because no one actually constructs a sampling distribution, how can its standard deviation be computed? Fortunately, there is a formula for estimating the SEM from data from a single sample, using the sample's standard deviation and its size. In the present example, the SEM equals 20, as shown in Figure 15.6. This statistic is an estimate of how much sampling error there would be from one sample mean to another in an infinite number of samples of 25 nursing school applicants.

We can now estimate the probability of drawing a sample with a certain mean. With a sample size of 25 and a population mean of 500, the chances are about 95 out of 100 that a sample mean would fall between the values of 460 and 540—2 SDs above and below the mean. Only 5 times out of 100 would the mean of a randomly selected sample of 25 applicants be greater than 540 or less than 460. In other words, only 5 times out of 100 would we be likely to draw a sample whose mean deviates from the population mean by more than 40 points.

Because the SEM is partly a function of sample size, we need only increase sample size to increase the accuracy of our estimate. Suppose that instead of using a sample of 25 applicants to estimate the population mean, we used a sample of 100. With this many students, the standard error of the mean would be 10, not 20—and the probability would be about 95 in 100 that a sample mean would be between 480 and 520. The chances of drawing a sample with a mean very different from that of the population are reduced as sample size increases because large numbers promote the likelihood that extreme cases will cancel each other out.

You may be wondering why you need to learn about these abstract statistical notions. Consider, though, that what we are talking about concerns how likely it is that research results are accurate. As a consumer, you need to evaluate how believable research evidence is so that you can decide whether to incorporate it into your nursing practice. The concepts underlying the standard error are important in such an evaluation and are related to issues we stressed in Chapter 12 on sampling. First, the more homogeneous the population is on the critical attribute (i.e., the smaller the standard deviation), the more likely it is that results calculated from a sample will be accurate. Second, the larger the sample size, the greater is the likelihood of accuracy. The concepts discussed in this section are the basis for statistical hypothesis testing.

Hypothesis Testing

Statistical inference consists of two major techniques: estimation of parameters and hypothesis testing. **Estimation procedures** are used to estimate a single population characteristic, such as a mean value (e.g., patients' mean temperature). Researchers usually are more interested in relationships between variables than in estimating the accuracy of a single sample value, however. For this reason, we focus on hypothesis testing.

Statistical **hypothesis testing** provides objective criteria for deciding whether research hypotheses should be accepted as true or rejected as false. Suppose we hypothesized that maternity patients exposed to a film on breastfeeding would breastfeed longer than mothers who did not see the film. We find that the mean number of days of breastfeeding is 131.5 for 25 experimental subjects and 125.1 for 25 control subjects. Should we conclude that the hypothesis is supported? True, group differences are in the predicted direction, but perhaps in another sample the group means would be nearly identical. Two explanations for the observed outcome are possible: (1) the film is truly effective in encouraging breastfeeding or (2) the difference in this sample was due to chance factors (e.g., differences in the two groups even before the film was shown, reflecting a selection bias).

The first explanation is the researcher's *research hypothesis*, and the second is the *null hypothesis*. The null hypothesis, it may be recalled, states that there is no relationship between the independent and dependent variables. Statistical hypothesis testing is basically a process of disproof or rejection. It cannot be demonstrated

The actual situation is that the null hypothesis is:

		True	False
The researcher calculates a test statistic and decides that the null hypothesis is:	True (Null accepted)	Correct decision	Type II error
	False (Null rejected)	Type I error	Correct decision

FIGURE 15.7 Outcomes of statistical decision making.

directly that the research hypothesis is correct. But it is possible to show, using theoretical sampling distributions, that the null hypothesis has a high probability of being incorrect, and such evidence lends support to the research hypothesis. Hypothesis testing helps researchers to make objective decisions about study results—that is, to decide which results likely reflect chance sample differences and which likely reflect true hypothesized effects in the population.

Researchers use **statistical tests** to test hypotheses. Although null hypotheses are accepted or rejected on the basis of sample data, the hypothesis is made about population values.

Type I and Type II Errors

Researchers decide whether to accept or reject the null hypothesis by determining how probable it is that observed relationships are due to chance. Because information about the population is not available, it cannot be asserted with certainty that the null hypothesis is or is not true. Researchers conclude that hypotheses are either *probably* true or *probably* false. Statistical inferences are based on incomplete information; there is always a risk of making an error.

Researchers can make two types of error, as summarized in Figure 15.7. Investigators make a **Type I error** by rejecting the null hypothesis when it is, in fact, true. For instance, if we concluded that the film was effective in promoting breastfeeding when, in fact, group differences were due to initial group differences, this would be a Type I error—a false-positive conclusion. In the reverse situation, we might conclude that observed differences in breastfeeding were due to sampling fluctuations when the film actually *did* have an effect. Acceptance of a false null hypothesis is called a **Type II error**—a false-negative conclusion.

Level of Significance

Researchers do not know when an error in statistical decision making has been made. The validity of a null hypothesis could be determined only by collecting data from the population, in which case there would be no need for statistical inference.

Researchers control the degree of risk in making a Type I error by selecting a **level of significance,** which is the term used to signify the probability of making a Type I error. The two most frequently used levels of significance (referred to as **alpha** or **α**) are .05 and .01. With a .05 significance level, we accept the risk that out of 100 samples, a true null hypothesis would be wrongly rejected five times. In 95 out of 100 cases, however, a true null hypothesis would be correctly accepted. With a .01 significance level, the risk of making a Type I error is lower: In only 1 sample out of 100 would we wrongly reject the null hypothesis. By convention, the minimal acceptable alpha level is .05.

Naturally, researchers would like to reduce the risk of committing both types of error. Unfortunately, lowering the risk of a Type I error increases the risk of a Type II error. The stricter the criterion for rejecting a null hypothesis, the greater the probability of accepting a false null hypothesis. However, researchers can reduce the risk of a Type II error simply by increasing their sample size.

The probability of committing a Type II error, referred to as **beta (β)**, can be estimated through *power analysis*, the same procedure we mentioned in Chapter 12 in connection with sample size. *Power*, the ability of a statistical test to detect true relationships, is the complement of beta—that is, power equals $1 - \beta$. The standard criterion for an acceptable risk for a Type II error is .20, and thus researchers ideally use a sample size that gives them a minimum power of .80.

> **TIP**
>
> In many studies, the risk of a Type II error is high because of small sample size, suggesting a need for greater use of power analysis. If a research report indicates that a research hypothesis was not supported, consider whether a Type II error might have occurred as a result of inadequate sample size.

Tests of Statistical Significance

Researchers testing hypotheses use study data to compute a **test statistic.** For every test statistic, there is a theoretical sampling distribution, analogous to the sampling distribution of means. Hypothesis testing uses theoretical distributions to establish *probable* and *improbable* values for the test statistics, which are, in turn, used as a basis for accepting or rejecting the null hypothesis.

A simple (if contrived) example will illustrate the process. Suppose we wanted to test the hypothesis that the average entrance examination score (on a hypothetical standardized examination) for students applying to nursing schools in Ontario is higher than that for applicants in all provinces, whose mean score is 500. The null hypothesis is that there is no difference in the mean population scores of students applying to nursing schools in Ontario versus elsewhere. Let us say that the mean score for a sample of 100 nursing school applicants in Ontario is 525, with a standard deviation of 100. Using statistical procedures, we can test the hypothesis that the mean of 525 is not merely a chance fluctuation from the population mean of 500.

In hypothesis testing, researchers assume that the null hypothesis is true and then gather evidence to disprove it. Assuming a mean of 500 for the entire applicant population, a sampling distribution can be constructed with a mean of 500 and an SD of 10. In this example, 10 is the standard error of the mean, calculated from a formula that used the sample standard deviation of 100 for a sample of 100 students. This is shown in Figure 15.8. On the basis of normal distribution characteristics, we can determine probable and improbable values of sample means from the population. If, as is assumed according to the null hypothesis, the population mean for Ontario applicants is 500, 95% of all sample means would fall between 480 and 520 because 95% of the cases are within 2 SDs of the mean. The obtained sample mean of 525 lies in the region considered *improbable* if the null hypothesis were true, with an alpha level of .05 as the criterion of improbability. The improbable range beyond 2 SDs corresponds to only 5% (100% − 95%) of the sampling distribution. We would thus reject the null hypothesis that the mean of the Ontario applicant population equals 500. We would not be justified in saying that we have proved the research hypothesis because the possibility of a Type I error remains.

Researchers reporting the results of hypothesis tests state whether their findings are **statistically significant.** The word *significant* does not mean important or meaningful. In statistics, the term *significant* means that obtained results are not likely to have been due to chance, at a specified level of probability. A **nonsignificant result** means that an observed difference or relationship could have been the result of a chance fluctuation.

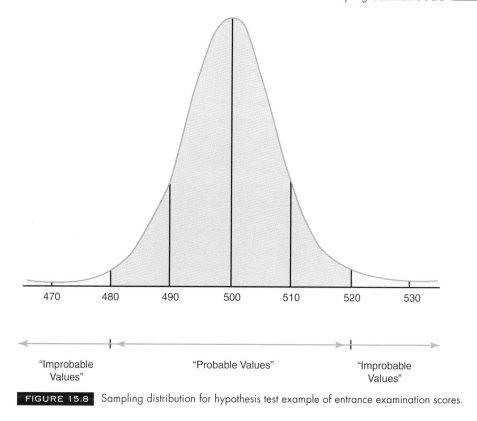

470   480   490   500   510   520   530

"Improbable
Values"

"Probable Values"

"Improbable
Values"

FIGURE 15.8   Sampling distribution for hypothesis test example of entrance examination scores.

TIP

Inferential statistics are usually more difficult to understand than descriptive statistics. It may help to keep in mind that inferential statistics are just a tool to help us evaluate whether the results are likely to be real and replicable, or simply spurious. As recommended in Chapter 4, you can overcome much of the obscurity of the results section by translating the basic thrust of research findings into everyday language.

Parametric and Nonparametric Tests

The bulk of the tests that we discuss in this chapter—and also most tests used by researchers—are **parametric tests.** Parametric tests have three attributes: (1) they focus on population parameters; (2) they require measurements on at least an interval scale; and (3) they involve other assumptions, such as the assumption that the variables in the analysis are normally distributed in the population.

Nonparametric tests, by contrast, do not estimate parameters and involve less restrictive assumptions about the shape of the distribution of the critical variables. Nonparametric tests are usually applied when the data have been measured on a nominal or ordinal scale. Parametric tests are more powerful than nonparametric tests and are generally preferred. Nonparametric tests are most useful when the research data cannot be construed as interval measures or when the data distribution is markedly skewed.

Overview of Hypothesis Testing Procedures

In the next section, a few statistical tests are discussed. The emphasis is on explaining their applications and on interpreting their meaning rather than on describing computations.

Each statistical test has a particular application and can be used only with certain kinds of data; however, the overall process of testing hypotheses is basically the same for all tests. The steps that researchers take are the following:

1. *Selecting an appropriate test statistic.* Researchers select a test based on such factors as the level of measurement of the variables and, if relevant, how many groups are being compared.

2. *Selecting the level of significance.* An α level of .05 is usually chosen, but sometimes the level is set more stringently at .01.

3. *Computing a test statistic.* Researchers then calculate a test statistic based on the collected data.

4. *Determining degrees of freedom.* The term **degrees of freedom** (*df*) refers to the number of observations free to vary about a parameter. The concept is too complex for elaboration here, but computing degrees of freedom is easy.

5. *Comparing the test statistic to a tabled value.* Theoretical distributions have been developed for all test statistics, and there are tables with distribution for specified degrees of freedom and levels of significance. The *tabled* value enables researchers to see whether the *computed* value of the statistic is beyond what is probable if the null hypothesis is true. If the absolute value of the computed statistic is larger than the tabled value, the results are statistically significant; if the computed value is smaller, the results are nonsignificant.

When a computer is used for the analysis, researchers follow only the first step and then give appropriate commands to the computer. The computer calculates the test statistic, the degrees of freedom, and the *actual* probability that the relationship being tested is due to chance. For example, the computer may print that the probability (*p*) of an experimental group doing better on a measure of postoperative recovery than the control group on the basis of chance alone is .025. This means that fewer than 3 times out of 100 (or only 25 times out of 1000) would a group difference of the size observed occur by chance. This computed probability can then be compared with the desired level of significance. In the present example, if the significance level were .05, the results would be significant because .025 is more stringent than .05. If .01 was the significance level, the results would be nonsignificant (sometimes abbreviated **NS**). Any computed probability level greater than .05 (e.g., .20) indicates a nonsignificant relationship (i.e., one that could have occurred on the basis of chance in more than 5 out of 100 samples).

BIVARIATE STATISTICAL TESTS

Researchers use a variety of statistical tests to make inferences about the validity of their hypotheses. The most frequently used bivariate tests are briefly described and illustrated below.

t Tests

A common research situation involves comparing scores on an outcome variable for two groups of people. The procedure used to test the statistical significance of a difference between the means of two groups is the parametric test called the *t* **test.**

Suppose we wanted to test the effect of early discharge of maternity patients on their perceived maternal competence. We administer a scale of perceived maternal competence 1 week after delivery to 10 primiparas who were discharged early (i.e., within 24 hours of delivery) and to 10 others who remained in the hospital longer. Some hypothetical data for this example are presented in Table 15.8. The mean scores for the two groups are 19.0 and 25.0, respectively. Is this difference a true

TABLE 15.8 ▶	FICTITIOUS DATA FOR *t* TEST EXAMPLE: SCORES ON A PERCEIVED MATERNAL COMPETENCE SCALE FOR TWO GROUPS OF MOTHERS	
REGULAR-DISCHARGE MOTHERS		**EARLY-DISCHARGE MOTHERS**
23		30
17		27
22		25
18		20
20		24
26		32
16		17
13		18
21		28
14		29
Mean = 19.0		Mean = 25.0
$t = 2.86$; $df = 18$; $p < .05$		

population difference—is it likely to be replicated in other samples of early-discharge and later-discharge mothers? Or is the group difference just the result of chance fluctuations in this sample? The 20 scores—10 for each group—vary from one person to another. Some variability reflects individual differences in perceived maternal competence. Some variability might be due to measurement error (e.g., the scale's low reliability), and so forth. The research question is: Is a portion of the variability attributable to the independent variable—time of discharge from the hospital? The *t* test allows us to answer this question objectively.

The value for the *t* statistic is calculated based on group means, variability, and sample size. The computed value of *t* for the data in Table 15.8 is 2.86. Next, degrees of freedom are calculated. Here, *df* equals the total sample size minus 2 (*df* = 20 − 2 = 18). Then, the tabled value for *t* with 18 *df* is ascertained. For an α level of .05, the tabled value of *t* is 2.10. *This value establishes an upper limit to what is probable if the null hypothesis is true.* Thus, the calculated *t* of 2.86, which is larger than the tabled value of the statistic, is improbable (i.e., statistically significant). We can now say that the primiparas discharged early had significantly lower perceptions of maternal competence than those who were not discharged early. The group difference in perceived maternal competence is sufficiently large that it is unlikely to reflect merely chance fluctuations. In fewer than 5 out of 100 samples would a difference in means this great be found by chance alone.

The situation just described requires an *independent groups t test*: mothers in the two groups were different people, independent of each other. There are situations in which this type of *t* test is not appropriate. For example, if means for a single group of people measured before and after an intervention were being compared, researchers would compute a *paired t test* (or a *dependent groups t test*) with a different formula.

⇒ Using a randomized controlled trial, Forchuk, MacClure, Van Beers, Smith, Csiernik, Hoch, and Jensen (2008) developed and tested an intervention to prevent homelessness among individuals discharged from psychiatric wards to shelters and "no fixed address." Participants were randomly assigned to either the intervention group, which involved assistance in finding housing, or the control group, which comprised usual care involving the referral to a social worker when deemed necessary by the health care team. The researchers used *t* tests to assess potential differences in sociodemographic data between intervention and control groups with no statistically significant differences found.

Analysis of Variance

Analysis of variance (ANOVA) is a parametric procedure used to test mean group differences of three or more groups. ANOVA decomposes the variability of a dependent variable into two components: variability attributable to the independent variable (i.e., group status) and variability due to all other sources (e.g., individual differences, measurement error). Variation *between* groups is contrasted with variation *within* groups to yield the statistic called an ***F* ratio.**

Suppose we wanted to compare the effectiveness of different instructional techniques to teach high school students about AIDS. One group of students is exposed to an interactive Internet course on AIDS, a second group is given special lectures, and a control group receives no special instruction. The dependent variable is students' scores on an AIDS knowledge test after the intervention. The null hypothesis is that the group population means for AIDS knowledge test scores are the same, whereas the research hypothesis predicts that they are different.

Test scores for 60 students are shown in Table 15.9, according to treatment group. As this table shows, there is variation from one student to the next within

TABLE 15.9 **FICTITIOUS DATA FOR ONE-WAY ANOVA: EFFECTS OF INSTRUCTIONAL MODE ON AIDS KNOWLEDGE TEST SCORES**

INTERNET GROUP (A)		LECTURE GROUP (B)		CONTROL GROUP (C)	
26	25	22	24	15	22
20	29	24	25	26	19
16	30	27	21	24	20
25	27	23	27	18	22
25	29	23	25	20	18
23	28	26	21	20	24
26	26	22	24	19	18
25	25	24	29	21	23
24	27	24	28	17	20
23	28	30	26	17	24
Mean	25.35		24.75		20.35

$F = 18.64$; $df = 2.57$; $p = .001$

a group, and there are also group differences. The mean test scores are 25.35, 24.75, and 20.35 for groups A, B, and C, respectively. These means are different, but are they significantly different—or do the differences reflect random fluctuations?

An ANOVA applied to these data yields an *F* ratio of 18.64. Two types of degree of freedom are calculated in ANOVA: between groups (number of groups minus 1) and within groups (total number of subjects minus the number of groups). In this example, *df* = 2 and 57. In a table of values for a theoretical *F* distribution, we would find that the value of *F* for 2 and 57 *df*, with an alpha level of .05, is 3.16. Because our obtained *F* value of 18.64 exceeds 3.16, we reject the null hypothesis that the population means are equal. The mean group differences would be obtained by chance in fewer than 5 samples out of 100. (Actually, the probability of achieving an *F* of 18.64 by chance is less than 1 in 1000.)

The data in our example support the hypothesis that the instructional interventions affected students' knowledge about AIDS, but we cannot tell from these results whether treatment A was significantly more effective than treatment B. **Multiple comparison procedures** (also called *post hoc* **tests**) are needed to isolate the differences between group means that are responsible for rejecting the overall ANOVA null hypothesis. Note that it is *not* appropriate to use a series of *t* tests (group A versus group B, group A versus group C, and group B versus group C) in this situation because this would increase the risk of a Type I error.

ANOVA can also be used to test the effect of two (or more) independent variables on a dependent variable (e.g., when a factorial experimental design has been used). Suppose we wanted to test whether the two instructional techniques discussed previously (Internet versus lecture) were equally effective in helping male and female students acquire knowledge about AIDS. We could set up a design in which males and females would be randomly assigned, separately, to the two modes of instruction. Some hypothetical data, shown in Table 15.10, reveal the following about two *main effects*: On average, people in the Internet group scored higher than those in the lecture group (25.35 versus 24.75), and female students scored higher than male

TABLE 15.10	FICTITIOUS DATA FOR TWO-WAY (2 × 2) ANOVA EXAMPLE: INSTRUCTIONAL MODE AND GENDER IN RELATION TO TEST SCORES						
	INSTRUCTIONAL MODE						
YEAR IN SCHOOL	Internet			Lecture			
Male	26 20	$\bar{X} = 23.3$		22 24	$\bar{X} = 24.5$		Male mean = 23.90
	16 25			27 33			
	25 23			23 26			
	26 25			22 24			
	24 23			24 30			
Female	25 29	$\bar{X} = 27.4$		24 25	$\bar{X} = 25.0$		Female mean = 26.20
	30 27			21 27			
	29 28			27 25			
	26 25			21 24			
	27 28			28 26			
Internet group mean	25.35	Lecture group mean	24.75				Grand mean = 25.05

students (26.20 versus 23.90). In addition, there is an *interaction effect:* Females scored higher in the Internet group, whereas males scored higher in the lecture group. By performing a *two-way ANOVA* on these data, it would be possible to ascertain the statistical significance of these differences.

A type of ANOVA known as **repeated-measures ANOVA** is used when the means being compared are means at different points in time (e.g., mean blood pressure at 2, 4, and 6 hours after surgery). This is analogous to a paired *t* test, extended to three or more points of data collection, because it is the same people being measured multiple times.

Example of an ANOVA

➢ In a randomized controlled trial, Johnston, Gagnon, Rennick, Rosmus, Patenaude, Ellis, Shapiro, Fillion, Ritchie, and Byron (2007) sought to determine whether 10 one-on-one coaching sessions based on audit with feedback and "think-aloud" interactions with an opinion leader could change attitudes and knowledge about pain in children and improve pain practices among pediatric nurses in six university-affiliated hospitals in Canada. Outcome data on the nurses' attitudes and knowledge about pain in children were collected preintervention, 2 weeks postintervention, and 6 months postintervention from participants in the experimental and control groups. Collected data were subsequently analyzed using repeated-measures ANOVA. The analysis revealed that nurses in the experimental group demonstrated a higher overall gain in knowledge scores, $F(1, 791) = 106.3$, $p < .0001$, and greater improvements in the rate of documented pain assessments (from 15% to 58%) than did nurses in the control group (who showed a decline from 24% to 9% on the latter outcome).

TIP

Experimental crossover designs (see Chapter 9) require either a dependent groups *t* test or a repeated-measures ANOVA because the same people are measured more than once after being randomly assigned to a different ordering of treatments. Repeated-measures ANOVA can also be used in studies that do not involve an experimental crossover design (e.g., in one-group preexperimental designs) if outcomes are measured more than once and the hypothesis concerns changes over time.

Chi-Squared Test

The **chi-squared** (χ^2) **test** is a nonparametric procedure used to test hypotheses about the proportion of cases that fall into various categories, as in a contingency table. Suppose we were interested in studying the effect of planned nursing instruction on patients' compliance with a medication regimen. The experimental group is instructed by nurses implementing a new instructional approach. Control group patients are cared for by nurses using the usual mode of instruction. The research hypothesis is that a higher proportion of people in the experimental group than in the control group will comply with the regimen. Some hypothetical data for this example are presented in Table 15.11.

The chi-squared statistic is computed by summing differences between the *observed frequencies* in each cell and the *expected frequencies*—the frequencies that would be expected if there were no relationship between the two variables. In this example, the value of the χ^2 statistic is 18.18, which we can compare with the value from a theoretical chi-squared distribution. For the chi-squared statistic, the *df* are equal to the number of rows minus 1 times the number of columns minus 1. In the present case, $df = 1 \times 1$, or 1. With 1 *df*, the value that must be exceeded to establish significance at the .05 level is 3.84. The obtained value of 18.18 is substantially larger than would be expected by chance. Thus, we can conclude that a significantly larger percentage of patients in the experimental group (60%) than in the control group (30%) were compliant.

TABLE 15.11	OBSERVED FREQUENCIES FOR A CHI-SQUARED EXAMPLE ON PATIENT COMPLIANCE		
	EXPERIMENTAL	CONTROL	TOTAL
Compliant	60	30	90
Noncompliant	40	70	110
Total	100	100	200

$$\chi^2 = 18.18; \, df = 1; \, p < .001$$

Example of a chi-squared test

⇝ Using a cross-sectional design, Stajduhar, Allan, Cohen, and Heyland (2008) explored the perspectives of seriously ill hospitalized Canadian patients and their family caregivers (FCG) from five tertiary care teaching hospitals across Canada for their preferences for location of death. Patients were categorized as either having cancer or not and asked about their preferences for location of death in the event of a drastic decline in their health status. Participants' family caregivers were asked a similar question pertaining to their preference for location of care of their loved one. Response categories for both included (a) home, (b) hospital, and (c) does not matter. Frequencies were used to examine preferences for location of death. Chi-squared tests were used to determine preference differences based on type of disease (cancer versus noncancer). The results revealed no statistically significant differences for location preferences between the patient ($\chi^2 = 0.54$, $p = .77$) and FCG groups ($\chi^2 = 2.40$, $p = .33$).

Correlation Coefficients

Pearson's r is both descriptive and inferential. As a descriptive statistic, r summarizes the magnitude and direction of a relationship between two variables. As an inferential statistic, r tests hypotheses about population correlations; the null hypothesis is that there is no relationship between two variables, that is, that $r = .00$.

Suppose we were studying the relationship between patients' self-reported level of stress (higher scores mean more stress) and the pH level of their saliva. With a sample of 50 patients, we find that $r = -.29$. This value indicates a tendency for people with high stress scores to have low pH levels. But we need to ask whether this finding can be generalized to the population. Does the coefficient of $-.29$ reflect a random fluctuation, observed only in this particular sample, or is the relationship significant? Degrees of freedom for correlation coefficients are equal to the number of participants minus 2—48 in this example. The tabled value for r with $df = 48$ and $\alpha = .05$ is .282. Because the absolute value of the calculated r is .29 and thus larger than .282, the null hypothesis can be rejected. There is a modest, significant relationship between patients' stress level and the acidity of their saliva.

Example of correlation coefficients

⇝ Bailey, Sabbagh, Loiselle, Boileau, and McVey (2009) studied relationships among informational support, anxiety, and satisfaction with care in family members of patients in an intensive care unit in Montreal, Quebec. They found, among other things, that informational support was significantly correlated with satisfaction with care ($r = .74$, $p < .001$) but not with anxiety levels.

Guide to Bivariate Statistical Tests

The selection of a statistical test depends on such factors as the number of groups and the levels of measurement of the variables. To aid you in evaluating the appropriateness of statistical tests used in studies, Table 15.12 summarizes major

TABLE 15.12 ▶ GUIDE TO WIDELY USED BIVARIATE STATISTICAL TESTS

NAME	TEST STATISTIC	PURPOSE	MEASUREMENT LEVEL*	
			IV	DV
Parametric Tests				
t test for independent groups	t	To test the difference between two independent group means	Nominal	Interval, ratio
t test for dependent groups	t	To test the difference between two dependent group means	Nominal	Interval, ratio
Analysis of variance	F	To test the difference among the means of three or more independent groups, or of more than one independent variable	Nominal	Interval, ratio
Repeated-measures ANOVA	F	To test the difference among means of three or more related groups or sets of scores	Nominal	Interval, ratio
Pearson's r	r	To test the existence of a relationship between two variables	Interval, ratio	Interval, ratio
Nonparametric Tests				
Chi-squared test	χ^2	To test the difference in proportions in two or more independent groups	Nominal	Nominal
Mann–Whitney U test	U	To test the difference in ranks of scores of two independent groups	Nominal	Ordinal
Kruskal–Wallis test	H	To test the difference in ranks of scores of three or more independent groups	Nominal	Ordinal
Wilcoxon-signed ranks test	T(Z)	To test the difference in ranks of scores of two related groups	Nominal	Ordinal
Friedman test	χ^2	To test the difference in ranks of scores of three or more related groups	Nominal	Ordinal
Phi coefficient	ϕ	To test the magnitude of a relationship between two dichotomous variables	Nominal	Nominal
Spearman's rank-order correlation	r_s	To test the existence of a relationship between two variables	Ordinal	Ordinal

*Measurement level of the independent variable (IV) and dependent variable (DV).

features of several tests. This table does not include every test you may encounter in research reports, but it does include the bivariate tests most often used by nurse researchers, including a few not discussed in this book.

TIP

Every time a report presents information about statistical tests such as those described in this section, it means that the researcher was testing hypotheses—whether those hypotheses were formally stated in the introduction or not.

MULTIVARIATE STATISTICAL ANALYSIS

Nurse researchers have become increasingly sophisticated, and many now use complex **multivariate statistics** to analyze their data. We use the term *multivariate* to refer to analyses dealing with at least three—but usually more—variables simultaneously. This evolution has resulted in better-quality evidence in nursing studies, but one unfortunate side effect is that it has become more challenging for novice consumers to understand research reports.

Given the introductory nature of this text, it is not possible to describe in detail the complex analytic procedures that now appear in nursing journals. However, we present some basic information that might assist you in reading reports in which two commonly used multivariate statistics are used: multiple regression and **analysis of covariance** (ANCOVA).

Multiple Regression

Correlations enable researchers to make predictions. For example, if the correlation between secondary school grades and nursing school grades were .60, nursing school admission committees could make predictions—albeit imperfect ones—about applicants' future performance. Because two variables are rarely perfectly correlated, researchers often strive to improve their ability to predict a dependent variable by including more than one independent variable in the analysis.

As an example, we might predict that infant birth weight is related to the amount of maternal–prenatal care. We could collect data on birth weight and number of prenatal visits and then compute a correlation coefficient to determine whether a significant relationship between the two variables exists (i.e., whether prenatal care would help predict infant birth weight). Birth weight is affected by many other factors, however, such as gestational period and mothers' smoking behaviour. Many researchers, therefore, perform **multiple regression analysis** (or *multiple correlation analysis*), which allows them to use more than one independent variable to explain or predict a dependent variable. In multiple regression, the dependent variables are interval-level or ratio-level variables. Independent variables (also called **predictor variables** in multiple regression) are either interval-level or ratio-level variables or dichotomous nominal-level variables, such as male/female.

When several independent variables are used to predict a dependent variable, the resulting statistic is the **multiple correlation coefficient,** symbolized as *R.* Unlike the bivariate correlation coefficient *r*, *R* does not have negative values. *R* varies from .00 to 1.00, showing the *strength* of the relationship between several independent variables and a dependent variable, but not *direction*.

There are several ways to evaluate *R*. One is to determine whether *R* is statistically significant—that is, whether the overall relationship between the independent variables and the dependent variables is likely to be real or the result of chance fluctuations. This is done through the computation of an F statistic that can be compared with tabled F values.

A second way of evaluating R is to determine whether the addition of new independent variables adds further predictive power. For example, we might find that the R between infant birth weight on the one hand and maternal weight and prenatal care on the other is .30. By adding a third independent variable—let us say maternal smoking behaviour—R might increase to .36. Is the increase from .30 to .36 statistically significant? In other words, does knowing whether the mother smoked during her pregnancy improve our understanding of the birth-weight outcome, or does the larger R value simply reflect factors peculiar to this sample? Multiple regression provides a way of answering this question.

The magnitude of R is also informative. Researchers would like to predict a dependent variable perfectly. In our example, if it were possible to identify all the factors that affect infants' weight, we could collect the relevant data to obtain an R of 1.00. Usually, the value of R in nursing studies is much smaller—seldom higher than .70. An interesting feature of the R statistic is that, when squared, it can be interpreted as the proportion of the variability in the dependent variable accounted for or explained by the independent variables. In predicting infant birth weight, if we achieved an R of .60 ($R^2 = .36$), we could say that the independent variables accounted for about one third (36%) of the variability in infants' birth weights. Two thirds of the variability, however, was caused by factors not identified or measured. Researchers usually report multiple correlation results in terms of R^2 rather than R.

Example of multiple regression

➤ Ing and Reutter (2003) studied sense of coherence (SOC) and other factors in the self-rated health of more than 6000 Canadian women. The SOC construct is a global orientation that enables a person to perceive world events as comprehensible and meaningful. Using multiple regression, the researchers found that SOC and several background characteristics were significant predictors of self-rated health. Overall, the R^2 between predictor variables and self-rated health was .15, $p < .001$.

We will use this study by Ing and Reutter (2003) to illustrate some additional features of multiple regression. First, multiple regressions yield information about whether each independent variable is related significantly to the dependent variable. In Table 15.13, the first column shows that the analysis used four independent variables to predict the health ratings: marital status, age, income, and SOC scores. (The first entry, "Constant," is a value we would need if we wanted to predict health ratings of women not in the sample, based on their scores on the predictor variables.) The next column shows the values for b, which are the *regression coefficients* associated with each predictor. These coefficients, which were computed from the raw study data, could be used to predict health ratings in other Canadian women; however, like the value for constant, they are not values you need to be concerned with in interpreting a regression table. The next column shows the standard error (SE) of the regression coefficients. When the regression coefficient (b) is divided by the standard error, the result is a value for the t statistic, which is used to determine the significance of individual predictors. In this table, the t values are not shown, but many regression tables in reports *do* present them. We can compute them, though, from information in the table; for example, the t value for the variable *age* is -2.67 ($-.08/.03 = -2.67$). This is highly significant, as shown in the last column: the probability (p) is less than 1 in 1000 (.000) that the relationship between age and health ratings is spurious. The results indicate that the older the woman, the lower the health ratings, as indicated by the negative regression coefficient. Income and SOC were also significantly related to self-rated health: women with higher income and higher SOC scores tended to have higher health ratings. Marital status was not significantly related to health rating (although this predictor narrowly missed being significant, $p = .062$).

TABLE 15.13 ▶ EXAMPLE OF MULTIPLE REGRESSION ANALYSIS: SELF-RATED HEALTH IN CANADIAN WOMEN, REGRESSED ON MARITAL STATUS, AGE, INCOME, AND SENSE OF COHERENCE

PREDICTOR VARIABLE*	b	SE	BETA (β)	p
Constant	2.57	0.07		<.001
Marital status: married or attached	−0.05	0.03	−0.02	.062
Age	−0.08	0.03	−0.20	<.001
Income	0.16	0.01	0.18	<.001
Sense of coherence	0.02	0.00	0.28	<.001
N = 6222 women				
F = 266.51	df = 4, 6217 p < .001 Adjusted R² = .15			

*Self-rated health (1 = poor to 5 = excellent); marital status (1 = married or attached, 0 = unattached); age (5-year cohorts from 20–24 to 60–64); income (1 = lowest income category to 5 = highest income category); sense of coherence scale (possible range = 0 to 78).

Adapted from Ing, J. D., & Reutter, L. (2003). Socioeconomic status, sense of coherence, and health in Canadian women. *Canadian Journal of Public Health, 94,* 224–228, Table II.

Multiple regression analysis indicates whether an independent variable is significantly related to the dependent variable *even after* the other predictor variables are controlled—a concept we explain more fully in the next section. In this example, SOC was a significant predictor of health ratings, even with the other three variables controlled. Thus, multiple regression, such as analysis of covariance (discussed next), is a means of controlling extraneous variables statistically.

The fourth column of Table 15.13 shows the value of the *beta* (β) *coefficients* for each predictor. Although it is beyond the scope of this textbook to explain beta coefficients in detail, suffice it to say that, unlike the *b* regression coefficients, betas are all in the same measurement units, and their absolute values are sometimes used to compare the relative importance of predictors. In this particular sample, and with these particular predictors, the variable *SOC* was the best predictor of health (β = .28) and the variable *age* was the second best predictor (β = −.20).

At the bottom of the table, we see that the value of *F* for the overall regression equation, with 4 and 6217 *df*, was 266.51, which is highly significant, $p < .001$. The value of R^2, after adjustments are made for sample size and number of predictors, is .15. Thus, 15% of the variance in self-rated health status is explained by the combined effect of the four predictors. The remaining 85% of variation in health is explained by other factors—variables not in the analysis, such as genetic factors, lifestyle behaviours, and so forth.

Analysis of Covariance

Analysis of covariance (ANCOVA), which is essentially a combination of ANOVA and multiple regression, is used to control extraneous variables statistically. This approach can be especially valuable in certain research situations, such as when a nonequivalent control group design is used. The initial lack of equivalence of the experimental and comparison groups in such studies is always a potential threat to internal validity. When control through randomization is lacking, ANCOVA offers the possibility of *post hoc* statistical control.

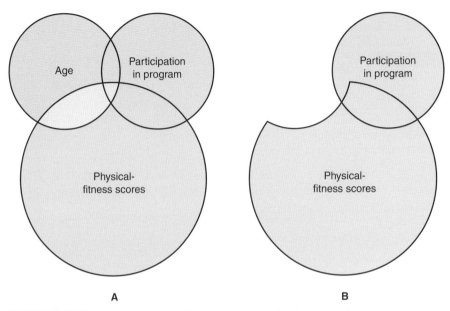

A   B

FIGURE 15.9   Schematic diagram illustrating the principle of analysis of covariance.

Because the concept of statistical control may mystify you, we will explain the underlying principle with a simple illustration. Suppose we were interested in testing the effectiveness of a special training program on physical fitness, using employees of two companies as subjects. Employees of one company receive the physical fitness intervention, and those of the second company do not. The employees' score on a physical fitness test is the dependent variable. The research question is: Can some of the group difference in performance on the physical fitness test be attributed to participation in the special program? Physical fitness is also related to other, extraneous characteristics of the study participants (e.g., their age)—characteristics that might differ between the two intact groups.

Figure 15.9 illustrates how ANCOVA works. The large circles represent total variability (i.e., the extent of individual differences) in physical fitness scores for both groups. A certain amount of variability can be explained by age differences: Younger people tend to perform better on the test than older ones. This relationship is represented by the overlapping small circle on the left in part A of Figure 15.9. Another part of the variability can be explained by participation in the physical fitness program, represented here by the overlapping small circle on the right. In part A, the fact that the two small circles (age and program participation) themselves overlap indicates that there is a relationship between these two variables. In other words, people in the experimental group are, on average, either older or younger than those in the comparison group. Because of this relationship, which could distort the results of the study, age should be controlled.

ANCOVA can do this by statistically removing the effect of the extraneous variable (age) on physical fitness, designated in part A of Figure 15.9 by the darkened area. Part B illustrates that the analysis would examine the effect of program participation on fitness scores *after* removing the effect of age (called a **covariate**). With the variability associated with age removed, we get a more precise estimate of the training program's effect on physical fitness. Note that even after removing variability resulting from age, there is still variability not associated with program participation (the bottom half of the large circle) that is not explained. This means that analytic precision could be further enhanced by controlling additional extraneous variables (e.g., nutritional habits, smoking status). ANCOVA can accommodate multiple extraneous variables.

ANCOVA tests the significance of differences between group means after adjusting scores on the dependent variable to eliminate the effect of covariates, using regression procedures. ANCOVA produces F statistics—one for evaluating the significance of the covariates and another for evaluating the significance of group differences—that can be compared with tabled values of F to determine whether to accept or reject the null hypothesis.

ANCOVA, like multiple regression analysis, is an extremely powerful and useful analytic technique for controlling extraneous influences on dependent measures. ANCOVA can be used with true experimental designs because randomization can never guarantee that groups are totally equivalent. Baseline measures of the dependent variables make particularly good covariates.

Example of ANCOVA

⮞ Using a randomized controlled trial, Downe-Wamboldt, Butler, Melanson, Coulter, Singleton, Keefe, and Bell (2007) wished to determine the effectiveness and efficiency of individualized, problem-solving counselling provided by nurses over the telephone in preventing depression in patients with cancer. Participants were randomly assigned to either the intervention group (receiving the counselling sessions during a 3-month interval plus usual care) or the control group (receiving usual care only) and outcome data were collected preintervention (baseline) and at 8 months from baseline. The primary outcome data collected included depression and psychosocial adjustment. ANCOVA was used to test differences between the groups, controlling for baseline coping scores (used as a covariate).

Other Multivariate Techniques

Other multivariate techniques are being used in nursing studies. We mention a few briefly to acquaint you with terms you might encounter in the research literature.

Discriminant Function Analysis

In multiple regression, the dependent variable being predicted is a measure on either the interval scale or the ratio scale. **Discriminant function analysis** is used to make predictions about membership in groups—that is, about a dependent variable measured on the nominal scale. For example, researchers might wish to use multiple independent variables to predict membership in such groups as compliant versus noncompliant cancer patients or patients with or without decubiti. In discriminant function analysis, as in multiple regression, the predictor variables and covariates are either interval-level or ratio-level measures or dichotomous nominal variables (e.g., smoker versus nonsmoker).

Logistic Regression

Logistic regression (or *logit analysis*) analyzes the relationships between multiple independent variables and a nominal-level dependent variable. It is thus used in situations similar to discriminant function analysis, but it employs a different statistical estimation procedure that many prefer for nominal-level dependent variables. Logistic regression transforms the probability of an event occurring (e.g., that a woman will practice breast self-examination or not) into its *odds* (i.e., into the ratio of one event's probability relative to the probability of a second event). After further transformations, the analysis examines the relationship of the independent variables to the transformed dependent variable. For each predictor, the logistic regression yields an **odds ratio** (OR), which is the factor by which the odds change for a unit change in the predictors.

Factor Analysis

Factor analysis is widely used by researchers who develop, refine, or validate complex instruments. The purpose of factor analysis is to reduce a large set of variables into a smaller, more manageable set. Factor analysis disentangles complex interrelationships among variables and identifies which variables go together as unified concepts. For example, suppose we developed 50 Likert statements to measure men's attitudes toward a vasectomy. It would not be appropriate to combine all 50 items to form a scale score because there are various dimensions to men's attitudes toward vasectomy. One dimension may relate to the issue of masculine identity, another may concern the loss of ability to reproduce, and so forth. These various dimensions should serve as the basis for scale construction, and factor analysis offers an objective, empirical method for doing so.

Multivariate Analysis of Variance

Multivariate analysis of variance (MANOVA) is the extension of ANOVA to more than one dependent variable. MANOVA is used to test the significance of differences between the means of two or more groups on two or more dependent variables considered simultaneously. For instance, if we wanted to compare the effect of two alternative exercise treatments on both blood pressure and heart rate, then a MANOVA would be appropriate. Covariates can also be included, in which case the analysis would be a **multivariate analysis of covariance** (MANCOVA).

Causal Modeling

Causal modeling involves the development and statistical testing of a hypothesized explanation of the causes of a phenomenon, usually with nonexperimental data. **Path analysis,** which is based on multiple regression, is a widely used approach to causal modeling. Alternative methods of testing causal models are also used by nurse researchers, the most important of which is **linear structural relations analysis,** more widely known as **LISREL.** Both LISREL and path analysis are highly complex statistical techniques whose utility relies on a sound underlying causal theory.

Guide to Multivariate Statistical Analyses

In selecting a multivariate analysis, researchers must attend to such issues as the number of independent variables, the number of dependent variables, the measurement level of all variables, and the desirability of controlling extraneous variables. Table 15.14 is an aid to help you evaluate the appropriateness of multivariate statistics used in research reports. This chart includes the major multivariate analyses used by nurse researchers.

TABLE 15.14   GUIDE TO WIDELY USED MULTIVARIATE STATISTICAL ANALYSES

NAME	PURPOSE	MEASUREMENT LEVEL*			NUMBER OF VERIABLES*		
		IV	DV	COV	IVs	DVs	COVs
Multiple correlation, regression	To test the relationship between two or more IVs and one DV; to predict a DV from two or more IVs	N, I, R	I, R		2+	1	
Analysis of covariance (ANCOVA)	To test the difference between the means of two or more groups, while controlling for one or more covariate	N	I, R	N, I, R	1+	1	1+
Multivariate analysis of variance (MANOVA)	To test the difference between the means of two or more groups for two or more DVs simultaneously	N	I, R		1+	2+	
Multivariate analysis of covariance (MANCOVA)	To test the difference between the means of two or more groups for two or more DVs simultaneously, while controlling for one or more covariate	N	I, R	N, I, R	1+	2+	1+
Factor analysis	To determine the dimensionality or structure of a set of variables						
Discriminant analysis	To test the relationship between two or more IVs and one DV; to predict group membership; to classify cases into groups	N, I, R	N		2+	1	
Logistic regression	To test the relationship between two or more IVs and one DV; to predict the probability of an event, to estimate relative risk (odds ratios)	N, I, R	N		2+	1	

*Measurement level of the independent variable (IV), dependent variable (DV), and covariates (COV): I, interval; N, nominal; R = ratio.

READING AND UNDERSTANDING STATISTICAL INFORMATION

Statistical findings are communicated in the "Results" section of research reports and are reported in the text as well as in tables (or, less frequently, figures). This section provides some assistance in reading and interpreting statistical information.

Tips on Reading Text With Statistical Information

The "Results" section of a research report presents various types of statistical information. First, there are descriptive statistics (such as those shown in Table 15.4), which typically provide readers with a basic overview of participants' characteristics. Information about the subjects' background enables readers to draw conclusions about the groups to which findings might be generalized. Second, researchers may provide statistical information about biases. For example, researchers sometimes compare the characteristics of people who did and did not agree to participate in the study (e.g., using t tests). Or, in a quasi-experimental design, statistics on the preintervention comparability of the experimental and comparison groups might be presented so that readers can evaluate internal validity. Inferential statistics relating to the research hypotheses are usually presented. Finally, supplementary analyses are sometimes included to help unravel the meaning of the results.

The text of research reports normally provides certain information about the statistical tests, including (1) which test was used, (2) the actual value of the calculated statistic, (3) the degrees of freedom, and (4) the level of statistical significance. Examples of how the results of various statistical tests would likely be reported in the text of a report are shown below.

t test:	$t = 1.68; df = 160; p = .09$
Chi-squared:	$\chi^2 = 16.65; df = 2; p < .001$
Pearson's r:	$r = .36; df = 100; p < .01$
ANOVA:	$F = 0.18; df = 1, 69$, NS

Note that the significance level is sometimes reported as the *actual* computed probability that the null hypothesis is correct, as in example 1. In this case, the observed group differences could be found by chance in 9 out of 100 samples; thus, this result is not significant because the differences have an unacceptably high chance of being spurious. The probability level is sometimes reported simply as falling below or above a significance level, as in examples 2 and 3. In both cases, the results are statistically significant because the probability of obtaining such results by chance alone is less than 1 in 100. When results do not achieve statistical significance at the desired level, researchers simply may indicate that the results were not significant (NS), as in example 4.

Statistical information usually is noted parenthetically in a sentence describing the findings, as in the following example: Patients in the experimental group had a significantly lower rate of infection than those in the control group ($\chi^2 = 7.99, df = 1, p < .01$). In reading research reports, you do not need to absorb the numeric values for the actual test statistic. For example, the actual value of χ^2 has no inherent interest. What is important is to grasp whether the statistical tests indicate that the research hypotheses were accepted as probably true (as established by significant results) or rejected as probably false (as established by nonsignificant results).

Tips on Reading Statistical Tables

Tables allow researchers to condense a lot of statistical information in a compact space and also prevent redundancy. Consider, for example, putting information from a correlation matrix (see Table 15.7) into the text: "The correlation between cardiac rehabilitation patients' anxiety and self-efficacy was $-.57$; the correlation between cardiac rehabilitation patients' self-efficacy and heart rate change was $-.61. . . .$"

Unfortunately, although tables are efficient, they may be daunting and difficult to decipher. Part of the problem is the lack of standardization of tables. There is no universally accepted method of presenting *t*-test information, for example, and so each table may present a new challenge. Another problem is that some researchers try to include an enormous amount of information in their tables; we deliberately used tables of relative simplicity as examples in this chapter.

We know of no magic solution for helping you to comprehend statistical tables, but we have some suggestions. First, read the text and the tables simultaneously—the text may help to unravel the tables. Second, before trying to understand the numbers in a table, try to glean as much information as possible from the words. Table titles and footnotes often communicate critical pieces of information. The table headings should be carefully reviewed because these indicate what the variables in the analyses are (often listed in the far left-hand column as row labels) and what statistical information is included (often specified in the top row as column headings). Third, you may find it helpful to consult the glossary of symbols in Box 15.1 to determine the meaning of a statistical symbol in a report table. Note

BOX 15.1 GLOSSARY OF SELECTED STATISTICAL SYMBOLS

This list contains some commonly used symbols in statistics. The list is in approximate alphabetical order, with English and Greek letters intermixed. Nonletter symbols have been placed at the end.

a	Regression constant, the intercept
α	Greek alpha; significance level in hypothesis testing, probability of Type I error
b	Regression coefficient, slope of the line
β	Greek beta, probability of a Type II error; also, a standardized regression coefficient (beta weights)
χ^2	Greek chi squared, a test statistic for several nonparametric tests
CI	Confidence interval around estimate of a population parameter
df	Degrees of freedom
η^2	Greek eta squared, index of variance accounted for in ANOVA context
f	Frequency (count) for a score value
F	Test statistic used in ANOVA, ANCOVA, and other tests
H_0	Null hypothesis
H_1	Alternative hypothesis; research hypothesis
λ	Greek lambda, a test statistic used in several multivariate analyses (Wilks' lambda)
μ	Greek mu, the population mean
M	Sample mean (alternative symbol for $\bar{X}$)
MS	Mean square, variance estimate in ANOVA
n	Number of cases in a subgroup of the sample
N	Total number of cases or sample members
p	Probability that observed data are consistent with null hypothesis
r	Pearson's product–moment correlation coefficient for a sample
r_s	Spearman's rank-order correlation coefficient
R	Multiple correlation coefficient
R^2	Coefficient of determination, proportion of variance in *dependent variable* attributable to *independent variables*
R_c	Canonical correlation coefficient
ρ	Greek rho, population correlation coefficient
SD	Sample standard deviation
SEM	Standard error of the mean
σ	Greek sigma (lowercase), population standard deviation
Σ	Greek sigma (uppercase), sum of
SS	Sum of squares
t	Test statistics used in *t* tests (sometimes called Student's *t*)
U	Test statistic for the Mann–Whitney *U* test
$\bar{X}$	Sample mean
x	Deviation score
Y'	Predicted value of *Y*, dependent variable in regression analysis
z	Standard score in a normal distribution
$\|\|$	Absolute value
$\leq$	Less than or equal to
$\geq$	Greater than or equal to
$\neq$	Not equal to

that not all symbols in Box 15.1 were described in this chapter; therefore, it may be necessary to refer to a statistics textbook, such as that of Polit (1996), for further information. We recommend that you devote some extra time to making sure you have grasped what the tables are conveying and that you write out a sentence or two that summarizes some of the tabular information in "plain English."

TIP

In tables, probability levels associated with the significance tests are sometimes presented directly (e.g., $p < .05$), as in Table 15.13. Here, the significance of each test is indicated in the last column, headed "p." However, researchers often indicate significance levels in tables through asterisks placed next to the value of the test statistic. By convention, one asterisk usually signifies $p < .05$, two asterisks signify $p < .01$, and three asterisks signify $p < .001$ (there is usually a key at the bottom of the table that indicates what the asterisks mean). Thus, a table might show: $t = 3.00$, $p < .01$ or $t = 3.00**$. The absence of an asterisk would signify a nonsignificant result.

CRITIQUING QUANTITATIVE ANALYSES

It may be difficult for you to critique statistical analyses. We hope this chapter has helped to demystify statistics, but we also recognize the limited scope of this presentation. Although it would be unreasonable to expect you to now be adept at evaluating statistical analyses, there are certain things you should routinely look for in reviewing research reports. Some specific guidelines are presented in Box 15.2.

Researchers generally perform many more analyses than can be reported in a journal article. You should determine whether the statistical information adequately describes the sample and reports the results of statistical tests for all hypotheses. You might also consider whether the report included unnecessary statistical information. Another presentational issue concerns the researcher's judicious use of tables to summarize statistical information.

BOX 15.2 GUIDELINES FOR CRITIQUING QUANTITATIVE ANALYSES

1. Does the report include any descriptive statistics? Do these statistics sufficiently describe the major characteristics of the researcher's data set?

2. Were the correct descriptive statistics used? (e.g., Were percentages reported when a mean would have been more informative?)

3. Does the report include any inferential statistical tests? If not, should it have (e.g., were groups compared without information on the statistical significance of group differences)?

4. Was a statistical test performed for each of the hypotheses or research questions?

5. Do the selected statistical tests appear to be appropriate (e.g., are the tests appropriate for the level of measurement of key variables)?

6. Were any multivariate procedures used? If not, should multivariate analyses have been conducted—would the use of a multivariate procedure strengthen the internal validity of the study?

7. Were the results of any statistical tests significant? Nonsignificant? What do the tests tell you about the plausibility of the research hypotheses? Can you draw any conclusions about the possibility that Type I or Type II errors were committed?

8. Was an appropriate amount of statistical information reported? Were important analyses omitted, or were unimportant analyses included?

9. Were tables used judiciously to summarize statistical information? Is information in the text and tables totally redundant? Are the tables clear, with a good title and carefully labelled headings?

10. Is the researcher sufficiently objective in reporting the results?

A thorough critique also addresses whether researchers used the appropriate statistics. Tables 15.12 and 15.14 provide summaries of the most frequently used statistical tests—although we do not expect that you will be able to determine the appropriateness of the tests used in a study without further statistical instruction. The major issues to consider are the number of independent and dependent variables, the levels of measurement of the research variables, the number of groups (if any) being compared, and the appropriateness of using a parametric test.

If researchers did not use a multivariate technique, you should consider whether the bivariate analysis adequately tests the relationship between the independent and dependent variables. For example, if a *t* test or ANOVA was used, could the internal validity of the study have been enhanced through the statistical control of extraneous variables, using ANCOVA? The answer will almost always be "yes," even when an experimental design was used.

As we noted in Chapter 9, statistical analyses and design issues are sometimes intertwined, in the sense that both analytic and design decisions can affect statistical conclusion validity. When sample size is low, when an independent variable is weakly defined (or when participation in an intervention is low), and when a weak statistical procedure is used in lieu of a more powerful one, then the risk of drawing the wrong conclusion about the research hypotheses is heightened. You should pay particular attention to the possibility of statistical conclusion validity problems when research hypotheses are not supported.

The main task for beginning consumers in reading the "Results" section of a research report is to understand the meaning of the statistical tests, but it is also important to consider the believability of the findings.

⏵ RESEARCH EXAMPLES AND CRITICAL THINKING ACTIVITIES

EXAMPLE 1 ■ Descriptive, Bivariate, and Multivariate Statistics

Aspects of a nursing study, featuring terms and concepts discussed in this chapter, are presented below, followed by some questions to guide critical thinking.

Study
"Effects of music therapy on physiological and psychological outcomes for patients undergoing cardiac surgery" (Sendelbach, Halm, Doran, Miller, and Gaillard, 2006)

Statement of Purpose
"To compare the effects of music therapy versus a quiet, uninterrupted rest period on pain intensity, anxiety, physiological parameters, and opioid consumption after cardiac surgery."

Research Design
A randomized clinical trial was conducted to address the research question with 86 patients from cardiovascular units in three hospitals. The participants were randomly assigned to either the experimental group, in which music was delivered on tape by headphone for 20 minutes twice per day from postoperation days (POD) (1 to 3), or the control group, in which patients received usual care (resting in bed for predetermined periods of time). Each group received its respective treatment between 8 AM and 10 AM in the morning and between 4 PM and 9 PM in the evening. For both groups, measures of pain intensity, anxiety, heart rate (HR), and blood pressure (BP) were obtained immediately before and after each 20-minute intervention period (i.e., while patients were listening to music or resting in bed). To ensure consistency in measurement, signs were placed on doors to the patients' rooms stating that the patient was currently listening to music/resting and to return later. Because of substantial missing data, only outcome data collected on POD 1 and POD AM were analyzed to address the study's purpose.

(Research Examples and Critical Thinking Activities continues on page 314)

Research Examples and Critical Thinking Activities (continued)

Descriptive Statistics

Statistical analyses were performed using a statistical package called SPSS (version 10.0). The researchers reported computed means, medians, standard deviations, and ranges for sample characteristics. For example, a mean of 63 years was obtained for participants' age, 69.8% of them were male, with 69.8% having had a coronary artery bypass surgery. Eighty-one percent of the sample had seldom used music therapy in the past.

Bivariate Descriptive Statistics

Researchers computed t tests for interval data and chi-squared tests for nominal data, to compare participants' characteristics in the experimental and control groups. The two groups were found to be equivalent on most characteristics with the exception of type of surgical procedure; the music therapy group had significantly more coronary artery bypass surgeries and valve replacement procedures than the control group ($p = .05$).

Bivariate Inferential Statistics

The researchers also used t tests to determine the effectiveness of music therapy when compared to usual care (the control group) on opioid consumption and physiological parameters such as blood pressure and heart rate; no significant differences were found between the two groups for opioid consumption, or systolic ($p = .17$) and diastolic blood pressure ($p = .11$), or for heart rate ($p = .76$).

The researchers used repeated measures ANOVA to test the effectiveness of music therapy on some of the dependent variables according to groups. Across time, anxiety ($p < .001$) and pain ($p = .009$) were found to be significantly lower in the music group than in the control group.

Conclusions

The researchers concluded that the greatest benefit of this intervention seems to be in the psychological impact of music therapy for these patients who underwent cardiac surgery.

CRITICAL THINKING SUGGESTIONS

1. Answer questions 1 through 7 from Box 15.2 (p. 312) regarding this study.

2. Also consider the following targeted questions, which may assist you in further assessing aspects of the study:
   a. Do you think the statistical conclusion validity of this study is high? Why or why not?
   b. In what way (if at all) do the choice of statistical tests in this study affect the quality of the study?
   c. One secondary study outcomes was the amount of opioid consumed by patients who had cardiac surgery. Which statistical test(s) would be appropriate for determining the intervention's effect on this outcome?

3. If the results of this study are valid and reliable, what may be their clinical relevance?

EXAMPLE 2 ■ Descriptive, Inferential, and Multivariate Statistics

1. Read the "Results" section from the study by Bryanton, Gagnon, Hatem, and Johnston in Appendix A of this book and then answer the relevant questions in Box 15.2 (p. 312).

Summary Points

➤ There are four major **levels of measurement:** (1) **nominal measurement**—the classification of attributes into mutually exclusive categories; (2) **ordinal measurement**—the ranking of objects based on their relative standing on an attribute; (3) **interval measurement**—indicating not only the ranking of objects but also the distance between them; and (4) **ratio measurement**—distinguished from interval measurement by having a rational zero point.

⇝ **Descriptive statistics** enable researchers to synthesize and summarize quantitative data.

⇝ In a **frequency distribution,** numeric values are ordered from lowest to highest, together with a count of the number (or percentage) of times each value was obtained.

⇝ Data for a variable can be completely described in terms of the shape of its distribution, central tendency, and variability.

⇝ The shape of a distribution can be **symmetric** or **skewed,** with one tail longer than the other; it can also be **unimodal** with one peak (i.e., one value of high frequency) or **multimodal** with more than one peak.

⇝ A **normal distribution** (bell-shaped curve) is symmetric, unimodal, and not too peaked.

⇝ Measures of **central tendency** indicate the average or typical value of a variable. The **mode** is the value that occurs most frequently in a distribution; the **median** is the point above which and below which 50% of the cases fall; and the **mean** is the arithmetic average of all scores. The mean is usually the preferred measure of central tendency because of its stability.

⇝ Measures of **variability**—how spread out the data are—include the range and standard deviation. The **range** is the distance between the highest and lowest scores, and the **standard deviation** indicates how much, on average, scores deviate from the mean.

⇝ A **contingency table** is a two-dimensional frequency distribution in which the frequencies of two nominal-level or ordinal-level variables are **cross-tabulated.**

⇝ **Correlation coefficients** describe the direction and magnitude of a relationship between two variables. The values range from -1.00 for a perfect negative correlation, to $.00$ for no relationship, to $+1.00$ for a perfect positive correlation. The most frequently used correlation coefficient is the **product–moment correlation coefficient** (**Pearson's r**), used with interval-level or ratio-level variables.

⇝ **Inferential statistics,** which are based on *laws of probability,* allow researchers to make inferences about a population based on data from a sample; they offer a framework for deciding whether the sampling error that results from sampling fluctuation is too high to provide reliable population estimates.

⇝ The **sampling distribution of the mean** is a theoretical distribution of the means of an infinite number of same-sized samples drawn from a population. Sampling distributions are the basis for inferential statistics.

⇝ The **standard error of the mean**—the standard deviation of this theoretical distribution—indicates the degree of average error of a sample mean; the smaller the standard error, the more accurate are the estimates of the population value based on the sample mean.

⇝ **Hypothesis testing** through statistical tests enables researchers to make objective decisions about relationships between variables.

⇝ The *null hypothesis* states that no relationship exists between the variables and that any observed relationship is due to chance or sampling fluctuations; rejection of the null hypothesis lends support to the research hypothesis.

⇝ A **Type I error** occurs if a null hypothesis is incorrectly rejected (false positives). A **Type II error** occurs when a null hypothesis is incorrectly accepted (false negatives).

⇝ Researchers control the risk of making a Type I error by establishing a **level of significance** (or **alpha** level), which specifies the probability that such an error will occur. The .05 level means that in only 5 out of 100 samples would the null hypothesis be rejected when it should have been accepted.

⇒ The probability of committing a Type II error, referred to as **beta** (β), can be estimated through *power analysis*. *Power*, the ability of a statistical test to detect true relationships, is the complement of beta (i.e., power equals $1 - \beta$). The standard criterion for an acceptable level of power is .80.

⇒ Results from hypothesis tests are either significant or nonsignificant; **statistically significant** means that the obtained results are not likely to be due to chance fluctuations at a given probability level (p **level**).

⇒ **Parametric statistical tests** involve the estimation of at least one parameter, the use of interval- or ratio-level data, and an assumption of normally distributed variables; **nonparametric tests** are used when the data are nominal or ordinal and the normality of the distribution cannot be assumed.

⇒ Two common statistical tests are the *t* **test** and **analysis of variance** (ANOVA), both of which can be used to test the significance of the difference between group means; ANOVA is used when there are more than two groups.

⇒ The most frequently used nonparametric test is the **chi-squared test,** which is used to test hypotheses about differences in proportions.

⇒ Pearson's *r* can be used to test whether a correlation is significantly different from zero.

⇒ **Multivariate statistics** are increasingly being used in nursing research to untangle complex relationships among three or more variables.

⇒ **Multiple regression** is a method for understanding the effect of two or more **predictor** (independent) **variables** on a dependent variable. The **multiple correlation coefficient** (*R*) can be squared to estimate the proportion of variability in the dependent variable accounted for by the predictors.

⇒ **Analysis of covariance** (ANCOVA) permits researchers to control extraneous variables (called **covariates**) before determining whether group differences are significant.

⇒ Other multivariate procedures used by nurse researchers include discriminant function analysis, logistic regression, factor analysis, multivariate analysis of variance (MANOVA), multivariate analysis of covariance (MANCOVA), path analysis, and LISREL.

STUDIES CITED IN CHAPTER 15*

*This reference list contains only those studies that were cited in this chapter. Citations pertaining to theoretical, methodological, or nonempirical work are included together in a separate section at the end of the book (beginning on page 399).

Bailey, J. J., Sabbagh, M., Loiselle, C. G., Boileau, J., & McVey, L. (2009). *Supporting families in the ICU: A descriptive correlational study of informational support, anxiety, and satisfaction with care.* Manuscript submitted for publication.

Bowen, A., Bowen, R., Maslany, G., & Muhajarine, N. (2008). Anxiety in a socially high-risk sample of pregnant women in Canada. *The Canadian Journal of Psychiatry*, *53*(7), 435–440.

Bryanton, J., Gagnon, A. J., Hatem, M., & Johnston, C. (2008). Predictors of early parenting self-efficacy: Results of a prospective cohort study. *Nursing Research, 57*(4), 252–259.

Downe-Wamboldt, B. L., Butler, L. J., Melanson, P. M., et al. (2007). The effects and expense of augmenting usual cancer clinic care with telephone problem-solving counseling. *Cancer Nursing*, *30*(6), 441–453.

Feeley, N., Gottlieb, L., & Zelkowitz, P. (2007). Mothers and fathers of very low birthweight infants: Similarities and differences in the first year after birth. *Journal of Obstetric, Gynecologic, and Neonatal Nursing, 36*(6), 558–567.

Forchuk, C., MacClure, S. K., Van Beers, M., et al. (2008). Developing and testing an intervention to prevent homelessness among individuals discharged from psychiatric wards to shelters and "No Fixed Address." *Journal of Psychiatric and Mental Health Nursing*, *15*(7), 569–575.

Fraser, S. N., Rodgers, W., & Daub, B. (2008). Psychosocial correlates of cardiovascular reactivity to anticipation of an exercise stress test prior to attending cardiac rehabilitation: A preliminary test. *Journal of Applied Biobehavioral Research, 13*(1), 20–41.

Ing, J. D., & Reutter, L. (2003). Socioeconomic status, sense of coherence and health in Canadian women. *Canadian Journal of Public Health, 94*(3), 224–228.

Janssen, P. A., Iker, C. E., & Carty, E. A. (2003). Early labour assessment and support at home: A randomized controlled trial. *Journal of Obstetrics and Gynaecology Canada, 25*(9), 734–741.

Johnston, C. C., Gagnon, A., Rennick, J., et al. (2007). One-on-one coaching to improve pain assessment and management practices of pediatric nurses. *Journal of Pediatric Nursing, 22*(6), 467–478.

Kim, S. E., Pérez-Stable, E. J., Wong, S., et al. (2008). Association between cancer risk perception and screening behaviour among diverse women. *Archives of Internal Medicine, 168*(7), 728–734.

King, K. M., Parry, M., Southern, D., Faris, P., & Tsuyuki, R. T. (2008). Women's recovery from Sternotomy-Extension (WREST-E) study: Examining long-term pain and discomfort following sternotomy and their predictors. *Heart, 94*(4), 493–497.

Loiselle, C. G., & Dubois, S. (2009). The impact of a multimedia cancer informational intervention as opposed to usual care on health care service use among individuals newly diagnosed with breast or prostate cancer. *Cancer Nursing, 32*(1), 37–44.

Nyamathi, A., Nahid, P., Berg, J., et al. (2008). Efficacy of nurse case-managed intervention for latent tuberculosis among homeless subsamples. *Nursing Research, 57*(1), 33–39.

Okoli, C. T., Hall, L. A., Rayens, M. K., & Hahn, E. J. (2007). Measuring tobacco smoke exposure among smoking and nonsmoking bar and restaurant workers. *Biology Research in Nursing, 9*(1), 81–89.

Ross-Kerr, J., Warren, S., Schalm, C., Smith, D., & Godkin, M. (2003, December). Multicultural aging. Adult day programs: Who needs them? *Journal of Gerontological Nursing, 29*(12), 11–17.

Sendelbach, S. E., Halm, M. A., Doran, K. A., Miller, E. H., & Gaillard, P. (2006). Effects of music therapy on physiological and psychological outcomes for patients undergoing cardiac surgery. *Journal of Cardiovascular Nursing, 21*(3), 194–200.

Stajduhar, K. L., Allan, D. E., Cohen, S. R., & Heyland, D. K. (2008). Preferences for location of death of seriously ill hospitalized patients: Perspectives from Canadian patients and their family caregivers. *Palliative Medicine, 22*(1), 85–88.

16 Analyzing Qualitative Data

On completing this chapter, you will be able to:

1. Distinguish prototypical qualitative analysis styles and understand the intellectual processes that play a role in qualitative analysis

2. Describe activities that qualitative researchers perform to manage and organize their data

3. Discuss the procedures used to analyze qualitative data, including both general procedures and those used in grounded theory, phenomenological, and ethnographic research

4. Evaluate researchers' descriptions of their analytic procedures and assess the adequacy of those procedures

5. Define new terms in the chapter

As we saw in Chapter 13, qualitative data are derived from narrative materials such as verbatim transcripts of in-depth interviews, fieldnotes from participant observation, and personal diaries. This chapter describes methods for analyzing such qualitative data.

INTRODUCTION TO QUALITATIVE ANALYSIS

Qualitative analysis is a labour-intensive activity that requires creativity, conceptual sensitivity, and sheer hard work. Qualitative analysis is more complex and difficult to do well than quantitative analysis because it is less formulaic. In this section, we discuss some general issues relating to qualitative analysis.

Qualitative Analysis: General Considerations

The purpose of data analysis, regardless of the type of data or the underlying research tradition, is to organize, provide structure to, and elicit meaning from the data. Data analysis is particularly challenging for qualitative researchers, for three major reasons. First, there are no universal rules for analyzing and summarizing qualitative data. The absence of standard analytic procedures makes it difficult to present findings in such a way that their validity is apparent. Some of the procedures described in Chapter 14 (e.g., member checking and investigator triangulation) are important tools for enhancing the trustworthiness not only of the data themselves but also of the analyses and interpretation of those data.

The second challenge of qualitative analysis is the enormous amount of work required. The qualitative analyst must organize and make sense of pages and pages of narrative materials. In a multiple method study by Polit, London, and Martinez (2000), the qualitative data consisted of transcribed, unstructured interviews with about 25 to 30 low-income women in four cities discussing life stressors and health problems over a 3-year period. The transcriptions ranged from 30 to 50 pages in length, resulting in thousands of pages that had to be read and reread and then organized, integrated, and interpreted.

The final challenge is reducing the data for reports. Quantitative results can often be summarized in two or three tables. Qualitative researchers, by contrast, must balance the need to be concise to adhere to journal requirements with the need to maintain the richness and evidentiary value of their data.

TIP

Qualitative analyses are often more difficult to do than quantitative ones, but qualitative findings are generally easier to understand than quantitative findings because the stories are often told in everyday language. However, qualitative analyses are harder to evaluate critically than quantitative analyses because readers cannot know first-hand if researchers adequately captured thematic patterns in the data.

Analysis Styles

Crabtree and Miller (1999) observed that there are nearly as many qualitative analysis strategies as there are qualitative researchers. However, they have identified three major styles that fall along a continuum. At one extreme is a style that is more systematic and standardized, and at the other is a style that is more intuitive, subjective, and interpretive. The three prototypical styles are as follows:

➢ **Template analysis style.** In this style, researchers develop a *template*—a category and analysis guide for sorting the narrative data. Researchers usually begin with a rudimentary template before collecting data, but the template undergoes constant revision as the data are gathered and analyzed. This style is most likely to be adopted by researchers whose research tradition is ethnography, ethology, discourse analysis, or ethnoscience.

➢ **Editing analysis style.** Researchers using an editing style act as interpreters who read through texts in search of meaningful segments. Once segments are identified and reviewed, researchers develop a category scheme and corresponding codes that can be used to sort and organize the data. The researchers then search for the patterns and structure that connect the thematic categories. Researchers whose research tradition is grounded theory, phenomenology, hermeneutics, or ethnomethodology use procedures within this analysis style.

➢ **Immersion/crystallization analysis style.** This style involves the analyst's total immersion in and reflection of the text materials, resulting in an intuitive crystallization of the data. This interpretive and subjective style is exemplified in personal case reports of a semianecdotal nature and is less frequently encountered in the nursing research literature than the other two styles.

Researchers seldom use terms such as template analysis style or editing style in their reports. However, King (1998) described the process of undertaking a template analysis, and his approach has been adopted by some nurse researchers undertaking descriptive qualitative studies.

Example of a template analysis
Sorensen, Waldorff, and Waldemar (2008) used a template to analyze their data in a Danish study of the effectiveness of a psychosocial intervention for patients with mild Alzheimer's disease and for their spousal caregivers. The study involved an analysis of individual, semistructured in-depth interviews, pre- and post-intervention, with 10 couples. Initial codes included: "Recognition of the changes before and after the intervention" and "Reactions to the impacts of the changes caused by the disease before and after the intervention" (p. 446).

The Qualitative Analysis Process

The analysis of qualitative data is an active and interactive process. Qualitative researchers typically scrutinize their data carefully and deliberatively. Insights cannot spring forth from the data unless the researchers are completely familiar with those data, and so they often read their narrative data over and over in search of meaning. Morse and Field (1995) note that qualitative analysis is "a process of fitting data together, of making the invisible obvious, of linking and attributing consequences to antecedents. It is a process of conjecture and verification, of correction and modification, of suggestion and defense" (p. 126). Morse and Field identified four cognitive processes that play a role in qualitative analysis:

⤇ *Comprehending.* Early in the analytic process, qualitative researchers strive to make sense of the data and to learn "what is going on." When comprehension is achieved, researchers are able to prepare a thorough description of the phenomenon under study, and new data do not add much to that description. Thus, comprehension is completed when saturation has been attained.

⤇ *Synthesizing.* Synthesizing involves a "sifting" of the data and inductively putting pieces together. At this stage, researchers get a sense of what is typical with regard to the phenomenon and of what variation is like. At the end of the synthesis process, researchers can make some general statements about the phenomenon and about study participants.

⤇ *Theorizing.* Theorizing involves a systematic sorting of the data. During the theorizing process, researchers develop alternative explanations of the phenomenon under study and then hold these explanations up to determine their "fit" with the data. The theorizing process continues to evolve until the best and most parsimonious explanation is obtained.

⤇ *Recontextualizing.* The process of *recontextualization* involves the further development of the theory such that its applicability to other settings or groups is explored.

Although the intellectual processes in qualitative analysis are not linear in the same sense as quantitative analysis, these four processes follow a rough progression over the course of the study in iterative cycles. Comprehension occurs primarily while in the field. Synthesis begins in the field but may continue well after the fieldwork has been completed. Theorizing and recontextualizing are processes that are difficult to undertake before synthesis has been completed.

QUALITATIVE DATA MANAGEMENT AND ORGANIZATION

Intellectual processes of qualitative analysis are supported and facilitated by early tasks that help to organize and manage the masses of narrative data.

Developing a Category Scheme

Qualitative researchers begin their analysis by organizing their data. The main organizational task is devising a method to classify and index the data.

Researchers must design a means of gaining access to parts of the data, without having to repeatedly reread the data set in its entirety. This phase of data analysis is essentially reductionist—data must be converted to smaller, more manageable units that can be retrieved and reviewed.

The most widely used procedure is to develop a category scheme and then to code the data according to the categories. A category system (or template) is sometimes drafted before data collection, but more typically the qualitative analyst develops categories based on a scrutiny of the actual data. In the previous example by Sorensen et al. (2008), the organizational template was developed after several readings of the interview data. The template was a starting point—the initial codes were then refined through the iterative analytic process.

There are, unfortunately, no straightforward or easy guidelines for this task. The development of a high-quality category scheme for qualitative data involves a careful reading of the data, with an eye to identifying underlying concepts and clusters of concepts. Depending on the aims of the study, the nature of the categories may vary in level of detail or specificity as well as in level of abstraction.

Researchers whose aims are primarily descriptive tend to use concrete categories. The category scheme may focus on actions or events or on different phases in the unfolding of an experience. In developing a category scheme, related concepts are often grouped together to facilitate the coding process.

Studies aimed at theory development are more likely to develop abstract and conceptual categories. In designing conceptual categories, researchers must break the data into segments, closely examine them, and compare them to other segments for similarities and dissimilarities to determine what type of phenomena are reflected in them and what the meaning of those phenomena are. Researchers ask questions about discrete events, incidents, or thoughts, such as the following:

➤ What is this?

➤ What is going on?

➤ What does it stand for?

➤ What else is like this?

➤ What is this distinct from?

Important concepts that emerge from close examination of the data are then given a label that forms the basis for a category scheme. These category names are abstractions, but the labels are usually sufficiently graphic that the nature of the material to which the label refers is clear—and often provocative.

Example of a conceptual category scheme
Box 16.1 shows the category scheme developed by Beck (2006) to categorize data from her Internet interviews on the anniversary of birth trauma. The coding scheme included four major thematic categories with subcodes. For example, an excerpt that described a mother's feelings of dread and anxiety during the days leading up to the anniversary of her traumatic birth experience would be coded under category 1A (i.e., "Plagued with an array of distressing thoughts and emotions" p. 386). Note that Beck's original coding scheme, shown in Box 16.1, was further developed and made more parsimonious during the analysis stage. For example, codes 2D, 2E, and 2F were collapsed into a larger category called "Various ways to make it through the day." Table 2 (p. 385) in the full report shows several significant statements that exemplify this broader category.

TIP

A high-quality category scheme is crucial to the analysis of qualitative data since researchers cannot retrieve the narrative information that has been collected without one. Unfortunately, research reports rarely present the category scheme for readers to review, but they may provide other information to help you evaluate its adequacy. For example, researchers may say that the scheme was reviewed by peers or developed and independently verified by two or more researchers to ensure intercoder reliability.

BOX 16.1 BECK'S (2006) CODING SCHEME FOR THE ANNIVERSARY OF BIRTH TRAUMA

Theme 1. The Prologue: An Agonizing Time
A.   Plagued with an array of distressing thoughts and emotions
B.   Physically taking a toll
C.   Clocks, calendars, and seasons playing key roles
D.   Ruminating about the day their babies had been born

Theme 2. The Actual Day: A Celebration of a Birthday or Torment of an Anniversary
A.   Concept of time taking centre stage
B.   Not knowing how to celebrate her child's birthday
C.   Tormented by powerful emotions
D.   Scheduled birthday party on a different day
E.   Consumed with technical details of the birthday party
F.   Need to physically get away on the birthday

Theme 3. The Epilogue: A Fragile State
A.   Surviving the actual anniversary took a heavy toll
B.   Needed time to recuperate
C.   Crippling emotions lingered
D.   Sense of relief

Theme 4. Subsequent Anniversaries: For Better or Worse
A.   Each birthday slightly easier to cope with
B.   No improvement noted
C.   Worrying about future birthdays
D.   Each anniversary is a lottery: a time bomb

Coding Qualitative Data

After a category scheme has been developed, the data are then read in their entirety and coded for correspondence to the identified categories. The process of coding qualitative material is not an easy one. Researchers may have difficulty in deciding which code is most appropriate, or they may not fully comprehend the underlying meaning of some aspect of the data. It may take a second or third reading of the material to grasp its nuances.

Moreover, researchers often discover in going through the data that the initial category scheme was incomplete or inadequate. It is not unusual for some themes to emerge that were not initially conceptualized. When this happens, it is risky to assume that the topic failed to appear in previously coded materials. That is, a concept might not be identified as salient until it has emerged a third or fourth time in the data. In such a case, it would be necessary to reread all previously coded material to have a truly complete grasp of that category.

Another issue is that narrative materials are generally not linear. For example, paragraphs from transcribed interviews may contain elements relating to three or four different categories embedded in a complex fashion.

Example of coding qualitative data
An example of a multitopic segment of an interview from Beck's (2006) phenomenological study of the anniversary of birth trauma is shown in Figure 16.1. The codes in the margin represent codes from the scheme presented in Box 16.1.

Manual Methods of Organizing Qualitative Data

Various procedures have been used to organize qualitative data. Before the advent of computer programs for managing qualitative data, the most usual procedure was to develop **conceptual files.** This approach involves creating a physical file for

"At some point a fetal scalp monitor was introduced then what seemed to be very shortly after that, my own OB came in and said my baby was in fetal distress and that a c-section was probably needed given that I was only 6 cms. This floored me in every imaginable way-emotionally, physically, and mentally. I'd labored in what I thought was "well mannered" for 12 hours. NO ONE had told me they were monitoring my baby. NO ONE told me they suspected she was in distress. Then BOOM, my baby is in trouble and my almost picture-perfect labor is gone. After that point, things became blurry because I can only see them through what I describe as an emotional fog. I lost it in front of everybody which I rarely do. — **2 A**

2 A — As they wheeled me into the theatre, I asked again where was my husband. They said he was on his way. They wheeled me in and told me to curl my back for the epidural. There were a few nurses there and I remember them talking about me as if I wasn't **2 A** there. Didn't they realize that I could hear them? The needle must have gone in 4 or 5 times. I was crying. I was scared and the epidural hurt a bloody lot. Some one please help me. I felt all alone. And I was thinking that I don't want another baby and go through this again. I recall thinking how much more pain do I have to put up with? Was my baby going to be all right? I needed reassurance but none was given. — **2 B**

Then another man took over the epidural and asked me to sit up and bend over while he put the needle in. I started to feel numb below my waist. I felt a pin prick and felt my tummy being pulled apart. It was awful as I couldn't see or feel anything. — **1 D**

1 A — So my trauma was a result of that emergency caesarean. It happened so fast. Of feeling so scared and alone and having to go through it all alone with out my husband there. The nurses didn't tell me anything about what was going on. I felt powerless. **3 C** I also felt the hospital staff could have given me some indication that I may have had to have an emergency caesarean instead of letting me think that I was going to have a natural labor. I also wished that the doctor herself could have come to see **1 C** how I was doing afterwards. I think it would have helped me a lot if she had come and talked about how I was doing and how I felt and why I had to have an emergency c-section. — **2 A**

4 B — All people kept telling me after my daughter was born was how lucky I was and that I could have lost her. I know I was lucky but telling that does not help how I felt. With them telling me that, I felt guilty for feeling the way I did. I wanted some attention too. I wanted to be looked after and listened to. I tried several times to bring up how **4 D** I felt but it was brushed away with the "I've been through that before and so what response." I really felt like I was in the wrong to feel the way I did because I had a healthy baby." — **4 C**

FIGURE 16.1   Coded excerpt from Beck's (2006) study.

each category, and then cutting out and inserting into the file all materials relating to that category. Researchers can then retrieve all of the content on a particular topic by reviewing the applicable file folder.

The creation of such conceptual files is a cumbersome and labour-intensive task, particularly when segments of the narrative materials have multiple codes (e.g., the excerpt shown in Figure 16.1). There would need to be, for example, three copies of the last paragraph—one for each file corresponding to the three codes used for this paragraph. Researchers must also be sensitive to the need to provide sufficient context that the cutup material can be understood. Thus, it is often necessary to include material preceding or following the directly relevant materials.

Computer Programs for Managing Qualitative Data

Traditional manual methods of organizing qualitative data have a long and respected history, but sophisticated computer programs for managing qualitative data are now widely used. These programs permit the entire data file to be entered onto the computer, each portion of an interview or observational record coded, and then portions of the text corresponding to specified codes retrieved and printed (or shown on a screen) for analysis. The current generation of programs also has features that go beyond simple indexing and retrieval—they offer possibilities for actual analysis and integration of the data.

Computer programs remove the drudgery of cutting and pasting pages and pages of narrative material. However, some people prefer manual indexing because it allows them to get closer to the data. Others have raised concerns about using programs for the analysis of qualitative data, objecting to having a process that is basically cognitive turned into an activity that is mechanical. Despite these issues, some qualitative researchers have switched to computerized data management because it frees up their time and permits them to pay greater attention to important conceptual issues.

Example of using computers to manage qualitative data
Thompson et al. (2008) studied the concept of busyness and how it relates to research utilization in nursing. A secondary data analysis of open-ended interviews, fieldnotes, and focus groups originally collected from four urban, tertiary level hospitals in Canada were entered into a computer program called N6 (a version of the widely used NUD*IST program) for coding and organization.

ANALYTIC PROCEDURES

Data *management* in qualitative research is reductionist in nature because it converts large masses of data into smaller, more convenient units. By contrast, qualitative data *analysis* is constructionist: it involves putting segments together into a meaningful conceptual pattern. Although there are several approaches to qualitative data analysis, some elements are common to several of them. We provide some general guidelines, followed by a description of the procedures used by ethnographers, phenomenologists, and grounded theory researchers.

It should be noted that qualitative researchers who conduct studies that are not based on a specific research tradition sometimes say that a **content analysis** was performed. Qualitative content analysis is the analysis of narrative data to identify prominent themes and patterns among the themes.

Example of a content analysis
Letourneau et al. (2007) explored Canadian mothers' perceived needs and resources, barriers, and preferences for support during postpartum depression. The authors used content analysis to analyze individual and group interview data—"A category system of key concepts and themes was used to code the interview data using inductive analysis (moving from particular experiences of participants to general themes or categories) . . . Codes were inclusive, useful, mutually exclusive, clear, and specific" (p. 443).

A General Analytic Overview

The analysis of qualitative materials generally begins with a search for recurring regularities or themes. DeSantis and Ugarriza (2000), in their thorough review of the way in which the term theme is used among qualitative researchers, offer this definition: "A **theme** is an abstract entity that brings meaning and identity to a current experience and its variant manifestations. As such, a theme captures and unifies the nature or basis of the experience into a meaningful whole" (p. 362).

Themes emerge from the data. They often develop within categories of data (i.e., within categories of the coding scheme used for indexing materials) but sometimes cut across them. For example, in Beck's (2006) anniversary of birth trauma study (see Figure 16.1), one theme that emerged was mothers' fragile state after the actual day of the anniversary was over, which included 3B (needed time to recuperate) and 3D (sense of relief).

The search for themes involves not only the discovery of commonalities but also a search for variation. Themes are never universal; researchers must attend not only to what themes arise but also to how they are patterned. Does the theme apply only to certain subsets of participants? In certain types of communities or in certain contexts? At certain periods? What are the conditions that precede an observed phenomenon, and what are the consequences of it? In other words, qualitative analysts must be sensitive to *relationships* within the data.

TIP

Major themes are often the subheadings used in the Results section of qualitative reports. For example, in their grounded theory study of the challenges faced by daughters caring for elderly, dying parents, Read and Wuest (2007) identified the central theme of *turmoil* (emotional, relational, and societal) as well as the substantive theory of *Relinquishing*, which were used to organize their Results section.

Researchers' search for themes and regularities in the data can sometimes be facilitated by charting devices that enable them to summarize the evolution of behaviours and processes. For example, for qualitative studies that focus on dynamic experiences (e.g., decision making), it is often useful to develop flow charts or time lines that highlight time sequences, major decision points, or events.

A further step involves validation to determine whether the themes inferred are an accurate representation of the phenomenon. Several validation procedures can be used, as discussed in Chapter 14. If more than one researcher is working on the study, sessions in which the themes are reviewed and specific cases discussed can be highly productive. Investigator triangulation cannot ensure thematic validity, but it can minimize idiosyncratic biases. It is also useful to undertake member checks—that is, to present the preliminary thematic analysis to some informants, who can be encouraged to offer comments to support or contradict the analysis.

At this point, some researchers introduce **quasi-statistics**—a tabulation of the frequency with which certain themes or patterns are supported by the data. The frequencies cannot be interpreted in the same way as frequencies generated in survey studies because of imprecision in the sampling of cases and enumeration of the themes. Nevertheless, as Becker (1970) pointed out:

> Quasi-statistics may allow the investigator to dispose of certain troublesome null hypotheses. A simple frequency count of the number of times a given phenomenon appears may make untenable the null hypothesis that the phenomenon is infrequent. A comparison of the number of such instances with the number of negative cases— instances in which some alternative phenomenon that would not be predicted by his theory appears—may make possible a stronger conclusion, especially if the theory was developed early enough in the observational period to allow a systematic search for negative cases. (p. 81)

It is important to remember that the application of quasi-statistics is very different from a multiple- or mixed-methods approach, which incorporates both qualitative and quantitative data collection and analysis methods to extend or enrich the research findings.

Example of tabulating qualitative data

Harrison et al. (2003) interviewed 47 women with a high-risk pregnancy to explore how satisfied they were with their personal involvement in health care decisions. The researchers tabulated some aspects of the women's experiences. For example, they noted that most women (n = 30 out of 47) wanted to be active partners in their care management decisions. Of these 30 women, 21 were satisfied with their active decisions, but 8 of the 21 had had to struggle with health professionals for increased involvement.

In the final analysis stage, researchers strive to weave the thematic pieces together into an integrated whole. The various themes need to be interrelated to provide an overall structure (such as a theory or integrated description) to the data. The integration task is a difficult one because it demands creativity and intellectual rigour to be successful.

TIP

Research reports vary in the amount of detail provided about qualitative analytic procedures. At one extreme, researchers say little more than "data were analyzed qualitatively." At the other extreme, researchers describe the steps they took to analyze their data and validate emerging themes. Most studies fall between the two extremes, but limited detail is more prevalent than abundant detail. Again, brevity is usually a deliberate decision on behalf of the researcher to allow as much space as possible for the Results given the report's word limit.

These general analytic procedures provide an overview of how qualitative researchers make sense of their data. However, variations in the goals and philosophies of qualitative researchers also lead to variations in analytic strategies. The next section describes data analysis in ethnographic studies.

Analysis of Ethnographic Data

Ethnographic analysis begins the moment the researcher sets foot in the field. Ethnographers are continually looking for *patterns* in the behaviour and thoughts of the participants, comparing one pattern against another, and analyzing many patterns simultaneously (Fetterman, 1989). As they analyze patterns of everyday life, ethnographers acquire a deeper understanding of the culture being studied. They analyze key events (e.g., social events) because these events provide a lens through which to view a culture. Maps, flow charts, and organizational charts are also useful analytic tools that help to crystallize and illustrate the data being collected.

Spradley's (1979) developmental research sequence is one method that is often used for data analysis in an ethnographic study. His method is based on the premise that language is the primary means that relates cultural meaning in a culture. The task of ethnographers is to describe cultural symbols and to identify their rules. His sequence of 12 steps, which includes both data collection and data analysis, is as follows:

1. Locating an informant
2. Interviewing an informant
3. Making an ethnographic record
4. Asking descriptive questions
5. Analyzing ethnographic interviews
6. Making a domain analysis
7. Asking structural questions
8. Making a taxonomic analysis
9. Asking contrast questions
10. Making a componential analysis
11. Discovering cultural themes
12. Writing the ethnography

Thus, in Spradley's method, there are four levels of data analysis: domain, taxonomic, componential, and theme. *Domain analysis* is the first level of analysis.

Domains, which are units of cultural knowledge, are broad categories that encompass smaller categories. There is no preestablished number of domains to be uncovered in an ethnographic study. During this first level of data analysis, ethnographers identify relational patterns among terms in the domains that are used by members of the culture. Ethnographers focus on the cultural meaning of terms and symbols (objects and events) used in a culture and their interrelationships.

In *taxonomic analysis*, ethnographers decide how many domains the data analysis will encompass. Will only one or two domains be analyzed in depth, or will a number of domains be studied less intensively? After making this decision, a **taxonomy**—a system of classifying and organizing terms—is developed to illustrate the internal organization of a domain and the relationship among the subcategories of the domain.

In *componential analysis*, ethnographers analyze data for similarities and differences among cultural terms in a domain. Finally, in *theme analysis*, cultural themes are uncovered. Domains are connected in cultural themes, which help to provide a holistic view of the culture being studied. The discovery of cultural meaning is the outcome.

Example of a study with a taxonomic analysis

Estabrooks et al. (2005) conducted a study that explored staff nurses' sources of practice knowledge, drawing on ethnographic data (individual and card sort interviews and fieldnotes) from four large, urban Canadian teaching hospitals in both adult and pediatric settings. Through taxonomic analysis, knowledge sources were categorized into four main groupings: social interactions, experiential knowledge, documentary sources, and *a priori* knowledge, with detailed structure elicited within each grouping.

Other approaches to ethnographic analysis have also been developed. For example, in her ethnonursing research method, Leininger (2001) provided ethnographers with a data analysis guide to help systematically analyze large amounts of data from their fieldwork. There are four phases to Leininger's ethnonursing data analysis guide. In the first phase, ethnographers collect, describe, and record data. The second phase involves identifying and categorizing descriptors. In the third phase, data are analyzed to discover repetitive patterns in their context. The fourth and final phase involves abstracting major themes and presenting findings.

Example of a study using Leininger's ethnonursing method

Martin et al. (2007) studied the experiences of Canadian health care staff implementing a mental health intervention aimed at transitioning patients from hospital into the community. Using Leininger's ethnonursing method, the researchers conducted focus groups with 49 staff. The themes that emerged included " . . . challenges in roles and responsibilities, relationships with others, the values and beliefs of clients, staff and community, resources, and the processes of care" (p. 105).

Phenomenological Analysis

Schools of phenomenology have developed different approaches to data analysis. Three frequently used methods of data analysis for descriptive phenomenology are the methods of Colaizzi (1978), Giorgi (1985), and Van Kaam (1966), all of whom are from the Duquesne school of phenomenology, based on Husserl's philosophy. Table 16.1 presents a comparison of the steps involved in these three methods of analysis. The basic outcome of all three methods is the description of the meaning of an experience, often through the identification of essential themes. The phenomenologist searches for common patterns shared by particular instances. However, there are some important differences among these three approaches. Colaizzi's method, for example, is the only one that calls for a validation of the

TABLE 16.1 ⊙ COMPARISON OF THREE PHENOMENOLOGICAL METHODS		
COLAIZZI (1978)	GIORGI (1985)	VAN KAAM (1966)
1. Read all protocols to acquire a feeling for them.	1. Read the entire set of protocols to get a sense of the whole.	1. List and group preliminarily the descriptive expressions, which must be agreed upon by expert judges. Final listing presents percentages of these categories in that particular sample.
2. Review each protocol and extract significant statements.	2. Discriminate units from participants' description of phenomenon being studied.	2. Reduce the concrete, vague, and overlapping expressions of the participants to more descriptive terms. (Intersubjective agreement among judges needed.)
3. Spell out the meaning of each significant statement (i.e., formulate meanings).	3. Articulate the psychological insight in each of the meaning units.	3. Eliminate elements not inherent in the phenomenon being studied or that represent blending of two related phenomena.
4. Organize the formulated meanings into clusters of themes. a. Refer these clusters back to the original protocols to validate them. b. Note discrepancies among or between the various clusters, avoiding the temptation of ignoring data or themes that do not fit.	4. Synthesize all of the transformed meaning units into a consistent statement regarding participants' experiences (referred to as the "structure of the experience"); can be expressed on a specific or general level.	4. Write a hypothetical identification and description of the phenomenon being studied.
5. Integrate results into an exhaustive description of the phenomenon under study.		5. Apply hypothetical description to randomly selected cases from the sample. If necessary, revise the hypothesized description, which must then be tested again on a new random sample.
6. Formulate an exhaustive description of the phenomenon under study in as unequivocal a statement of identification as possible.		6. Consider the hypothesized identification as a valid identification and description once preceding operations have been carried out successfully.
7. Ask participants about the findings thus far as a final validating step.		

results by returning to study participants (i.e., member checking). Giorgi's analysis relies solely on the researcher. His view is that it is inappropriate to either return to the participants to validate the findings or to use external judges to review the analysis. Van Kaam's method requires that intersubjective agreement be reached with other expert judges.

Example of a study using Colaizzi's method

Struthers, Eschiti, and Patchell (2008) explored the experience of being an Anishinabe man healer within the dominant Western biomedical culture. The name Anishinabe refers to the various tribes and bands of the Ojibway First Nations people who reside in Canada and the United States. Four traditional indigenous healers were interviewed by the first author, who also collected fieldnotes and journaled the experience. The second author conducted the analysis, following the methods described by Colaizzi and Van Manen, including integrating the results into an exhaustive description that is then formulated into a statement of identification of its fundamental structure, and then validating the analysis by returning to each participant/researcher for comment.

A second school of phenomenology is the Utrecht school. Phenomenologists using this Dutch approach combine characteristics of descriptive and interpretive phenomenology. Van Manen's (1990) method is an example of this combined approach in which researchers try to grasp the essential meaning of the experience being studied. According to Van Manen, themes can be uncovered from descriptions of an experience by three different means: (1) the holistic approach, (2) the selective or highlighting approach, and the (3) detailed or line-by-line approach. In the *holistic approach*, researchers view the text as a whole and try to capture its meanings. In the *selective approach*, researchers underline, highlight, or pull out statements or phrases that seem essential to the experience under study. In the *detailed approach*, researchers analyze every sentence. Once the themes have been identified, they become the objects of reflecting and interpreting through follow-up interviews with participants. Through this process, the essential themes are discovered. In addition to identifying themes from participants' descriptions, Van Manen's method also encourages gleaning thematic descriptions from artistic sources (e.g., from poetry, novels, and other art forms).

Example of a study using Van Manen's method

Spence and Smythe (2008) conducted a phenomenological study of the essential meaning of being a nurse. Van Manen's thematic approach was used to analyze the data from written stories describing "feeling like a nurse" by nine registered nurses in New Zealand, since " . . . stories point the way to meaning that resides in primordial experience. When a person recalls a specific experience, the feelings, mood, action, and context are all there, inextricably linked" (p. 245).

Some qualitative researchers—especially phenomenologists—use *metaphors* as an analytic strategy. A metaphor, a figurative comparison, can be a powerfully creative and expressive tool for qualitative analysts (Carpenter, 2008). As a literary device, metaphors can permit greater insight and understanding in qualitative data analysis in addition to helping link together parts to the whole. A Danish research team studying women's perceptions of risk related to osteoporosis described a building metaphor that emerged from the women's own descriptions.

Example of a metaphor

"A body at risk would deviate from the norm comparable to the foundations of a normal and solid house. The path of future risk could be followed through the crumbling building material of the skeleton, leading to the collapse of the upright position. Since the changes were viewed as irreparable, the conclusion would be that the foundations could not be trusted. As the ultimate endpoint, the body would no longer have the capacity of being a safe home for the person" (Reventlow et al., 2008, p. 107).

A third school of phenomenology is the interpretive approach of Heideggerian hermeneutics. Central to analyzing data in a hermeneutic study is the notion of the **hermeneutic circle.** The circle (which is itself a metaphor) signifies a methodologic process in which, to reach understanding, there is continual movement between the parts and the whole of the text being analyzed. To interpret a text is to understand the possibilities that can be revealed by the text. Gadamer (1975) stressed that to interpret a text, researchers cannot separate themselves from the meanings of the text. Ricoeur (1981) broadened this notion of text to include not just the written text but also any human action or situation.

Example of Gadamerian hermeneutics

Lyneham, Parkinson, and Denholm (2008) studied the experience of intuitive knowing in the clinical setting. Fourteen Australian emergency nurses with 4.5 to 30 years clinical experience were individually interviewed on their experiences of intuition in their practice. Guided by this approach, "the data were viewed from a Gadamerian fusion of the participant's horizons, and a hermeneutical analysis, establishing that intuition was a reality within the participant's practice" (p. 103).

Diekelmann, Allen, and Tanner (1989) have proposed a seven-stage process of data analysis in hermeneutics that involves collaborative effort by a team of researchers. The goal of this process is to describe shared practices and common meanings. Diekelmann and colleagues' stages include the following:

1. Reading all interviews or texts for an overall understanding.
2. Preparing interpretive summaries of each interview.
3. Analyzing selected transcribed interviews or texts by a research team.
4. Resolving any disagreements on interpretation by going back to the text.
5. Identifying recurring themes that reflect common meanings and shared practices of everyday life by comparing and contrasting the texts.
6. Identifying emergent relationships among themes.
7. Presenting a draft of the themes, along with exemplars from texts, to the team; incorporating responses and suggestions into the final draft.

According to Diekelmann and colleagues, the discovery (step 6) of a **constitutive pattern**—a pattern that expresses the relationships among relational themes and is present in all the interviews or texts—forms the highest level of hermeneutical analysis. A situation is constitutive when it gives actual content or style to a person's self-understanding or to a person's way of being in the world.

Example of Diekelmann's hermeneutic analysis

Arthur, Unwin, and Mitchell (2007) used Diekelmann's method to explore English teenagers' experiences of local health services during pregnancy and early parenthood. The researchers analyzed data collected through individual semistructured interview with eight participants, " . . . ensuring that coding, categorizing, and thematasizing remained consistent between researchers" (p. 673). Themes that emerged included Are you being served?; Standing on your own two feet; and The scariest things.

Another data analytic approach for hermeneutic phenomenology is offered by Benner (1994). Her interpretive analysis consists of three interrelated processes: the search for paradigm cases, thematic analysis, and analysis of exemplars. **Paradigm cases** are "strong instances of concerns or ways of being in the world" (Benner, 1994, p. 113). Paradigm cases are used early in the analytic process as a strategy for gaining understanding. Thematic analysis is done to compare and contrast similarities across cases. Lastly, paradigm cases and thematic analysis can be enhanced by *exemplars* that illuminate aspects of a paradigm case or theme. The presentation of paradigm cases and exemplars in research reports allows readers to play a role in consensual validation of the results by deciding whether the cases support the researchers' conclusions.

Example of Benner's hermeneutic analysis
Mahrer-Imhof, Hoffman, and Froelicher (2007) conducted an interpretive phenomenological study of the impact of cardiac disease on Swiss couples' relationships. The researchers interviewed couples, who had experienced hospitalization for an acute cardiac event and subsequently participated in an outpatient rehabilitation program within the past year, both individually and as a couple (dyad). Using Benner's interpretive method, paradigm cases were uncovered and thematic analyses undertaken. Three relational patterns of coping emerged and exemplars were described to support their conclusion that " . . . couples experience cardiac disease as a call to change, and attempt to deal with the illness experience jointly" (p. 519).

Grounded Theory Analysis

As noted in Chapter 10, there are two major approaches to substantive grounded theory analysis. One grounded theory approach was developed by Glaser and Strauss (1967) and another by Strauss and Corbin (1998).

Glaser and Strauss' Grounded Theory Method

Grounded theory in both systems of analysis uses the **constant comparative** method of data analysis. This method involves a comparison of elements present in one data source (e.g., in one interview) with those identified in another. The process is continued until the content of each source has been compared to the content in all sources. In this fashion, commonalities are identified.

The concept of fit is an important element in Glaser and Strauss' grounded theory analysis. **Fit** is the process of identifying characteristics of one piece of data and comparing them with those of other data to determine whether they are similar. Fit is used to sort and reduce data; it enables researchers to determine whether data can be placed in the same category or if they can be related to one another (but data should not be forced or distorted to fit the developing category).

Coding in Glaser and Strauss' grounded theory approach is used to conceptualize data into patterns or concepts. The substance of the topic being studied is conceptualized through **substantive codes,** whereas **theoretical codes** provide insights into how the substantive codes relate to each other.

In the Glaser and Strauss approach, there are two types of substantive codes: open and selective. **Open coding,** used in the first stage of analysis, captures what is going on in the data. Open codes may be the actual words used by participants. Through open coding, data are broken down into incidents, and their similarities and differences are examined. During open coding, researchers ask, "What category or property of a category does this incident indicate?" (Glaser, 1978, p. 57).

There are three levels of open coding that vary in level of abstraction. **Level I codes** (or *in vivo codes*) are derived directly from the language of the substantive area. They have vivid imagery and "grab." Table 16.2 presents five level I codes from interviews in Beck's (2002) grounded theory study on mothering twins, and excerpts associated with those codes.

As researchers constantly compare new level I codes with previously identified ones, they condense them into broader categories—**level II codes.** For example, in Table 16.2, Beck's five level I codes were collapsed into the level II code, "Reaping the blessings." **Level III codes** (or theoretical constructs) are the most abstract codes. These constructs "add scope beyond local meanings" (Glaser, 1978, p. 70) to the generated theory. Collapsing level II codes aids in identifying constructs.

TABLE 16.2 ▶ COLLAPSING LEVEL I CODES INTO THE LEVEL II CODE OF *"REAPING THE BLESSINGS"* (BECK, 2002)

QUOTE	LEVEL I CODE
I enjoy just watching the twins interact so much. Especially now that they are mobile. They are not walking yet but they are crawling. I will tell you they are already playing. Like one will go around the corner and kind of peek around and they play hide and seek. They crawl after each other.	Enjoying Twins
With twins it's amazing. She was sick and she had a fever. He was the one acting sick. She didn't seem like she was sick at all. He was. We watched him for like 6–8 hours. We gave her the medicine and he started calming down. Like WOW! That is so weird. 'Cause you read about it but it's like, Oh come on! You know that doesn't really happen and it does. It's really neat to see.	Amazing
These days it's really neat 'cause you go to the store or you go out and people are like, "Oh, they are twins, how nice." And I say, "Yeah they are. Look, look at my kids."	Getting Attention
I just feel blessed to have two. I just feel like I am twice as lucky as a mom who has one baby. I mean that's the best part. It's just that instead of having one baby to watch grow and change and develop and become a toddler and school age child you have two.	Feeling Blessed
It's very exciting. It's interesting and it's fun to see them and how the twin bond really is. There really is a twin bond. You read about it and you hear about it but until you experience it, you just don't understand. One time they were both crying and they were fed. They were changed and burped. There was nothing wrong. I couldn't figure out what was wrong. So I said to myself, "I am just going to put them together and close the door." I put them in my bed together and they patty caked their hands and put their noses together and just looked at each other and went right to sleep.	Twin Bonding

Example of open codes in grounded theory analysis

Mills, Francis, and Bonner (2008) used a grounded theory approach to explore Australian rural nurses' experiences of professional mentoring. Using data collected through interviews with nine participants, the researchers identified an overall core variable of *cultivating and growing* containing an aspect termed *live my work* which " . . . describes the motivation for experienced rural nurses to create and sustain supportive relationships with new or novice rural nurses" (p. 602). An aspect of this process, *getting to know a stranger*, is derived from a participant's own words (*in vivo*).

Open coding ends when the core category is discovered, and then selective coding begins. The **core category** is a pattern of behaviour that is relevant or problematic for study participants. In **selective coding** (which can also have three levels of abstraction), researchers code only those data that are related to the core variable. One kind of core variable is a **basic social process** (BSP), which evolves over time in two or more phases. All BSPs are core variables, but not all core variables have to be BSPs.

Glaser (1978) provided nine criteria to help researchers decide on a core category:

1. It must be central, meaning that it is related to many categories.
2. It must reoccur frequently in the data.
3. It takes more time to saturate than other categories.
4. It relates meaningfully and easily to other categories.
5. It has clear and grabbing implications for formal theory.

6. It has considerable carry-through.

7. It is completely variable.

8. It is a dimension of the problem.

9. It can be any kind of theoretical code.

Theoretical codes help the grounded theorist to weave the broken pieces of coded data back together again. Glaser (1978) proposed 18 families of theoretical codes that researchers can use to conceptualize how substantive codes relate to each other. Five examples of the 18 families include the following:

⇝ *Process*: stages, phases, passages, and transitions

⇝ *Type*: kinds, styles, and forms

⇝ *Strategy*: tactics, techniques, and manoeuverings

⇝ *Cutting point*: boundaries, critical junctures, and turning points

⇝ *The six Cs*: causes, contexts, contingencies, consequences, covariances, and conditions

Example of theoretical codes

Furlong and Wuest (2008) undertook a grounded theory approach to understand how caregivers manage their self-care needs while caring for a family member with Alzheimer's disease. The Canadian study interviewed nine spousal caregivers with a beginning open-ended question such as "Tell me about how you care for yourself" (p. 1663). Through the three levels of coding, a core variable theory and basic social process of *finding normalcy for self* was uncovered. The researchers applied Glaser's six Cs as well as additional theoretical codes (i.e., process, degrees, dimensions, types, and strategies) to complete the analysis.

Throughout coding and analysis, grounded theory researchers document their ideas about the emerging conceptual scheme in *memos*. Memos preserve ideas that may initially not seem productive but may later prove valuable once further developed. Memos also encourage researchers to reflect on and describe patterns in the data, relationships between categories, and emergent conceptualizations.

Glaser and Strauss' grounded theory method is concerned with the *generation* of categories and hypotheses rather than testing them. The product of the typical grounded theory analysis is a theoretical model that explains a pattern of behaviour that is both relevant and/or problematic for the people in the study. Once the basic problem emerges, the grounded theorist goes on to discover the process these participants experience in coping with or resolving this problem.

Example of a Glaser and Strauss' grounded theory analysis

Figure 16.2 presents the model developed by Beck (2002) in her grounded theory study that conceptualized "Releasing the pause button" as the core category and the process through which mothers of twins progressed as they attempted to resume their lives after giving birth. According to this model, the process involves four phases: "Draining power," "Pausing own life," "Striving to reset," and "Resuming own life" (p. 593). Beck used 10 coding families in her theoretical coding for the "Releasing the pause button" process. The family *cutting point* provides an illustration. Three months seemed to be the turning point for mothers, when life started to become more manageable. Here is an excerpt from an interview that Beck coded as a cutting point: "Three months came around and the twins sort of slept through the night and it made a huge, huge difference" (p. 604).

Strauss and Corbin's Grounded Theory Method

The Strauss and Corbin (1998) approach to grounded theory analysis differs from the original Glaser and Strauss method with regard to method and outcomes. Table 16.3 summarizes major analytic differences between these two methods.

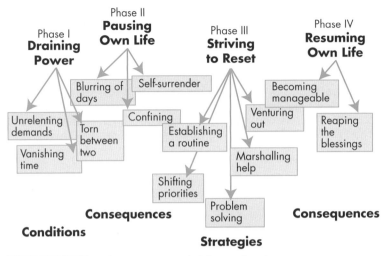

FIGURE 16.2   Beck's (2002) grounded theory of mothering twins.

Glaser (1978) stressed that to generate a grounded theory, the basic problem must emerge from the data—it must be discovered. The theory is, from the very start, grounded in the data, rather than starting with a preconceived problem. Strauss and Corbin, however, argued that the research itself is only one of four possible sources of the research problem. Research problems can, for example, come from the literature or from researchers' personal and professional experience.

The Strauss and Corbin method involves three types of coding: open, axial, and selective. In **open coding,** data are broken down into parts and compared for similarities and differences. Similar actions and events are grouped together into categories. In open coding, the researcher focuses on generating categories and their properties. In **axial coding,** the analyst systematically develops categories and links them with subcategories. Strauss and Corbin (1998) term this process of relating categories and their subcategories as "axial because coding occurs around the axis of a category, linking categories at the level of properties and dimensions" (p. 123). **Selective coding** is a process in which the findings are integrated and refined. The first step in integrating the findings is to decide on the **central category** (or core category), which is the main theme of the research. Recommended techniques to facilitate identifying the central category are writing the storyline, using diagrams, and reviewing and organizing memos.

TABLE 16.3   COMPARISON OF GLASER & STRAUSS AND STRAUSS & CORBIN'S METHODS

	GLASER AND STRAUSS	STRAUSS AND CORBIN
Initial data analysis	Breaking down and conceptualizing data involves comparison of incident to incident so patterns emerge	Breaking down and conceptualizing data includes taking apart a single sentence, observation, and incident
Types of coding	Open, selective, theoretical	Open, axial, selective
Connections between categories	18 coding families	Paradigm model (conditions, contexts, action/interactional strategies, and consequences)
Outcome	Emergent theory (discovery)	Conceptual description (verification)

The outcome of the Strauss and Corbin approach is a full conceptual description. The original grounded theory method (Glaser & Strauss, 1967), by contrast, generates a theory that explains how a basic social problem that emerged from the data is processed in a social setting.

Example of a Strauss and Corbin grounded theory analysis
O'Brien, Evans, and White-McDonald (2002) used the Strauss and Corbin method in their study of women's coping with severe nausea and vomiting during pregnancy. Interviews with 24 women admitted to a large tertiary care hospital in western Canada were read and coded by at least two researchers. Lines, paragraphs, and words were coded and emerging categories were discussed and finalized by consensus. "Data were then reconstructed by linking categories and subcategories within a set of relationships so that the context in which the experience occurred could be described (axial coding). A concept (i.e., core category) around which all emerging categories could be related was selected" (p. 304). The core category was the process of increasingly complete isolation to cope with unrelenting and severe symptoms.

CRITIQUING QUALITATIVE ANALYSES

The task of evaluating a qualitative analysis is not an easy one, even for experienced researchers. The difficulty lies mainly in the fact that readers must accept largely on faith that researchers exercised good judgment and insight in coding the narrative materials, developing a thematic analysis, and integrating the materials into a meaningful whole. This is because researchers are seldom able to include more than a handful of examples of actual data in a research report and because the process of inductively abstracting meaning from data is difficult to describe.

In a critique of qualitative analysis, a primary task usually is determining whether researchers took sufficient steps to validate inferences and conclusions. A major focus of a critique of qualitative analyses, then, is whether the researchers have adequately documented the analytic process. The report should provide information about the approach used to analyze the data. For example, a report for a grounded theory study should indicate whether the researchers used the Glaser and Strauss method or the Strauss and Corbin method.

Quantitative analyses can be evaluated in terms of the adequacy of specific analytic decisions (e.g., did the researcher use the appropriate statistical test?). Critiquing analytic decisions is substantially less clearcut in a qualitative study. For example, it typically would be inappropriate to critique a phenomenological analysis for following Giorgi's approach rather than Colaizzi's approach. Both are respected methods of conducting a phenomenological study and analyzing the resulting data (although phenomenologists themselves may have cogent reasons for preferring one approach over the other).

One aspect of a qualitative analysis that *can* be critiqued, however, is whether the researchers have documented that they have used one approach consistently and have been faithful to the integrity of its procedures. For example, if researchers say they are using the Glaser and Strauss approach to grounded theory analysis, they should not also include elements from the Strauss and Corbin method. An even more serious problem occurs when, as sometimes happens, the researchers "muddle" traditions. For example, researchers who describe their study as a grounded theory study should not have a presentation of *themes* because grounded theory analysis does not yield themes. Furthermore, researchers who attempt to blend elements from two traditions may not have a clear grasp of the analytic precepts of either one. For example, a researcher who claims to have undertaken an ethnography using a grounded theory approach to analysis may not be well informed about the underlying goals and philosophies of these two traditions.

Some further guidelines that may be helpful in evaluating qualitative analyses are presented in Box 16.2.

BOX 16.2 GUIDELINES FOR CRITIQUING QUALITATIVE ANALYSES

1. Given the nature of the data, was the data analysis approach appropriate for the research design?
2. Is the category scheme described? If so, does the scheme appear logical and complete? Does there seem to be unnecessary overlap or redundancy in the categories?
3. Were manual methods used to index and organize the data, or was a computer program used?
4. Does the report adequately describe the process by which the actual analysis was performed? Does the report indicate whose approach to data analysis was used (e.g., Glaser and Strauss or Strauss and Corbin, in grounded theory studies)? Was this method consistently and appropriately applied?
5. What major themes or processes emerged? If excerpts from the data are provided, do the themes appear to capture the meaning of the narratives—that is, does it appear that the researcher adequately interpreted the data and conceptualized the themes? Is the analysis parsimonious—could two or more themes be collapsed into a broader and perhaps more useful conceptualization?
6. What evidence does the report provide that the analysis is accurate and replicable?
7. Were data displayed in a manner that allows you to verify the researcher's conclusions? Was a conceptual map, model, or diagram effectively displayed to communicate important processes?
8. Was the context of the phenomenon adequately described? Does the report give you a clear picture of the social or emotional world of study participants?
9. Did the analysis yield a meaningful and insightful picture of the phenomenon under study? Is the resulting theory or description trivial or obvious?

RESEARCH EXAMPLES AND CRITICAL THINKING ACTIVITIES

EXAMPLE 1 ■ Analysis in a Grounded Theory Study

Aspects of a grounded theory study, featuring terms and concepts discussed in this chapter, are presented below, followed by some questions to guide critical thinking.

Study

"'Tied down'—The process of becoming bedridden through gradual local confinement" (Zegelin, 2008)

Statement of Purpose

The purpose of this study was to understand the causes and types of being bedridden.

Method

The author used Strauss and Corbin's grounded theory methods to explore the complexity of the development of the bedridden state. She conducted interviews with 32 elderly bedridden persons in a mix of long-term or home care in Germany. The timeframe for being bedridden ranged from 2 weeks to 4 years. Although 32 interviews were undertaken, saturation was achieved after 28—"Survey, coding and analysis were used alternatively in this study and the results were each checked again in the field and the continued progression of the study was then determined by the data itself (theory-led selection)" (p. 2296).

Analysis

Data analysis was ongoing as new interviews were conducted. Constant comparison among concepts and incidents was used to identify relevant processes, connections, and contextual conditions. "In constant comparison, various factors such as location, age, sex, status of illness, and length of recumbency could be contrasted with each other" (p. 2296). A phase model of being bedridden was developed, which served as a frame of reference and the primary finding.

Key Findings

- The data revealed phases of development and a range of factors influencing the state of becoming bedridden.

- The five phases were "instability," "incident," "immobility in the room," "local confinement," and "bedridden" (p. 2297).

- The fourth stage, "local confinement," involved being in one place and dependent on others for switching between their bed or wheelchair—being "tied down" or "chained up" (p. 2298). Most of the interviewees were at this phase.

CRITICAL THINKING SUGGESTIONS

1. Answer questions 1 through 9 from Box 16.2 (p. 336) regarding this study.

2. Also answer the following targeted question, which may assist you in further assessing aspects of this study:

   a. Zegelin comments that there is no existing research on this topic. Why do you think she chose a grounded theory approach in light of this?

3. If the results of this study are trustworthy, what are some of the uses to which the findings might be put into clinical practice?

EXAMPLE 2 ■ Analysis in an Ethnographic Study

Aspects of an ethnographic nursing study, featuring terms and concepts discussed in this chapter, are presented below, followed by some questions to guide critical thinking.

Study

"Sources of practice knowledge among nurses" (Estabrooks et al., 2005)

Statement of Purpose

The purpose of this study was to explore and identify nurses' sources of practice knowledge.

Method

This report was based on two large studies that used an ethnographic case study design to examine factors that influence nurses' use of research in their practice. The cases for the first study were five pediatric units, and those for the second were two adult patient care units, drawn from four tertiary level hospitals in Alberta and Ontario. Data included transcribed individual and focus group interviews with nurses in the hospitals, as well as fieldnotes from participant observation. Card-sorting interviews were also conducted to uncover the structure of the knowledge sources domain. In each setting, data were collected by a research assistant (a master's prepared nurse), who spent 6 months on the unit.

Analysis

Interview transcripts and fieldnotes were entered into the computer program called NUD*IST for subsequent coding and analysis. Data were coded using a line-by-line process. Initial codes, which were based on a reading of the first interviews, were reviewed by the research team until consensus on the coding scheme was achieved. Spradley's procedures were used to develop a taxonomy. "The process was a dynamic one, involving repeated re-categorization of initial categories, and further sorting and analysis of each large (and saturated) category" (p. 462).

Key Findings

Nurses' sources of practice knowledge were categorized into four broad groupings, and these groupings formed the structure of the taxonomy.

- The category of *social interactions* dominated the findings; these interactions are processes through which nurses communicate and exchange information between and among each other, other health care professionals, and patients.

(Research Examples and Critical Thinking Activities continues on page 338)

Research Examples and Critical Thinking Activities (continued)

- *Experiential knowledge*, the second category, is knowledge gained during the regular course of nursing practice.

- *Documentary sources* included written and printed materials, including unit-based sources (e.g., patients' charts) and off-unit sources (e.g., material in journals, on the Internet); use of these latter sources was limited.

- *A priori knowledge* is knowledge that a nurse brings to the unit, including knowledge gained in nursing school and from prior experiences.

CRITICAL THINKING SUGGESTIONS

1. Answer questions 1 through 9 from Box 16.2 (p. 336) regarding this study.

2. Also answer the following targeted questions, which may assist you in further assessing aspects of this study:
   a. Comment on the amount of data that had to be analyzed in this study.
   b. What parts of Spradley's analytic method appear to have been followed in this study? What was the *domain* in this study?

3. If the results of this study are trustworthy, what are some of the uses to which the findings might be put into clinical practice?

EXAMPLE 3 ■ Analysis in a Phenomenological Study

1. Read the "Method" and "Findings" sections from the study by Woodgate, Ateah, and Secco in Appendix B of this book, and then answer the relevant questions in Box 16.1 (p. 322).

2. Also consider the following targeted questions, which may further sharpen your critical thinking skills and assist you in assessing aspects of the study's merit:
   a. Comment on the applicability of Van Manen's method in open-ended questioning and data analysis.
   b. Describe the steps involved in "selective highlighting."

Summary Points

⇒ Qualitative analysis is a challenging, labour-intensive activity, guided by few standardized rules.

⇒ Although there are no universal strategies, three prototypical analytic styles have been identified: (1) a **template analysis style** that involves the development of an analysis guide (*template*) to sort the data; (2) an **editing analysis style** that involves an interpretation of the data on which a **category scheme** is based; and (3) an **immersion/crystallization style** that is characterized by the analyst's total immersion in and reflection of text materials.

⇒ Qualitative analysis typically involves four intellectual processes: comprehending, synthesizing, theorizing, and **recontextualizing** (exploration of the developed theory vis-à-vis its applicability to other settings or groups).

⇒ The first major step in analyzing qualitative data is to organize and index the data for easy retrieval, typically by coding the content according to a category scheme.

⇒ Traditionally, researchers have organized their coded data by developing **conceptual files,** which are physical files in which excerpts of data relevant to specific categories are placed. Now, however, computer programs are widely used to perform basic indexing functions and to facilitate data analysis.

⇒ The actual analysis of data begins with a search for patterns, regularities, or **themes** in the data, which involves the discovery not only of commonalities across subjects but also of natural variation in the data.

⇒ Another analytic step generally involves a validation of the thematic analysis. Some researchers use **quasi-statistics,** a tabulation of the frequency with which certain themes or relations are supported by the data.

⇒ In a final analytic step, analysts try to weave thematic strands together into an integrated picture of the phenomenon under investigation.

⇒ In ethnographies, analysis begins as the researcher enters the field. Ethnographers continually search for *patterns* in the behaviour and expressions of study participants.

⇒ One approach to analyzing ethnographic data is Spradley's method, which involves four levels of data analysis: *domain analysis* (identifying **domains,** or units of cultural knowledge); *taxonomic analysis* (selecting key domains and constructing **taxonomies** or systems of classification); *componential analysis* (comparing and contrasting terms in a domain); and a *theme analysis* (to uncover cultural themes).

⇒ Leininger's method for ethnonursing research involves four phases: collecting and recording data; categorizing descriptors; searching for repetitive patterns; and abstracting major themes.

⇒ There are various approaches to phenomenological analysis, including the descriptive methods of Colaizzi, Giorgi, and Van Kaam, in which the goal is to find common patterns of experiences shared by particular instances.

⇒ In Van Manen's approach, which involves efforts to grasp the essential meaning of the experience being studied, researchers search for themes using a *holistic approach* (viewing text as a whole); a *selective approach* (pulling out key statements and phrases); or a *detailed approach* (analyzing every sentence).

⇒ Central to analyzing data in a hermeneutic study is the notion of the **hermeneutic circle,** which signifies a methodological process in which there is continual movement between the parts and the whole of the text under analysis.

⇒ In hermeneutics, there are several choices for data analysis. Diekelmann's method calls for the discovery of a **constitutive pattern,** which expresses the relationships among themes. Benner's approach consists of three processes: searching for **paradigm cases,** thematic analysis, and analysis of *exemplars.*

⇒ Grounded theory uses the **constant comparative** method of data analysis.

⇒ One approach to grounded theory is the Glaser and Strauss method, in which there are two broad types of codes: **substantive codes** (in which the empirical substance of the topic is conceptualized) and **theoretical codes** (in which the relationships among the substantive codes are conceptualized).

⇒ Substantive coding involves **open coding** to capture what is going on in the data, and then **selective coding** (in which only variables relating to a core category is coded). The **core category,** a behaviour pattern that has relevance for participants, is sometimes a **basic social process** (BSP) that involves an evolutionary process of coping or adaptation.

⇒ In the Glaser and Strauss method, open codes begin with **level I** (*in vivo*) **codes,** which are collapsed into a higher level of abstraction in **level II codes.** Level II codes are then used to formulate **level III codes,** which are theoretical constructs.

⇒ The Strauss and Corbin method is an alternative grounded theory method whose outcome is a full conceptual description. This approach to grounded theory analysis involves three types of coding: open coding (in which categories are generated), **axial coding** (where categories are linked with subcategories), and selective coding (in which the findings are integrated and refined).

➢ Some researchers identify neither a specific approach nor a specific research tradition; rather, they might say that they used qualitative **content analysis** as their analytic method.

STUDIES CITED IN CHAPTER 16*

*This reference list contains only those studies that were cited in this chapter. Citations pertaining to theoretical, methodologic, or nonempirical work are included together in a separate section at the end of the book (beginning on page 399).

Arthur, A., Unwin, S., & Mitchell, T. (2007). Teenage mothers' experiences of maternity services: A qualitative study. *British Journal of Midwifery, 15*(11), 672–677.

Becker, H. S. (1970). *Sociological work*. Chicago: Aldine.

Beck, C. T. (2002). Releasing the pause button: Mothering twins during the first year of life. *Qualitative Health Research, 12*, 593–608.

Beck, C. T. (2006). Anniversary of birth trauma: Failure to rescue. *Nursing Research, 55*(6), 381–390.

Benner, P. (1994). The tradition and skill of interpretive phenomenology in studying health, illness, and caring practices. In P. Benner (Ed.), *Interpretive phenomenology* (pp. 99–127). Thousand Oaks, CA: Sage.

Carpenter, J. (2008). Metaphors in qualitative research: Shedding light or casting shadows? *Research in Nursing & Health, 31*(3), 274–282.

Colaizzi, P. (1978). Psychological research as the phenomenologist views it. In R. Valle & M. King (Eds.), *Existential phenomenological alternatives for psychology*. New York: Oxford University Press.

Crabtree, B. F., & Miller, W. L. (Eds.). (1999). *Doing qualitative research* (2nd ed.). Newbury Park, CA: Sage.

DeSantis, L., & Ugarriza, D. N. (2000). The concept of theme as used in qualitative nursing research. *Western Journal of Nursing Research, 22*, 351–372.

Diekelmann, N., Allen, D., & Tanner, C. (1989). *The NLN criteria for appraisal of baccalaureate programs: A critical hermeneutic analysis*. New York: NLN Press.

Estabrooks, C. A., Rutakumwa, W., O'Leary, K. A., et al. (2005). Sources of practice knowledge among nurses. *Qualitative Health Research, 15*(4), 460–476.

Fetterman, D. M. (1998). *Ethnography: Step by step* (2nd ed.) Newbury Park, CA: Sage.

Furlong, K. E., & Wuest, J. (2008). Self-care behaviors of spouses caring for significant others with Alzheimer's disease: The emergence of self-care worthiness as a salient condition. *Qualitative Health Research, 18*(12), 1662–1672.

Gadamer, H. G. (1975). *Truth and method*. (G. Borden & J. Cumming, Trans.). London: Sheed and Ward.

Giorgi, A. (1985). *Phenomenology and psychological research*. Pittsburgh: Duquesne University Press.

Glaser, B. G., & Strauss, A. L. (1967). *The discovery of grounded theory: Strategies for qualitative research*. Chicago: Aldine.

King, N. (1998). Template analysis. In C. Cassell & G. Symon (Eds.), *Qualitative methods and analysis in organizational research* (pp. 118–134). London: Sage.

Leininger, M. (2001). *Culture care diversity and universality: A theory of nursing*. Boston: Jones and Bartlett.

Letourneau, N., Duffett-Leger, L., Stewart, M., et al. (2007). Canadian mothers' perceived support needs during postpartum depression. *Journal of Obstetric, Gynecologic, & Neonatal Nursing, 36*(5), 441–449.

Lyneham, J., Parkinson, C., & Denholm, C. (2008). Intuition in emergency nursing: A phenomenological study. *International Journal of Nursing Practice, 14*(2), 101–108.

Mahrer-Imhof, R., Hoffmann, A., & Froelicher, E. S. (2007). Impact of cardiac disease on couples' relationships. *Journal of Advanced Nursing, 57*(5), 513–521.

Martin, M. L., Jensen, E., Coatsworth-Puspoky, R., Forchuk, C., Lysiak-Globe, T., & Beal, G. (2007). Integrating an evidenced-based research intervention in the discharge of mental health clients. *Archives of Psychiatric Nursing, 21*(2), 101–111.

Mills, J., Francis, K., & Bonner, A. (2008). Getting to know a stranger—rural nurses' experiences of mentoring: A grounded theory. *International Journal of Nursing Studies, 45*(4), 599–607.

Morse, J. M., & Field, P. A. (1995). *Qualitative research methods for health professionals* (2nd ed.). Thousand Oaks, CA: Sage.

O'Brien, B., Evans, M., & White-McDonald, E. (2002). Isolation from "being alive": coping with severe nausea and vomiting of pregnancy. *Nursing Research, 51*(5), 302–8.

Polit, D. F., London, A., & Martinez, J. M. (2000). *Food security and hunger in poor, mother-headed families in four U.S. cities*. New York: MDRC.

Read, T., & Wuest, J. (2007). Daughters caring for dying parents: A process of relinquishing. *Qualitative Health Research*, *17*(7), 932–944.

Reventlow, S. D., Overgaard, I. S., Hvas, L., & Malterud, K. (2008). Metaphorical mediation in women's perceptions of risk related to osteoporosis: A qualitative interview study. *Health, Risk & Society*, *10*(2), 103–115.

Ricoeur, P. (1981). *Hermeneutics and the social sciences*. (J. Thompson, Trans. & Ed.). New York: Cambridge University Press.

Sorensen, L. V., Waldorff, F. B., & Waldemar, G. (2008). Early counseling and support for patients with mild Alzheimer's disease and their caregivers: A qualitative study on outcome. *Aging & Mental Health*, *12*(4), 444–450.

Spradley, J. P. (1979). *The ethnographic interview*. New York: Holt, Rinehart, and Winston.

Spence, D., & Smythe, E. (2008). Feeling like a nurse: Recalling the spirit of nursing. *Journal of Holistic Nursing*, *26*(4), 243–252.

Strauss, A. L., & Corbin, J. M. (1998). *Basics of qualitative research: Techniques and procedures for developing grounded theory* (2nd ed.). Thousand Oaks, CA: Sage.

Struthers, R., Eschiti, V. S., & Patchell, B. (2008). The experience of being an Anishinabe man healer: Ancient healing in a modern world. *Journal of Cultural Diversity*, *15*(2), 70–75.

Thompson, D. S., O'Leary, K., Jensen, E., Scott-Findlay, S., O'Brien-Pallas, L., & Estabrooks, C. A. (2008). The relationship between busyness and research utilization: It is about time. *Journal of Clinical Nursing*, *17*(4), 539–548.

Van Kaam, A. (1966). *Existential foundations of psychology*. Pittsburgh: Duquesne University Press.

Van Manen, M. (1990). *Researching lived experience*. New York: State University of New York.

Zegelin, A. (2008). "Tied down"—The process of becoming bedridden through gradual local confinement. *Journal of Clinical Nursing*, *17*(17), 2294–2301.

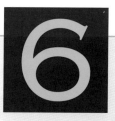

Critical Appraisal and Utilization of Nursing Research

17 Critiquing Research Reports

On completion of this chapter, you will be able to:

1. Describe aspects of a study's findings important to consider in developing an interpretation of quantitative and qualitative findings

2. Evaluate researchers' interpretation of their results

3. Describe the purpose and dimensions of a research critique

4. Conduct a comprehensive critique of a qualitative or quantitative research report

5. Define new terms in the chapter

Throughout this book, we have provided questions and suggestions for critiquing various aspects of nursing research reports. This chapter describes the purpose of a research critique and offers further tips on how to evaluate research reports. An important aspect of a research critique is the reviewer's interpretation of the study findings. Therefore, we begin this chapter by offering some suggestions on interpreting study results.

INTERPRETING STUDY RESULTS

The analysis of research data provides the study *results*, which need to be evaluated and interpreted—often a challenging task. *Interpretation* should take into account the study's aims, its theoretical underpinnings, the existing body of related research, and the limitations of the research methods used. The interpretive task involves a consideration of the following:

➢ The credibility and accuracy of the results

➢ The meaning of the results

➢ The importance of the results

➢ The extent to which the results can be generalized or have potential use in other contexts

➢ The implications for practice, theory, or research

In this section, we review issues relating to these interpretive aspects for quantitative and qualitative research reports.

Interpreting Quantitative Results

Quantitative research results often offer readers more interpretive opportunities than qualitative ones—in large part because a quantitative report summarizes most of the study data (e.g., in statistical tables), whereas qualitative reports contain only illustrative examples of the data. When reading quantitative reports, you will need to give careful thought to the possible meaning behind the numbers. Your interpretations can then be compared to those of the researchers, who discuss their views on the meaning and implications of the study results in the "Discussion" section of their reports.

The Credibility of Quantitative Results

One of the first tasks in interpreting quantitative results is assessing their accuracy. A thorough assessment of the credibility of the results relies on critical thinking skills and on your understanding of research methods. The evaluation should be based on an analysis of evidence, not on "gut feelings." Both external and internal evidence can be brought to bear. External evidence comes primarily from the body of prior research. If the results are consistent, the credibility of the findings is enhanced. If the results are inconsistent with prior research, possible reasons for the discrepancy should be sought. What was different about the way the data were collected, the sample was selected, key variables were operationalized, and so forth? You should also consider whether the findings are consistent with common sense and with your own clinical experiences.

Internal evidence for the accuracy of the findings comes from an evaluation of the methods used. You will need to evaluate carefully all the major methodologic decisions made in executing the study to determine whether alternative decisions might have yielded different results. This issue is discussed later in this chapter.

A critical analysis of the research methods and conceptualization almost inevitably indicates some limitations. These limitations must be taken into account in interpreting the results and in contrasting your interpretation with that of the researchers themselves.

The Meaning of Quantitative Results

Quantitative results are usually in the form of test statistic values and probability levels, which do not in and of themselves confer meaning. The statistical results must be translated conceptually and interpreted. In this section, we discuss the interpretation of research outcomes within a statistical hypothesis-testing context.

> **TIP**
>
> Many research reports do not formally state hypotheses, but rather present research questions or purpose statements (see Chapter 6). However, every time researchers use an inferential statistic (e.g., a *t* test), they are using statistics to test a hypothesis. Research hypotheses being tested often relate to the following: the groups being compared are significantly different or study variables are significantly related to one another. When hypotheses are not stated but statistical tests are performed, you have to infer the hypotheses.

Interpreting Hypothesized Significant Results. When statistical tests support the researcher's hypotheses, the task of interpreting the results may be straightforward because the rationale for the hypotheses typically offers an explanation of what the findings mean. However, hypotheses can be correct even when the researcher's explanation of what is going on is not. As a reviewer, you need to evaluate whether the researchers went beyond the data in interpreting the results. For example, suppose a nurse researcher hypothesized that a relationship exists between a pregnant woman's level of anxiety about the labour and delivery experience and the number of children she has already borne. The study data reveal that a negative relationship between anxiety levels and parity does exist ($r = -.40$; $p < .05$). The researcher concludes that childbirth experience reduces anxiety. Is this conclusion supported by the data? The conclusion seems logical, but, in fact, there is nothing within the data that leads to this interpretation. An important, indeed critical, research precept is: correlation does not mean causation. The finding that two variables are related offers no evidence about which of the two variables—if either—caused the other. Alternative explanations for the findings should always be considered. If competing interpretations can be excluded on the basis of the data or previous research findings, so much the better, but interpretations should always be given adequate competition.

Throughout the interpretation process, you should bear in mind that the support of research hypotheses through statistical testing never constitutes proof of their validity. Hypothesis testing is probabilistic, and it is always possible that obtained relationships were due to chance.

Example of corroboration of a hypothesis

Using a randomized controlled trial, Fillion et al. (2008) studied the effect of a brief intervention combining stress management and physical activity, on various outcomes including fatigue among women with breast cancer. In support of one of their hypotheses, at 3-months, a significant reduction in fatigue was found for the experimental group when compared to the control group.

This study is a good example of reliance on a robust research design, a randomized controlled trial (RCT), to rule out possible competing explanations for the results. If researchers had used a weaker design (e.g., non-experimental), they would have encountered various challenges in interpreting their findings and having confidence in the study's conclusions.

Interpreting Nonsignificant Results. Nonsignificant results pose interpretive problems. Standard statistical procedures are geared toward disconfirmation of the null hypothesis. Failure to reject a null hypothesis (i.e., obtaining results indicating no relationship between the independent and dependent variables) could occur for either of two reasons: (1) because the null hypothesis is true (i.e., there really is no relationship among research variables) or (2) because the null hypothesis is false (i.e., a true relationship exists but the data failed to show it). Neither you nor the researchers know which is right. In the first situation (a true null hypothesis), the problem is likely to lie in the conceptualization that led the researcher to posit the hypotheses. The second situation (a false null hypothesis), by contrast, generally reflects methodologic limitations, such as internal validity problems, a small or atypical sample, or a weak statistical procedure. Thus, the interpretation must consider both substantive and methodologic reasons for nonsignificant results.

Whatever the underlying cause, there is never justification for interpreting a retained null hypothesis as proof of the absence of a relationship among variables. The safest interpretation is that nonsignificant findings represent a lack of evidence for either truth or falsity of the hypothesis.

Note, however, that there is a decided bias against publishing the results of studies in which the results are nonsignificant. This reflects the concern of those making publication decisions that nonsignificant results are likely to reflect methodologic limitations.

Example of nonsignificant results

In a randomized clinical trial with a 2×2 factorial design, Lespérance and colleagues (2007) studied the effects of interpersonal psychotherapy (IPT) on depression in 284 patients with coronary artery disease recruited from nine Canadian academic centres. The researchers hypothesized that patients receiving IPT show significantly lower depression than those receiving usual care. However, this hypothesis was not supported. Group differences pertaining to the main outcome variable were not significant ($p = .06$)

Because statistical procedures are designed to provide support for the *rejection* of null hypotheses, they are not well suited for testing actual research hypotheses about the *absence* of relationships between variables or about *equivalence* between groups. Yet sometimes this is exactly what researchers want to do—and this is especially true in clinical situations in which the goal is to determine whether one practice is just as effective as another. When the actual *research* hypothesis is null (i.e., a prediction of no group difference or no relationship), stringent additional strategies must be used to provide supporting evidence. For one thing, it is imperative to perform a power analysis to demonstrate that the risk of a Type II error is small. There may also be clinical standards that can be used to corroborate that nonsignificant— but predicted—results can be accepted as consistent with the research hypothesis.

Example of nonsignificant results supporting a hypothesis

In a two-centre randomized equivalence trial, Beaver et al. (2009) examined the effectiveness of traditional hospital follow-up versus telephone follow-up by clinical nurse specialists on psychological morbidity among women with breast cancer having completed treatment. The researchers hypothesized that the group receiving telephone follow-ups would experience no more psychological morbidity, specifically anxiety, than the group receiving hospital follow-ups. Their hypothesis was supported; differences between the two groups were not significant.

Interpreting Unhypothesized Significant Results. Although this does not often happen, there are situations in which researchers obtain significant results that are the opposite of the research hypothesis—that is, *unhypothesized significant results.* For example, a researcher might predict a negative relationship between patient satisfaction with nursing care and the length of stay in the hospital, but a significant *positive* relationship might be found. In such cases, it is less likely that the methods are flawed than that the reasoning or theory is incorrect. In attempting to explain such findings, you should pay particular attention to the results of previous research and alternative theories. It is also useful to consider, however, whether there is anything unusual about the sample that might have led participants to behave or respond atypically.

Example of unhypothesized significant results

Willem, Buelens, and DeJongue (2007) studied nurses' job satisfaction and factors that might affect their level of satisfaction. One hypothesis was that the more formalization there is in a hospital, the less satisfied nurses are with task requirements, organizational policies, and interaction among colleagues. However, formalization was found to be significantly associated with *higher* job satisfaction.

Interpreting Mixed Results. The interpretive process is often complicated by *mixed results*: some hypotheses are supported by the data, whereas others are not. Or a hypothesis may be accepted when one measure of the dependent variable is used but rejected with a different measure. When only some results run counter to a conceptual scheme or prior findings, the research methods likely deserve critical scrutiny. Differences in the validity and reliability of the various measures may account for such discrepancies, for example. On the other hand, mixed results may suggest that a theory needs to be qualified, or that certain constructs within the theory need to be reconceptualized.

Example of mixed results

Using a single-blind randomized crossover design, Johnston et al. (2008) studied the effect of kangaroo mother care (KMC) on pain from heel lance in preterm neonates between 28 and 32 weeks of gestation. Repeated-measures analysis of covariance was used to evaluate group differences between the experimental group and the control group. The researchers found mixed results as KMC was shown to significantly lower pain at 90 seconds postintervention but not at 30, 60, or 120 seconds. Although the researchers suggested that KMC has a slightly delayed effective response, its ineffectiveness at 120 seconds raises questions about sustained effects.

The Importance of Quantitative Results

In quantitative studies, results supporting the hypotheses are described as being significant. A careful analysis of study results involves an evaluation of whether, in addition to being statistically significant, they are important.

The fact that statistical significance was attained in testing the hypothesis does not necessarily mean the results were of value. Statistical significance indicates that the results were unlikely to be due to chance. This means that the observed group differences or relationships were probably real—but not necessarily important. With large samples, even modest relationships can be statistically significant. For instance, with a sample of 500 participants, a correlation coefficient of .10 is significant at the .05 level, but a relationship of this magnitude might have little practical value. As a reviewer, therefore, you should pay attention to the numeric values obtained in an analysis in addition to the significance level when assessing the implications of the findings.

Conversely, the absence of statistically significant results does not mean that the results are unimportant—although, because of problems in interpreting nonsignificant results, the case is more complex. Suppose we compared two methods of making a clinical assessment (e.g., pain) and retained the null hypothesis (i.e., found no statistically significant differences between the two methods). If the study involved a small sample, the nonsignificant results would be ambiguous. If a very large sample was used, however, the probability of a Type II error would be low. It might then be concluded that the two procedures yield equally accurate assessments. If one of these procedures were more efficient, less stressful, or less costly than the other, the nonsignificant findings could, indeed, be clinically important.

It should be noted that, especially in an evidence-based practice environment, research findings do not necessarily need to reveal new insights to be important. To build a strong base of knowledge upon which practice decisions are made, findings that can be replicated are quite important.

The Generalizability of Quantitative Results

Another aspect of quantitative results that you should assess is their generalizability. The aim of most nursing research is to develop evidence for use in nursing practice. Therefore, an important interpretive question is whether the intervention will work or whether the observed relationships will hold in other settings, with other people. Part of the interpretive process involves asking the question: To what groups, environments, and conditions can the results of the study be applied?

The Implications of Quantitative Results

After you have formed conclusions about the accuracy, meaning, importance, and generalizability of the results, you are ready to draw inferences about their implications. You might consider the implications of the findings with respect to theory development or future research (What should other researchers working in this area do—what is the right "next step?") However, you are most likely to consider the implications for nursing practice. (How, if at all, should the results be used by other nurses in their practice—or by me in my own work as a nurse?) Of course, if you have reached the conclusion that the results have limited credibility or importance, they may be of little utility to your practice.

Interpreting Qualitative Results

It is usually difficult for readers of qualitative research reports to interpret qualitative findings thoroughly because authors have to be selective in the amount and types of data included in the report. Nevertheless, you should strive to consider the same five interpretive dimensions for a qualitative study as for a quantitative one.

The Credibility of Qualitative Results

As with the case of quantitative reports, you should question whether the results of a qualitative inquiry are believable. It is reasonable to expect authors of qualitative reports to provide evidence of the credibility of the findings, as described in Chapter 14—although this does not always happen. Because readers of qualitative reports are exposed to only a portion of the data, they must rely on researchers' efforts to corroborate findings through such mechanisms as peer debriefings, member checks, audits, and triangulation.

TIP

Even when peer debriefings or member checks have been undertaken, you should realize that they do not unequivocally establish evidence that the results are believable. For example, member checks may not always be effective in controlling bias. Perhaps some participants are too polite to disagree with the researcher's interpretations. Or perhaps they become intrigued with a conceptualization that they themselves would have never developed on their own—a conceptualization that is not necessarily accurate.

In thinking about the believability of qualitative results—as with quantitative results—it is advisable to adopt the posture of a person who needs to be persuaded about the researcher's conceptualization and to expect the researcher to marshal solid evidence with which to persuade you. It is also appropriate to consider whether the researcher's conceptualization of the phenomenon is consistent with common clinical experiences and insights.

The Meaning of Qualitative Results

In qualitative studies, interpretation and analysis of the data occur virtually simultaneously: researchers interpret the data as they categorize them, develop a thematic analysis, and integrate the themes into a unified whole. Efforts to validate the qualitative analysis validate interpretations as well. Thus, unlike quantitative analyses, the meaning of the data flows from qualitative analysis.

Nevertheless, prudent qualitative researchers hold their interpretations up for closer scrutiny—self-scrutiny as well as review by peers and outside reviewers. Thus, for qualitative researchers as well as quantitative researchers, it is important to consider possible alternative explanations for the findings and to take into account methodologic or other limitations that could have affected study results.

Example of researcher self-scrutiny during analysis
Clarke, Butler, and Esplen (2008) conducted a qualitative study guided by grounded theory to understand the experiences of BRCA1/2 carriers in communicating genetic information to their offspring. Data were collected from 24 women during 12 videotaped supportive–expressive group intervention sessions. The researchers independently reviewed verbatim transcripts of the sessions and subsequently held meetings to ensure a high degree of consistency in interpretation.

The Importance of Qualitative Results

Qualitative research is especially productive when it is used to describe and explain poorly understood phenomena. But the amount of prior research on a topic is not a sufficient barometer for deciding whether the findings can make a contribution to nursing knowledge. The phenomenon must be one that merits rigorous scrutiny. For example, some people prefer the colour green and others like red. Colour preference may not, however, be a sufficiently important topic for an in-depth inquiry. Thus, you must judge whether the topic under study is important or trivial.

In a critical evaluation of a study's importance, you should also consider whether the findings themselves are trivial. Perhaps the topic is worthwhile, but you may feel after reading the report that nothing has been learned beyond what is common sense or everyday knowledge—which can result when the data are too "thin" or when the conceptualization is shallow. Catchy labels are often attached to themes and processes studied, but you should ask yourself whether the labels have really captured an insightful construct.

The Transferability of Qualitative Results

Although qualitative researchers do not strive for generalizability, the application of the results to other settings and contexts must be considered. If the findings are only relevant to the people who participated in the study, they cannot be useful to nursing practice. Thus, in interpreting qualitative results, you should consider how transferable the findings are. In what other types of settings and contexts would you expect the phenomenon under study to be manifested in a similar fashion? Of course, to make such an assessment, the author of the report must have described in sufficient detail the context in which the data were collected. Because qualitative studies are context bound, it is only through a careful analysis of the key parameters of the study context that the transferability of results can be assessed.

The Implications of Qualitative Results

If the findings are judged to be believable and important and you are satisfied with their interpretation, you can consider potential implications. As with quantitative studies, the implications can be multidimensional. First, you can consider the implications for further research: Should a similar study be undertaken in a new setting? Can the study be expanded in productive ways? Do the results reveal an important construct that merits formal measurement? Does the emerging theory suggest hypotheses that could be tested through controlled research? Second, do the findings have implications for nursing practice? For example, could the health care needs of a subculture (e.g., the homeless) be identified and addressed more effectively as a result of the study? Finally, do the findings shed light on fundamental processes that can be incorporated into nursing theory?

RESEARCH CRITIQUES
⏵

If nursing practice is to be based on research evidence, the worth of related studies must be critically appraised. Consumers may mistakenly believe that if a research report was accepted for publication, the study must be completely sound. Unfortunately, this is not necessarily the case. Indeed, most studies have limitations, and thus no single study offers definitive answers to research questions. Nevertheless, the methods of disciplined inquiry continue to provide us with the best possible means of answering certain questions. Evidence is accumulated not by an individual researcher conducting a single study but rather through the conduct of several studies addressing the same or similar questions and through the subsequent critical appraisal of these studies by others. Thus, consumers who can thoughtfully critique research reports also play a key role in the advancement of nursing knowledge.

Purposes of a Research Critique

A research **critique** is not just a summary of a study but rather a careful appraisal of its merits and flaws. Regardless of the scope or purpose of a critique, its function is not to hunt for and expose mistakes. A good critique objectively identifies areas of adequacy and inadequacy, virtues as well as faults. Sometimes, the need for this balance is obscured by the terms *critique* and *critical appraisal*, which connote unfavourable observations. The merits of a study are as important as its limitations in coming to conclusions about the worth of its findings. Therefore, a research critique should reflect a thoughtful, objective, and balanced consideration of the study's validity and significance.

Critiques can vary in scope, length, and form, depending on the underlying purpose. Three main types of critiques that are relevant to nursing research include those:

❧ undertaken by students to demonstrate their skills;

❧ conducted by other researchers (**peer reviewers**) to assist journal editors with publication decisions;

❧ conducted by researchers whose intent is to evaluate the strength of evidence of related studies as part of an integrative review (including meta-analyses and metasyntheses).

All three types attach great importance to whether the study focused on a problem of importance to nursing, but additional concerns depend on the type of critique. For example a meta-analyst would focus more on the quality of the evidence than on ethical aspects of the studies reviewed. The emphases in a critique depend on the overall purpose of conducting it.

In this chapter we focus primarily on the type of critique that students undertake. We briefly describe the two other main types of critiques, because you may one day be part of an integrative review team or be called upon to be a peer reviewer.

Student Critiques

As a student, you are likely to be asked to prepare a critique of a research report as a course requirement. Such critiques are usually expected to be comprehensive, with attention paid to all five dimensions of a report (substantive and theoretical, methodologic, ethical, interpretive, and presentational). The purpose of such a critique is to cultivate critical thinking, to induce you to use and demonstrate newly acquired skills in research methods, and to prepare you for a rewarding professional career in which research will almost surely play a role. Writing research critiques is an important step on the path to developing an evidence-based practice.

Although student critiques are comprehensive, involving the evaluation of all aspects of a report, there are a few critiquing questions that are less relevant for students than for others. For example, students are typically not required to be sufficiently knowledgeable about the substantive content of a report to critically evaluate the thoroughness of its literature review. Students also may not be expected to evaluate the qualifications of a research team, an issue that might have greater salience in other types of critiques.

Much of the remainder of this chapter presents materials that are relevant to comprehensive reviews such as those you are likely to undertake. Appendices C and D—which contain a quantitative and qualitative research report, respectively—also include comprehensive critiques that you can use as models.

Peer Reviews

Most nursing journals that publish research reports have a policy of independent, anonymous (sometimes called **blind**) **reviews** by two or more peers who are experts in the field. By anonymous, we mean that the peer reviewers do not know the identity of the authors, and authors do not learn the identity of reviewers. Journals that have such a policy are called **refereed journals,** and are generally more prestigious than *nonrefereed journals*. The journals *Canadian Journal of Nursing Research (CJNR)* and *Nursing in Research & Health* and many other journals cited in this book are refereed journals. Peer reviewers develop written critiques and make a recommendation about whether or not to publish the report.

Example of categories of recommendation for peer reviewers

The *Canadian Journal of Nursing Research (CJNR)* asks reviewers to make one of four recommendations to the editor pertaining to a manuscript under review: (1) acceptable as it is, (2) acceptable with minor revisions, (3) acceptable with major revisions, and (4) not at all acceptable. The reviewers also are asked to rate the manuscript, if acceptable, in terms of publication priority: low, medium, or high.

Peer reviewers' critiques can address a wide array of concerns, but they typically are brief and focus primarily on key substantive and methodologic issues. Reviewers may also comment on prominent presentational deficiencies (e.g., a confusing table) and noteworthy ethical issues. Peer reviewers' comments may be written in narrative, essay form or may take the form of a bulleted list of the study's strengths and weaknesses. Researchers typically revise their manuscripts based on the reviewers' critiques addressing, to the extent possible, the reviewers suggestions for improvement.

Critiques for Assessing a Body of Literature

Critiques of individual studies are sometimes undertaken as part of a formal, systematic evaluation of multiple studies on a topic. Such reviews are often undertaken with the aim of developing practice guidelines or drawing conclusions about the state of knowledge on which practice can be based. As described in Chapter 7, there are various ways of integrating findings on a topic from the research literature, including meta-analyses (for quantitative research) and metasyntheses (for qualitative ones). In both cases, reviewers must draw conclusions about what is known about a topic or phenomenon, and must consider the quality of the studies included in the review.

Chapter 18, which focuses on the utilization of nursing research for evidence-based practice, discusses the important role of systematic, integrative reviews. These reviews, rather than being comprehensive, focus on the methodologic dimension of studies and on the study findings. A person undertaking an integrative review as part of an EBP effort is not typically concerned with, for example, the thoroughness of the literature review in individual reports because it has no bearing on the quality of study's *evidence*.

Integrative reviews and critiques of a body of research typically do not involve written critiques of individual studies. More often, the people doing such reviews use a formal instrument for evaluating each study, often with quantitative ratings of different aspects of the study, so that appraisals across studies ("scores") can be compared. Many such instruments have been developed for use with quantitative research, as we discuss in Chapter 18.

Although less has been done to develop formal scoring systems for evaluating the quality of evidence in qualitative research, work in this area has begun. One example is the system developed by Cesario, Morin, and Santa-Donato (2002) as part of a project to develop clinical guidelines by the Association of Women's Health, Obstetric, and Neonatal Nurses (AWHONN). Another tool is the Primary

Research Appraisal Tool, which was developed by Canadian nurse researchers for determining a study's eligibility to be included in a meta-analysis (Paterson, Thorne, Canam, & Jillings, 2001).

Dimensions of a Research Critique

This section offers guidance primarily to those preparing detailed, comprehensive critiques. The goal of such critiques is to evaluate thoroughly the decisions the researcher made in conceptualizing, designing, and executing the study and in interpreting and communicating the results. Each researcher, in addressing the same or a similar research question, makes different decisions about how a study should be done, and researchers who have made different *methodologic decisions* may arrive at different answers to the same research question. It is precisely for this reason that you, as a consumer, must be knowledgeable about research methods. You must be able to evaluate research decisions so that you can determine how much faith should be put in the study findings. You must ask: What other approaches could have been used to study this research problem? And, If another approach had been used, would the results have been more credible or replicable? In other words, you need to evaluate the impact of the researcher's decisions on the study's ability to reveal the "truth."

Much of this book has been designed to acquaint you with a range of methodologic options for the conduct of research—options on how to design a study, collect and analyze data, select a sample, and so forth. We hope a familiarity with these options will provide you with the tools to challenge a researcher's decisions when it is appropriate to do so.

As previously noted, a comprehensive review involves an appraisal of five dimensions of a research report, each of which is discussed below. Specific critiquing guidelines for quantitative and qualitative studies are presented later in the chapter.

Substantive and Theoretical Dimension

In preparing a critique, you need to assess whether the study was sound in terms of the significance of the problem, the appropriateness of the conceptual framework, and the insightfulness of the analysis and interpretation. The research problem should have clear relevance to some aspect of nursing.

Another issue that has both substantive and methodologic implications is the congruence between the study question and the methods used to address it. There must be a good fit between the research problem on the one hand and the research methods on the other. Questions that deal with poorly understood phenomena, with processes, with the dynamics of a situation, or with in-depth description, for example, are usually best addressed with flexible designs, unstructured methods of data collection, and qualitative analysis. Questions that involve the measurement of well-defined variables, cause-and-effect relationships, or the effectiveness of some specific intervention, however, are better suited to more structured, quantitative approaches using designs that maximize research control.

A final issue to consider is whether the researcher has appropriately placed the research problem into a larger theoretical context. As noted in Chapter 8, researchers do little to enhance the value of a study if the connection between the research problem and a conceptual framework is contrived. But a research problem that is genuinely framed as a part of a larger intellectual problem can often make an especially important contribution to nursing knowledge.

Methodologic Dimension

Researchers make a number of important decisions regarding how best to answer their research questions or test their research hypotheses. It is your job as consumer to evaluate critically the consequences of those decisions. In fact, the heart of a research critique lies in the appraisal of the researchers' methodologic decisions. The quality of evidence that a study yields is inextricably linked to the researchers' choice of methods and strategies for study design and for collecting and analyzing data.

One thing to keep in mind in assessing a study's methods is that, because of practical constraints, researchers almost always make compromises between what is ideal and what is feasible. For example, a quantitative researcher might ideally like to have a sample of 500 participants, but financial resources may prohibit a sample larger than 200. A qualitative researcher might recognize that 3 years of fieldwork would yield an especially rich understanding of the phenomenon under study, but cannot afford to devote this much time. In doing a critique, you cannot realistically demand that researchers attain methodologic perfection, but you must evaluate the consequences of not doing so.

Ethical Dimension

In performing a comprehensive critique, you should consider whether there is evidence of ethical violations. If there are any potential ethical problems, you will need to consider the impact of those problems on the scientific merit of the study as well as on participants' well-being.

Sometimes ethical transgressions are inadvertent. For example, privacy and confidentiality can sometimes be compromised when interviews are conducted in participants' homes and other family members are nearby. In other cases, researchers are aware of potential ethical problems but consciously decide that the violation is minor in relation to the knowledge gained. For example, researchers may decide not to obtain informed consent from the parents of adolescents who are attending a family planning clinic because it might discourage adolescents to take part in the study thus leading to a biased sample of clinic users. It could also violate minors' right to confidential treatment at the clinic. When researchers knowingly elect not to follow ethical principles outlined in Chapter 5, the decision itself, the researchers' rationale, and the likely effect of the decision of the study's rigour should be evaluated.

TIP

Sometimes ethical transgressions, if still acceptable to ethics review committees, actually strengthen the methodological rigour of the study, and so you may need to "pit" one dimension of the critique against another.

Interpretive Dimension

Research reports conclude with a "Discussion," "Conclusions," or "Implications" section. In this final section, researchers offer an interpretation of the findings, consider whether the findings are congruent with a conceptual framework or earlier research, and discuss what the findings might imply for nursing.

As a reviewer, you should be somewhat wary if the "Discussion" section fails to point out any limitations. Researchers are in the best position to detect and assess the impact of sampling deficiencies, practical constraints, data quality problems, and so forth, and it is a professional responsibility to alert readers to these difficulties. Moreover, when researchers note methodologic or other shortcomings, readers know that these limitations were considered in interpreting the results.

Example of researcher-noted limitations

McCay and colleagues (2007) studied the effects of a 12-week group intervention designed to enhance healthy self-concept on engulfment and self-stigmatization in patients with a first episode of schizophrenia. Using a randomized clinical trial, the researchers randomly assigned participants to either the experimental group or the control group and measured the dependent variables: self-concept, self-esteem, self-efficacy, engulfment, self-stigmatization, quality of life, and hope. Although the researchers found significant differences between groups related to quality of life, hope, and engulfment, they found no statistically significant differences related to the other primary dependent variables. These results were attributed to several limitations highlighted by the researchers, a high attrition rate of 26.9% with a small sample size of 67. These significantly diminish the power of statistical testing. In addition, participants who dropped out of the study were found to be significantly different from those who remained in the study.

Of course, researchers are unlikely to note all relevant shortcomings of their work. Thus, the inclusion of comments about study limitations in the "Discussion" section, although important, does not relieve you of the responsibility of appraising methodologic decisions. Your task as reviewer is to contrast your own interpretation and assessment of limitations with those of the researchers, to challenge conclusions that do not appear to be warranted by the results, and to indicate how the study's evidence could have been enhanced.

It may be especially difficult for you to determine the validity of qualitative researchers' interpretations. To help readers understand the lens from which they interpreted their data, qualitative researchers ideally should mention whether they kept fieldnotes or a journal of their actions and emotions during the investigation, discuss their own behaviour and experiences in relation to the participants' experiences, and acknowledge any effects of their presence on data quality. You should look for such information in critiquing qualitative reports and drawing conclusions about the interpretations.

Your critique should also draw conclusions about the stated implications of the study. Some researchers offer unfounded recommendations on the basis of modest results. Some guidelines for evaluating researchers' interpretation and implications are offered in Box 17.1.

Presentation and Stylistic Dimension

Although the worth of the study is primarily reflected in the dimensions discussed thus far, the manner in which the information is communicated in the research report is also fair game in a comprehensive critical appraisal. Box 17.2 summarizes points that should be taken into account in evaluating the presentation of a research report.

An important consideration is whether the research report has provided sufficient information for a thoughtful critique of the other dimensions. For example, if the report does not describe how participants were selected, reviewers cannot comment on the adequacy of the sample, but they can criticize the report's failure to include information on sampling. When vital pieces of information are missing, researchers leave readers little choice but to assume the worst because this would lead to the most cautious interpretation of the worth of the evidence.

The writing in a research report, as in any published document, should be clear, grammatical, concise, and well organized. Unnecessary jargon should be minimized. Inadequate organization is another flaw in some reports: logical development of thoughts is critical to good communication of scientific information. Tables and figures should highlight key points and should be capable of "standing alone," without forcing readers to scrutinize the text to grasp what they mean.

Styles of writing do differ for qualitative and quantitative reports, and it is unreasonable to apply the standards considered appropriate for one paradigm to the other. Quantitative research reports are typically written in a more formal,

---

BOX 17.1 GUIDELINES FOR CRITIQUING THE "DISCUSSION" SECTION OF A RESEARCH REPORT

(▶)

Interpretation of the Findings

1. Are all important results discussed? If not, what is the likely explanation for omissions?

2. Does the report discuss the limitations of the study and possible effects of the limitations on the results?

3. Are interpretations consistent with results? Do the interpretations take limitations into account? Do the interpretations suggest distinct biases?

4. What types of evidence are offered in support of the interpretation, and is that evidence persuasive? Are results interpreted in light of findings from other studies? Are results interpreted in terms of the study hypotheses and the conceptual framework?

5. In qualitative studies, are the findings interpreted within an appropriate social or cultural context?

6. Are alternative explanations for the findings mentioned, and is the rationale for their rejection presented?

7. In quantitative studies, does the interpretation distinguish between practical and statistical significance?

8. Are any unwarranted interpretations of causality made?

9. Are generalizations made that are not warranted?

Implications of the Findings and Recommendations

10. Do the researchers discuss the study's implications for clinical practice, nursing education, nursing administration, or nursing theory, or make specific recommendations?

11. If yes, are the stated implications appropriate, given the study's limitations and given the body of evidence from other studies? Are there important implications that the report neglected to include?

---

impersonal fashion, using either the third person or passive voice to connote objectivity. Qualitative studies are likely to be written in a more literary style, using the first or second person and active voice to connote proximity and intimacy with the phenomenon under study. Regardless of style, as a reviewer you must be alert to indications of overt biases, exaggerations, emotionally laden comments or melodramatic language.

BOX 17.2 GUIDELINES FOR CRITIQUING THE PRESENTATION OF A RESEARCH REPORT

(▶)

1. Does the report include a sufficient amount of detail to permit a thorough critique of the study's substantive, methodologic, ethical, and interpretive dimensions? Does the report neglect to include key aspects of the study's methods?

2. Is the report understandable to those with moderate research skills, or is it unnecessarily abstruse? Is research jargon or clinical jargon used when simpler language could have improved communication to a broad audience of nurses?

3. Does the report suggest any overt biases on the part of the researcher? Does the researcher convey the tentative nature of research findings (e.g., avoiding words like "demonstrated" or "proved")?

4. Is the report well organized, or is the presentation confusing? Is there a logical, orderly presentation of ideas? Are transitions smooth, and is the report characterized by continuity of thought and expression?

5. Is the report well written and grammatical?

6. Does the report avoid sexist language? Does the report suggest any insensitivity to racial, ethnic, or cultural groups?

7. Does the report title adequately capture key concepts and the target population? Does the abstract adequately summarize the research problem, study methods, and key findings?

In summary, a research report should be an account of how and why a problem was studied and what results were obtained. The report should be accurate, clearly written, cogent, and concise. It should reflect scholarship, but not pedantry, and it should be written in a manner that stimulates the reader's interest and curiosity.

GUIDELINES FOR CRITIQUING RESEARCH REPORTS

Most chapters in this book have presented guidelines for evaluating various research decisions and aspects of research reports. The guidelines present detailed questions, whose primary function is to encourage you to read particular sections of research reports carefully and critically. Hopefully, these questions help reinforce the methodologic content of this book. However, you would seldom be expected to answer all of these questions in an overall critique of a research report. If you did this, the critique would be far longer than the report itself!

This section presents an abridged set of critiquing questions to assist you in evaluating quantitative and qualitative reports. We can begin by offering a few general suggestions. First, you will need to read the report you are critiquing at least twice, and you may need to read parts of it several times. It may be helpful to skim the section titled "Reading and Summarizing Research Reports" in Chapter 4, which offers suggestions on how to carefully and actively read research reports. Obviously, the first step in preparing a critique is to understand what the report is saying.

It is sometimes helpful to create a preliminary list of the aspects of the study that you thought were well done and those you viewed as problematic, without worrying too much initially about the organization of your thoughts. Once you have a preliminary list, you can organize it by arranging the items or bullets into a structure corresponding to the major sections of the report. You can then revise and augment your list by using the guidelines provided in this section.

When you are ready to write the critique, it may be useful to begin by preparing an abstract or introductory summary that will give you—and the person reading your critique—an overall "road map." The abstract should succinctly state what your final conclusions are about, the merits of the study and the degree of confidence placed in the study findings. Then in the body of the critique, you need to document the specific features that led you to those conclusions. It is important to remember that assuming the posture of a skeptic is key. Just as a careful clinician seeks evidence from research that certain practices are effective, you as a reviewer should demand evidence from the report that the researchers' decisions were sound.

Some additional broad tips for preparing a formal, written research critique are presented in Box 17.3.

Critiquing Quantitative Reports

Table 17.1 presents guidelines for critiquing quantitative research reports. They are organized using the IMRAD format, following the structure of most research reports (i.e., Introduction, Method, Results, and Discussion). The first column identifies the section of the report for which the questions are relevant. The next column provides cross-references to the more detailed guidelines in the earlier chapters of the book. And the final column lists some key critiquing questions that have broad applicability to quantitative studies.

A few comments about these guidelines are in order. First, the wording of the questions call for a yes or no answer (although for some, you may answer "Yes, *but* . . . ").

BOX 17.3 GENERAL GUIDELINES FOR CONDUCTING A WRITTEN RESEARCH CRITIQUE

▶

1. The function of a critique is not to *describe* a study or to *summarize* the content of the report. A research critique should provide an appraisal of the worth of the study itself and the merits of the report.
2. Be sure to comment on the study's strengths *and* weaknesses. The critique should be a balanced analysis of the study's value, noting positive as well as negative aspects.
3. Avoid vague generalizations—give specific examples of the study's strengths and limitations, providing direct references or quotes with page numbers.
4. Justify your criticisms. Offer a rationale for how a limitation affected the quality of the study, and suggest an alternative approach that could have eliminated the problem—but be sure that your suggestions are practical.
5. Be as objective as possible. Try not to be overly critical of a study simply because, for example, your worldview is inconsistent with the underlying paradigm or because your field of specialization is different from that of the researchers.
6. If you are writing a critique that the report authors themselves will receive, be sensitive to your tone and the sharpness of your criticisms, and avoid sarcasm.

In all cases, the desirable answer is "yes"—that is, a "no" suggests a possible limitation, and a "yes" suggests a strength. Therefore, the more "yeses" a study gets, the stronger it is likely to be. Thus, these guidelines can cumulatively suggest a global assessment: a report of 25 "yeses" is likely to be superior to one with only 10.

It is also important to realize that not all "yeses" are equal. Some elements are far more important in drawing conclusions about the rigour of a study than others. For example, the inadequacy of a literature review is less damaging to the validity of the study findings than the use of a design with weak internal validity. In general, the questions addressing the researchers' methodologic decisions (i.e., the questions under "Method," as well as questions relating to the statistical analysis) are especially important in evaluating the integrity of a study.

Although the questions in Table 17.1 elicit yes or no responses, your critique will obviously need to do more than point out what the study did and did not do. Each relevant issue needs to be discussed—and you will need to supply supporting evidence for your conclusions. For example, if you answered "no" to the question about whether the design minimized threats to the study's internal validity, your critique should elaborate on why you said this—for example, by pointing out that the design was vulnerable to self-selection bias because the groups being compared were not comparable at the outset. Each time you answer a question negatively, it might be profitable to review the more detailed questions presented in earlier chapters of the book.

TIP

Many questions in these guidelines may not lead to entirely clear answers. Even experts sometimes disagree about the best methodologic strategies to use. Thus, you should not be afraid to "stick out your neck" to express an evaluative opinion, but be sure to base your comments on sound methodologic principles discussed in this book.

These simplified guidelines carry, however, a number of short-comings. In particular, they are generic and critiquing cannot really use a one-size-fits-all list of questions. Critiquing questions that are relevant to certain types of studies

TABLE 17.1 ⊙	GUIDE TO AN OVERALL CRITIQUE OF A QUANTITATIVE RESEARCH REPORT	
ASPECT OF THE REPORT	DETAILED CRITIQUING GUIDELINES	BASIC QUESTIONS FOR A CRITIQUE
Title		➣ Is the title clear, suggesting the research problem and the study population?
Abstract		➣ Does the abstract clearly and concisely summarize the main features of the report?
Introduction Statement of the problem	Box 6.1, page 104	➣ Is the problem stated unambiguously, and is it easy to identify? ➣ Does the problem statement make clear the concepts and the population under study? ➣ Does the problem have significance for nursing? ➣ Is there a good match between the research problem and the paradigm and methods used? Is a quantitative approach appropriate?
Literature review	Box 7.1, page 121	➣ Is the literature review thorough, up-to-date, and based mainly on primary sources? ➣ Does the review summarize knowledge on the dependent and independent variables and the relationship between them? ➣ Does the literature review lay a solid basis for the new study?
Conceptual/theoretical framework	Box 8.1, page 138	➣ Are key concepts adequately defined conceptually? ➣ Is there a conceptual/theoretical framework, and is it appropriate? If not, is the absence of one justified?
Hypotheses or research questions	Box 6.1, page 104	➣ Are research questions and/or hypotheses explicitly stated? If not, is their absence justified? ➣ Are questions and hypotheses appropriately worded? ➣ Are the questions/hypotheses consistent with the literature review and the conceptual framework?
Method Research design	Box 9.1, page 166	➣ Was the most rigorous possible design used, given the study purpose? ➣ Were appropriate comparisons made to enhance interpretability of the findings? ➣ Was the number of data collection points appropriate? ➣ Did the design minimize threats to the internal and external validity of the study?
Population and sample	Box 12.1, page 223	➣ Was the population identified and described? Was the sample described in sufficient detail? ➣ Was the best possible sampling design used to enhance the sample's representativeness? ➣ Was the sample size adequate? Was a power analysis used to estimate sample size needs?

(table continues on page 360)

| | GUIDE TO AN OVERALL CRITIQUE OF A QUANTITATIVE | |
| TABLE 17.1 ▶ | RESEARCH REPORT (Continued) | |

ASPECT OF THE REPORT	DETAILED CRITIQUING GUIDELINES	BASIC QUESTIONS FOR A CRITIQUE
Data collection and measurement	Box 13.2, page 243; Box 13.4, page 250; Box 13.5, page 252; Box 14.1, page 271	➤ Are the operational and conceptual definitions congruent? ➤ Were key variables operationalized using the best possible method (e.g., interviews and observations)? ➤ Were the specific instruments adequately described, and were they good choices? ➤ Did the report provide evidence that the data collection methods yielded data that were high on reliability and validity?
Procedures	Box 13.6, page 253; Box 5.2, page 86	➤ If there was an intervention, was it adequately described, and was it properly implemented? ➤ Were data collected in a manner that minimized bias? Were data collection staff appropriately trained? ➤ Were appropriate procedures used to safeguard the rights of study participants?
Results Data analysis	Box 15.2, page 312	➤ Were analyses undertaken to address each research question or test each hypothesis? ➤ Were appropriate statistical methods used, given the level of measurement of the variables, number of groups being compared, and so forth? ➤ Was the most powerful analytic method used? (e.g., Did the analysis help to control for extraneous variables?)
Findings	Box 15.2, page 312	➤ Were the findings adequately summarized, with good use of tables and figures? ➤ Do the findings provide strong evidence regarding the research questions? Were Type I and Type II errors minimized?
Discussion Interpretation of the findings	Box 17.1, page 356	➤ Are all major findings interpreted and discussed within the context of prior research and/or the study's conceptual framework? ➤ Are the interpretations consistent with the results and with the study's limitations? ➤ Does the report address the issue of the generalizability of the findings?
Implications/ recommendations	Box 17.1, page 356	➤ Do the researchers discuss the implications of the study for clinical practice or further research—and are those implications reasonable and complete?

(table continues on page 361)

ASPECT OF THE REPORT	DETAILED CRITIQUING GUIDELINES	BASIC QUESTIONS FOR A CRITIQUE
Global issues		
Presentation	Box 17.2, page 356	❧ Was the report well written, well organized, and sufficiently detailed for critical analysis?
		❧ Were you able to understand the study? Was the report written in a manner that makes the findings accessible to practicing nurses?
Summary assessment		❧ Despite any identified limitations, do the study findings appear to be valid—do you have confidence in the *truth* value of the results?
		❧ Does the study contribute any meaningful evidence that can be used in nursing practice or that is useful to the nursing discipline?

(e.g., experiments) do not fit into a set of general questions for all quantitative studies. For example, we have not included a question about whether participants or research staff were blinded to experimental treatments because this question would not be relevant to most studies, which are nonexperimental. Furthermore, many supplementary questions would be needed to thoroughly assess certain types of research—for example, mixed-method studies. Thus, you will need to use judgment about whether the guidelines are sufficiently comprehensive for the type of study you are critiquing.

Another word of caution is that we developed these guidelines based on our years of experience as researchers and research methodologists. They do not represent a rigorously developed set of questions that can be used for a formal EBP-type critique. They should, however, facilitate your beginning efforts to critically appraise nursing studies.

Critiquing Qualitative Reports

Table 17.2 presents guidelines for you to use in critiquing qualitative research reports. These guidelines, similar to those in Table 17.1, are organized using the IMRAD format. Although qualitative reports are somewhat less likely than quantitative ones to follow this format, many of them do. In any event, it would still be possible to organize your critique using this structure, regardless of how the report is organized. Table 17.2 also presents, for each section, a series of questions and cross-references to more in-depth critiquing questions.

The comments about the guidelines for quantitative studies presented in the previous section are also relevant for critiquing qualitative ones. In particular, the difficulty with a "one-size-fits-all" approach is also salient for critiques of qualitative studies. Supplementary questions may be needed to fully critique studies within specific qualitative research traditions. Additional questions would be relevant for comprehensive critiques of, say, grounded theory studies (e.g., Did the categories describe the full range or continuum of the process?).

In undertaking a critique of a qualitative study, you should keep in mind that richness and thoroughness of description are especially important. Rich detail is required in the description of the methods in part because of the lack of standardization in qualitative studies—readers need to have sufficient information with which to judge the researchers' approach. For example, in a quantitative study, it might be sufficient to say that the data analysis involved a series of *t*-tests, whereas in a qualitative report, it is important to know, for example, how the data were

TABLE 17.2   GUIDE TO AN OVERALL CRITIQUE OF A QUALITATIVE
RESEARCH REPORT

ASPECT OF THE REPORT	DETAILED CRITIQUING GUIDELINES	BASIC QUESTIONS FOR A CRITIQUE
Title		⤳ Is the title clear, suggesting the key phenomenon and the group or community under study?
Abstract		⤳ Does the abstract clearly and concisely summarize the main features of the report?
Introduction Statement of the problem	Box 6.1, page 104	⤳ Is the phenomenon of interest clearly identified? ⤳ Is the problem stated unambiguously, and is it easy to identify? ⤳ Does the problem have significance for nursing? ⤳ Is there a good match between the research problem and the paradigm and methods used? Is a qualitative approach appropriate?
Literature review	Box 7.1, page 121	⤳ Does the report summarize the existing body of knowledge related to the problem or phenomenon of interest? ⤳ Is the literature review adequate? ⤳ Does the literature review lay a solid basis for the new study?
Conceptual underpinnings	Box 8.1, page 138	⤳ Are key concepts adequately defined conceptually? ⤳ Is the philosophical basis, underlying tradition, conceptual framework, or ideological orientation made explicit, and is it appropriate for the problem?
Research questions	Box 6.1, page 104	⤳ Are research questions explicitly stated? If not, is their absence justified? ⤳ Are the questions consistent with the study's philosophical basis, underlying tradition, conceptual framework, or ideological orientation?
Method Research design and research tradition	Box 10.1, page 185	⤳ Is the identified research tradition (if any) congruent with the methods used to collect and analyze data? ⤳ Was an adequate amount of time spent in the field or with study participants? ⤳ Did the design unfold in the field, allowing researchers to capitalize on early understandings? ⤳ Was there evidence of reflexivity in the design? ⤳ Was there an adequate number of contacts with study participants?
Sample and setting	Box 12.2, page 223	⤳ Was the group or population of interest adequately described? Were the setting and sample described in sufficient detail? ⤳ Was the approach used to gain access to the site or to recruit participants appropriate? ⤳ Was the best possible method of sampling used to enhance information richness and address the needs of the study? ⤳ Was the sample size adequate? Was saturation achieved?

(table continues on page 363)

ASPECT OF THE REPORT	DETAILED CRITIQUING GUIDELINES	BASIC QUESTIONS FOR A CRITIQUE
Data collection	Box 13.2, page 243; Box 13.4, page 250	➳ Were the methods of gathering data appropriate? Were data gathered through two or more methods to achieve triangulation? ➳ Did the researcher ask the right questions or make the right observations, and were they recorded in an appropriate fashion? ➳ Was a sufficient amount of data gathered? Was the data of sufficient depth and richness?
Procedures	Box 13.6, page 253; Box 5.2, page 86	➳ Were data collection and recording procedures adequately described, and do they appear appropriate? ➳ Were data collected in a manner that minimized bias or behavioral distortions? Were data collection staff appropriately trained? ➳ Were appropriate procedures used to safeguard the rights of study participants?
Enhancement of rigour	Box 14.2, page 271	➳ Were methods used to enhance the trustworthiness of the data (and analysis), and was the description of those methods adequate? ➳ Were the methods used to enhance credibility appropriate and sufficient? ➳ Did the researcher document research procedures and decision processes sufficiently that findings are auditable and confirmable?
Results Data analysis	Box 16.1, page 322	➳ Were the data management (e.g., coding) and data analysis methods sufficiently described? ➳ Was the data analysis strategy compatible with the research tradition and with the nature and type of the data gathered? ➳ Did the analysis yield an appropriate "product" (e.g., a theory, taxonomy, or thematic pattern)? ➳ Did the analytic procedures suggest the possibility of biases?
Findings	Box 16.1, page 322	➳ Were the findings effectively summarized, with good use of excerpts? ➳ Do the themes adequately capture the meaning of the data? Does it appear that the researcher satisfactorily conceptualized the themes or patterns in the data? ➳ Did the analysis yield an insightful, provocative, and meaningful picture of the phenomenon under investigation?
Theoretical integration	Box 16.1, page 322	➳ Are the themes or patterns logically connected to each other to form a convincing and integrated whole? ➳ Were figures, maps, or models used effectively to summarize conceptualizations? ➳ If a conceptual framework or ideological orientation guided the study, are the themes or patterns linked to it in a cogent manner?

(table continues on page 364)

		GUIDE TO AN OVERALL CRITIQUE OF A QUALITATIVE RESEARCH REPORT (Continued)
ASPECT OF THE REPORT	DETAILED CRITIQUING GUIDELINES	BASIC QUESTIONS FOR A CRITIQUE
Discussion Interpretation of the findings	Box 17.1, page 356	➤ Are the findings interpreted within an appropriate social or cultural context? ➤ Are major findings interpreted and discussed within the context of prior studies? ➤ Are the interpretations consistent with the study's limitations? ➤ Does the report address the issue of the transferability of the findings?
Implications/ recommendations	Box 17.1, page 356	➤ Do the researchers discuss the implications of the study for clinical practice or further inquiry—and are those implications reasonable?
Global issues Presentation	Box 17.2, page 356	➤ Was the report well written, well organized, and sufficiently detailed for critical analysis? ➤ Was the description of the methods, findings, and interpretations sufficiently rich and vivid?
Summary assessment		➤ Do the study findings appear to be trustworthy—do you have confidence in the *truth* value of the results? ➤ Does the study contribute any meaningful evidence that can be used in nursing practice or that is useful to the nursing discipline?

TABLE 17.2

coded, how coding categories were combined, who did the coding, and whether there was intercoder agreement. Vivid description is also needed in presenting results in qualitative studies because without descriptive clarity and eloquence, readers cannot grasp the nuances and complexities of the phenomenon under study. Qualitative studies can be a "gold mine for clinical insights" (Kearney, 2001, p. 146) only when the presentation is richly detailed and powerfully narrated.

As noted earlier, formal systems have been proposed to evaluate the quality of evidence in qualitative studies, and these approaches are typically not organized according to sections of a report but rather according to a number of cross-cutting themes. For example, Cesario and her colleagues (2002), who were involved with the AWHONN practice guideline development project, used five broad categories that were suggested by Burns (1989) for rating the quality of qualitative studies: descriptive vividness, methodologic congruence, analytic precision, theoretical connectedness, and heuristic relevance. Our guidelines cover most of the same issues and questions raised in the rating system but with a less abstract structure.

RESEARCH EXAMPLES AND CRITICAL THINKING ACTIVITIES

EXAMPLE 1 ■ Interpretation of Quantitative Findings

1. Read the "Discussion" section from the study by Bryanton and colleagues (2008) in Appendix A of this book and then answer the relevant questions in Box 17.1 (p. 356).

EXAMPLE 2 ■ **Interpretation of Qualitative Findings**

1. Read the "Discussion" section from Woodgate, Ateah, and Secco (2008) in Appendix B of this book, and then answer the relevant questions in Box 17.1 (p. 356).

2. Also consider the following targeted questions, which may further sharpen your critical thinking skills and assist you in assessing aspects of the study's merit:
   a. Suggest two future studies that researchers could conduct based on the findings of the Woodgate et al.'s (2008) study. One study should be quantitative and one study should be qualitative.
   b. Suggest a qualitative study that would increase the transferability of Woodgate et al.'s findings.

EXAMPLE 3 ■ **Critique of a Quantitative Study**

Read the full study by Moore and colleagues (2009) in Appendix C, and then address the following activities and questions.

1. Before reading our critique, which accompanies the full report, either write your own critique or prepare a list of what you think are the major strengths and weaknesses of the study. Then contrast your critique or list with ours. Remember that you (or your instructor) do not necessarily have to agree with all points made in our critique and that you may identify strengths and weaknesses that we overlooked.

2. Using the guidelines in Table 17.1 (p. 359), how many "yes" ratings would you give to the study? Compare your "score" with that of other classmates.

3. In selecting studies to include in this textbook, we avoided choosing weak ones—which would have been much easier to critique. To push your critical thinking, we offer some "pretend" scenarios below in which the researchers may have made different methodologic decisions than those reported by Moore et al. (2009). Write a paragraph or two critiquing these "pretend" decisions, pointing out how these alternatives would have affected the quality of the study.
   a. Pretend that the researchers had been unable to randomize participants to treatments. The design, in other words, would be a posttest-only preexperiment, with the three tested interventions (saline washouts, commercial washouts, or no washouts, i.e., usual care) not randomly assigned to participants.
   b. Pretend that the total sample size was only 30 (i.e., 10 participants per group).

EXAMPLE 4 ■ **Critique of a Qualitative Study**

Read the full study by Bottorff and colleagues (2008) in Appendix D, and then address the following activities and questions.

1. Before reading our critique, which accompanies the full report, either write your own critique or prepare a list of what you think are the major strengths and weaknesses of the study. Then contrast your critique or list with ours. Remember that you (or your instructor) do not necessarily have to agree with the points made in our critique and that you may identify strengths and weaknesses that we overlooked.

2. Using the guidelines in Table 17.2 (p. 362), how many "yes" ratings would you give to the study? Compare your "score" with that of other classmates.

3. As noted in Example 3, we purposely selected good-quality studies to feature in this textbook. In the questions below, we offer some "pretend" scenarios with different methodologic decisions than those made by Bottorff et al. (2008). Write a paragraph or two critiquing these "pretend" decisions, pointing out how these alternatives would have affected the quality of the study.
   a. Pretend that Bottorff et al. (2008) had used structured questionnaires rather than interviews to gather their data.
   b. Pretend that the researchers had done a descriptive qualitative study, not in the ethnographic tradition.

Summary Points

· ·

⇝ The *interpretation* of research findings is a search for the broader meaning and implications of the results of an investigation.

⇝ Interpretation of both qualitative and quantitative results typically involves: (1) analyzing the credibility of the results; (2) determining their meaning; (3) considering their importance; (4) determining the generalizability or transferability of the findings; and (5) assessing the implications in regard to nursing practice, theory, and future research.

⇝ A research **critique** is a careful, critical appraisal of the strengths and limitations of a study to draw conclusions about the worth of the evidence and its significance to nursing.

⇝ Critiques are done for a variety of purposes, including critiques by students to demonstrate their research skills; assessments by **peer reviewers** to assist journal editors with publication decisions; and critiques done as part of an integrated review.

⇝ Peer reviewers who critique studies for a **refereed journal** often do **blind reviews** in which the reviewers do not learn the identity of the researchers, and *vice versa*.

⇝ Critiques of individual studies done in an effort to come to conclusions about a body of literature (e.g., those done by a meta-analyst) often involve the use of a structured instrument or scale to rate aspects of study quality.

⇝ A reviewer preparing a comprehensive review should consider five major dimensions of the study: the substantive and theoretical, methodologic, ethical, interpretive, and presentation and stylistic dimensions.

⇝ Researchers designing a study must make a number of important *methodologic decisions* that affect the quality and rigour of the research. Consumers preparing a critique must evaluate these decisions to determine how much faith can be placed in the results.

⇝ When undertaking a critique, it is appropriate to assume the posture of a sceptic who demands evidence from the report that the conclusions are credible and significant.

STUDIES CITED IN CHAPTER 17*

This reference list contains only those studies that were cited in this chapter. Citations pertaining to theoretical, methodologic, or nonempirical work are included together in a separate section at the end of the book (beginning on page 399).

Beaver, K., Tysver-Robinson, D., Campbell, M., et al. (2009). Comparing hospital and telephone follow-up after treatment for breast cancer: Randomized equivalence trial. *British Medical Journal, 338*, Article 3147. Retrieved March 16, 2009, from http://www.pubmedcentral.nih.gov/articlerender.fcgi?artid=2628299

Bottorff, J. L., Oliffe, J. L., Halpin, M., Phillips, M., McLean, G., & Mroz, L. (2008). Women and prostate cancer support groups: The gender connect? *Social Science and Medicine, 66*(5), 1217–1227.

Bryanton, J., Gagnon, A. J., Hatem, M., & Johnston, C. (2008). Predictors of early parenting self-efficacy: Results of a prospective cohort study. *Nursing Research, 57*(4), 252–259.

Burns, N. (1989). Standards for qualitative research. *Nursing Science Quarterly, 2*, 254–260.

Cesario, S., Morin, K., & Santa-Donato, A. (2002). Evaluating the level of evidence of qualitative research. *Journal of Obstetrics, Gynecologic, & Neonatal Nursing, 31*, 708–714.

Clarke, S., Butler, K., & Esplen, M. J. (2008). The phases of disclosing BRCA1/2 genetic information to offspring. *Psychooncology, 17*(8), 797–803.

Fillion, L., Gagnon, P., Leblond, F., et al. (2008). A brief intervention for fatigue management in breast cancer survivors. *Cancer Nursing, 31*(2), 145–159

Johnston, C. C., Filion, F., Campbell-Yeo, M., et al. (2008). Kangaroo mother care diminishes pain from heel lance in very preterm neonates: A crossover trial. *BioMed Central Pediatrics, 8*, 13.

Kearney, M. H. (2001). Levels and applications of qualitative research evidence. *Research in Nursing & Health, 24*, 145–153.

Lespérance, F., Frasure-Smith, N., & Koszycki, D., et al. (2007). Effects of citalopram and interpersonal psychotherapy on depression in patients with coronary artery disease: The Canadian Cardiac Randomized Evaluation of Antidepressant and Psychotherapy Efficacy (CREATE) trial. *Journal of the American Medical Association, 297*(4), 367–379.

McCay, E., Beanlands, H., Zipursky, R., et al. (2007). A randomised controlled trial of a group intervention to reduce engulfment and self-stigmatisation in first episode schizophrenia. *Australian e-Journal for the Advancement of Mental Health, 6*(3), 1–9.

Moore, K. N., Hunter, K. F., McGinnis, R., et al. (2009). Do catheter washouts extend patency time in long-term indwelling urethral catheters? A randomized controlled trial of acidic washout solution, normal saline washout, or standard care. *Journal of Wound, Ostomy and Continence Nursing, 36*(1), 82–90.

Paterson, B. L., Thorne, S. E., Canam, C., & Jillings, C. (2001). *Meta-study of qualitative health research.* Thousand Oaks, CA: Sage.

Willem, A., Buelens, M., & DeJongue, I. (2007). Impact of organizational structure on nurses' job satisfaction. *International Journal of Nursing Studies, 44*(6), 1011–1020.

Woodgate, R. L., Ateah, C., & Secco, L. (2008). Living in a world of our own: The experience of parents who have a child with autism. *Qualitative Health research, 18*(8), 1075–1083.

18 Using Research in Evidence-Based Nursing Practice

On completion of this chapter, you will be able to:

1. Distinguish research utilization (RU) and evidence-based practice (EBP) and discuss their current status within nursing

2. Identify barriers to EBP and strategies for improving it

3. Identify several models that have relevance for EBP and describe the general steps in an EBP project

4. Discuss the role that integrative reviews play in EBP and describe basic steps in undertaking such a review

5. Critique an integrative review

6. Define new terms in the chapter

Most nurse researchers would like to have their findings incorporated into nursing protocols and curricula, and most nurses in clinical settings are aware of the benefits of research-based practice. There is a growing interest in basing nursing actions on solid evidence confirming that the actions are clinically appropriate, cost-effective, and beneficial for clients. In this chapter, we discuss various issues related to the use of nursing research to support evidence-based practice.

RESEARCH UTILIZATION AND EVIDENCE-BASED PRACTICE

▶

The term *research utilization* is sometimes used synonymously with **evidence-based practice (EBP).** There is overlap between the two concepts, but they are, in fact, distinct. EBP, the broader of the two terms, involves making clinical decisions based on the best possible evidence. The best evidence usually comes from rigorous research, but EBP also uses other sources of information. A basic feature of EBP is that it de-emphasizes decision making based on custom or authority opinion. Rather, the emphasis is on identifying the best available research evidence and *integrating* it with clinical expertise, patient input, and existing resources.

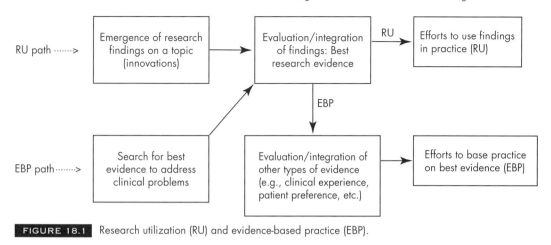

FIGURE 18.1 Research utilization (RU) and evidence-based practice (EBP).

Broadly speaking, **research utilization (RU)** refers to the use of findings from a disciplined study or set of studies in a practical application that is unrelated to the original research. In RU projects, the goal is to translate empirically based knowledge into real-world applications. Figure 18.1 provides a basic schema of how RU and EBP are interrelated. This section further explores and distinguishes the two concepts.

The Utilization of Nursing Research

During the 1980s and early 1990s, RU became an important buzzword (see Graham et al., 2006; Thompson, Estabrooks, & Degner, 2006, for further reading on the various terms used in this field). Several changes in nursing education and nursing research were prompted by the desire to develop a knowledge base for nursing practice. Nursing schools increasingly began to include courses on research methods so that students would become skilful research consumers, and researchers shifted their focus to clinical problems. These changes, coupled with the completion of several large RU projects, played a role in sensitizing the nursing community to the desirability of using research as a basis for practice; the changes were not enough, however, to lead to widespread integration of research findings into the delivery of nursing care. RU, as the nursing community has come to recognize, is a complex and nonlinear phenomenon that poses professional challenges.

The Research Utilization Continuum

As Figure 18.1 indicates, the starting-point of RU is new knowledge and new ideas that emerge from research. When studies are completed, knowledge on a topic accumulates and works its way into use—to varying degrees and at differing rates.

Theorists who have studied knowledge development and the diffusion of ideas recognize a continuum in terms of the specificity of the use to which research findings are put. At one end is **instrumental utilization** (Caplan & Rich, 1975), which refers to discrete, identifiable attempts to base specific actions on research findings. For example, a series of studies in the 1960s and 1970s demonstrated that the optimal placement time of a glass thermometer for accurate oral temperature determination is 9 minutes. When nurses specifically altered their behaviour from shorter placement times to the empirically based recommendation of 9 minutes, this constituted instrumental utilization.

Research findings can, however, be used in a more diffuse manner—in a way that promotes cumulative awareness or understanding. Caplan and Rich (1975) refer to this end of the utilization continuum as **conceptual utilization**. As an example, a nurse may read a qualitative research report describing *courage* among individuals with chronic illness as a dynamic process that includes efforts to accept reality and to develop problem-solving skills. The nurse may be reluctant to alter his or her own behaviour based on the results, but the study may make the nurse more observant in working with patients with chronic illnesses; it may also lead to informal efforts to promote problem-solving skills. Conceptual utilization, then, refers to situations in which users are influenced in their thinking about an issue based on research findings but do not put the findings to any specific use.

The middle ground of this continuum involves the partial use of research findings on nursing actions, reflecting what Weiss (1980) has termed knowledge creep and decision accretion. *Knowledge creep refers to an evolving* "percolation" of research ideas and findings. *Decision accretion* refers to the manner in which momentum for a decision builds over a period of time based on accumulated information gained through readings, discussions, and so forth. Increasingly, however, nurses *are* making conscious decisions to use research in their clinical practice, and the EBP movement has contributed to this change.

Estabrooks (1999) studied RU by collecting survey data from 600 Canadian nurses. She found evidence to support three distinct types of RU: (1) *indirect RU*, involving changes in nurses' thinking—analogous to conceptual utilization; (2) *direct RU*, involving the direct use of findings in giving patient care—analogous to instrumental utilization; and (3) *persuasive utilization*, involving the use of findings to persuade others to make changes in policies or practices relevant to nursing care.

These varying ways of thinking about RU suggest that both qualitative and quantitative research can play key roles in improving nursing practice. Estabrooks (2001) has argued that the process of using research findings in practice is essentially the same for both quantitative and qualitative research, but she claims that qualitative research may have a privileged position: clinicians do not need a background in statistics to understand qualitative research, and thus using qualitative results is more readily accomplished.

Research Utilization in Nursing Practice

During the 1980s and 1990s, there was considerable concern that nurses had failed to use research findings as a basis for making clinical decisions. This concern was based on early studies suggesting that nurses were not always aware of research results or did not use results in their practice. For example, Helen Shore (1972), a Canadian nurse, was one of the first to study this problem; she studied the adoption of six nursing practices presented in a nursing institute and learned that whereas there were some "adopters," there were also "laggards" who resisted new ideas. Ketefian (1975) reported on nurses' oral temperature determination practices. As noted, there was solid evidence that the optimal placement time with glass thermometers is 9 minutes. In Ketefian's study, only 1 out of 87 nurses reported the correct placement time, suggesting that these practicing nurses were unaware of or ignored the research findings. Other studies in the 1980s (e.g., Kirchhoff, 1982) were similarly discouraging.

In 1990, Coyle and Sokop investigated practicing nurses' adoption of 14 strong, empirically based innovations that had been reported in the literature. A sample of 113 nurses from 10 hospitals completed questionnaires that measured the nurses' awareness and use of the findings. There was wide variation across the 14 innovations, with awareness of them ranging from 34% to 94%. Each innovation was categorized according to the stage of adoption: awareness (indicating knowledge of the innovation); persuasion (indicating the nurses' belief that nurses *should* use the innovation in practice); occasional use in practice; and regular use in practice. Only 1 of the 14 studies was at the regular use stage of adoption, but 6 were in the persuasion stage—possibly an early indication of the importance of nursing unit culture that is being discussed in the literature today (see, e.g., Scott & Pollock, 2008).

In 1995, a study by Varcoe and Hilton with 183 Canadian nurses found that 9 of the 10 research-based practices investigated were used by 50% or more of the acute care nurses at least sometimes. Similar results have been reported in a survey of nearly 1000 nurses from 25 hospitals in Scotland (Rodgers, 2000). A more recent study by Hek and Shaw (2006) explored the views of new nursing graduates in relation to research-based practice. Approximately 50% of the sample indicated that research was "embedded" in their workplace practice, and could offer specific examples, such as "conference feedback to staff" and "research activity on the ward."

Example from Hek and Shaw's study
This interesting snapshot of 58 newly graduated nurses in England also explored their self-reported "preparedness for practice" over time. Respondents were interviewed at 3 and 12 months on their views of the preregistration training they received. At 3 months, they "· · · felt that they had received too much teaching about research, were not interested in the subject and struggled to see its relevance to clinical practice" (p. 473). However, at 12 months, their view of research had changed from being a "peripheral subject" to being something "often talked about" (p. 474) and visible in their workplace.

The results of the recent studies are more encouraging than the earlier ones because they suggest that, on average, practicing nurses are aware of many research findings, are persuaded that the innovations should be used, and are beginning to use them, at least on occasion.

Efforts to Improve Utilization of Nursing Research

The desire to reduce the gap between nursing research and nursing practice has led to formal attempts to bridge the gap. The best known of several early nursing RU projects is the **Conduct and Utilization of Research in Nursing** (CURN) **project,** a 5-year project awarded to the Michigan Nurses Association in the 1970s. CURN's major objective was to increase the use of research findings in nursing practice by disseminating research findings, facilitating organizational changes, and encouraging collaborative clinical research. CURN project staff saw RU as primarily an organizational process, with the commitment of organizations that employ nurses as essential to the RU process (Horsley, Crane, & Bingle, 1978). The CURN project team concluded that RU by practicing nurses is feasible, but only if the research is relevant to practice and if the results are broadly disseminated. The CURN project generated considerable international interest. For example, the Cross Cancer Institute in Edmonton, Alberta, used the CURN model as a framework to integrate research findings into nursing practice (Alberta Association of Registered Nurses, 1997).

During the 1980s and 1990s, utilization projects were undertaken by a growing number of hospitals and organizations, and project descriptions began to appear in the nursing research literature worldwide. These projects were usually institutional attempts to implement changes in nursing practice on the basis of research findings and to evaluate the effects of the innovation. For example, Logan et al. (1999) described a project implemented at three Ottawa health care settings during a time of multiple restructuring changes. The **Ottawa Model of Research Use,** which we describe in a later section, was applied in an effort to increase evidence-based decision making in the three project sites. Multiple approaches aimed at research transfer were used, with a major emphasis on educational activities such as workshops.

These early utilization projects often did not have the hoped-for impact on the use of research in nursing practice, but during the 1990s, the call for RU began to be superseded by the push for EBP.

Evidence-Based Nursing Practice

The RU process begins with an empirically based innovation or new idea that gets scrutinized for possible adoption in practice settings. EBP, by contrast, begins with a search for information about how best to solve specific problems (see Figure 18.1). Findings from rigorous research are considered the best source of information, but EBP also draws on other sources of evidence.

The EBP movement has given rise to considerable debate. Supporters of EBP argue that a rational approach is needed to provide the best possible care to the most people, with the most cost-effective use of resources. Critics worry that the advantages of EBP are exaggerated and that clinical judgments and patient inputs are being devalued. Although there is a need for close scrutiny of how the EBP journey unfolds, it is an indisputable path that health care professions will tread in the 21st century.

Overview of the EBP Movement

In the 1970s, British epidemiologist Archie Cochrane published an influential book that drew attention to the dearth of solid evidence about the effects of health care. He called for efforts to make research summaries available to health care decision makers. This eventually led to the development of the Cochrane Centre in Oxford in 1992 and the **Cochrane Collaboration,** with centres established in 15 locations throughout the world. The aim of the collaboration is to help people make good decisions about health care by preparing, maintaining, and disseminating systematic reviews of the effects of health care interventions.

At about the same time as the Cochrane Collaboration got underway, a group from McMaster Medical School developed a clinical learning strategy they called evidence-based medicine (EBM). Dr. David Sackett, a pioneer of EBM at McMaster, defined evidence-based medicine as "the conscientious, explicit, and judicious use of current best evidence in making decisions about the care of individual patients. Evidence-based medicine means integrating individual clinical expertise with the best available external evidence from systematic research" (Sackett, Rosenberg, Gray, Haynes, & Richardson, 1996, p. 71). The EBM movement has shifted over time to a broader conception of using best evidence by all health care practitioners (not just doctors) in a multidisciplinary team.

Types of Evidence and Evidence Hierarchies

There is no consensus about what constitutes good evidence for EBP, but there is general agreement that findings from rigorous studies are paramount. In the early years of the EBP movement, there was a strong bias toward reliance on evidence from randomized clinical trials (RCTs)—a bias that led to some resistance to EBP by nurses who felt that evidence from qualitative and non-RCT studies would be ignored.

Positions about what constitutes useful evidence have broadened (see Rycroft-Malone et al., 2004; Scott-Findlay & Pollock, 2004, for further reading on the debate over the definition of evidence), but there have nevertheless been efforts to develop **evidence hierarchies** that rank studies according to the strength of evidence they provide. Several such hierarchies have been developed, many based on the one proposed by Archie Cochrane. Most hierarchies put meta-analyses of RCT studies at the pinnacle and other types of nonresearch evidence (e.g., clinical expertise) at the base. As one example, Stetler et al. (1998) developed a six-level evidence hierarchy. The levels (from strongest to weakest) are as follows: (I) meta-analyses of RCTs; (II) individual experimental studies; (III) quasi-experimental studies or matched case-control studies; (IV) nonexperimental studies (e.g., correlational studies, qualitative studies); (V) RU studies, quality improvement projects, case reports; and (VI) opinions of respected authorities and of expert committees.

To date, there have been relatively few published RCT studies in nursing, and even fewer published meta-analyses of RCT nursing studies. Therefore, evidence from other types of research will play an important role in evidence-based nursing practice. Many clinical questions of importance to nurses can best be answered with rich descriptive and qualitative data from levels IV and V studies. In this effort, nursing academics are now challenging the traditional, medically driven hierarchy of evidence (e.g., Thorne, 2008), and calling for greater rigor in conducting and reporting qualitative research (see, e.g., Nelson, 2008).

Nurses and other health care professionals must be able to locate research evidence, evaluate it, and integrate it with clinical judgment and patient preferences to determine the most clinically effective solutions to health problems. Note that an important feature of EBP is that it does not necessarily imply practice changes; the best evidence may confirm that existing practices are effective and cost-efficient.

Barriers to Research Utilization and EBP in Nursing

Studies done in Canada and in many other countries have explored nurses' perceptions of barriers to RU and have yielded remarkably similar results about constraints clinical nurses face (e.g., Gerrish & Clayton, 2004; Graham, Logan, Davies, & Nimrod, 2004; Hutchinson & Johnston, 2004; McCleary & Brown, 2003a).

Research-Related Barriers

For some nursing problems, research knowledge is at a rudimentary level. Research findings may not warrant use in practice if studies are flawed or small in number. Thus, one impediment to RU is that, for some problems, a solid base of trustworthy study results has not been developed.

As we have stressed throughout this text, most studies have flaws of one type or another; therefore, if nurses were to wait for "perfect" studies before basing clinical decisions on research evidence, they would have a long wait. Replication is essential: when repeated efforts to address a research question in different settings yield similar results, there can be greater confidence in the evidence. Single studies rarely provide an adequate basis for making practice changes. Therefore, another utilization constraint is the dearth of published replications. A further aspect is the notion of *efficacy* versus *effectiveness* in clinical intervention studies, or research under "ideal" versus "ordinary" conditions. While many studies report results that are efficacious, the true test is whether the same results can be produced and sustained in a real-world setting (see Feldstein & Glasgow, 2008, for an interesting approach to this issue within public health).

As a consumer, you should evaluate the extent to which researchers have adopted strategies to enhance RU/EBP. These include working collaboratively with clinicians, communicating clearly so that practicing nurses can evaluate studies, and describing clinical implications in the "Discussion" section of their reports.

Nurse-Related Barriers

Nurses are increasingly sophisticated and able to appreciate research findings. Indeed, a Scottish survey suggests that nurses may have better skills to carry out literature reviews and evaluate research evidence than other health care professionals in primary care (O'Donnell, 2004). However, studies have also found that nurses prefer to use knowledge gained through personal experiences and interactions with coworkers rather than through textbooks and journal articles (e.g., Estabrooks, Chong, Brigidear, & Profetto-McGrath, 2005; Gerrish & Clayton, 2004; Spenceley, O'Leary, Chizawsky, Ross, & Estabrooks, 2008).

Nurses' education and research skills have consistently been found to constrain the use of research evidence in practice (e.g., McCleary & Brown, 2003b). Many clinical nurses have not had formal instruction in research and may lack the skills to evaluate a study. Courses on research methods are now offered in most baccalaureate nursing programs, but the ability to critique a study is not necessarily sufficient for effectively incorporating research evidence into daily decision making.

Nurses' attitudes toward research and their motivation to engage in EBP have also been identified as potential barriers. Studies have found that the more positive the attitude, the more likely is the nurse to use research in practice. Fortunately, there is growing evidence from international surveys that many nurses value nursing research and want to be involved in research-related activities.

Organizational Barriers

Many of the impediments to using research in practice stem from the organizations that train and employ nurses (see Cummings, Estabrooks, Midodzi, Wallin, & Hayduk, 2007; Scott-Findlay & Estabrooks, 2006, for further reading on the influence of the organizational context on RU). Organizations, perhaps to an even greater degree than individuals, resist change unless there is a strong organizational perception that there is something fundamentally wrong with the status quo. To challenge tradition and accepted practices, a spirit of intellectual curiosity and openness must prevail.

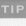

TIP

Every nurse can play a role in using research evidence. Here are some strategies:

➤ *Read widely.* Professionally accountable nurses keep abreast of new developments. You should read journals relating to your specialty, including research reports in them.

➤ *Attend professional conferences.* Many nursing conferences include presentations of studies that have clinical relevance. At a conference, you can meet researchers and explore practice implications.

➤ *Learn to expect evidence that a procedure is effective.* Every time you are told about a standard nursing procedure, you have a right to ask, why? Nurses should develop expectations that their clinical decisions are based on sound rationales.

➤ *Become involved in a journal club.* Many organizations that employ nurses sponsor journal clubs that meet to review studies that have potential relevance to practice.

➤ *Pursue and participate in RU/EBP projects.* Sometimes ideas for RU or EBP projects come from staff nurses (e.g., ideas may emerge in a journal club). Studies have found that nurses who are involved in research-related activities (e.g., data collection efforts) develop more positive attitudes toward research and EBP.

In many practice settings, administrators have systems to reward competence in nursing practice, but few have instituted a system to reward nurses for critiquing studies, using research in practice, or discussing research findings with clients. Thus, organizations have failed to motivate nurses for RU/EBP. Organizations may also be reluctant to expend resources for RU/EBP projects. Resources may be required for outside consultants, staff release time, library materials, and so forth. With the push toward cost containment in health care settings, resource constraints may pose a barrier to change—unless cost containment is an explicit project goal.

EBP will become part of organizational norms only if there is a commitment on the part of managers and administrators. Strong leadership in health care organizations is essential to making EBP happen.

THE PROCESS OF USING RESEARCH IN NURSING PRACTICE

In the years ahead, many of you are likely to be engaged in individual and institutional efforts to use research as a basis for clinical decisions. This section describes how that might be accomplished. We begin with a description of some RU and EBP models developed by nurses.

Models for Evidence-Based Nursing Practice

A number of different models of RU have been developed by nurse researchers in Canada, the United States, the United Kingdom, and other countries during the past few decades (see Estabrooks, Thompson, Lovely, & Hofmeyer, 2006). These models, which offer guidelines for designing and implementing RU and EBP projects in practice settings, include the following:

⇒ Stetler Model of RU (Stetler, 1994, 2001)

⇒ Iowa Model of Research in Practice (Titler et al., 1994, 2001)

⇒ PARiHS (Promoting Action on Research Implementation in Health Services) framework (Kitson, Ahmed, Harvey, Seers, & Thompson, 1996; Kitson et al., 2008)

⇒ Ottawa Model of Research Use (Logan & Graham, 1998)

⇒ Evidence-Based Multidisciplinary Practice Model (Goode & Piedalue, 1999)

⇒ Model for Change to EBP (Rosswurm & Larrabee, 1999)

The most prominent of these have been the Stetler, Iowa, and Ottawa Models as well as the PARiHS framework. The first two models were originally developed in an environment that emphasized RU and have been updated to incorporate EBP processes.

The Stetler Model

According to a recent study by Canadian researchers Estabrooks and colleagues (2004), Cheryl Stetler continues to be one of the most often-cited authors in the RU field. The **Stetler Model** (originally developed with Marram in 1976 and then refined in 1994) has an underlying assumption that RU can be undertaken not only by organizations but also by individual clinicians and managers. The model was designed to facilitate critical thinking about the application of research findings in practice. The updated model is based on many of the same assumptions and strategies as the original but provides "an enhanced approach to the overall application of research in the service setting" (Stetler, 2001, p. 273). Stetler's model, presented graphically in Figure 18.2, involves five sequential phases of an EBP effort:

1. *Preparation.* In this phase, nurses define the underlying purpose of the project; search for and select sources of research evidence; consider external factors that can influence potential application and internal factors that can diminish objectivity; and affirm the clinical significance of solving the perceived problem.

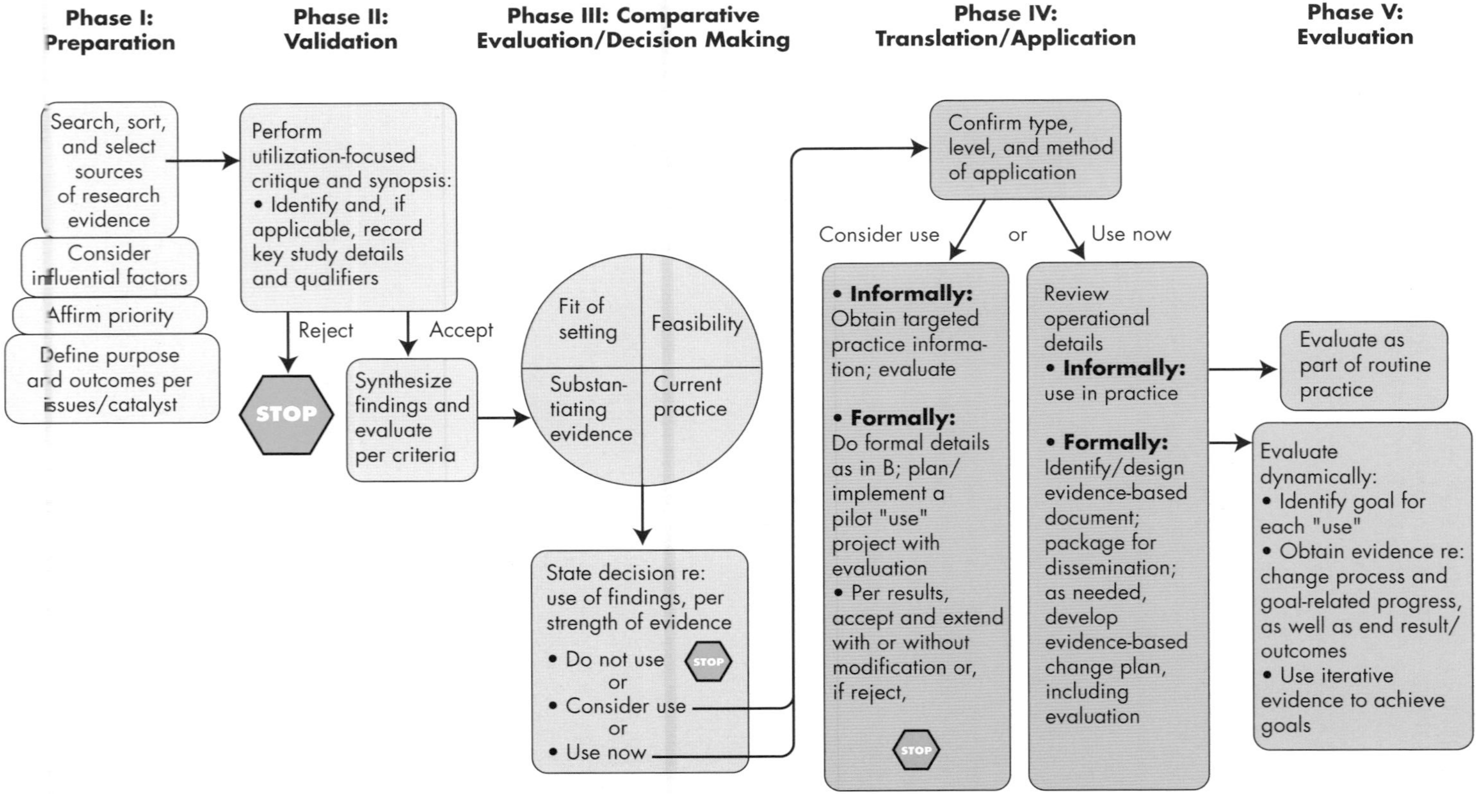

FIGURE 18.2 Stetler Model of Research Utilization to Facilitate Evidence-Based Practice. (Adapted from Stetler, C. B. [1994]. Refinement of the Stetler/Marram model for application of research findings into practice. *Nursing Outlook, 42,* 15–25.)

BOX 18.1 CRITERIA FOR COMPARATIVE EVALUATION PHASE OF STETLER'S MODEL

▶

1. Fit of Setting
Similarity of sample's characteristics to your client population
Similarity of study's environment to the one in which you work

2. Feasibility
Potential risks of implementation to patients, staff, and the organization
Readiness for change among those who would be involved in a change in practice
Resource requirements and availability

3. Current Practice
Congruency of the study with your theoretical basis for current practice behaviour

4. Substantiating Evidence
Availability of confirming evidence from other studies
Availability of confirming evidence from a meta-analysis or integrative review

---

Adapted from Stetler, C. B. (1994). Refinement of the Stetler/Marram model for application of research findings into practice. *Nursing Outlook, 42,* 15–25.

2. *Validation.* The second phase involves a utilization-focused critique of each evidence source, focusing on whether it is sufficiently sound for potential use in practice. The process stops at this point if the evidence sources are rejected.

3. *Comparative evaluation and decision making.* This phase involves a synthesis of findings and the application of four criteria that are used to determine the desirability and feasibility of applying findings from validated sources to nursing practice. These criteria (fit of setting, feasibility, current practice, and substantiating evidence) are summarized in Box 18.1. The end result of this phase is to make a decision about using the evidence.

4. *Translation/application.* This phase involves confirming how the findings will be used (e.g., formally or informally), spelling out the operational details of the application, and then implementing the plan. The latter might involve the development of a guideline or plan of action, possibly including a proposal for formal organizational change.

5. *Evaluation.* In the final phase, the application would be evaluated. Informal versus formal use of the innovation would lead to different evaluative strategies.

Although the Stetler Model was designed as a tool for individual practitioners, it has also been the basis of formal RU and EBP projects by groups of nurses.

Example of an application of the Stetler Model
Bishop (2007) applied the five phrases of the Stetler Model to screening for postpartum depression in primary care settings.

The Iowa Model

Efforts to use research evidence to improve nursing practice are often addressed by groups of nurses interested in a critical practice issue, using a model such as the Iowa Model of Research in Practice (Titler et al., 1994). This model, like the Stetler Model, was revised recently and renamed the **Iowa Model of Evidence-Based Practice to Promote Quality Care** (Titler et al., 2001). The current version of the Iowa Model, shown in Figure 18.3, acknowledges that a formal RU/EBP project begins with a *trigger*—an impetus to explore possible changes to practice. The start-point can be either (a) a *knowledge-focused trigger* that emerges from awareness of an innovation (and thus follows a more traditional RU path, as in the top

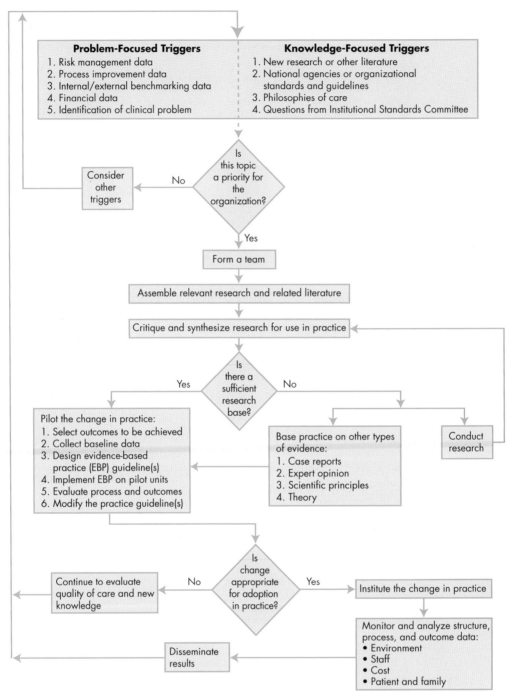

FIGURE 18.3 Iowa Model of Evidence-Based Practice to Promote Quality Care (Adapted from Titler et al. [2001]. The Iowa Model of evidence-based practice to promote quality care. *Critical Care Nursing Clinics of North America, 13,* 497–509.)

panel of Figure 18.3) or (b) a *problem-focused trigger* that has its roots in a clinical or organizational problem (and thus follows a path that more closely resembles an EBP intent). The model outlines a series of activities with three decision points:

1. Deciding whether the problem is a sufficient priority for the organization exploring possible changes; if yes, a team is formed to proceed with the project;
2. Deciding whether there is a sufficient research base; if yes, the innovation is piloted in the practice setting (if no, the team would either search for other sources of evidence or conduct its own research); and
3. Deciding whether the change is appropriate for adoption in practice; if yes, a change would be instituted and monitored.

Examples of application of the Iowa Model
Numerous EBP projects are underway at the University of Iowa, including an initiative focused on pain management in acute care and outpatient settings and another focused on facilitation of pet visitation in acute care settings (*http://www.uihealthcare.com/depts/nursing/rqom/evidencebasedpractice/currentprojects.html*).

The Ottawa Model of Research Use (OMRU)

The OMRU, developed by Logan and Graham (1998), consists of six key components interrelated through the process of evaluation. The six components deal with "the practice environment, the potential research adopter (administrators and clinical staff), the evidence-based innovation (the research intended for use in practice), strategies for transferring the innovation into practice, adoption/use of the evidence, and health and other outcomes" (Logan et al., 1999, p. 39). Systematic assessment, monitoring, and evaluation (AME) are central to the OMRU and are applied to each of the six components before, during, and after any effort to transfer research findings. The data gathered through AME serves several purposes:

⇒ to determine potential barriers to and supports for research use associated with the practice environment (structural, social, patients, and others);

⇒ to consider the knowledge, attitudes, and skills possessed by potential adopters;

⇒ to offer direction for choosing and tailoring transfer strategies to surmount the recognized barriers and enhance strategies that were deemed supportive; and

⇒ to evaluate the evidence-based innovation used and the influence it had on the outcomes of interest.

Example of an application of the Ottawa Model
Stacey et al. (2008) used the OMRU to guide the evaluation of a decision support intervention with health care professionals, which aimed to improve services for clients at an Australian cancer call centre.

The PARiHS Framework

The Promoting Action on Research Implementation in Health Services (PARiHS) framework was developed by Kitson and colleagues from the National Institute of Nursing in Oxford in 1996. This organizational model proposes that successful implementation of evidence into practice is a three-way interaction of: (1) the nature of the evidence (i.e., research, clinical experience, and patient preference); (2) the quality of the context (i.e., culture, leadership, and evaluation); and (3) expert facilitation (i.e., characteristics, role, and style). It offers a three-dimensional view, where optimal implementation is achieved along a continuum of "high to low" evidence and context. Kitson and colleagues recently summarized progress in the model to date, calling for greater testing and refinement (Kitson et al., 2008).

Example of an application of the PARiHS framework
Wright et al. (2007) applied the PARiHS framework to continence care in rehabilitation settings with older persons in Ireland, with a focus on defining and understanding contextual indicators (i.e., culture, leadership, and evaluation) that may facilitate or impede EBP.

Activities in a Research Utilization or EBP Project

As the various models of RU/EMP imply, formal efforts to use research to improve nursing practice involves a series of activities, decisions, and assessments. In this section, we discuss some of the major activities that are typical in an RU/EBP project. The three models described in the previous section are used as a basis for discussing key activities to support RU and EBP.

Selecting a Topic or Problem

As noted in the Iowa Model, there are two types of stimulus for an EBP or RU endeavour—identification of a clinical practice problem needing solution and discovery of an innovation in the literature. Problem-focused triggers may arise in the normal course of clinical practice or in the context of quality improvement efforts. This approach is likely to have staff support if the problem is one that numerous nurses have encountered, and it is likely to have considerable clinical relevance because a specific clinical situation generated interest in the problem in the first place.

Gennaro, Hodnett, and Kearney (2001) advise nurses following this approach to begin by clarifying the practice problem that needs to be solved and framing it as a question. The goal can be to find the most effective way to anticipate a problem (how to diagnose it) or the best way to solve a problem (how to intervene). Clinical practice questions may well take the form of "What is the best way to . . . "—for example, "What is the best way to manage hospitalized children's pain?"

A second catalyst for an RU/EBP project is the research literature, that is, knowledge-focused triggers. For example, a utilization project could emerge as a result of discussions within a journal club. In this approach, a preliminary assessment needs to be made of the clinical relevance of the research. The central issue is whether a significant nursing problem will be solved by making some change. Five questions relating to clinical relevance (shown in Box 18.2) can be applied to

---

BOX 18.2 CRITERIA FOR EVALUATING THE CLINICAL RELEVANCE OF A BODY OF RESEARCH

1. Does the research have the potential to help solve a problem that is currently being faced by practitioners?
2. Does the research have the potential to help with clinical decision making with respect to (a) making appropriate observations, (b) identifying client risks or complications, or (c) selecting an appropriate intervention?
3. Are clinically relevant theoretical propositions tested by the research?
4. If the research involves an intervention, does the intervention have potential for implementation in clinical practice? Do nurses have control over the implementation of such interventions?
5. Can the measures used in the study be used in clinical practice?

Adapted from Tanner, C. A. (1987). Evaluating research for use in practice: Guidelines for the clinician. *Heart & Lung, 16,* 424–430.

a research report or set of related reports. If the answer is yes to any of these questions, the next step can be pursued.

With both types of triggers, it is important to ensure that there is a consensus about the importance of the problem and the need for change. Titler and colleagues (2001) include as the first decision point in their model the resolution of whether the topic is a priority for the organization considering practice changes. They advise that the following issues be taken into account when initiating an EBP project: the topic's fit with the organization's strategic plan, magnitude of the problem, number of people invested in the problem, support of nurse leaders and of those in other disciplines, costs, and possible barriers to change.

TIP

The method of selecting a topic does not appear to have any bearing on the success of an RU/EBP project. What is important, however, is that the nurses who will implement an innovation are involved in the topic selection and that key stakeholders are "on board."

Assembling and Evaluating Evidence

Once a clinical practice question has been selected and a team has been formed to work on the project, the next step is to search for and assemble evidence on the topic. Chapter 7 provided information about locating research information, and Chapter 17 discussed research critiques, but some additional issues are relevant.

In doing a literature review for a new study, the central goal is to discover how best to advance knowledge. For EBP or RU projects, which typically have as end products prescriptive practice protocols or clinical guidelines, literature reviews are typically much more rigorous and formalized. The emphasis is on gathering comprehensive information on the topic, weighing pieces of evidence, and integrating information to draw conclusions about the evidence base. *Integrative reviews* thus play a crucial role in developing an EBP. If nurses are to glean best practices from research findings, they must take into account as much of the evidence as possible, organized and synthesized in a rigorous manner.

High-quality integrative reviews are a critical tool for RU/EBP, and if the project team has the skills to complete one, this is valuable. It is, however, unlikely that every clinical organization will be able to assemble the skills needed to do a high-quality critical review of research literature on a chosen topic. Fortunately, many researchers and organizations have taken on the responsibility of preparing integrative reviews and making them available for EBP.

Cochrane reviews are an especially important resource (see Grimshaw, Santesso, Cumpston, Mayhew, & McGowan, 2006). These reports, which are based mainly on meta-analyses, describe the background and objectives of the review; the methods used to search for, select, and evaluate studies; the main results; and, importantly, the reviewers' conclusions. Cochrane reviews are checked and updated regularly.

Example of a Cochrane review

Dobbins et al. (2009) completed a Cochrane review to critically appraise the evidence relating to the effectiveness of school-based interventions promoting physical activity and fitness in children aged 6 to 18 years. Data from 26 studies involving students from Australia, South America, Europe, and North America were included in the review. The authors concluded that although the interventions showed positive effect on only a limited number of outcome measures (i.e., duration of physical activity, television viewing, VO_2 max, and blood cholesterol), ongoing school-based physical activity intervention is currently recommended.

Another important resource for integrative reviews is the Agency for Healthcare Research and Quality (AHRQ) in the United States. This agency awarded twelve 5-year contracts in 1997 to establish EBP Centres at institutions in the United States and Canada (e.g., at McMaster University), and new 5-year contracts were awarded in 2002. Each centre issues *evidence reports* that are based on rigorous integrative reviews of relevant scientific literature; dozens of these reports are now available to help "improve the quality, effectiveness, and appropriateness of clinical care" (AHRQ website, *http://www.ahrq.gov/*). In Canada, the Ontario Ministry of Health and Long-Term Care sponsored the Effective Public Health Practice Project (EPHPP), a project that also undertakes and disseminates integrative reviews on a broad array of health topics (*http://www.hamilton.ca/ phcs/ephpp*).

If an integrative review has been prepared, it is possible that a formal evidence-based clinical guideline has been developed and can be used directly in an RU/EBP project. AHRQ, for example, has developed such guidelines on pain management, continence, and other problems of relevance to nurses (*http://www.guidelines.gov/*). Nursing organizations have also developed clinical practice guidelines on several topics. For example, the Registered Nurses Association of Ontario (RNAO) launched its Nursing Best Practice Guidelines (NBPG) Project in 1999. Funded as a multiyear project by the Ontario Ministry of Health and Long Term Care, the project team has developed 29 guidelines to date from gerontology to emergency care, available at *http://www.rnao.org/bestpractices* (Virani & Grinspun, 2007) with an additional four guidelines currently in progress.

In some cases, it may be possible to develop a new practice guideline based on a published integrative review. However, it is always wise to make sure that the review is up-to-date and that new findings published after the review are taken into consideration. Moreover, even a published integrative review needs to be critiqued and the validity of its conclusions assessed. Of course, there are many clinical questions for which integrative reviews are not available, and so the RU/EBP team might need to prepare its own integrative review. Some information about conducting and critiquing integrative reviews is presented later in this chapter.

An integrative review or synthesis of research evidence is used by the RU/EBP team to draw conclusions about the sufficiency of the research base for guiding clinical practice. Adequacy of research evidence depends on such factors as the consistency of findings across studies, the quality and rigour of the studies, the strength of observed effects, the transferability of the findings to clinical settings, and cost-effectiveness.

Conclusions about a body of evidence can lead to different decisions for further action. First, if the research base is small—or if there is a large base with ambiguous conclusions—the team might decide to pursue a different problem. A second option (preferable in the EBP environment) is to assemble other types of evidence (e.g., through consultation with experts or surveys of clients) and assess whether that evidence suggests a practice change. Finally, another possibility is to pursue an original clinical study to directly address the practice question, thereby gathering new evidence and contributing to the base of practice knowledge. This last course may well be impractical for many and would clearly result in years of delay before any further conclusions could be drawn.

A solid research base also could point in different directions. The evidence might, for example, support existing practices—which might lead to an analysis of why the practice question emerged and what might make existing practices work better. Another possibility is that there would be compelling evidence that a clinical change is warranted, which would lead to the activities described next.

Assessing Implementation Potential

Some models of RU/EBP move directly from the conclusion that evidence supports a change in practice to the pilot testing of the innovation. Others include steps to first evaluate the appropriateness of the innovation within the specific organizational context; in some cases, such an assessment (or aspects of it) may be warranted even before embarking on efforts to assemble best evidence. We think a preliminary assessment of the **implementation potential** of an innovation is often sensible.

In determining the implementation potential of an innovation in a particular setting, several issues should be considered, particularly the transferability of the innovation, the feasibility of implementing it, and the cost/benefit ratio. Box 18.3 presents some assessment questions for these categories.

➤ *Transferability.* The main question relating to transferability is whether it makes good sense to implement the innovation in the new practice setting. If there is some aspect of the practice setting that is fundamentally incongruent with the innovation in terms of its philosophy, types of client served, personnel, or

---

BOX 18.3 CRITERIA FOR EVALUATING THE IMPLEMENTATION POTENTIAL OF AN INNOVATION UNDER SCRUTINY

Transferability of the Findings

1. Will the innovation "fit" in the proposed setting?
2. How similar are the target populations in the research and in your setting?
3. Is the philosophy of care underlying the innovation fundamentally different from the philosophy prevailing in your setting? How entrenched is the prevailing philosophy?
4. Is there a sufficiently large number of clients in your setting who could benefit from the innovation?
5. Will the innovation take too long to implement and evaluate?

Feasibility

1. Will nurses have the freedom to carry out the innovation? Will they have the freedom to terminate the innovation if it is considered undesirable?
2. Will the implementation of the innovation interfere inordinately with current staff functions?
3. Does the administration support the innovation? Is the organizational climate conducive to RU?
4. Is there a fair degree of consensus among the staff and among the administrators that the innovation could be beneficial and should be tested? Are there major pockets of resistance or uncooperativeness that could undermine efforts to implement and evaluate the innovation?
5. To what extent will the implementation of the innovation cause friction within your organization? Does the utilization project have the support and cooperation of departments outside the nursing department?
6. Are the skills needed to carry out the utilization project (both the implementation and the clinical evaluation) available in the nursing staff? If not, how difficult will it be to collaborate with or to secure the assistance of others with the necessary skills?
7. Does your organization have the equipment and facilities necessary for the innovation? If not, is there a way to obtain the needed resources?
8. If nursing staff need to be released from other practice activities to learn about and implement the innovation, what is the likelihood that this will happen?
9. Are appropriate measuring tools available for a clinical evaluation of the innovation?

Cost/Benefit Ratio of the Innovation

1. What are the risks to which clients would be exposed during the implementation of the innovation and what are the potential benefits to clients?
2. What are the risks of maintaining current practices (i.e., the risks of *not* trying the innovation)?
3. What are the material costs of implementing the innovation? What are the costs in the short term during utilization, and what are the costs in the long run, if the change is to be institutionalized?
4. What are the material costs of *not* implementing the innovation (i.e., could the new procedure result in some efficiencies that could lower the cost of providing service)?
5. What are the potential nonmaterial costs and benefits of implementing the innovation to the organization (e.g., in terms of lower staff morale, staff turnover, absenteeism)?

administrative structure, it may not be prudent to try to adopt the innovation, even if it has been shown to be effective in other contexts.

➤ *Feasibility.* The feasibility questions in Box 18.3 address various practical concerns about the availability of staff and resources, the organizational climate, the availability of external assistance, and the potential for clinical evaluation. An important issue here is whether nurses will have (or share) control over the innovation. When nurses do not have full control over the new procedure, it is important to recognize the interdependent nature of the project and to proceed as early as possible to establish necessary cooperative arrangements.

➤ *Cost/benefit ratio.* A critical part of any decision to proceed with an RU/EBP project is a careful assessment of the costs and benefits of the innovation. The *cost–benefit assessment* should encompass likely costs and benefits to various groups, including clients, staff, and the overall organization. Clearly, the most important factor is the client. If the degree of risk in introducing a new procedure is high, then the potential benefits must be great, and the knowledge base must be very sound. A cost–benefit assessment should consider the opposite side of the coin as well: the costs and benefits of *not* implementing the innovation. It is sometimes easy to forget that the status quo bears its own risks and that failure to change, especially when such change is based on rigourous evidence, is also costly.

If the assessment suggests that there might be problems in testing the innovation within that particular practice setting, the team might consider devising a plan to improve the implementation potential (e.g., seeking external resources if costs are the inhibiting factor).

Developing, Implementing, and Evaluating the Innovation

If the implementation criteria are met, the next phase of the project would involve the following activities:

➤ Developing a written EBP guideline or protocol based on the synthesis of the evidence, preferably a guideline that is clear and user-friendly and that uses such devices as flow charts and decision trees;

➤ Training relevant staff in the use of the new guideline and, if necessary, "marketing" the innovation to users so that it is given a fair test;

➤ Developing an evaluation plan (e.g., identifying outcomes to be achieved, determining how many clients to involve, deciding when and how often to take measurements);

➤ Collecting baseline data relating to those outcomes, to develop a counterfactual against which the outcomes of the innovation would be assessed;

➤ Trying out the guideline in some units or with a sample of clients; and

➤ Evaluating the pilot project, in terms of both process (e.g., how was the innovation received, to what extent were the guidelines actually followed, what implementation problems were encountered?) and outcomes (in terms of clinical outcomes and cost effectiveness).

Evaluation data should be gathered over a sufficiently long period (typically, 6 to 12 months) to allow for a true test of a "mature" innovation. The end result of this process is a decision about whether to adopt the innovation, to modify it for ongoing use, or to revert to prior practices.

Examples of Evidence-Based Nursing Projects

Many EBP and RU projects are underway in practice settings, and some that have been described in the nursing literature offer information about planning and implementing such an endeavour. For example, Thurston and King (2004) described their use of Russworm and Larrabee's EBP model with 10 nursing teams in a regionwide mentorship program aimed at enabling clinical nurses to understand and implement an evidence-based approach to practice. As another example, Clarke et al. (2005) collaborated in a 2-year project to evaluate the use of computer-assisted strategies for implementing clinical practice guidelines for prevention and optimal treatment of pressure ulcers.

The Association of Women's Health, Obstetric, and Neonatal Nurses (AWHONN) has conducted several major RU/EBP projects as part of its Research-Based Practice program. Each project has resulted in the development and testing of evidence-based nursing protocols. For example, one project is focusing on a smoking cessation counselling strategy for pregnant women in clinical settings (Maloni, Albrecht, Thomas, Halleran, & Jones, 2003), and another is focusing on the management of cyclic perimenstrual pain and discomfort (Collins-Sharp, Taylor, Thomas, Killeen, & Dawood, in press). And yet another group, under the leadership of neonatal clinical nurse specialist Carolyn H. Lund, undertook a 4-year project designed to develop and evaluate an evidence-based clinical practice guideline for assessment and routine care of neonatal skin (Lund et al., 2001a, 2001b). The project also sought to educate nurses about the scientific basis for the recommended skin care practices and designed procedures to facilitate using the guideline in practice.

INTEGRATIVE REVIEWS

EBP relies on meticulous integration and critical evaluation of research evidence on a topic. This section is not specifically designed to teach you how to do an integrative review because the conduct of such reviews requires methodologic sophistication (see Whittemore & Knafl, 2005). However, it is important for you to have some skills in critiquing and appraising integrative reviews so that you can decide how much confidence to place in the reviewers' conclusions. To critique integrative reviews, you will need to learn a bit about how they are done.

Steps in Doing an Integrative Review

An **integrative review** is in itself a systematic inquiry that follows many of the same rules as those for primary studies. In other words, those doing an integrative review develop research questions or hypotheses, devise a sampling plan and data collection strategy, collect relevant data, and analyze and interpret those data.

It should be noted that integrative reviews are sometimes done by individuals, but it is far preferable to have at least two reviewers. Multiple reviewers not only share the workload but also help to minimize subjectivity. Reviewers should have substantive and clinical knowledge of the problem and sufficiently strong methodologic skills to evaluate study quality.

Research Questions and Hypotheses in Integrative Reviews

An integrative review begins with a problem statement and a research question or hypothesis. In critiquing an integrative review, you should determine whether the problem statement and questions are clearly worded and sufficiently specific, whether the variables or phenomena under study are adequately defined, and whether the population has been stated. Whether the review is a traditional narrative review, a meta-analysis, or a metasynthesis, the reviewers should clearly communicate their purpose and their rationale for undertaking it.

Example of a rationale from a metasynthesis
Price (2009) outlined the following rationale for undertaking her study—"A meta-synthesis of existing qualitative research on early professional socialization and career choice in nursing has the potential to inform future research and theoretical development which may be used to develop future recruitment and retention strategies required to address the critical and growing shortage of nurses" (p. 12).

Questions for an integrative review can be narrow, focusing, for example, on a particular type of intervention, or more inclusive, examining a range of alternative interventions or practices. In the above example, Price (2009) described an integrative review guided by the question, "What factors and experiences (personal, social and organizational) influence socialization to the nursing profession and the choice of nursing as a career?" (p. 12). The broader the question, the more complex and costly the integrative review becomes. In some cases, the broader the question, the less appropriate it is to integrate studies—just as in primary research, there must be an identifiable independent and dependent variable (for quantitative studies) or phenomenon (in qualitative studies).

Sampling in Integrative Reviews

In an integrative review, the "sample" involves primary studies that have addressed the same or a similar research question. In most cases, the reviewers try first to identify the full population of relevant studies, only some of which (a sample) may actually be used in the review.

Reviewers must make a number of upfront decisions regarding the sample, which they should share in their review so that readers can evaluate the rigour and generalizability of their conclusions. Sampling decisions include the following:

⮞ What are the exclusion and/or inclusion criteria for the search?

⮞ Will both published and unpublished reports be assembled?

⮞ What databases and other retrieval mechanisms will be used to locate the sample?

⮞ What key words or search terms will be used to identify relevant studies?

Example of sampling decisions for an integrative review
Spenceley et al. (2008) used a sampling timeframe of empirical research studies published between 1985 and 2006, in addition to other inclusion criteria, to reduce the initial sample from 165 to 32 articles used in the final review of studies exploring sources of information used by nurses to inform practice.

Eligibility criteria cover substantive, methodologic, and practical factors. Substantively, the criteria must stipulate what specific variables (or phenomena) are going to be studied. For example, if the review is integrating material about the effectiveness of a nursing intervention, what outcomes (dependent variables) must the researchers have studied? Another substantive issue concerns the study population. For example, will certain age groups of study participants (e.g., children, the elderly) be excluded? Methodologically, the criteria might specify that (for example) only studies that used an experimental design would be included. From a practical standpoint, the criteria might exclude, for example, reports written in a language other than English, or reports published before a certain date.

There is some disagreement about whether reviewers should limit their sample to published studies or cast as wide a net as possible and include *grey literature*— that is, studies with a more limited distribution, such as dissertations, unpublished reports, and so on. Some people use only published reports in peer-reviewed journals, as a proxy for study rigour. Conn et al. (2003) conducted a study on this matter, however, and concluded that the exclusion of grey literature can lead to certain types of biases, such as overestimating effects.

In searching for a comprehensive sample of research reports, reviewers usually need to use techniques more exhaustive than simply doing a computerized literature search of key databases, and this is especially true if the sample is to include grey literature. Five search methods described in path-breaking work by Cooper (1984) include the *ancestry approach* ("footnote chasing" of cited studies), the *decadency approach* (searching forward in citation indexes for subsequent references to key studies), online searches (including Internet searches), informal contacts at research conferences, and the more traditional searches of bibliographic databases.

Example of a search strategy for an integrative review
Gifford et al. (2007) did an integrative review of studies on managerial leadership and nurses' use of research evidence. They noted that "Selected databases were searched from January 1995 to January 2006 . . . The search strategy was executed for all databases using the same keywords and mapped subject headings (MeSH) for each database. Online searches of authors known to publish in the areas of leadership or RU were conducted (e.g., Estabrooks, Hicks, Kitson, Stetler, Upeniek), and reference lists from retrieved articles were manually searched" (p. 128).

When a potential pool of studies has been identified, reviewers then screen them for appropriateness. Typically, many located studies are discarded because they turn out not to be relevant or do not meet the eligibility criteria. Yet another reason for excluding studies from the initial pool (particularly for meta-analyses) is that some provide insufficient information to perform the necessary analyses. All decisions relating to exclusions (preferably made by at least two reviewers to ensure objectivity) should be well documented and justified.

Evaluating Primary Studies for Integrative Reviews

In any integrative review, each study must be evaluated to determine how much confidence to place in the findings. Strong studies need to be given more weight than weaker ones in coming to conclusions about the state of knowledge. There are different strategies for doing this, however. Some reviewers use methodologic quality as an exclusion criterion—for example, excluding non-RCT studies or studies with a low-quality rating. Others, however, include studies regardless of quality but incorporate information about quality into the analysis.

Example of excluding low-quality studies in an integrative review
In the previous example, Gifford et al. (2007) reviewed the included studies according to various methodological criteria—"Using the checklists and appraisal techniques discussed by Greenhalgh et al. (2004), the quality of papers was classified as 'excellent', 'some limitations', or 'many limitations'. Excellent quality was assigned when no major confounders or flaws were found in the quality assessment. 'Many limitations' was assigned when the number of confounders or flaws represented greater than half of the criteria" (p. 130).

For metasyntheses, Paterson et al. (2001) have developed the Primary Research Appraisal Tool as a systematic means of reviewing and evaluating qualitative studies. This protocol covers such aspects of a qualitative study as the sampling procedure, data gathering strategy, data analysis, researcher credentials, and researcher reflexivity. At the end of the process, the reviewer makes a decision to include the qualitative study in the metasynthesis or to reject it.

In meta-analyses, the evaluation usually involves a quantitative rating of the scientific merit of each study. AHRQ (2002) has published a guide that describes and evaluates various systems and instruments to rate the strength of evidence in quantitative medical and health studies. On the basis of a comprehensive review of the literature, the authors identified 121 instruments or systems, only 19 of which fully address quality domains AHRQ deemed to be essential. One of these

19 was developed by a British team working at the Royal College of Nursing Institute at the University of Oxford (Sindhu, Carpenter, & Seers, 1997). Deeks et al. (2003) reviewed 194 instruments for assessing the rigour of nonexperimental intervention studies and recommended only 6 for future use; one of these was developed by a team from Ontario that included nurse researchers (Thomas, Ciliska, Dobbins, & Micucci, 2004).

Quality assessments in integrative reviews should involve ratings by two or more qualified individuals. If there are disagreements between the two raters, there should be a discussion until a consensus has been reached, or, if necessary, a third rater should be asked to help resolve the difference. Indexes of interrater reliability are often calculated to demonstrate to readers that rater agreement was adequate.

Extracting and Recording Data for Integrative Reviews

The next step in an integrative review is to extract and record relevant information about study characteristics, methods, and findings. Reviewers often use a written protocol to record such information. The goal of this task is to produce a *data set*, and procedures similar to those used in creating a data set with raw data from individual participants also apply. Examples of the type of methodologic information that reviewers record for each study include type of research design and sample size. Characteristics of the study participants (e.g., age, gender) are usually recorded, as well as information about the data source (e.g., year of publication, country where the study took place). For a meta-analysis, all information would be numerically coded for statistical analysis.

Finally, and most important, information about the results must be extracted and recorded. In a narrative review, results are usually noted with a verbal summary or simple classification (e.g., nonsignificant versus significant group difference). In a metasynthesis, the information to be recorded includes the key metaphors, themes, or categories from each study. In a meta-analysis, as we subsequently discuss, the information to be recorded might include group means and standard deviations, and, most important, the **effect size,** that is, the index summarizing the magnitude of the relationship between the independent and dependent variables.

As with ratings of quality, extraction and coding of information ideally should be completed by two or more people, at least for a portion of the studies in the sample. This allows for an assessment of interrater agreement, which should be sufficiently high to persuade readers of the review that the recorded information is accurate.

Example of interrater agreement
In the same example, Gifford et al. (2007), two authors independently screened potential studies using a three-stage process where "Uncertainties regarding inclusion were discussed with a third reviewer until consensus was reached" (p. 129).

Analyzing Data in Integrative Reviews

In narrative integrative reviews, reviewers interpret the pattern of findings, draw conclusions about the evidence, and derive implications for practice and further research. There are various methods of qualitatively analyzing the data for narrative reviews, although many reviewers appear to rely primarily on judgments and do not make clear the rules of inference they used. Stetler and her colleagues (1998) have argued that analysis and synthesis in narrative integrative reviews should be a group process and that a whole review team should meet to discuss their conclusions after reviewing synopsized studies.

In a metasynthesis, data analysis involves transforming individual findings into a new conceptualization. Noblit and Hare (1988) provide one approach to metasynthesis. Their method consists of making a list of key metaphors from each study and determining their relation to each other. Are the metaphors, for example, directly comparable (reciprocal)? Are they in opposition to each other (refutational)? Next, the studies' metaphors are translated into each other. Noblit and Hare noted that "translations are especially unique syntheses because they protect the particular, respect holism, and enable comparison. An adequate translation maintains the central metaphors and/or concepts of each account in their relation to other key metaphors or concepts in that account" (1988, p. 28). This synthesis of qualitative studies creates a whole that is more than the sum of the parts of the individual studies.

Example of data analysis in a metasynthesis

Aagaard and Hall (2008) used Noblit and Hare's approach in their metasynthesis of 14 qualitative studies on mothers' experiences having a preterm infant in the neonatal intensive care unit. Five key metaphors were revealed in the analysis: "from their baby to my baby," "striving to be a real normal mother," "from foreground to background," "from silent vigilance to advocacy," and "from continuously answering questions through chatting to sharing of knowledge" (p. 26).

Meta-analysts analyze their data quantitatively using objective, standardized procedures. The essence of a meta-analysis is the calculation of a common metric—an *effect size*—for every study. The effect size represents the magnitude of the impact of an intervention on an outcome, or the degree of association between variables. Formulas for effect size differ depending on the nature of the statistical test used in the original analysis. The simplest formula to understand is the effect size for the difference between two means (e.g., an experimental group versus a control group). In this situation, the effect size for an outcome variable equals the mean for one group, minus the mean for the second group, divided by the overall standard deviation. Effect sizes for individual studies are then pooled across studies and averaged to yield estimates of population effects. These average effect sizes yield information about not only the *existence* of a relationship between variables but also the *magnitude*. Meta-analysts can, for example, draw conclusions about how big an effect an intervention has (with a specified probability of accuracy), which can yield estimates of the intervention's cost-effectiveness.

Meta-analysts can also examine whether there are **moderator effects** (or **subgroup effects**), that is, whether the relationship between an independent variable and a dependent variable is *moderated* by a third variable. For example, effect sizes can be computed separately for key subgroups (e.g., men versus women, children versus adolescents) to determine whether effects or relationships differ for segments of a population or variants of an intervention.

Some meta-analysts exclude studies that fail to meet a specified level of quality. Others prefer to retain methodologically weak studies in the data set, and then to "downweight" them in the analysis. For example, weights proportional to the quality rating can be assigned so that more rigorous studies "count" more in developing estimates of effects. Another approach is to conduct **sensitivity analyses**. This involves doing the statistical analyses twice, first including low-quality studies and then excluding them to see if including them changes the conclusions, or comparing the effect sizes for low-quality studies versus higher-quality studies.

TIP

It is difficult to provide explicit guidance on whether an effect size is "large" because it depends on the circumstances. However, it might help to know that effect sizes for comparing two group means are in standard deviation units. Thus, an effect size of 1.0 in an experimental–control group comparison would mean that the experimental group's average score was a full standard deviation higher (or lower) than that for the control group. This would be considered a very large effect size. An effect size of .50 typically would be considered a moderate effect.

Example of subgroup analysis in a meta-analysis
Hill Rice and Stead (2008) completed a Cochrane review on the effectiveness of nursing-delivered smoking cessation interventions. The meta-analysis of 42 studies indicated that there was reasonable evidence that these interventions were effective. However, subgroup analysis suggested that the effect was weaker if the intervention was brief and provided by nurses without expertise in health promotion.

Evaluating the Body of Evidence

The emphasis on EBP has led to the development of systems not only for appraising and rating individual studies but also for evaluating the strength of a body of evidence. The report by AHRQ (2002) identified seven such systems as being especially useful, four of which were specifically created for use in developing practice guidelines. As an example, one system was developed by the Institute for Clinical Systems Improvement (ICSI), a collaboration of 17 medical groups in Minnesota (Greer, Mosser, Logan, & Halaas, 2000). ICSI has used its system to develop numerous practice guidelines and technology assessment reports. An example of an ICSI guideline developed in 2004 is "The Assessment and Management of Acute Pain" (*http://www.icsi.org/*).

The AHRQ report identified three domains that are important in systems to grade the strength of a body of evidence on a topic: (1) *quality*—the aggregate of quality ratings for individual studies; (2) *quantity*—the magnitude of effect, number of studies, and aggregate sample size; and (3) *consistency*—the extent to which similar findings are reported using similar and different study designs. The ICSI system addresses all three domains.

Meta-analysts do not typically apply a formal system such as the one developed by ICSI to the body of evidence under review. However, their conclusions should include comments about the three domains of quality, quantity, and consistency.

The Written Integrative Review

Reports for integrative reviews typically follow the same format as a research report for a primary study. That is, there is typically an "Introduction" section, a "Method" section, a "Results" section, and a "Discussion" section. An abstract summarizing the major features of the review project is important. The "Method" section should be thorough: readers of the review need to be able to assess the validity of the findings by understanding and critiquing the procedures the reviewers used.

A well-written and thorough "Conclusion" or "Discussion" section is especially crucial in integrative reviews. The discussion should include an overall summary of the findings, the reviewers' assessment of the strength and limitations of the body of evidence, what further research should be undertaken to extend the evidence base, and what the implications of the review are for clinicians and patients.

The review should also discuss the consistency of findings across studies and provide an interpretation of why there might be inconsistency. Did the samples, research designs, or data collection strategies in the studies differ in important ways? Or do differences reflect substantive differences, such as variation in the interventions or outcomes themselves?

Dissemination efforts for integrative reviews are even more important than for primary studies. Ideally, the review should be made available in a variety of formats and to a wide audience.

Critiquing Integrative Reviews

Like primary studies, integrative reviews should be thoroughly critiqued before the findings are deemed trustworthy and relevant to clinicians. Box 18.4 offers guidelines for evaluating integrative reviews.

Although these guidelines are fairly broad, not all questions apply equally well to all integrative reviews. For example, the question on subgroups under the "Data

BOX 18.4 GUIDELINES FOR CRITIQUING INTEGRATIVE REVIEWS

The Problem

Does the review clearly state the research problem and/or research questions? Is the topic of the review important for the nursing profession? Is the scope of the review appropriate? Are concepts, variables, or phenomena adequately defined?

Search Strategy

Does the review clearly describe the criteria for selecting primary studies, and are those criteria reasonable? Are the databases the reviewers used identified, and are they appropriate? Are key words identified, and are they appropriate? Did the reviewers use adequate supplementary efforts to identify relevant studies, including unpublished studies?

The Sample

Did the search strategy yield an adequate sample of studies? Did the studies include an adequate sample of participants? If an original report was lacking key information, did the reviewers attempt to contact the original researchers for additional information—or did the study have to be excluded? If studies were excluded for reasons other than insufficient information, did the reviewers provide a rationale for the decision? Did the reviewers retrieve primary source materials (i.e., the actual study reports), or did they draw their data from secondary sources?

Quality Appraisal

Did the reviewers determine the methodologic comparability of the studies in the review? Did the reviewers use appropriate procedures for appraising the quality of individual studies? Were formal criteria used in the appraisal, and were those criteria explicit? Were the criteria appropriate for the type of studies in the sample? Did two or more raters do the appraisals, and was interrater reliability reported?

The Data Set

Were two or more coders used to extract and record information for analysis? Was adequate information extracted about substantive, methodologic, and administrative aspects of the study? Was sufficient information extracted to permit subgroup analysis (if appropriate)? In a meta-analysis, was it possible to compute effect sizes for a sufficient number of studies in the sample?

Data Analysis

Do the reviewers explain their method of pooling and integrating their data? In a meta-synthesis, do the reviewers describe the techniques they used to compare the findings of each study, and do they explain their method of interpreting their data? Was the analysis of data objective and thorough? Were appropriate procedures used to address differences in methodologic quality among studies in the sample? Were appropriate subgroup analyses undertaken—or was the absence of subgroup analyses justified?

Conclusions

Did the reviewers draw reasonable conclusions about the quality, quantity, and consistency of evidence? In a metasynthesis, did the synthesis achieve a fuller understanding of the phenomenon to advance knowledge? Are limitations of the review noted? Are implications for nursing practice and further research clearly stated?

Analysis" questions is relevant primarily for integrative reviews of quantitative studies. Moreover, questions in Box 18.4 are not necessarily comprehensive. Supplementary questions might be needed for certain types of review.

In drawing conclusions about an integrative review, one issue is to evaluate whether the reviewer did a good job in pulling together and summarizing the evidence, as suggested by the questions in Box 18.4. Another aspect, however, is drawing inferences about how you might use the evidence in your own practice. It is not the reviewer's job, for example, to consider such issues as barriers to making use of the evidence, acceptability of an innovation, and costs and benefits of change in various settings. These are issues for practicing nurses seeking to maximize the effectiveness of their actions and decisions.

▶ RESEARCH EXAMPLES AND CRITICAL THINKING ACTIVITIES

EXAMPLE 1 ■ A Metasynthesis Using Paterson et al.'s Framework

Aspects of a metasynthesis, featuring terms and concepts discussed in this chapter, are presented below, followed by some questions to guide critical thinking.

Study

"Becoming a nurse: A meta-study of early professional socialization and career choice in nursing" (Price, 2009)

Purpose

The purpose of the study was to provide a meta-study of early professional socialization and career choice in nursing, in order to develop possible future recruitment and retention strategies.

Eligibility Criteria

A study was included if it explored the concept of "professional socialization in nursing" or "nurses' career choice decisions" from a qualitative approach, including individual interviews, focus group interviews, and observation. Studies were excluded if the methods were not clearly defined or applied surveys using open-ended questions.

Search Strategy

Price searched existing literature from 1990 to 2007 in six electronic databases: CINAHL, PsychINFO, Sociological Abstracts, PubMed, Medline, and Embase, as well as hand-searching the reference lists. Studies without abstracts and unpublished theses were excluded.

Sample

Of the 871 studies initially retrieved, 10 met the final inclusion and exclusion criteria. These included three descriptive studies, one phenomenological study, two grounded theory studies, and four ethnographies. The combined sample of participants included 159 mothers from the United States, Australia, England, Sweden, and Denmark.

Data Extraction and Analysis

Paterson et al.'s framework for qualitative metasynthesis was applied to extract details from each study including: purpose, sample, sampling procedures, theoretical approaches, methodology, methods, and key findings. Thematic analysis was used involving first- and second-level coding: "The first level of coding arose from the themes identified in the primary studies. Second level coding involved exploring similarities and differences in codes within and between studies. Once the studies were coded, data were categorized, with individual units being brought together into categories having similar content/meaning until all the data were accounted for. Once categorization was complete each set of categories was examined for relationships and themes both within and between each set. Findings were then grouped according to similar themes" (p. 14).

Key Findings

- Discovery of an overarching meta-theme—"realizing and redefining role expectations" (p. 14).
- Identification of three main themes—"influence of ideals," "paradox of caring," and "role of others" (p. 15–17).

Discussion

Price concluded that early socialization experiences are fundamental to "an individual's view of nursing, self-identification with nurse attributes, and the decision to enter the profession" and can be positively influenced by role models like mentors and peers (p. 18). Depictions of nursing as a career need to be realistic and contemporary for successful retention of new nurses long-term.

CRITICAL THINKING SUGGESTIONS

1. Answer appropriate questions from Box 18.4 (p. 391) regarding this study.
2. Also consider the following targeted questions, which may assist you in further assessing aspects of the study:
   a. Comment on the author undertaking sole review in the critical appraisal process.
   b. Comment on the author's choice not to search the grey literature with this kind of topic.
3. If the results of this study are valid and reliable, what are some of the uses to which the findings might be put into clinical practice?

EXAMPLE 2 ■ A Metasynthesis Using Noblit and Hare's Approach

Aspects of a metasynthesis, featuring terms and concepts discussed in this chapter, are presented below, followed by some questions to guide critical thinking.

Study
"Mothers' experiences of having a preterm infant in the neonatal care unit: A meta-synthesis" (Aagaard & Hall, 2008)

Purpose
The purpose of the study was to synthesize qualitative studies on the phenomenon of mothers' experiences of having a preterm infant in the neonatal intensive care unit (NICU).

Eligibility Criteria
A study was included if the phenomenon under investigation was the experience of having a preterm baby in NICU and if a qualitative approach was used, regardless of research tradition. Studies were excluded if the sample only included the experience of having a full-term baby in NICU.

Search Strategy
The authors searched the following databases for studies published after 2000 with the keywords "preterm," "mother," and "neonatal intensive care": PubMed, CINAHL, Web of Science, and PsychINFO, as well as the references listed in the studies found.

Sample
Fourteen studies met the sample inclusion and exclusion criteria. The fourteen studies included six descriptive studies, four phenomenological studies, one grounded theory study, one Foucauldian, and two ethnographies. The combined sample of participants included 159 mothers from the United States, Australia, England, Sweden, and Denmark.

Data Extraction and Analysis
Noblit and Hare's (1988) comparative approach was used to compare study findings. The original metaphors, themes, concepts, and phrases from each of the 14 studies were reciprocally translated, one into the other, revealing five interrelated metaphors.

Key Findings
The five interrelated metaphors were:

- Mother–baby relationship: From their baby to my baby;
- Maternal development: A striving to be a real mother;
- A turbulent neonatal environment: From foreground to background;
- Maternal caregiving and role reclaiming strategies: From silent vigilance to advocacy; and
- Mother–nurse relationship: From continuously answering questions through chatting to sharing of knowledge.

(Research Examples and Critical Thinking Activities continues on page 394)

Research Examples and Critical Thinking Activities (Continued)

Discussion

Aagaard and Hall concluded that the metasynthesis provides nurses with a comprehensive picture of the experience of having a preterm infant in NICU. The authors argue that while the nursing focus is understandably on providing the best possible care to the infant, additional support should be provided to the mother (through the use of a care delivery plan, guided participation, and chat) to develop and strengthen maternal competence during a time of "uncertain motherhood."

CRITICAL THINKING SUGGESTIONS

1. Answer appropriate questions from Box 18.4 (p. 391) regarding this study.
2. Also consider the following targeted questions, which may assist you in further assessing aspects of the study:
   a. Comment on the authors' decision to include studies from countries outside of North America.
   b. Comment on the authors' decision to include studies from various qualitative research traditions.
3. If the results of this study are trustworthy, what are some of the uses to which the findings might be put into clinical practice?

Summary Points

- ⇝ **Research utilization** (RU) and **evidence-based practice** (EBP) are overlapping concepts that concern efforts to use research as a basis for clinical decisions. RU starts with research findings that get evaluated for possible use in practice. EBP starts with a search for the best possible evidence for a clinical problem, with emphasis on research-based evidence.

- ⇝ RU exists on a continuum, with direct utilization of some specific innovation at one end (**instrumental utilization**) and more diffuse situations in which users are influenced in their thinking about an issue based on some research (**conceptual utilization**) at the other end.

- ⇝ Several major utilization projects have been implemented (e.g., the **Conduct and Utilization of Research in Nursing**—or CURN—**project**), which have demonstrated that RU can be increased but which have also shed light on barriers to utilization.

- ⇝ EBP, which de-emphasizes clinical decision making based on custom or ritual, integrates the best available research evidence with other sources of data, including clinical expertise and patient preferences.

- ⇝ In nursing, EBP and RU efforts often face various barriers, including methodologically weak or unreplicated studies, nurses' limited training in research and EBP, lack of organizational support, resource constraints, and limited communication and collaboration between practitioners and researchers.

- ⇝ Many models of RU and EBP have been developed, including models for individual clinicians (e.g., the **Stetler Model**) and models for organizations or groups of clinicians (e.g., the **Iowa Model of Evidence-Based Practice to Promote Quality Care,** the **Ottawa Model** of **Research Use**).

- ⇝ Most models of utilization involve the following steps: selecting a topic or problem; assembling and evaluating evidence; assessing the **implementation potential** of an evidence-based innovation; implementing the innovation and evaluating outcomes; and deciding whether to adopt or modify the innovation or revert to prior practices.

⇒ Assessing implementation potential includes the dimensions of transferability of findings, the feasibility of using the findings in the new setting, and the cost/benefit ratio of a new practice.

⇒ EBP relies on integration of research evidence on a topic through **integrative reviews,** which are rigorous, systematic inquiries with many similarities to original primary studies.

⇒ Integrative reviews can involve either qualitative, narrative approaches to integration (including metasynthesis of qualitative studies), or quantitative (meta-analytic) methods.

⇒ Integrative reviews typically involve the following activities: developing a question or hypothesis; assembling a review team; searching for and selecting a sample of studies to be included in the review; doing quality assessments of the studies; extracting and recording data from the sampled studies; analyzing the data; and writing up the review.

⇒ Quality assessments (which may involve formal quantitative ratings) are sometimes used to exclude weak studies from integrative reviews but can also be used in **sensitivity analyses** to determine whether including or excluding weaker studies changes conclusions.

⇒ Meta-analysis involves the computation of an **effect size** (which quantifies the magnitude of relationship between the independent and dependent variables) for every study in the sample, and averaging across studies. Meta-analysts can also test for **moderator** (or **subgroup**) **effects,** that is, whether effects are moderated by a third variable.

STUDIES CITED IN CHAPTER 18*

*This reference list contains only those studies that were cited in this chapter. Citations pertaining to theoretical, methodologic, or nonempirical work are included together in a separate section at the end of the book (beginning on page 399).

Aagaard, H., & Hall, E. O. C. (2008). Mothers' experiences of having a preterm infant in the neonatal care unit: A meta-synthesis. *Journal of Pediatric Nursing, 23*(3), e26–e36.

Alberta Association of Registered Nurses. (1997). *Nursing research dissemination and utilization.* Retrieved October, 2003, from Alberta Association of Registered Nurses Website, *http://www. nurses. ab.ca/publications/*papers/html

Bishop, K. K. (2007). Utilization of the Stetler Model: Evaluating the scientific evidence on screening for postpartum depression risk factors in a primary care setting. *Kentucky Nurse, 55*(1), 7.

Caplan, N., & Rich, R. F. (1975). *The use of social science knowledge in policy decisions at the national level.* Ann Arbor, MI: Institute for Social Research, University of Michigan.

Clarke, H. F., Bradley, C., Whytock, S., Handfield, S., van der Wal, R., & Gundry, S. (2005). Pressure ulcers: implementation of evidence-based nursing practice. *Journal of Advanced Nursing, 49*(6), 578–90.

Cochrane, A. L. (1972). *Effectiveness and Efficiency: random reflections on health services.* London: Nuffield Provincial Hospitals Trust.

Collins Sharp, B. A., Taylor, D. L., Thomas, K. K., Killeen, M. B., & Dawood, M. Y. (2002). Cyclic perimenstrual pain and discomfort: the scientific basis for practice. *Journal of Obstetric, Gynecologic and Neonatal Nursing, 31*(6), 637–649.

Conn, V. S., Valentine, J. C., Cooper, H. M., & Rantz, M. J. (2003). Grey literature in meta-analyses. *Nursing Research, 52,* 256–261.

Cooper, H. (1984). *The integrative research review: A social science approach.* Beverly Hills, CA: Sage.

Coyle, L. A, & Sokop, A. G. (1990). Innovation adoption behavior among nurses. *Nursing Research, 39*(3), 176–80.

Cummings, G. G., Estabrooks, C. A., Midodzi, W. K., Wallin, L., & Hayduk, L. (2007). Influence of organizational characteristics and context on research utilization. *Nursing Research, 56*(4 Suppl.), S24–S39.

Deeks, J. J., Dinnes, J., D'Amico, R., et al. (2003). Evaluating non-randomized intervention studies. *Health Technology Assessment, 7,* 1–173.

Dobbins, M., De Corby, K., Robeson, P., Husson, H., & Tirilis, D. (2009). School-based physical activity programs for promoting physical activity and fitness in children and adolescents aged 6–18. *Cochrane Database of Systematic Reviews,* Issue 1. Art. No.: CD007651. DOI: 10.1002/ 14651858.CD007651.

Estabrooks C. A. (1999). The conceptual structure of research utilization. *Research in Nursing and Health, 22*(3), 203–16.

Estabrooks, C. A., Chong, H., Brigidear, K., & Profetto-McGrath, J. (2005). Profiling Canadian nurses' preferred knowledge sources for clinical practice. *Canadian Journal of Nursing Research, 37*(2), 118–40.

Estabrooks, C. A., Thompson, D. S., Lovely, J. J., & Hofmeyer, A. (2006). A guide to knowledge translation theory. *The Journal of Continuing Education in the Health Professions, 26*(1), 25–36.

Estabrooks, C. A. (2004). Thoughts on evidence-based nursing and its science: A Canadian perspective. *Worldviews on Evidence-Based Nursing, 1*, 88–91.

Estabrooks, C. E. (2001). Research utilization and qualitative research. In J. M. Morse, J. M. Swanson, & A. J. Kuzel (Eds), *The nature of qualitative evidence* (pp. 275–298). Thousand Oaks, CA: Sage.

Feldstein, A. C., & Glasgow, R. E. (2008). A practical, robust implementation and sustainability model (PRISM) for integrating research findings into practice. *The Joint Commission Journal on Quality and Patient Safety, 34*(4), 228–243.

Gerrish, K., & Clayton, J. (2004). Promoting evidence-based practice: An organizational approach. *Journal of Nursing Management, 12*, 114–123.

Gifford, W., Davies, B., Edwards, N., Griffin, P., & Lybanon, V. (2007). Managerial leadership for nurses' use of research evidence: An integrative review of the literature. *Worldviews on Evidence-Based Nursing, 4*(3), 126–145.

Goode, C., & Piedalue, F. (1999). Evidence based clinical practice. *Journal of Nursing Administration, 29*(6), 15–21.

Graham, I. D., Logan, J., Davies, B., & Nimrod, C. (2004). Changing the use of electronic fetal monitoring and labor support: A case study of barriers and facilitators. *Birth*, 31, 293–301.

Graham, I. D., Logan, J., Harrison, M. B., et al. (2006). Lost in knowledge translation: Time for a map? *Journal of Continuing Education in the Health Professions, 26*(1), 13–24.

Greer, N., Mosser, G., Logan, G., & Halaas, G. W. (2000). A practical approach to evidence grading. *Joint Commission Journal on Quality Improvement, 26*, 700–712.

Grimshaw, J. M., Santesso, N., Cumpston, M., Mayhew, A., & McGowan, J. (2006). Knowledge for knowledge translation: The role of the Cochrane Collaboration. *The Journal of Continuing Education in the Health Professions, 26*(1), 55–62.

Hek, G., & Shaw, A. (2006). The contribution of research knowledge and skills to practice: An exploration of the views and experiences of newly qualified nurses. *Journal of Research in Nursing, 11*(6), 473–482.

Hill Rice, V., & Stead, L. F. (2008). Nursing interventions for smoking cessation. *Cochrane Database of Systematic Reviews*, Issue 1. Art. No.: CD001188. DOI: 10.1002/14651858.CD001188.pub3.

Horsley, J. A., Crane, J., & Bingle, J. D. (1978). Research utilization as an organizational process. *Journal of Nursing Administration*, 8, 4–6.

Hutchinson, A. M., & Johnston, L. (2004). Bridging the divide: A Survey of nurses' opinions regarding barriers to, and facilitation of, research utilization in the practice setting. *Journal of Clinical Nursing*, 13, 304–315.

Kent, B., & Fineout-Overholt, E. (2008). Using meta-synthesis to facilitate evidence-based practice. *Worldviews on Evidence-Based Nursing, 5*(3), 160–162.

Ketefian, S. (1975). Application of selected nursing research findings into nursing practice: a pilot study. *Nursing Research, 24*(2), 89–92.

Kirchhoff, KT. (1982). Visiting policies for patients with myocardial infarction: a national survey. *Heart & Lung, 11*(6), 571–6.

Kitson, A., Ahmed, L. B., Harvey, G., Seers, K., & Thompson, D. R. (1996). From research to practice: One organisational model for promoting research-based practice. *Journal of Advanced Nursing, 23*(3), 430–440.

Kitson, A., Rycroft-Malone, J., Harvey, G., McCormack, B., Seers, K., & Titchen, A. (2008). Evaluating the successful implementation of evidence into practice using the PARiHS framework: Theoretical and practical challenges. *Implementation Science*, 3, 1.

Logan, J., & Graham, I. (1998). Toward a comprehensive interdisciplinary model of health care research use. *Science Communication*, 20, 227–246.

Logan, J., Harrison, M. B., Graham, I. D., Dunn, K., & Bissonnette, J. (1999). Evidence-based pressure-ulcer practice: The Ottawa Model of Research Use. *Canadian Journal of Nursing Research*, 31, 37–52.

Lund, C. H., Kuller, J., Lane, A. T., Lott, J. W., Raines, D. A., & Thomas, K. K. (2001). Neonatal skin care: Evaluation of the AWHONN/NANN research-based practice project on knowledge and skin care practices. *Journal of Obstetric, Gynecologic, & Neonatal Nursing, 30*, 30–40.

Lund, C. H., Osborne, J. W., Kuller, J., Lane, A. T., Lott, J. W., & Raines, D. A. (2001). Neonatal skin care: Clinical outcomes of the AWHONN/NANN evidence-based clinical practice guideline. *Journal of Obstetric, Gynecologic, & Neonatal Nursing*, 30, 41–51.

Maloni, J. A., Albrecht, S. A., Thomas, K. K., Halleran, J., & Jones, R. (2003). Implementing evidence-based practice: Reducing risk for low birth weight through pregnancy smoking cessation. *Journal of Obstetric, Gynecology, & Neonatal Nursing*, 32, 676–682.

McCleary, L., & Brown, G. T. (2003a). Barriers to paeditriac nurses' research utilization. *Journal of Advanced Nursing, 42,* 364–372.

McCleary, L., & Brown, G. T. (2003b). Association between nurses' education about research and their research use. *Nurse Education Today, 23,* 556–565.

Nelson, A. M. (2008). Addressing the threat of evidence-based practice to qualitative inquiry through increasing attention to quality: A discussion paper. *International Journal of Nursing Studies, 45*(2), 316–322.

Noblit, G., & Hare, R. D. (1988). *Meta-ethnography: Synthesizing qualitative studies.* Newbury Park, CA: Sage.

O'Donnell, C. A. (2004). Attitudes and knowledge of primary care professionals toward evidence-based practice. *Journal of Evaluation in Clinical Practice, 10,* 197–205.

Price, S. L. (2009). Becoming a nurse: A meta-study of early professional socialization and career choice in nursing. *Journal of Advanced Nursing, 65*(1), 11–19.

Rodgers, S. E. (2000). The extent of nursing research utilization in general medical and surgical wards. *Journal of Advanced Nursing, 32,* 182–193.

Rosswurm, M. A., & Larrabee, J. H. (1999). A model for change to evidence-based practice. *Image: Journal of Nursing Scholarship, 31,* 317–322.

Rycroft-Malone, J., Seers, K., Titchen, A., Harvey, G., Kitson, A., & McCormack, B. (2004). What counts as evidence in evidence-based practice? *Journal of Advanced Nursing, 47*(1), 81–90.

Sackett, D. L., Rosenberg, W., Gray, J. A., Haynes, R., & Richardson, W. (1996). Evidence based medicine: What it is and what it isn't. *British Medical Journal, 312,* 71–72.

Scott, S. D., & Pollock, C. (2008). The role of nursing unit culture in shaping research utilization behaviours. *Research in Nursing & Health, 31*(4), 298–309.

Scott-Findlay, S., & Estabrooks, C. A. (2006). Mapping the organizational culture research in nursing: A literature review. *Journal of Advanced Nursing, 56*(5), 498–513.

Scott-Findlay, S., & Pollock, C. (2004). Evidence, research, knowledge: A call for conceptual clarity. *Worldviews on Evidence-Based Nursing, 1*(2), 92–97.

Shore, H. L. (1972). Adopters and laggards. *Canadian Nurse, 68*(7), 36–9.

Sindhu, F., Carpenter, L., & Seers, K. (1997). Development of a tool to rate the quality assessment of randomized controlled trials using a Delphi technique. *Journal of Advanced Nursing, 25,* 1262–1268.

Spenceley, S. M., O'Leary, K. A., Chizawsky, L. L. K., Ross, A. J., & Estabrooks, C. A. (2008). Sources of information used by nurses to inform practice: An integrative review. *International Journal of Nursing Studies, 45*(6), 954–970.

Stacey, D., Chambers, S. K., Jacobsen, M. J., & Dunn, J. (2008). Overcoming barriers to cancer-helpline professionals: Providing decision support for callers: An implementation study. *Oncology Nursing Forum, 35*(6), 961–969.

Stetler, C. B. (1994). Refinement of the Stetler/Marram model for application of research findings into practice. *Nursing Outlook, 42,* 15–25.

Stetler, C. B. (2001). Updating the Stetler Model of Research Utilization to facilitate evidence-based practice. *Nursing Outlook, 49,* 272–279.

Stetler, C. B., Morsi, D., Rucki, S., et al. (1998). Utilization-focused integrative reviews in a nursing service. *Applied Nursing Research, 11,* 195–206.

Thompson, G. N., Estabrooks, C. A., & Degner, L. F. (2006). Clarifying the concepts in knowledge transfer: A literature review. *Journal of Advanced Nursing, 53*(6), 691–701.

Thorne, S. (2008). The role of qualitative research within an evidence-based context: Can meta-synthesis be the answer? A discussion paper. *International Journal of Nursing Studies,* doi:10.1016/j.ijnurstu.2008.05.001.

Thorne, S., Jensen, L., Kearney, M. H., Noblit, G., & Sandelowski, M. (2004). Qualitative metasynthesis: Reflections on methodological orientation and ideological agenda. *Qualitative Health Research, 14,* 1342–1354.

Thurston, N. E., & King, K. M. (2004). Implementing evidence-based practice: Walking the talk. *Applied Nursing Research, 17,* 239–247.

Titler, M. G., Kleiber, C., Steelman, V., et al. (1994). Infusing research into practice to promote quality care. *Nursing Research, 43,* 307–313.

Titler, M. G., Kleiber, C., Steelman, V., et al. (2001). The Iowa model of evidence-based practice to promote quality care. *Critical Care Nursing Clinics of North America, 13,* 497–509.

Varcoe, C., & Hilton, A. (1995). Factors affecting acute-care nurses' use of research findings. *Canadian Journal of Nursing Research, 27*(4), 51–71.

Virani, T., & Grinspun, D. (2007). RNAO's best practice guidelines program: Progress report on a phenomenal journey. *Advances in Skin & Wound Care, 20*(10), 528–535.

Weiss, C. (1980). Knowledge creep and decision accretion. *Knowledge: Creation, Diffusion, Utilization, 1,* 381–404.

Whittemore, R., & Knafl, K. (2005). The integrative review: Updated methodology. *Journal of Advanced Nursing, 52*(5), 546–553.

Wright, J., McCormack, B., Coffey, A., & McCarthy, G. (2007). Evaluating the context within which continence care is provided in rehabilitation units for older people. *International Journal of Older People Nursing, 2*(1), 9–19.

World Wide Web Sites

❧ AHCPR/AHRQ Clinical Practice Guidelines
   http://www.ahrq.gov/ and *http://www.guidelines.gov/*

❧ The Cochrane Collaboration
   http://www.cochrane.org/

❧ Evidence Based Clinical Practice (McMaster University, Hamilton, Ontario)
   http://www-hsl.mcmaster.ca/ebcp

❧ Health Care Guidelines
   http://evidence.ahc.umn.edu/health_care_guidelines.htm

❧ Registered Nurses Association of Ontario Best Practice Guidelines
   http://www.rnao.org/bestpractices

❧ University of Alberta University of Alberta's "Evidence-Based Medicine Tool Kit"
   http://www.med.ualberta.ca/ebm/ebm.htm

❧ University of Iowa's Evidence Based Practice Center
   http://www.uihealthcare.com/depts/nursing/rqom/evidencebasedpractice/toolkit.html

❧ University of Sheffield (United Kingdom), "Netting the Evidence"
   http://www.shef.ac.uk/scharr/ir/netting/

Methodologic and Theoretical References

Agency for Healthcare Research and Quality. (2002). *Systems to rate the strength of scientific evidence.* Washington, DC: Author.

Baker, C., Wuest, J., & Stern, P. N. (1992). Method slurring: The grounded theory/phenomenology example. *Journal of Advanced Nursing, 17,* 1355–1360.

Baldwin, K. M., & Nail, L. M. (2000). Opportunities and challenges in clinical nursing research. *Journal of Nursing Scholarship, 32,* 163–166.

Barker, J. H. (2008). Q-methodology: An alternative approach to research in nurse education. *Nurse Education Today, 28,* 917–925.

Beck, C. T. (1990). The research critique: General criteria for evaluating a research report. *Journal of Obstetric, Gynecologic, and Neonatal Nursing, 19,* 18–22.

Beck, C. T. (1993). Qualitative research: The evaluation of its credibility, fittingness, and auditability. *Western Journal of Nursing Research, 15,* 263–266.

Beck, C. T. (1997). Use of meta-analysis as a teaching strategy in nursing research courses. *Journal of Nursing Education, 36,* 87–90.

Beck, C. T. (2005). Benefits of participants in Internet interviews. Women helping women. *Qualitative Health Research, 15,* 411–422.

Biggs, A. (2008). Orem's self-care deficit nursing theory: Update on the state of the art and science. *Nursing Science Quarterly, 21*(3), 200–216.

Canadian Institutes of Health Research. (2007). *CIHR guidelines for health research involving Aboriginal People.* Ottawa, ON: Author.

Canadian Institutes of Health Research, Natural Sciences and Engineering Research Council of Canada, and Social Sciences and Humanities Research Council of Canada. (1998, with 2000, 2002, and 2005 amendments). *Tri-council policy statement: Ethical conduct for research involving humans.* Ottawa, ON: Minister of Supply and Services.

Canadian Institutes of Health Research, Natural Sciences and Engineering Research Council of Canada, and Social Sciences and Humanities Research Council of Canada. (1998, with 2000, 2002, and 2005 amendments). *Tri-council policy statement: Integrity in research and scholarship.* Ottawa, ON: Minister of Supply and Services.

Canadian Nurses Association. (2002). *Ethical guidelines for nurses in research involving human subjects.* Ottawa, ON: Author.

Canadian Nurses Association. (2002). *Position statement: Evidence-based decision-making and nursing practice.* Ottawa, ON: Author.

Canadian Nurses Association. (2008). *Code of ethics for registered nurses.* Ottawa, ON: Author.

Canadian Nurses Association. (2008). *Position statement: Practice: The code of ethics for registered nurses.* Ottawa, ON: Author.

Carpenter, J. (2008). Metaphors in qualitative research: Shedding light or casting shadows? *Research in Nursing & Health, 31,* 274–282.

Chiovitti, R. F., & Piran, N. (2003). Rigour and grounded theory research. *Journal of Advanced Nursing, 44,* 427–435.

Creswell, J. W. (1998). *Qualitative inquiry and research design: Choosing among five traditions.* Thousand Oaks, CA: Sage.

Cummings, G. G., Estabrooks, C. A., Midodzi, W. K., Wallin, L., & Hayduk, L. (2007). Influence of organizational characteristics and context on research utilization. *Nursing Research, 56*(4, Suppl.), S24–S39.

Degner, L. F. (2002, October 2). *Pathfinding for nursing science in the 21st century.* Paper presented at the Think Tank Meeting of Canadian Nurse Scientists, sponsored by the Nursing Policy Division of Health Canada, Toronto, Canada.

Denzin, N. K. (2009). *The research act: A theoretical introduction to sociological methods.* New York: McGraw-Hill.

Denzin, N. K., & Lincoln, Y. S. (Eds.). (2000). *Handbook of qualitative research* (2nd ed.). Thousand Oaks, CA: Sage.

Donaldson, S. K. (2000). Breakthroughs in scientific research: The discipline of nursing, 1960–1999. *Annual Review of Nursing Research, 18,* 247–311.

Downs, F. S. (1999). How to cozy up to a research report. *Applied Nursing Research, 12,* 215–216.

Estabrooks, C. A., Thompson, D. S., Lovely, J. E., & Hofmeyer, A. (2006). A guide to knowledge translation theory. *The Journal of Continuing Education in the Health Professions, 26*(1), 25–36.

Fawcett, J. (2004). *Contemporary nursing knowledge: Analysis and evaluation of conceptual models of nursing* (2nd ed.). Philadelphia: F. A. Davis.

Fawcett, J., & Garity, J. (2008). *Evaluation research for evidence-based nursing practice.* Philadelphia: F. A. Davis.

Feldstein, A. C., & Glasgow, R. E. (2008). A practical, robust implementation and sustainability model (PRISM) for integrating research findings into practice. *The Joint Commission Journal on Quality and Patient Safety, 34*(4), 228–243.

Ferguson, L. (2004). External validity, generalizability, and knowledge utilization. *Journal of Nursing Scholarship, 36,* 16–22.

Fink, A. (1998). *Conducting research literature reviews: From paper to the Internet.* Thousand Oaks, CA: Sage.

Flicker, S., Haans, D., & Skinner, H. (2004). Ethical dilemmas in research on Internet communities. *Qualitative Health Research, 14,* 124–134.

Frank-Stromberg, M., & Olsen, S. J. (Eds.). (2004). *Instruments for clinical health care.* Sudbury, MA: Jones & Bartlett.

Gennaro, S., Hodnett, E., & Kearney, M. (2001). Making evidence-based practice a reality in your institution. *Maternal Child Nursing, 26,* 236–244.

Giddings, L. S., & Grant, B. M. (2007). A Trojan horse of positivism? A critique of mixed methods research. *Advances in Nursing Science, 30,* 52–60.

Giorgi, A. (1989). Some theoretical and practical issues regarding the psychological and phenomenological method. *Saybrook Review, 7,* 71–85.

Glaser, B. G. (1992). *Basics of grounded theory analysis.* Mill Valley, CA: Sociology Press.

Glaser, B. G. (2001). *The grounded theory perspective: Conceptualization contrasted with description.* Mill Valley, CA: Sociology Press.

Glaser, B. G. (2003). *The grounded theory perspective II: Description's remodeling of grounded theory methodology.* Mill Valley, CA: Sociology Press.

Glaser, B. G. (2005). *The grounded theory perspective III: Theoretical coding.* Mill Valley, CA: Sociology Press.

Glaser, B., & Strauss, A. L. (1971). *Status passage: A formal theory.* Mill Valley, CA: Sociology Press.

Graham, I. D., Logan, J., Davies, B., & Nimrod, C. (2004). Changing the use of electronic fetal monitoring and labor support: A case study of barriers and facilitators. *Birth, 31,* 293–301.

Graham, I. D., Logan, J., Harrison, M. B., et al. (2006). Lost in knowledge translation: Time for a map? *Journal of Continuing Education in the Health Professions, 26*(1), 13–24.

Grimshaw, J. M., Santesso, N., Cumpston, M., Mayhew, A., & McGowan, J. (2006). Knowledge for knowledge translation: The role of the Cochrane Collaboration. *The Journal of Continuing Education in the Health Professions, 26,* 55–62.

Grinspun, D., Virani, T., & Bajnok, I. (2001–2002). Nursing best practice guidelines: The RNAO (Registered Nurses Association of Ontario) project. *Hospital Quarterly, 5*(2), 56–60.

Guba, E. G. (Ed.). (1990). *The paradigm dialog.* Newbury Park, CA: Sage.

Hall, J. M., & Stevens, P. E. (1991). Rigor in feminist research. *Advances in Nursing Science, 13,* 16–29.

Heidegger, M. (1962). *Being and time.* New York: Harper & Row.

Holtzclaw, B. J., & Hanneman, S. K. (2002). Use of nonhuman biobehavioral models in critical care nursing research. *Critical Care Nursing Quarterly, 24,* 30–40.

Husserl, E. (1962). *Ideas: General introduction to pure phenomenology.* New York: MacMillan.

Interagency Advance Panel on Research Ethics. (2008, December). *Tri-council policy statement: Ethical conduct for research involving humans* (Draft 2nd ed.). Retrieved September 9, 2009 from http://pre.ethics.gc.ca

Jaccard, J., & Becker, M. A. (2001). *Statistics for the behavioral sciences* (4th ed.). Belmont, CA: Wadsworth.

Janesick, V. J. (2004). *Stretching exercises for qualitative researchers.* Thousand Oaks, CA: Sage.

Kearney, M. H. (1998). Ready-to-wear: Discovering grounded formal theory. *Research in Nursing & Health, 21,* 179–186.

Kent, B., & Fineout-Overholt, E. (2008). Using meta-synthesis to facilitate evidence-based practice. *Worldviews on Evidence-Based Nursing, 5*(3), 160–162.

Kerlinger, F. N. (1986). *Foundations of behavioral research* (3rd ed.). New York: Holt, Rinehart & Winston.

Kitson, A., Ahmed, L. B., Harvey, G., Seers, K., & Thompson, D. R. (1996). From research to practice: One organisational model for promoting research-based practice. *Journal of Advanced Nursing, 23*(3), 430–440.

Kitson, A., Rycroft-Malone, J., Harvey, G., McCormack, B., Seers, K., & Titchen, A. (2008). Evaluating the successful implementation of evidence into practice using the PARiHS framework: Theoretical and practical challenges. *Implementation Science, 3,* 1.

Lather, P. (1991). *Getting smart: Feminist research and pedagogy within the postmodern.* New York: Routledge.

Leininger, M. (1991). *Culture care diversity and universality: A theory of nursing.* New York: National League for Nursing.

Lemieux-Charles, L., & Champagne, F. (Eds). (2004). *Using knowledge and evidence in health care: Multidisciplinary perspectives.* Toronto: UofT Incorporated.

Lincoln, Y. S., & Guba, E. G. (1985). *Naturalistic inquiry.* Newbury Park, CA: Sage.

Lipowski, E. E. (2008). Developing great research questions. *American Journal of Health-System Pharmacy, 65*(1), 1667–1670.

Loiselle, C. G., Bottorff, J. L., Butler, L., & Degner, L. F. (2004). PORT—Psychosocial Oncology Research Training: A newly funded strategic initiative in health research. *Cancer Journal of Nursing Research, 36*(1), 159–164.

Mapp, T. (2008). Understanding phenomenology: The lived experience. *British Journal of Midwifery, 16*(5), 308–311.

Marriner-Tomey, A. M. & Alligood, M. R. (2006). *Nursing theorists and their work* (6th ed.). St. Louis, MO: Elsevier Mosby.

Martin, P. S. (1997). Writing a useful literature review for a quantitative research project. *Applied Nursing Research, 10,* 159–162.

McCall, R. B. (2000). *Fundamental statistics for behavioral sciences* (8th ed.). Belmont, CA: Wadsworth.

Mishel, M. H. (1988). Uncertainty in illness. *Image—The Journal of Nursing Scholarship, 20*, 225–232.

Mishel, M. H. (1990). Reconceptualization of the uncertainty in illness theory. *Image—The Journal of Nursing Scholarship, 22*, 256–262.

Morse, J. M. (1991). Approaches to qualitative-quantitative methodological triangulation. *Nursing Research, 40*, 120–122.

Morse, J. M. (1991). *Qualitative nursing research: A contemporary dialogue*. Newbury Park, CA: Sage.

Morse, J. M. (1999). Myth #93: Reliability and validity are not relevant to qualitative inquiry. *Qualitative Health Research, 9*, 717–718.

Morse, J. M. (1999). Qualitative methods: The state of the art. *Qualitative Health Research, 9*, 393–406.

Nelson, A. M. (2008). Addressing the threat of evidence-based practice to qualitative inquiry through increasing attention to quality: A discussion paper. *International Journal of Nursing Studies, 45*, 316–322.

Neuman, B., & Fawcett, J. (2010). *The Neuman systems model* (5th ed.). Upper Saddle River, NJ: Prentice-Hall.

Nightingale, F. (1859). *Notes on nursing: What it is and what it is not*. Philadelphia: J. B. Lippincott.

Nunnally, J., & Bernstein, I. H. (1994). *Psychometric theory* (3rd ed.). New York: McGraw-Hill.

Olesen, V. (2000). Feminism and models of qualitative research at and into the millenium. In N. K. Denzin, & Y. S. Lincoln (Eds.). *Handbook of qualitative research* (2nd ed., pp. 215–255). Thousand Oaks, CA: Sage.

Orem, D. E., Taylor, S. G., Renpenning, K. M., & Eisenhandler, S. A. (2003). *Self-care theory in nursing: Selected papers of Dorothea Orem*. New York: Springer.

Parse, R. R. (1999). *Illuminations: The human becoming theory in practice and research*. Sudbury, MA: Jones & Bartlett.

Pender, N. J., Murdaugh, C., & Parsons, M. A. (2006). *Health promotion in nursing practice* (5th ed.). Upper Saddle River, NJ: Prentice-Hall.

Polit, D. F. (1996). *Data analysis and statistics for nursing research*. Stamford, CT: Appleton & Lange.

Polit, D. F., & Beck, C. T. (2004). *Nursing research: Principles and methods* (7th ed.). Philadelphia: Lippincott Williams & Wilkins.

Polit, D. F., & Hungler, B. P. (2004). *Nursing research: Principles and methods* (7th ed.). Philadelphia: Lippincott Williams & Wilkins.

Polit, D. F., & Tatano Beck, C. (2008). *Nursing research: Generating and assessing evidence for nursing practice* (8th ed.). Philadelphia: Wolters Kluwer Health/Lippincott Williams & Wilkins.

Punch, M. (1994). Politics and ethics in qualitative research. In N. K. Denzin & Y. S. Lincoln (Eds.), *Handbook of qualitative research*. Thousand Oaks, CA: Sage.

Reed, P. G., Shearer, N., & Nicoll, L. H. (2003). *Perspectives on nursing theory* (4th ed.). Philadelphia: Lippincott Williams & Wilkins.

Rew, L., Bechtel, D., & Sapp, A. (1993). Self-as-instrument in qualitative research. *Nursing Research, 42*, 300–301.

Rosenfeld, P., Duthie, E., Bier, J., et al. (2000). Engaging staff nurses in evidence-based research to identify nursing practice problems and solutions. *Applied Nursing Research, 13*, 197–203.

Roy, C. (2008). *The Roy adaptation model* (3rd ed.). Upper Saddle River, NJ: Prentice-Hall.

Rycroft-Malone, J., Seers, K., Titchen, A., Harvey, G., Kitson, A., & McCormack, B. (2004). What counts as evidence in evidence-based practice? *Journal of Advanced Nursing, 47*(1), 81–90.

Sandelowski, M. (2000). Combining qualitative and quantitative sampling, data collection, and analysis techniques in mixed-method studies. *Research in Nursing & Health, 23*, 246–255.

Sandelowski, M. (2004). Using qualitative research. *Qualitative Health Research, 14*, 1366–1386.

Sandelowski, M. (2008). Reading, writing and systematic review. *Journal of Advanced Nursing, 64*(1), 104–110.

Sandelowski, M., & Barroso, J. (2002). Finding the findings in qualitative studies. *Journal of Nursing Scholarship, 34*, 213–219.

Sandelowski, M., & Barroso, J. (2003). Creating metasummaries of qualitative findings *Nursing Research, 52*, 226–233.

Sandelowski, M., Docherty, S., & Emden, C. (1997). Qualitative metasynthesis: Issues and techniques. *Research in Nursing & Health, 20*, 365–371.

Scott, S. D., & Pollock, C. (2008). The role of nursing unit culture in shaping research utilization behaviours. *Research in Nursing & Health, 31*(4), 298–309.

Scott-Findlay, S., & Estabrooks, C. A. (2006). Mapping the organizational culture research in nursing: A literature review. *Journal of Advanced Nursing, 56*(5), 498–513.

Scott-Findlay, S., & Pollock, C. (2004). Evidence, research, knowledge: A call for conceptual clarity. *Worldviews on Evidence-Based Nursing, 1*(2), 92–97.

Sidani, S., & Epstein, D. R. (2003). Enhancing the evaluation of nursing care effectiveness. *Canadian Journal of Nursing Research, 35*(3), 26–38.

Silva, M. C. (1995). *Ethical guidelines in the conduct, dissemination, and implementation of nursing research*. Washington, DC: American Nurses Association.

Smith, J. L. (2007). Critical discourse analysis for nursing research. *Nursing Inquiry, 14*(1), 60–70.

Spearman, S. A., Duldt, B. W., & Brown, S. (1993). Research testing theory: A selective review of Orem's self-care theory. *Journal of Advanced Nursing, 18*(10), 1626–1631.

Spenceley, S. M., O'Leary, K. A., Chizawsky, L. L. K., Ross, A. J., & Estabrooks, C. A. (2008). Sources of information used by nurses to inform practice: An integrative review. *International Journal of Nursing Studies, 45*, 954–970.

Thomas, B. H., Ciliska, D., Dobbins, M., & Micucci, B. A. (2004). A process for systematically reviewing the literature: Providing the research evidence for public health nursing interventions. *Worldviews on Evidence Based Nursing, 1*, 176–184.

Thompson, G. N., Estabrooks, C. A., & Degner, L. F. (2006). Clarifying the concepts in knowledge transfer: A literature review. *Journal of Advanced Nursing, 53*(6), 691–701.

Thorne, S. (2008). The role of qualitative research within an evidence-based context: Can metasynthesis be the answer? A discussion paper. *International Journal of Nursing Studies, 46*(4), 569–575. DOI:10.1016/j.ijnurstu.2008.05.001.

Thorne, S. E. (2008). Meta-synthesis. In L. M. Given (Ed.), *The Sage encyclopedia of qualitative research methods*. Los Angeles: Sage.

Thorne, S., Kirkham, S. R., & MacDonald-Emes, J. (1997). Interpretive description: A noncategorical qualitative alternative for developing nursing knowledge. *Research in Nursing & Health, 20*, 169–177.

Titler, M. G., & Everett, L. Q. (2001). Translating research into practice. Considerations for critical care investigators. *Critical Care Nursing Clinics of North America, 13*(4), 587–604.

Tomey, A., & Alligood, M. (2009). *Nursing theorists and their work* (7th ed.). St. Louis, MO: C.V. Mosby.

Tornquist, E. M., Funk, S. G., Champagne, M. T., & Wiese, R. A. (1993). Advice on reading research: Overcoming the barriers. *Applied Nursing Research, 6*, 177–183.

Van Manen, M. (1997). *Researching lived experience: Human science for an action sensitive pedagogy*. London, ON: Althouse.

Van Manen, M. (2006). Writing qualitatively or the demands of writing. *Qualitative Health Research, 16*, 713–722.

Waltz, C. F., Strickland, O. L., & Lenz, E. R. (2005). *Measurement in nursing research* (3rd ed.). Philadelphia: F. A. Davis.

Welkowitz, J., Ewen, R. B., & Cohen, J. (2000). *Introductory statistics for the behavioral sciences* (5th ed.). New York: Harcourt College.

Whittemore, R., & Knafl, K. (2005). The integrative review: Updated methodology. *Journal of Advanced Nursing, 52*, 546–553.

Wuest, J. (2007). Grounded theory: The method. In P. Munhall (Ed.), *Nursing research: A qualitative perspective* (pp. 239–272). Sudbury, MA: Jones & Bartlett.

Glossary

abstract A brief description of a completed or proposed study, usually located at the beginning of the report or proposal.

accessible population The population of people available for a particular study; often a nonrandom subset of the target population.

accidental sampling Selection of the most readily available persons as study participants; also called *convenience sampling*.

acquiescence response set A bias in self-report instruments, especially in psychosocial scales, created when study participants characteristically agree with statements ("yea-say") independent of their content.

*****adjusted mean** The mean group value for the dependent variable, after statistically removing the effect of covariates.

after-only design An experimental design in which data are collected from subjects only after an experimental intervention has been introduced.

alpha (α) (1) In tests of statistical significance, the level designating the probability of committing a Type I error; (2) in estimates of internal consistency, a reliability coefficient, as in Cronbach's alpha.

*****alternative hypothesis** In hypothesis testing, a hypothesis different from the one being tested—usually, different from the null hypothesis.

analysis The process of organizing and synthesizing data so as to answer research questions and test hypotheses.

analysis of covariance (ANCOVA) A statistical procedure used to test mean differences among groups on a dependent variable, while controlling for one or more extraneous variables (covariates).

analysis of variance (ANOVA) A statistical procedure for testing mean differences among three or more groups by comparing variability between groups to variability within groups.

*****analysis triangulation** The use of two or more analytic techniques to analyze the same set of data.

anonymity Protection of participants in a study such that even the researcher cannot link individuals with the information provided.

applied research Research designed to find a solution to an immediate practical problem.

assent The affirmative agreement of a vulnerable subject (e.g., a child) to participate in a study.

associative relationship An association between two variables that cannot be described as causal (i.e., one variable *causing* the other).

assumption A basic principle that is accepted as being true based on logic or reason, but without proof or verification.

asymmetric distribution A distribution of data values that is skewed, that is, has two halves that are not mirror images of each other.

*****attribute variables** Preexisting characteristics of study participants, which the researcher simply observes or measures.

attrition The loss of participants over the course of a study, which can create bias and undermine internal validity by changing the composition of the sample—particularly if more participants are lost from one group (e.g., experimentals) than another (e.g., controls).

*****audio-CASI (computer-assisted self-interview)** An approach to collecting self-report data in which respondents listen to questions being read over headphones and respond by entering information directly onto a computer.

auditability The extent to which an external reviewer or reader can follow a qualitative researcher's steps and decisions and draw conclusions about the analysis and interpretation of the data.

audit trail The systematic documentation of material that allows an independent auditor of a qualitative study to draw conclusions about the trustworthiness of the data.

auto-ethnography Ethnographic studies in which researchers study their own culture or group.

axial coding The second level of coding in a grounded theory study using the Strauss and Corbin approach, involving the process of categorizing, recategorizing, and condensing all first-level codes by connecting a category and its subcategories.

*back-translation The translation of a translated text back into the original language, so that a comparison of the original and back-translated version can be made.

baseline data Data collected before an intervention, including pretreatment data from a measure of the dependent variable.

basic research Research designed to extend the knowledge base in a discipline for the sake of knowledge production or theory construction, rather than for solving an immediate problem.

basic social process (BSP) The central social process emerging through an analysis of grounded theory data.

before–after design An experimental design in which data are collected from research subjects before and after the introduction of an experimental intervention.

beneficence A fundamental ethical principle that seeks to prevent harm and exploitation of, and maximize benefits for, study participants.

beta (β) (1) In multiple regression, the standardized coefficients indicating the relative weights of the independent variables in the regression equation; (2) in statistical testing, the probability of a Type II error.

between-subjects design A research design in which there are separate groups of people being compared (e.g., smokers and non-smokers).

bias Any influence that produces a distortion in the results of a study.

bimodal distribution A distribution of data values with two peaks (high frequencies).

bivariate statistics Statistics derived from analyzing two variables simultaneously to assess the empirical relationship between them.

"blind" review The review of a manuscript or proposal such that neither the author nor the reviewer is identified to the other party.

blinding The masking or withholding of information (e.g., from research subjects, research personnel, or reviewers) to reduce the possibility of certain biases.

borrowed theory A theory borrowed from another discipline to guide nursing practice or research.

bracketing In phenomenological inquiries, the process of identifying and holding in abeyance any preconceived beliefs and opinions about the phenomena under study.

bricolage The tendency in qualitative research to assemble a complex array of data from a variety of sources, using a variety of methods.

*calendar question A question used to obtain retrospective information about the chronology of events and activities in people's lives.

*canonical analysis A statistical procedure for examining the relationship between two or more independent variables *and* two or more dependent variables.

carry-over effect The influence that one treatment can have on subsequent treatments.

case-control design A nonexperimental research design involving the comparison of a "case" (i.e., a person with the condition under scrutiny, such as lung cancer) and a matched control (a similar person without the condition).

case study A research method involving a thorough, in-depth analysis of an individual, group, institution, or other social unit.

categorical variable A variable with discrete values (e.g., gender) rather than values along a continuum (e.g., weight).

category system In observational studies, the prespecified plan for organizing and recording the behaviours and events under observation; in qualitative studies, the system used to sort and organize narrative data.

causal modeling The development and statistical testing of an explanatory model of hypothesized causal relationships among phenomena.

causal (cause-and-effect) relationship A relationship between two variables such that the presence or absence of one variable (the "cause") determines the presence or absence, or value, of the other (the "effect").

cell (1) The intersection of a row and column in a table with two or more dimensions; (2) in an experimental design, the representation of an experimental condition in a schematic diagram.

census A survey covering an entire population.

central (core) category The main theme of the research in a Strauss and Corbin grounded theory analysis.

central tendency A statistical index of the "typicalness" of a set of scores, derived from the centre of the score distribution; indexes of central tendency include the mode, median, and mean.

chi-squared test A nonparametric test of statistical significance used to assess whether a relationship exists between two nominal-level variables. Symbolized as χ^2.

clinical relevance The degree to which a study addresses a problem of significance to the practice of nursing.

clinical research Research designed to generate knowledge to guide clinical practice in nursing and other health care fields.

clinical trial A study designed to assess the safety and effectiveness of a new clinical treatment, sometimes involving several phases, one of which (Phase III) is a randomized clinical trial using an experimental design and, often, a large and heterogeneous sample of subjects.

closed-ended question A question that offers respondents a set of mutually exclusive and jointly exhaustive alternative response options, from which the one most closely approximating the "right" answer must be chosen.

*cluster analysis A multivariate statistical procedure used to cluster people or things based on patterns of association.

*cluster randomization The random assignment of intact groups of subjects—rather than individual subjects—to treatment conditions.

cluster sampling A form of sampling in which large groupings ("clusters") are selected first (e.g., nursing schools), with successive subsampling of smaller units (e.g., nursing students).

code of ethics The fundamental ethical principles established by a discipline or institution to guide researchers' conduct in research with human (or animal) subjects.

*codebook A record documenting categorization and coding decisions.

coding The process of transforming raw data into standardized form for data processing and analysis; in quantitative research, the process of attaching numbers to categories; in qualitative research, the process of identifying recurring words, themes, or concepts within the data.

coefficient alpha (Cronbach's alpha) A reliability index that estimates the internal consistency or homogeneity of a measure composed of several items or subparts.

coercion In a research context, the explicit or implicit use of threats (or excessive rewards) to gain people's cooperation in a study.

cohort study A kind of trend study that focuses on a specific subpopulation (which is often an age-related subgroup) from which different samples are selected at different points in time (e.g., the cohort of nursing students who graduated between 2005 and 2009).

comparison group A group of subjects whose scores on a dependent variable are used to evaluate the outcomes of the group of primary interest (e.g., nonsmokers as a comparison group for smokers); term often used in lieu of control group when the study design is not a true experiment.

*computer-assisted personal interviewing (CAPI) In-person interviewing in which the interviewers read questions from, and enter responses onto, a laptop computer.

*computer-assisted telephone interviewing (CATI) Interviewing done over the telephone in which the interviewers read questions from, and enter responses onto, a computer.

concealment A tactic involving the unobtrusive collection of research data without participants' knowledge or consent, used to obtain an accurate view of naturalistic behaviour when the known presence of an observer would distort the behaviour of interest.

concept An abstraction based on observations of—or inferences from—behaviours or characteristics (e.g., stress, pain).

conceptual definition The abstract or theoretical meaning of the concepts being studied.

conceptual file A manual method of organizing qualitative data, by creating file folders for each category in the coding scheme and inserting relevant excerpts from the data.

conceptual model Interrelated concepts or abstractions assembled together in a rational scheme by virtue of their relevance to a common theme; sometimes called *conceptual framework*.

conceptual utilization The use of research findings in a general, conceptual way to broaden one's thinking about an issue, without putting the knowledge to any specific, documentable use.

concurrent validity The degree to which scores on an instrument are correlated with some external criterion, measured at the same time.

*__confidence interval__ The range of values within which a population parameter is estimated to lie.

*__confidence level__ The estimated probability that a population parameter lies within a given confidence interval.

confidentiality Protection of participants in a study such that individual identities are not linked to information provided and are never publicly divulged.

confirmability A criterion for evaluating the quality of qualitative research, referring to the objectivity or neutrality of the data or the analysis and interpretation.

*__confirmatory factor analysis__ A factor analysis, based on maximum likelihood estimation, designed to confirm a hypothesized measurement model.

consent form A written agreement signed by a study participant and a researcher concerning the terms and conditions of voluntary participation in a study.

constant comparison A procedure often used in a grounded theory analysis wherein newly collected data are compared in an ongoing fashion with data obtained earlier, to refine theoretically relevant categories.

constitutive pattern In hermeneutic analysis, a pattern that expresses the relationships among relational themes and is present in all the interviews or texts.

construct An abstraction or concept that is deliberately invented (constructed) by researchers for a scientific purpose (e.g., health locus of control).

construct validity The degree to which an instrument measures the construct under investigation.

consumer An individual who reads, reviews, and critiques research findings and who attempts to use and apply the findings in his or her practice.

*__contact information__ Information obtained from study participants in longitudinal studies that facilitates their relocation at a future date.

*__contamination__ The inadvertent, undesirable influence of one experimental treatment condition on another treatment condition.

content analysis The process of organizing and integrating narrative, qualitative information according to emerging themes and concepts.

content validity The degree to which the items in an instrument adequately represent the universe of content for the concept being measured.

content validity index (CVI) An indicator of the degree to which an instrument is content valid, based on average ratings of a panel of experts.

contingency table A two-dimensional table that permits a crosstabulation of the frequencies of two categorical variables.

continuous variable A variable that can take on an infinite range of values along a specified continuum (e.g., height).

control The process of holding constant possible influences on the dependent variable under investigation.

control group Subjects in an experiment who do not receive the experimental treatment and whose performance provides a baseline against which the effects of the treatment can be measured (see also *comparison group*).

convenience sampling Selection of the most readily available persons as participants in a study; also called *accidental sampling*.

*__convergent validity__ An approach to construct validation that involves assessing the degree to which two methods of measuring a construct are similar (i.e., converge).

core variable (category) In a grounded theory study, the central phenomenon that is used to integrate all categories of the data.

correlation An association or connection between variables, such that variation in one variable is related to variation in another.

correlation coefficient An index summarizing the degree of relationship between variables, typically ranging from +1.00 (for a perfect positive relationship) through 0.0 (for no relationship) to −1.00 (for a perfect negative relationship).

correlation matrix A two-dimensional display showing the correlation coefficients between all pairs of a set of study variables.

correlational research Research that explores the interrelationships among variables of interest without any active intervention by the researcher.

cost–benefit analysis An evaluation of the monetary costs of a program or intervention relative to the monetary gains attributable to it.

*counterbalancing The process of systematically varying the order of presentation of stimuli or treatments to control for ordering effects, especially in a crossover design.

counterfactual The condition or group used as a basis of comparison in a study.

covariate A variable that is statistically controlled (held constant) in analysis of covariance. The covariate is typically an extraneous, confounding influence on the dependent variable or a preintervention measure of the dependent variable.

covert data collection The collection of information in a study without participants' knowledge.

*Cramér's V An index describing the magnitude of the relationship between nominal-level data, used when the contingency table to which it is applied is larger than 2 × 2.

credibility A criterion for evaluating data quality in qualitative studies, referring to confidence in the truth of the data.

criterion sampling A sampling approach in qualitative research that involves selecting cases that meet a predetermined criterion of importance.

criterion variable The criterion against which the effect of an independent variable is tested; sometimes used instead of *dependent variable*.

criterion-related validity The degree to which scores on an instrument are correlated with some external criterion.

*critical case sampling A sampling approach used by qualitative researchers involving the purposeful selection of cases that are especially important or illustrative.

critical ethnography An ethnography that focuses on raising consciousness in the group or culture under study in the hope of effecting social change.

critical incident technique A method of obtaining data from study participants by in-depth exploration of specific incidents and behaviours related to the topic under study.

*critical region The area in the sampling distribution representing values that are "improbable" if the null hypothesis is true.

critical theory An approach to viewing the world that involves a critique of society, with the goal of envisioning new possibilities and effecting social change.

critique An objective, critical, and balanced appraisal of a research report's various dimensions (e.g., conceptual, methodologic, ethical).

Cronbach's alpha A widely used reliability index that estimates the internal consistency or homogeneity of a measure composed of several subparts; also called *coefficient alpha*.

crossover design An experimental design in which one group of subjects is exposed to more than one condition or treatment in random order; sometimes called a *repeated-measures design*.

cross-sectional design A study design in which data are collected at one point in time; sometimes used to infer change over time when data are collected from different age or developmental groups.

cross tabulation A determination of the number of cases occurring when two variables are considered simultaneously (e.g., gender—male/female– crosstabulated with smoking status—smoker/nonsmoker). The results are typically presented in a table with rows and columns divided according to the values of the variables.

data The pieces of information obtained in the course of a study (singular is *datum*).

data analysis The systematic organization and synthesis of research data and, in most quantitative studies, the testing of research hypotheses using those data.

data collection The gathering of information to address a research problem.

data collection protocols The formal procedures researchers develop to guide the collection of data in a standardized fashion in most quantitative studies.

data saturation See *saturation*.

data set The total collection of data on all variables for all study participants.

data source triangulation The use of multiple data sources for the purpose of validating conclusions.

debriefing Communication with study participants after participation is complete regarding various aspects of the study.

deception The deliberate withholding of information, or the provision of false information, to study participants, usually to reduce potential biases.

deductive reasoning The process of developing specific predictions from general principles (see also *inductive reasoning*).

degrees of freedom (*df*) A concept used in statistical testing, referring to the number of sample values free to vary (e.g., with a given sample mean, all but one value would be free to vary); degrees of freedom is often $N - 1$, but different formulas are relevant for different tests.

*Delphi technique A method of obtaining written judgments from a panel of experts about an issue of concern; experts are questioned individually in several rounds, with a summary of the panel's views circulated between rounds, to achieve some consensus.

*demonstration A test of an innovative intervention, often on a large scale, to determine its effectiveness and the desirability of making practice or policy changes.

dependability A criterion for evaluating data quality in qualitative data, referring to the stability of data over time and over conditions.

dependent variable The variable hypothesized to depend on or be caused by another variable (the *independent variable*); the outcome variable of interest.

descriptive phenomenology A type of phenomenology, developed by Husserl, that emphasizes the careful description of ordinary conscious experience of everyday life.

descriptive research Research studies that have as their main objective the accurate portrayal of the characteristics of persons, situations, or groups, and/or the frequency with which certain phenomena occur.

descriptive statistics Statistics used to describe and summarize data (e.g., means, standard deviations).

descriptive theory A broad characterization that thoroughly accounts for a single phenomenon.

determinism The belief that phenomena are not haphazard or random, but rather have antecedent causes; an assumption in the positivist paradigm.

*deviation score A score computed by subtracting the mean of a set of scores from an individual score.

dichotomous variable A variable having only two values or categories (e.g., sex).

directional hypothesis A hypothesis that makes a specific prediction about the direction and nature of the relationship between two variables.

discourse analysis A qualitative tradition, from the discipline of sociolinguistics, that seeks to understand the rules, mechanisms, and structure of conversations.

*discrete variable A variable with a finite number of values between two points.

discriminant function analysis A statistical procedure used to predict group membership or status on a categorical (nominal level) variable on the basis of two or more independent variables.

*discriminant validity An approach to construct validation that involves assessing the degree to which a single method of measuring two constructs yields different results (i.e., discriminates the two).

disproportionate sample A sample in which the researcher samples differing proportions of study participants from different population strata to ensure adequate representation from smaller strata.

domain In ethnographic analysis, a unit or broad category of cultural knowledge.

double-blind experiment An experiment in which neither the subjects nor those who administer the treatment know who is in the experimental or control group.

*dummy variable Dichotomous variables created for use in many multivariate statistical analyses, typically using codes of 0 and 1 (e.g., female = 1, male = 0).

ecological psychology A qualitative tradition that focuses on the environment's influence on human behaviour and attempts to identify principles that explain the interdependence of humans and their environmental context.

editing analysis style An approach to the analysis of qualitative data, in which researchers read through texts in search of meaningful segments and develop a categorization scheme that is used to sort and organize the data.

effect size A statistical expression of the magnitude of the relationship between two variables, or the magnitude of the difference between two groups, with regard to some attribute of interest.

*eigenvalue In factor analysis, the value equal to the sum of the squared weights for each factor.

electronic database Bibliographic files that can be accessed by computer for the purpose of conducting a literature review.

element The most basic unit of a population from which a sample is drawn—typically humans in nursing research.

eligibility criteria The criteria used to designate the specific attributes of the target population, and by which people are selected for participation in a study.

emergent design A design that unfolds in the course of a qualitative study as the researcher makes ongoing design decisions reflecting what has already been learned.

*emergent fit A concept in grounded theory that involves comparing new data and new categories with previously existing conceptualizations (e.g., from the literature).

emic perspective A term used by ethnographers to refer to the way members of a culture themselves view their world; the "insider's view."

empirical evidence Evidence rooted in objective reality and gathered using one's senses as the basis for generating knowledge.

*endogenous variable In path analysis, a variable whose variation is determined by other variables within the model.

error of measurement The deviation between true scores and obtained scores of a measured characteristic.

*error term The mathematic expression (typically in a regression analysis) that represents all unknown or immeasurable attributes that can affect the dependent variable.

estimation procedures Statistical procedures that have as their goal the estimation of population parameters based on sample statistics.

*eta squared In ANOVA, a statistic calculated to indicate the proportion of variance in the dependent variable explained by the independent variables, analogous to R^2 in multiple regression.

ethics A system of moral values that is concerned with the degree to which research procedures adhere to professional, legal, and social obligations to the study participants.

ethnography A branch of human inquiry, associated with the field of anthropology, that focuses on the culture of a group of people, with an effort to understand the worldview of those under study.

ethnomethodology A branch of human inquiry, associated with sociology, that focuses on the way in which people make sense of their everyday activities and come to behave in socially acceptable ways.

ethnonursing research The study of human cultures, with a focus on a group's beliefs and practices relating to nursing care and related health behaviours.

etic perspective A term used by ethnographers to refer to the "outsider's" view of the experiences of a cultural group.

evaluation research Research that investigates how well a program, practice, or policy is working.

event sampling In observational studies, a sampling plan that involves the selection of integral behaviours or events.

evidence hierarchy A ranked arrangement of the validity and dependability of evidence based on the rigour of the design that produced it.

evidence-based practice A practice that involves making clinical decisions on the best available evidence, with an emphasis on evidence from disciplined research.

ex post facto research Nonexperimental research conducted after variations in the independent variable have occurred in the natural course of events and, therefore, any causal explanations are inferred "after the fact."

exclusion criteria The criteria that specify characteristics that a population does *not* have.

*exogenous variable In path analysis, a variable whose determinants lie outside the model.

experiment A study in which the researcher controls (manipulates) the independent variable and—in a true experiment— randomly assigns subjects to different conditions.

experimental group Subjects in a study who receive the experimental treatment or intervention.

experimental intervention (experimental treatment) See *intervention*; *treatment*.

*exploratory factor analysis A factor analysis undertaken to determine the underlying dimensionality of a set of variables.

exploratory research A study that explores the dimensions of a phenomenon or that develops or refines hypotheses about relationships between phenomena.

*external criticism In historical research, the systematic evaluation of the authenticity and genuineness of data.

external validity The degree to which study results can be generalized to settings or samples other than the one studied.

extraneous variable A variable that confounds the relationship between the independent and dependent variables and that needs to be controlled either in the research design or through statistical procedures to clarify relationships.

extreme case sampling A sampling approach used by qualitative researchers that involves the purposeful selection of the most extreme or unusual cases.

extreme response set A bias in self-report instruments, especially in psychosocial scales, created when participants select extreme response alternatives (e.g., "strongly agree"), independent of the item's content.

F-ratio The statistic obtained in several statistical tests (e.g., ANOVA) in which variation attributable to different sources (e.g., between groups and within groups) is compared.

face validity The extent to which a measuring instrument looks as though it is measuring what it purports to measure.

factor analysis A statistical procedure for reducing a large set of variables into a smaller set of variables with common characteristics or underlying dimensions.

*factor extraction The first phase of a factor analysis, which involves the extraction of as much variance as possible through the successive creation of linear combinations of the variables in the analysis.

*factor loading In factor analysis, the weight associated with a variable on a given factor.

*factor rotation The second phase of factor analysis, during which the reference axes for the factors are moved such that variables more clearly align with a single factor.

*factor score A person's score on a latent variable (factor).

factorial design An experimental design in which two or more independent variables are simultaneously manipulated, permitting a separate analysis of the main effects of the independent variables, plus the interaction effects of those variables.

feasibility study A small-scale test to determine the feasibility of a larger study (see also *pilot study*).

feminist research Research that seeks to understand, typically through qualitative approaches, how gender and a gendered social order shapes women's lives and their consciousness.

field diary A daily record of events and conversations in the field; also called a *log*.

field notes The remarks taken by researchers describing the unstructured observations

they have made in the field and their interpretation of those observations.

field research Research in which the data are collected "in the field" from individuals in their normal roles, with the aim of understanding the practices, behaviours, and beliefs of individuals or groups as they normally function in real life.

fieldwork The activities undertaken by researchers (usually qualitative researchers) to collect data out in the field (i.e., in natural settings outside the research environment).

findings The results of the analysis of research data.

*Fisher's exact test A statistical procedure used to test the significance of the difference in proportions, used when the sample size is small or cells in the contingency table have no observations.

fit In grounded theory analysis, the process of identifying characteristics of one piece of data and comparing them with the characteristics of another datum to determine similarity.

fittingness In an assessment of the transferability of findings from a qualitative study, the degree of congruence between the research sample and another group or setting of interest.

fixed alternative question A question that offers respondents a set of prespecified responses, from which the respondent must choose the alternative that most closely approximates the correct response.

focus group interview An interview with a group of individuals assembled to answer questions on a given topic.

focused interview A loosely structured interview in which an interviewer guides the respondent through a set of questions using a topic guide; also called a *semistructured interview*.

follow-up study A study undertaken to determine the outcomes of individuals with a specified condition or who have received a specified treatment.

forced-choice question A question that requires respondents to choose between two statements that represent polar positions or characteristics.

formal grounded theory A theory developed at a highly abstract level of theory by compiling several substantive grounded theories.

framework The conceptual underpinnings of a study; often called a *theoretical framework* in studies based on a theory, or a *conceptual framework* in studies rooted in a specific conceptual model.

frequency distribution A systematic array of numeric values from the lowest to the highest, together with a count of the number of times each value was obtained.

frequency polygon Graphic display of a frequency distribution in which dots connected by a straight line indicate the number of times score values occur in a data set.

***Friedman test** A nonparametric analog of ANOVA, used with paired-groups or repeated-measures situations.

full disclosure The communication of complete information to potential study participants about the nature of the study, the right to refuse participation, and the likely risks and benefits that would be incurred.

functional relationship A relationship between two variables in which it cannot be assumed that one variable caused the other, but it can be said that one variable changes values in relation to changes in the other variable.

gaining entrée The process of gaining access to study participants in qualitative field studies through the cooperation of key actors in the selected community or site.

generalizability The degree to which the research methods justify the inference that the findings are true for a broader group than study participants; in particular, the inference that the findings can be generalized from the sample to the population.

***"going native"** A pitfall in qualitative research wherein a researcher becomes too emotionally involved with participants, and therefore loses the ability to observe rationally and objectively.

grand theory A broad theory aimed at describing large segments of the physical, social, or behavioural world; also called a *macrotheory*.

grand tour question A broad question asked in an unstructured interview to gain a general overview of a phenomenon on the basis of which more focused questions are subsequently asked.

***graphic rating scale** A scale in which respondents are asked to rate something (e.g., a concept or an issue) along an ordered bipolar continuum (e.g., "excellent" to "very poor").

grounded theory An approach to collecting and analyzing qualitative data that aims to develop theories and theoretical propositions grounded in real-world observations.

Hawthorne effect The effect on the dependent variable resulting from subjects' awareness that they are participants under study.

hermeneutic circle In hermeneutics, the qualitative circle signifies a methodologic process in which, to reach understanding, there is continual movement between the parts and the whole of the text that are being analyzed.

hermeneutics A qualitative research tradition, drawing on interpretive phenomenology, that focuses on the lived experiences of humans and on how they interpret those experiences.

heterogeneity The degree to which objects are dissimilar (i.e., characterized by high variability) with respect to some attribute.

***hierarchical multiple regression** A multiple regression analysis in which predictor variables are entered into the equation in steps that are prespecified by the analyst.

***histogram** A graphic presentation of frequency distribution data.

historical research Systematic studies designed to discover facts and relationships about past events.

history threat The occurrence of events external to an intervention (or other independent variable) but occurring concurrent with it, which can affect the dependent variable and threaten the study's internal validity.

homogeneity (1) In terms of the reliability of an instrument, the degree to which its subparts are internally consistent (i.e., are measuring the same critical attribute); (2) more generally, the degree to which objects are similar (i.e., characterized by low variability).

homogenous sampling A sampling approach used by qualitative researchers involving the deliberate selection of cases with limited variation.

hypothesis A prediction, usually a statement of predicted relationships between variables.

hypothesis testing A statistical procedure that involves the comparison of empirically observed sample findings with theoretically expected findings that would be expected if the null hypothesis were true.

impact analysis An evaluation of the effects of a program or intervention on outcomes of interest, net of other factors influencing those outcomes.

implementation analysis In an evaluation, a description of the process by which a program or intervention was implemented in practice.

implementation potential The extent to which an innovation is amenable to implementation in a new setting, an assessment of which is usually made in an evidence-based practice (or research utilization) project.

implied consent Consent to participate in a study that a researcher assumes has been given based on certain actions of the participant (such as returning a completed questionnaire).

IMRAD format The organization of a research report into four sections: the Introduction, Methods, Research, and Discussion sections.

*incidence rate The rate of new "cases" with a specified condition, determined by dividing the number of new cases over a given period of time by the number at risk of becoming a new case (i.e., free of the condition at the outset of the time period).

independent variable The variable that is believed to cause or influence the dependent variable; in experimental research, the manipulated (treatment) variable.

inductive reasoning The process of reasoning from specific observations to more general rules (see also *deductive reasoning*).

inferential statistics Statistics that permit inferences on whether relationships observed in a sample are likely to occur in the larger population.

informant A term used to refer to those individuals who provide information to researchers about a phenomenon under study (usually in qualitative studies).

informed consent An ethical principle that requires researchers to obtain the voluntary participation of subjects, after informing them of possible risks and benefits.

inquiry audit An independent scrutiny of qualitative data and relevant supporting documents by an external reviewer to determine the dependability and confirmability of qualitative data.

insider research Research on a group or culture—usually in an ethnography—by a member of the group or culture.

Institutional Review Board (IRB) In the United States, the name for the group of individuals from an institution who convene to review proposed and ongoing studies with respect to ethical considerations.

instrument The device used to collect data (e.g., questionnaire, test, observation schedule).

instrumental utilization Clearly identifiable attempts to base some specific action or intervention on the results of research findings.

*instrumentation threat The threat to the internal validity of the study that can arise if the researcher changes the measuring instrument between two points of data collection.

integrative review A review of research that amasses comprehensive information on a topic, weighs pieces of evidence, and integrates information to draw conclusions about the state of knowledge.

*intensity sampling A sampling approach used by qualitative researchers involving the purposeful selection of intense (but not extreme) cases.

*intention to treat A principle for analyzing data that involves the assumption that each person received the treatment to which he or she was assigned; contrary to *on-protocol analysis*.

interaction effect The effect of two or more independent variables acting in combination (interactively) on a dependent variable rather than as unconnected factors.

intercoder reliability The degree to which two coders, operating independently, agree in their coding decisions.

interdisciplinary In a team or in research, involves more than one discipline working together to produce a unified perspective on a problem or issue. This can ultimately lead to the creation of new knowledge.

internal consistency The degree to which the subparts of an instrument are all measuring the same attribute or dimension, as a measure of the instrument's reliability.

*internal criticism In historical research, an evaluation of the worth of the historical evidence.

internal validity The degree to which it can be inferred that the experimental treatment (or independent variable), rather than extraneous factors, is responsible for observed effects.

interpretation The process of making sense of the results of a study and examining their implications.

interpretive phenomenology An approach to phenomenology in which interpreting and understanding—and not just describing—human experience is stressed; also called *hermeneutics.*

interrater (interobserver) reliability The degree to which two raters or observers, operating independently, assign the same ratings or values for an attribute being measured or observed.

*interrupted time series design. See *time series* **design.**

*interval estimation A statistical estimation approach in which the researcher establishes a range of values that are likely, within a given level of confidence, to contain the true population parameter.

interval measurement A level of measurement in which an attribute of a variable is rank-ordered on a scale that has equal distances between points on that scale (e.g., Celsius degrees).

intervention An experimental treatment or manipulation.

intervention protocol In experimental research, the specification of exactly what the treatment and the alternative condition (the counterfactual) will be, and how treatments are to be administered.

*intervention research A systematic research approach distinguished not so much by a particular research methodology as by a distinctive *process* of planning, developing, implementing, testing, and disseminating interventions.

interview A method of data collection in which one person (an interviewer) asks questions of another person (a respondent); interviews may be conducted face-to-face, by telephone, or via the use of a computer program.

interview schedule The formal instrument, used in structured self-report studies, that specifies the wording of all questions to be asked of respondents.

intuiting The second step in descriptive phenomenology, which occurs when researchers remain open to the meaning attributed to the phenomenon by those who experienced it.

inverse relationship A relationship characterized by the tendency of high values on one variable to be associated with low values on the second variable; also called a *negative relationship.*

investigator triangulation The use of two or more researchers to analyze and interpret a data set to enhance the validity of the findings.

item A single question on a test or questionnaire, or a single statement on an attitude or other scale (e.g., a final examination might consist of 100 items).

*item analysis A type of analysis used to assess whether items are tapping the same construct and are sufficiently discriminating.

joint interview An interview in which two or more people are interviewed simultaneously, typically using either a semistructured or an unstructured interview.

*jottings Short notes jotted down quickly in the field so as to not distract researchers from their observations or their role as participating members of a group.

journal article A report appearing in professional journals such as *Nursing Research.*

journal club A group that meets (often in clinical settings) to discuss and critique research reports appearing in journals, sometimes to assess the potential use of the findings in practice.

judgmental sampling A type of nonprobability sampling method in which the researcher selects study participants based on personal judgment about who will be most representative or informative; also called *purposive sampling.*

*Kendall's tau A correlation coefficient used to indicate the magnitude of a relationship between ordinal-level variables.

key informant A person well-versed in the phenomenon of research interest and who is willing to share the information and insight with the researcher.

keyword An important concept or term used to search for references on a topic (e.g., in an electronic bibliographic database).

known-groups technique A technique for estimating the construct validity of an instrument through an analysis of the degree to which the instrument separates groups predicted to differ based on known characteristics or theory.

*Kruskal–Wallis test A nonparametric test used to test the difference between three or more independent groups, based on ranked scores.

*Kuder–Richardson (KR-20) formula A method of calculating an internal consistency reliability coefficient for a scaled set of items when the items are dichotomous.

*latent variable An unmeasured variable that represents an underlying, abstract construct (usually in the context of a LISREL analysis).

*law A theory that has accrued such persuasive empirical support that it is accepted as true (e.g., Boyle's law of gases).

*least-squares estimation A commonly used method of statistical estimation in which the solution minimizes the sums of squares of error terms; also called OLS (*ordinary least squares*).

level of measurement A system of classifying measurements according to the nature of the quantitative information and the type of mathematical operations to which they are amenable; the four levels are nominal, ordinal, interval, and ratio.

level of significance The risk of making a Type I error in a statistical analysis, established by the researcher beforehand (e.g., the .05 level). A number that expresses the probability that the result of a given experiment or study could have occurred purely by chance.

life history A narrative self-report about a person's life experiences vis-à-vis a theme of interest.

*life table analysis A statistical procedure used when the dependent variable represents a time interval between an initial event (e.g., onset of a disease) and an end event (e.g., death); also called *survival analysis*.

Likert scale A composite measure of attitudes involving the summation of scores on a set of items that are rated by respondents for their degree of agreement or disagreement.

*linear regression An analysis for predicting the value of a dependent variable by determining a straight-line fit to the data that minimizes the sum of squared deviations from the line.

LISREL The widely used acronym for linear structural relation analysis, typically used for testing causal models.

literature review A critical summary of research on a topic of interest, often prepared to put a research problem in context.

log In participant observation studies, the observer's daily record of events and conversations that took place.

logical positivism The philosophy underlying the traditional scientific approach; see also *positivist paradigm*.

logistic regression A multivariate regression procedure that analyzes relationships between multiple independent variables and categorical dependent variables; also called *logit analysis*.

*logit The natural log of the odds, used as the dependent variable in logistic regression; short for logistic probability unit.

longitudinal study A study designed to collect data at more than one point in time, in contrast to a cross-sectional study.

macrotheory A broad theory aimed at describing large segments of the physical, social, or behavioural world; also called a *grand theory*.

main effects In a study with multiple independent variables, the effects of a single independent variable on the dependent variable.

*manifest variable An observed, measured variable that serves as an indicator of an underlying construct (i.e., a latent variable), usually in the context of a LISREL analysis.

manipulation An intervention or treatment introduced by the researcher in an experimental or quasi-experimental study to assess its impact on the dependent variable.

*manipulation check In experimental studies, a test to determine whether the manipulation was implemented as intended.

*Mann-Whitney *U* test A nonparametric statistic used to test the difference between two independent groups, based on ranked scores.

MANOVA See *multivariate analysis of variance*.

matching The pairing of subjects in one group with those in another group, based on their similarity on one or more dimension, to enhance the overall similarity of comparison groups.

maturation threat A threat to the internal validity of a study that results when changes to the outcome measure (dependent variable) result from the passage of time.

*maximum likelihood estimation An estimation approach (sometimes used in lieu of the least-squares approach) in which the estimators are ones that estimate the parameters most likely to have generated the observed measurements.

maximum variation sampling A sampling approach used by qualitative researchers involving the purposeful selection of cases with a wide range of variation.

*McNemar test A statistical test for comparing differences in proportions when values are derived from paired (nonindependent) groups.

mean A descriptive statistic that is a measure of central tendency, computed by summing all scores and dividing by the number of subjects.

measurement The assignment of numbers to objects according to specified rules to characterize quantities of an attribute.

*measurement model In LISREL, the model that stipulates the hypothesized relationships among the manifest and latent variables.

median A descriptive statistic that is a measure of central tendency, representing the exact middle value in a score distribution; the value above and below which 50% of the scores lie.

*median test A nonparametric statistical test involving the comparison of median values of two independent groups to determine whether the groups are from populations with different medians.

mediating variable A variable that mediates or acts like a "go-between" in a chain linking two other variables (e.g., coping skills mediate the relationship between stressful events and anxiety).

member check A method of validating the credibility of qualitative data through debriefings and discussions with informants.

meta-analysis A technique for quantitatively integrating the findings from multiple studies on a given topic.

meta-matrix A device sometimes used in mixed-method studies that permits researchers to recognize important patterns and themes across data sources and to develop hypotheses.

metasynthesis The theories, grand narratives, generalizations, or interpretive translations produced from the integration or comparison of findings from multiple qualitative studies.

method triangulation The use of multiple methods of data collection about the same phenomenon to enhance the validity of the findings.

methodologic notes In observational field studies, the researcher's notes about the methods used in collecting data.

methodologic research Research designed to develop or refine methods of obtaining, organizing, or analyzing data.

methods (research) The steps, procedures, and strategies for gathering and analyzing data in a research investigation.

middle-range theory A theory that focuses on only a piece of reality or human experience involving a selected number of concepts (e.g., theories of stress).

minimal risk Anticipated risks that are no greater than those ordinarily encountered in daily life or during the performance of routine tests or procedures.

*missing values Values missing from a data set for some study participants, due, for example, to refusals, researcher error, or skip patterns in an instrument.

*mixed-mode strategy An approach to collecting survey data in which efforts are first made to conduct the interview by telephone, but then in-person interviewing is used if a telephone interview cannot be completed.

modality A characteristic of a frequency distribution describing the number of peaks (i.e., values with high frequencies).

mode A descriptive statistic that is a measure of central tendency; the score or value that occurs most frequently in a distribution of scores.

model A symbolic representation of concepts or variables and interrelationships among them.

moderator effect The effect that a third variable (a *moderator variable*) has on the relationship between the independent and dependent variables.

mortality threat A threat to the internal validity of a study, referring to the differential loss of participants (attrition) from different groups.

Multidisciplinary In a team or in research, involves more than one discipline offering their distinct perspectives on a problem or issue

multimethod (mixed-method) research Generally, research in which multiple approaches are used to address a problem; often used to designate studies in which both qualitative and quantitative data are collected and analyzed.

multimodal distribution A distribution of values with more than one peak (high frequency).

*multiple classification analysis A variant of multiple regression and ANCOVA that yields group means on the dependent variable adjusted for the effects of covariates.

multiple comparison procedures Statistical tests, normally applied after an ANOVA indicates statistically significant group differences, that compare different pairs of groups; also called *post hoc tests*.

multiple correlation coefficient An index (symbolized as R) that summarizes the degree of relationship between two or more independent variables and a dependent variable.

multiple regression analysis A statistical procedure for understanding the simultaneous effects of two or more independent (predictor) variables on a dependent variable.

multistage sampling A sampling strategy that proceeds through a set of stages from larger to smaller sampling units (e.g., from states, to nursing schools, to faculty members).

***multitrait–multimethod matrix method** A method of establishing the construct validity of an instrument that involves the use of multiple measures for a set of subjects; the target instrument is valid to the extent that there is a strong relationship between it and other measures purporting to measure the same attribute (convergence) and a weak relationship between it and other measures purporting to measure a different attribute (discriminability).

multivariate analysis of variance (MANOVA) A statistical procedure used to test the significance of differences between the means of two or more groups on two or more dependent variables, considered simultaneously.

multivariate statistics Statistical procedures designed to analyze the relationships among three or more variables; commonly used multivariate statistics include multiple regression, analysis of covariance, and factor analysis.

N The symbol designating the total number of subjects (e.g., "the total N was 500").

n The symbol designating the number of subjects in a subgroup or cell of a study (e.g., "each of the four groups had an n of 125, for a total N of 500").

narrative analysis A type of qualitative approach that focuses on the story as the object of the inquiry.

***natural experiment** A nonexperimental study that takes advantage of some naturally occurring event or phenomenon (e.g., an earthquake) that is presumed to have implications for people's behaviour or condition, typically by comparing people exposed to the event with those not exposed.

naturalistic paradigm An alternative paradigm to the traditional positivist paradigm that holds that there are multiple interpretations of reality, and that the goal of research is to understand how individuals construct reality within their context; often associated with qualitative research.

naturalistic setting A setting for the collection of research data that is natural to those being studied (e.g., homes, places of work, and so forth).

***needs assessment** A study designed to describe the needs of a group, a community, or an organization, usually as a guide to policy planning and resource allocation.

negative case analysis A method of refining a hypothesis or theory in a qualitative study that involves the inclusion of cases that appear to disconfirm earlier hypotheses.

negative relationship A relationship between two variables in which there is a tendency for higher values on one variable to be associated with lower values on the other (e.g., as temperature increases, people's productivity may decrease); also called an *inverse relationship*.

negative results Research results that fail to support the researcher's hypotheses.

negatively skewed distribution An asymmetric distribution of data values with a disproportionately high number of cases having high values—that is, falling at the upper end of the distribution; when displayed graphically, the tail points to the left.

***net effect** The effect of an independent variable on a dependent variable after controlling for the effect of one or more covariates through multiple regression or ANCOVA.

network sampling The sampling of participants based on referrals from others already in the sample; also called *snowball sampling* and *nominated sampling*.

***nocebo effect** Adverse side effect experienced by those receiving a placebo treatment.

nominal measurement The lowest level of measurement involving the assignment of characteristics into categories (e.g., males, category 1; females, category 2).

nominated sampling A sampling method in which researchers ask early informants to make referrals to other study participants;

called *snowball sampling* and *network sampling*.

nondirectional hypothesis A research hypothesis that does not stipulate in advance the expected direction of the relationship between variables.

nonequivalent control group design A quasi-experimental design involving a comparison group that was not developed on the basis of random assignment, but from whom preintervention data usually are obtained to assess the initial equivalence of the groups.

nonexperimental research Studies in which the researcher collects data without introducing an intervention.

nonparametric statistical tests A class of inferential statistical tests that do not involve rigourous assumptions about the distribution of critical variables; most often used with nominal or ordinal data.

nonprobability sampling The selection of sampling units (e.g., participants) from a population using nonrandom procedures, as in convenience, judgmental, and quota sampling.

*nonrecursive model A causal model that predicts reciprocal effects (i.e., a variable can be both the cause of and an effect of another variable).

nonresponse bias A bias that can result when a nonrandom subset of people invited to participate in a study fail to participate.

nonsignificant result The result of a statistical test indicating that group differences or a relationship between variables could have occurred as a result of chance at a given level of significance; sometimes abbreviated as *NS*.

normal distribution A theoretical distribution that is bell shaped, symmetric, and not too peaked or flat; also called a *normal curve*.

norms Test performance standards, based on test score information from a large, representative sample.

null hypothesis A hypothesis stating no relationship between the variables under study; used primarily in statistical testing as the hypothesis to be rejected.

nursing research Systematic inquiry designed to develop knowledge about issues or phenomena important to the nursing profession and discipline.

objectivity The extent to which two independent researchers would arrive at similar judgments or conclusions (i.e., judgments not biased by personal values or beliefs).

*oblique rotation In factor analysis, a rotation of factors such that the reference axes are allowed to move to acute or oblique angles, and hence the factors are allowed to be correlated.

observational notes An observer's in-depth descriptions about events and conversations observed in naturalistic settings.

observational research Studies in which data are collected by observing and recording behaviours or activities of interest.

observed (obtained) score The actual score or numeric value assigned to a person on a measure.

odds The ratio of two probabilities, namely, the probability of an event occurring to the probability that it will not occur.

odds ratio (OR) The ratio of one odds to another odds; used in logistic regression as a measure of association and as an estimate of relative risk.

*on-protocol analysis A principle for analyzing data that includes data only from those members of a treatment group who actually received the treatment; contrary to an *intention-to-treat* analysis.

*one-tailed test A test of statistical significance in which only values at one extreme (tail) of a distribution are considered in determining significance; used when the researcher can predict the direction of a relationship (see *directional hypothesis*).

open coding The first level of coding in a grounded theory study, referring to the basic descriptive coding of the content of the narrative data.

open-ended question A question in an interview or questionnaire that does not restrict respondents' answers to preestablished alternatives.

operational definition The definition of a concept or variable in terms of the procedures by which it is to be measured.

operationalization The process of translating research concepts into measurable phenomena.

*oral history An unstructured self-report technique used to gather personal recollections of events and their perceived causes and consequences.

ordinal measurement A level of measurement that rank-orders phenomena or attributes along some dimension (e.g., socioeconomic status).

ordinary least-squares (OLS) regression Regression analysis that uses the least-squares criterion for estimating the parameters in the regression equation.

*orthogonal rotation In factor analysis, a rotation of factors such that the reference axes are kept at a right angle, and hence the factors remain uncorrelated.

outcome analysis An evaluation of what happens with regard to outcomes of interest after implementing a program or intervention, without using an experimental design to assess net effects; see also *impact analysis*.

outcome measure A term sometimes used to refer to the dependent variable, that is, the measure that captures the outcome of an intervention.

outcomes research Research designed to document the effectiveness of health care services and the end results of patient care.

p **value** In statistical testing, the probability that the obtained results are due to chance alone; the probability of committing a Type I error.

pair matching See *matching*.

panel study A type of longitudinal study in which data are collected from the same people (a *panel*) at two or more points in time, often in the context of a survey.

paradigm A way of looking at natural phenomena that encompasses a set of philosophical assumptions and that guides one's approach to inquiry.

paradigm case In a hermeneutic analysis following the precepts of Benner, a strong exemplar of the phenomenon under study, often used early in the analysis to gain understanding of the phenomenon.

parameter A characteristic of a population (e.g., the mean age of all Canadian citizens).

parametric statistical tests A class of inferential statistical tests that involve (a) assumptions about the distribution of the variables, (b) the estimation of a parameter, and (c) the use of interval or ratio measures.

participant See *study participant*.

participant observation A special approach to collecting observational data in which researchers immerse themselves in the world of study participants and participate in that world insofar as possible.

participatory action research A research approach with an ideological perspective based on the premise that the use and production of knowledge can be political and used to exert power.

path analysis A regression-based procedure for testing causal models, typically using nonexperimental data.

*path coefficient The weight representing the impact of one variable on another in a path analytic causal model.

*path diagram A graphic representation of the hypothesized linkages and causal flow among variables in a causal relationship.

Pearson's *r* A widely used correlation coefficient designating the magnitude of the relationship between two variables measured on at least an interval scale; also called the *product–moment correlation*.

peer debriefing Sessions with peers to review and explore various aspects of a study—typically in a qualitative study.

peer reviewer A person who reviews and critiques a research report or proposal, who himself or herself is a researcher (usually working on similar types of research problems as those under review), and who makes a recommendation about publishing or funding the research.

perfect relationship A correlation between two variables such that the values of one variable permit perfect prediction of the values of the other; designated as 1.00 or 1.00.

persistent observation In qualitative research, the researcher's intense focus on the aspects of a situation that are relevant to the phenomena being studied.

*person triangulation The collection of data from different levels of persons, with the aim of validating data through multiple perspectives on the phenomenon.

personal interview A face-to-face interview between an interviewer and a respondent.

personal notes In field studies, written comments about the observer's own feelings during the research process.

phenomenology A qualitative research tradition, with roots in philosophy and psychology, that focuses on the lived experience of humans.

phenomenon The abstract concept under study, most often used by qualitative researchers in lieu of the term "variable."

*phi coefficient A statistical index describing the magnitude of the relationship between two dichotomous variables.

*photo elicitation An interview stimulated and guided by photographic images.

pilot study A small-scale version, or trial run, done in preparation for a major study.

placebo A sham or pseudo-intervention, often used as a control condition.

placebo effect Changes in the dependent variable attributable to the placebo condition.

*point estimation A statistical estimation procedure in which the researcher uses information from a sample to estimate the single value (statistic) that best represents the value of the population parameter.

*point prevalence rate The number of people with a condition or disease divided by the total number at risk, multiplied by the number of people for whom the rate is being established (e.g., per 1000 population).

population The entire set of individuals or objects having some common characteristics (e.g., all RNs in South Africa); sometimes called a *universe*.

positive relationship A relationship between two variables in which there is a tendency for high values on one variable to be associated with high values on the other (e.g., as physical activity increases, pulse rate also increases).

positive results Research results that are consistent with the researcher's hypotheses.

positively skewed distribution An asymmetric distribution of values with a disproportionately high number of cases having low values—that is, falling at the lower end of the distribution; when displayed graphically, the tail points to the right.

positivist paradigm The traditional paradigm underlying the scientific approach, which assumes that there is a fixed, orderly reality that can be objectively studied; often associated with quantitative research.

poster session A session at a professional conference in which several researchers simultaneously present visual displays summarizing their studies, while conference attendees circulate around the room perusing the displays.

post hoc test A test for comparing all possible pairs of groups following a significant test of overall group differences (e.g., in an ANOVA).

postpositivist paradigm A modification of the traditional positivist paradigm that acknowledges the impossibility of total objectivity; postpositivists appreciate the impediments to knowing reality with certainty and therefore seek *probabilistic* evidence.

posttest The collection of data after introducing an experimental intervention.

posttest-only design An experimental design in which data are collected from subjects only after the experimental intervention has been introduced; also called an *after-only design*.

power A research design's ability to detect relationships that exist among variables.

power analysis A procedure for estimating either the likelihood of committing a Type II error or sample size requirements.

prediction The use of empirical evidence to make forecasts about how variables will behave in a new setting and with different individuals.

predictive validity The degree to which an instrument can predict some criterion observed at a future time.

predictor variables In a regression analysis (and other multivariate analyses), the independent variables entered into the analysis to predict the dependent variable.

preexperimental design A research design that does not include mechanisms to compensate for the absence of either randomization or a control group.

pretest (1) The collection of data before the experimental intervention; sometimes called *baseline data*; (2) the trial administration of a newly developed instrument to identify flaws or assess time requirements.

pretest–posttest design An experimental design in which data are collected from research subjects both before and after introducing the experimental intervention; also called a *before–after design*.

*prevalence study A study undertaken to determine the prevalence rate of some condition (e.g., a disease or behaviour, such as smoking) at a particular point in time.

primary source First-hand reports of facts, findings, or events; in research, the primary source is the original research report prepared by the investigator who conducted the study.

*principal investigator (PI) The person who is the lead researcher and who will have primary responsibility for overseeing the project.

probability sampling The selection of sampling units (e.g., participants) from a population using random procedures, as in simple random sampling, cluster sampling, and systematic sampling.

*probing Eliciting more useful or detailed information from a respondent in an interview than was volunteered in the first reply.

problem statement The statement of the research problem, often phrased in the form of a research question.

process analysis An evaluation focusing on the process by which a program or intervention gets implemented and used in practice.

process consent In a qualitative study, an ongoing, transactional process of negotiating consent with study participants, allowing them to play a collaborative role in the decision making regarding their continued participation.

product–moment correlation coefficient (r) A widely used correlation coefficient, designating the magnitude of the relationship between two variables measured on at least an interval scale; also called *Pearson's r*.

*projective technique A method of measuring psychological attributes (values, attitudes, personality) by providing respondents with unstructured stimuli to which to respond.

prolonged engagement In qualitative research, the investment of sufficient time during data collection to have an in-depth understanding of the group under study, thereby enhancing data credibility.

*proportional hazards model A model applied in multivariate analyses in which independent variables are used to predict the risk (hazard) of experiencing an event at a given point in time.

proportionate sample A sample that results when the researcher samples from different strata of the population in proportion to their representation in the population.

proposal A document specifying what the researcher proposes to study; it communicates the research problem, its significance, planned procedures for solving the problem, and, when funding is sought, how much the study will cost.

prospective design A study design that begins with an examination of presumed causes (e.g., cigarette smoking) and then goes forward in time to observe presumed effects (e.g., lung cancer).

psychometric assessment An evaluation of the quality of an instrument, based primarily on evidence of its reliability and validity.

psychometrics The theory underlying principles of measurement and the application of the theory in the development of measuring tools.

purposive (purposeful) sampling A non-probability sampling method in which the researcher selects participants based on personal judgment about which ones will be most representative or informative; also called *judgmental sampling*.

Q sort A data collection method in which participants sort statements into a number of piles (usually 9 or 11) along a bipolar dimension (e.g., most like me/least like me; most useful/least useful).

qualitative analysis The organization and interpretation of nonnumeric data for the purpose of discovering important underlying dimensions and patterns of relationships.

qualitative data Information collected in narrative (nonnumeric) form, such as the transcript of an unstructured interview.

*qualitative outcome analysis (QOA) An approach to address the gap between qualitative research and clinical practice, involving the identification and evaluation of clinical interventions based on qualitative findings.

qualitative research The investigation of phenomena, typically in an in-depth and holistic fashion, through the collection of rich narrative materials using a flexible research design.

quantitative analysis The manipulation of numeric data through statistical procedures for the purpose of describing phenomena or assessing the magnitude and reliability of relationships among them.

quantitative data Information collected in a quantified (numeric) form.

quantitative research The investigation of phenomena that lend themselves to precise measurement and quantification, often involving a rigourous and controlled design.

quasi-experiment A study involving an intervention in which subjects are not randomly assigned to treatment conditions, but the researcher exercises certain controls to enhance the study's internal validity.

quasi-statistics An "accounting" system used to assess the validity of conclusions derived from qualitative analysis.

questionnaire A method of gathering self-report information from respondents through self-administration of questions in a paper-and-pencil or computerized format.

quota sampling The nonrandom selection of participants in which the researcher pre-specifies characteristics of the sample to increase its representativeness.

r The symbol for a bivariate correlation coefficient, summarizing the magnitude and direction of a relationship between two variables.

R The symbol for a multiple correlation coefficient indicating the magnitude (but not direction) of the relationship between the dependent variable and multiple independent variables taken together.

R^2 The squared multiple correlation coefficient, indicating the proportion of variance in the dependent variable accounted for or explained by a group of independent variables.

random assignment The assignment of subjects to treatment conditions in a manner determined by chance alone; also called *randomization*.

random number table A table displaying hundreds of digits (from 0 to 9) set up in such a way that each number is equally likely to follow any other.

random sampling The selection of a sample such that each member of a population has an equal probability of being included.

randomization The assignment of subjects to treatment conditions in a manner determined by chance alone; also called *random assignment*.

*randomized block design An experimental design involving two or more factors (independent variables), only one of which in experimentally manipulated.

randomized clinical trial (RCT) A full experimental test of a new treatment, involving random assignment to treatment groups and, typically, a large and diverse sample (also known as a Phase III clinical trial).

randomness An important concept in quantitative research, involving having certain features of the study established by chance rather than by design or personal preference.

range A measure of variability, computed by subtracting the lowest value from the highest value in a distribution of scores.

rating scale A scale that requires ratings of an object or concept along a continuum.

ratio measurement A level of measurement with equal distances between scores and a true meaningful zero point (e.g., weight).

raw data Data in the form in which they were collected, without being coded or analyzed.

reactivity A measurement distortion arising from the study participant's awareness of being observed, or, more generally, from the effect of the measurement procedure itself.

*readability The ease with which research documents (e.g., a questionnaire) can be read by people with varying reading skills, often empirically determined through readability formulas.

*receiver operating characteristic curve (ROC curve) A method used in developing and refining screening instruments to determine the best cut-off point for "caseness."

*recursive model A path model in which the causal flow is unidirectional, without any feedback loops; opposite of a nonrecursive model.

refereed journal A journal in which decisions about the acceptance of manuscripts are made based on recommendations from peer reviewers.

reflective notes Notes that document a qualitative researcher's personal experiences, reflections, and progress in the field.

reflexive journal A journal maintained by qualitative researchers during data collection and data analysis to document their self-analysis of both how they affected the research and how the research affected them.

reflexivity In qualitative studies, critical self-reflection about one's own biases, preferences, and preconceptions.

regression analysis A statistical procedure for predicting values of a dependent variable based on the values of one or more independent variables.

relationship A bond or a connection between two or more variables.

*relative risk An estimate of risk of "caseness" in one group compared to another, computed by dividing the rate for one group by the rate for another.

reliability The degree of consistency or dependability with which an instrument measures the attribute it is designed to measure.

reliability coefficient A quantitative index, usually ranging in value from .00 to 1.00, that provides an estimate of how reliable an instrument is; it is computed through such procedures as Cronbach's alpha technique, the split-half technique, the test–retest approach, and interrater approaches.

Repeated-measures design An experimental design in which one group of subjects is exposed to more than one condition or treatment in random order; also called a *crossover design*.

replication The deliberate repetition of research procedures in a second investigation for the purpose of determining if earlier results can be repeated.

representative sample A sample whose characteristics are comparable to those of the population from which it is drawn.

research Systematic inquiry that uses orderly, disciplined methods to answer questions or solve problems.

research control See *control*.

research design The overall plan for addressing a research question, including specifications for enhancing the study's integrity.

Research Ethics Board (REB) A group established within Canadian universities, hospitals, and other institutions where research is conducted to ensure that ethical principles are applied to research involving human subjects.

research hypothesis The actual hypothesis a researcher wants to test (as opposed to the *null hypothesis*), stating the anticipated relationship between two or more variables.

research methods The techniques used to structure a study and to gather and analyze information in a systematic fashion.

research misconduct Fabrication, falsification, plagiarism, or other practices that seriously deviate from those that are commonly accepted within the scientific community for proposing, conducting, or reporting research.

research problem A situation involving an enigmatic, perplexing, or conflictful condition that can be investigated through disciplined inquiry.

research proposal See *proposal*.

research question A statement of the specific query the researcher wants to answer to address a research problem.

research report A document summarizing the main features of a study, including the research question, the methods used to address it, the findings, and the interpretation of the findings.

research utilization The use of some aspect of a study in an application unrelated to the original research.

researcher credibility The faith that can be put in a researcher, based on his or her training, qualifications, and experience.

*residuals In multiple regression, the error term or unexplained variance.

respondent In a self-report study, the study participant responding to questions posed by the researcher.

response rate The rate of participation in a study, calculated by dividing the number of persons participating by the number of persons sampled.

response set bias The measurement error introduced by the tendency of some individuals to respond to items in characteristic ways (e.g., always agreeing), independently of the items' content.

results The answers to research questions, obtained through an analysis of the collected data; in a quantitative study, the information obtained through statistical tests.

retrospective design A study design that begins with the manifestation of the dependent variable in the present (e.g., lung cancer) and then searches for the presumed cause occurring in the past (e.g., cigarette smoking).

risk/benefit ratio The relative costs and benefits, to an individual subject and to society at large, of participation in a study; also, the relative costs and benefits of implementing an innovation.

rival hypothesis An alternative explanation, competing with the researcher's hypothesis, to account for the results of a study.

sample A subset of a population, selected to participate in a study.

sample size The total number of study participants participating in a study.

sampling The process of selecting a portion of the population to represent the entire population.

sampling bias Distortions that arise when a sample is not representative of the population from which it was drawn.

sampling distribution A theoretical distribution of a statistic (e.g., a mean), using the values of the statistic computed from an infinite number of samples as the data points in the distribution.

sampling error The fluctuation of the value of a statistic from one sample to another drawn from the same population.

sampling frame A list of all the elements in the population from which the sample is drawn.

sampling plan The formal plan specifying a sampling method, a sample size, and procedures for recruiting subjects.

saturation The collection of data in a qualitative study to the point at which a sense of closure is attained because new data yield redundant information.

scale A composite measure of an attribute, involving the combination of several items that have a logical and empirical relationship to each other, resulting in the assignment of a score to place people on a continuum with respect to the attribute.

*****scatter plot** A graphic representation of the relationship between two variables.

scientific merit The degree to which a study is methodologically and conceptually sound.

scientific method A set of orderly, systematic, controlled procedures for acquiring dependable, empirical–and typically quantitative–information; the methodologic approach associated with the positivist paradigm.

screening instrument An instrument used to determine whether potential subjects for a study meet eligibility criteria (or for determining whether a person has a specified condition).

secondary analysis A form of research in which the data collected by one researcher are reanalyzed, usually by another investigator, to answer new research questions.

secondary source Second-hand accounts of events or facts; in a research context, a description of a study or studies prepared by someone other than the original researcher.

selective coding A level of coding in a grounded theory study that begins after the core category is discovered and involves systematically integrating relationships between the core category and other categories and validating those relationships.

selection threat (self-selection) A threat to the internal validity of the study resulting from preexisting differences between groups under study; the differences affect the dependent variable in ways extraneous to the effect of the independent variable.

self-determination A person's ability to voluntarily decide whether or not to participate in a study.

self-report A method of collecting data that involves a direct report of information by the person who is being studied (e.g., by interview or questionnaire).

semantic differential A technique used to measure attitudes that asks respondents to rate a concept of interest on a series of bipolar rating scales.

semistructured interview An interview in which the researcher has listed topics to cover rather than specific questions to ask.

sensitivity The ability of screening instruments to correctly identify a "case" (i.e., to correctly diagnose a condition).

sensitivity analysis In a meta-analysis, a method to determine whether conclusions are sensitive to the quality of the studies included.

*****sequential clinical trial** A clinical trial in which data are continuously analyzed and "stop rules" are used to decide when the evidence about the intervention's efficacy is sufficiently strong that the experiment can be stopped.

setting The physical location and conditions in which data collection takes place in a study.

significance level The probability that an observed relationship could be caused by chance (i.e., as a result of sampling error); significance at the .05 level indicates the probability that a relationship of the observed magnitude would be found by chance only 5 times out of 100.

*****sign test** A nonparametric test for comparing two paired groups based on the relative ranking of values between the pairs.

simple random sampling The most basic type of probability sampling, wherein a sampling frame is created by enumerating all members of a population and then selecting a sample from the sampling frame through completely random procedures.

*****simultaneous multiple regression** A multiple regression analysis in which all predictor variables are entered into the equation simultaneously; sometimes called *direct* or *standard* multiple regression.

*****single-subject experiment** A study that tests the effectiveness of an intervention with a single subject, typically using a time series design.

site The overall location where a study is undertaken.

skewed distribution The asymmetric distribution of a set of data values around a central point.

snowball sampling The selection of participants through referrals from earlier participants; also called *network sampling* or *nominated sampling*.

social desirability response set A bias in self-report instruments created when participants have a tendency to misrepresent their opinions in the direction of answers consistent with prevailing social norms.

*Solomon four-group design An experimental design that uses a before–after design for one pair of experimental and control groups, and an after-only design for a second pair.

*space triangulation The collection of data on the same phenomenon in multiple sites to enhance the validity of the findings.

*Spearman–Brown prophecy formula An equation for making corrections to a reliability estimate calculated by the split-half technique.

Spearman's rank-order correlation (Spearman's rho) A correlation coefficient indicating the magnitude of a relationship between variables measured on the ordinal scale.

specificity The ability of a screening instrument to correctly identify noncases.

split-half technique A method for estimating internal consistency reliability by correlating scores on half of the instrument with scores on the other half.

standard deviation The most frequently used statistic for measuring the degree of variability in a set of scores.

standard error The standard deviation of a theoretical sampling distribution, such as a sampling distribution of means.

*standard scores Scores expressed in terms of standard deviations from the mean, with raw scores transformed to have a mean of zero and a standard deviation of one; also called z scores.

statement of purpose A broad declarative statement of the overall aims/goals of a study.

statistic An estimate of a parameter, calculated from sample data.

statistical analysis The organization and analysis of quantitative data using statistical procedures, including both descriptive and inferential statistics.

statistical conclusion validity The degree to which conclusions about relationships and differences from a statistical analysis of the data are legitimate.

statistical control The use of statistical procedures to control extraneous influences on the dependent variable.

statistical inference The process of inferring attributes about the population based on information from a sample, using laws of probability.

statistical power The ability of the research design and analysis to detect true relationships among variables.

statistical significance A term indicating that the results from an analysis of sample data are unlikely to have been caused by chance, at some specified level of probability.

statistical test An analytic tool that estimates the probability that obtained results from a sample reflect true population values.

*stepwise multiple regression A multiple regression analysis in which predictor variables are entered into the equation in steps, in the order in which the increment to R is greatest.

stipend A monetary payment to individuals participating in a study to serve as an incentive for participation and/or to compensate for time and expenses.

strata Subdivisions of the population according to some characteristic (e.g., males and females); singular is *stratum*.

stratified random sampling The random selection of study participants from two or more strata of the population independently.

*structural equations Equations representing the magnitude and nature of hypothesized relations among sets of variables in a theory.

structured data collection An approach to collecting information from participants, either through self-report or observations, in which the researcher determines response categories in advance.

study participant An individual who participates and provides information in a study.

subgroup effect The differential effect of the independent variable on the dependent variable for various subsets of the sample.

subject An individual who participates and provides data in a study; term used primarily in quantitative research.

substantive theory In grounded theory, a theory that is grounded in data from a single study on a specific substantive area (e.g., postpartum depression); in contrast to *formal theory*.

summated rating scale A composite scale with multiple items, each of which is scored; item scores are added together to yield a total score that distributes people along a continuum (e.g., a Likert scale).

survey research Nonexperimental research in which information regarding the activities, beliefs, preferences, and attitudes of people is gathered by direct questioning.

*****survival analysis** A statistical procedure used when the dependent variable represents a time interval between an initial event (e.g., onset of a disease) and an end event (e.g., death); also called *life table analysis*.

symmetric distribution A distribution of values with two halves that are mirror images of each other; a distribution that is not skewed.

systematic sampling The selection of study participants such that every *k*th (e.g., every 10th) person (or element) in a sampling frame or list is chosen.

table of random numbers See *random number table*.

tacit knowledge Information about a culture that is so deeply embedded that members do not talk about it or may not even be consciously aware of it.

target population The entire population in which the researcher is interested and to which he or she would like to generalize the results of a study.

taxonomy In an ethnographic analysis, a system of classifying and organizing terms and concepts, developed to illuminate the internal organization of a domain and the relationship among the subcategories of the domain.

template analysis style An approach to qualitative analysis in which a preliminary template or coding scheme is used to sort the narrative data.

test statistic A statistic used to test for the statistical significance of relationships between variables; the sampling distributions of test statistics are known for circumstances in which the null hypothesis is true; examples include chi-square, *F*-ratio, *t*, and Pearson's *r*.

test–retest reliability Assessment of the stability of an instrument by correlating the scores obtained on repeated administrations.

*****testing threat** A threat to a study's internal validity that occurs when the administration of a pretest or baseline measure of a dependent variable results in changes on the variable, apart from the effect of the independent variable.

theme A recurring regularity emerging from an analysis of qualitative data.

theoretical notes In field studies, notes detailing the researcher's interpretations of observed behaviour.

theoretical sampling In qualitative studies, the selection of sample members based on emerging findings as the study progresses to ensure adequate representation of important themes.

theory An abstract generalization that presents a systematic explanation about the relationships among phenomena.

theory triangulation The use of competing theories or hypotheses in the analysis and interpretation of data.

thick description A rich and thorough description of the research context in a qualitative study.

think aloud method A qualitative method used to collect data about cognitive processes (e.g., problem solving, decision making), involving the use of audio recordings to capture people's reflections on decisions as they are being made or problems as they are being solved.

time sampling In observational research, the selection of time periods during which observations will take place.

time series design A quasi-experimental design involving the collection of data over an extended time period, with multiple data collection points both before and after an intervention.

time triangulation The collection of data on the same phenomenon or about the same people at different points in time to enhance the validity of the findings.

topic guide A list of broad question areas to be covered in a semistructured interview or focus group interview.

transferability The extent to which findings can be transferred to other settings or groups—often used in qualitative research and analogous to generalizability in quantitative research.

treatment The experimental intervention under study; the condition being manipulated.

treatment group The group receiving the intervention being tested; the experimental group.

trend study A form of longitudinal study in which different samples from a population are studied over time with respect to some phenomenon (e.g., annual Gallup polls on abortion attitudes).

triangulation The use of multiple methods to collect and interpret data about a phenomenon so as to converge on an accurate representation of reality.

true score A hypothetical score that would be obtained if a measure were infallible.

trustworthiness The degree of confidence qualitative researchers have in their data, assessed using the criteria of credibility, transferability, dependability, and confirmability.

t-test A parametric statistical test for analyzing the difference between two means.

*two-tailed tests Statistical tests in which both ends of the sampling distribution are used to determine improbable values.

Type I error An error created by rejecting the null hypothesis when it is true (i.e., the researcher concludes that a relationship exists when in fact it does not—a false positive).

Type II error An error created by accepting the null hypothesis when it is false (i.e., the researcher concludes that *no* relationship exists when in fact it does—a false negative).

typical case sampling An approach to sampling in qualitative research involving the selection of participants who highlight what is typical or average.

unimodal distribution A distribution of values with one peak (high frequency).

unit of analysis The basic unit or focus of a researcher's analysis; in nursing research, the unit of analysis is typically the individual study participant.

univariate descriptive study A study that gathers information on the occurrence, frequency of occurrence, or average value of the variables of interest, one variable at a time, without focusing on interrelationships among variables.

univariate statistics Statistical procedures for analyzing a single variable for purposes of description.

unstructured interview An oral self-report in which the researcher asks a respondent questions without having a predetermined plan regarding the content or flow of information to be gathered.

unstructured observation The collection of descriptive information through direct observation that is not guided by a formal, prespecified plan for observing, enumerating, or recording the information.

validity The degree to which an instrument measures what it is intended to measure.

validity coefficient A quantitative index, usually ranging in value from .00 to 1.00, that provides an estimate of how valid an instrument is.

variability The degree to which values on a set of scores are dispersed.

variable An attribute of a person or object that varies, that is, takes on different values (e.g., body temperature, age, heart rate).

variance A measure of variability or dispersion, equal to the standard deviation squared.

vignette A brief description of an event, person, or situation about which respondents are asked to describe their reactions.

visual analog scale A scaling procedure used to measure certain clinical symptoms (e.g., pain, fatigue) by having people indicate on a straight line the intensity of the symptom.

vulnerable subjects Special groups of people whose rights in research studies need special protection because of their inability to provide meaningful informed consent or because their circumstances place them at higher-than-average risk of adverse effects; examples include young children, the mentally retarded, and unconscious patients.

weighting A correction procedure used to arrive at population values when a disproportionate sampling design has been used.

*Wilcoxon signed ranks test A nonparametric statistical test for comparing two paired groups based on the relative ranking of values between the pairs.

*Wilk's lambda An index used in discriminant function analysis to indicate the proportion of variance in the dependent variable unaccounted for by predictors; $\lambda = 1 - R^2$.

within-subjects design A research design in which a single group of subjects is compared under different conditions or at different points in time (e.g., before and after surgery).

*z score A standard score, expressed in terms of standard deviations from the mean.

APPENDIX A.
Predictors of Early Parenting Self-efficacy: Results of a Prospective Cohort Study

Janet Bryanton
Anita J. Gagnon
Marie Hatem
Celeste Johnston

➤ **Background:** Parenting self-efficacy has been identified as one determinant of positive parenting. The literature is inconsistent regarding the predictors of parenting self-efficacy, and there is limited evidence regarding these predictors in the early postpartum period.

➤ **Objectives:** To determine the factors predictive of parenting self-efficacy at 12 to 48 hr after childbirth and at 1 month postpartum.

➤ **Method:** Six-hundred fifty-two women were recruited consecutively from the postpartum units of two general hospitals on Prince Edward Island, Canada. Data were collected at 12 to 48 hr postpartum using self-report and chart review. On the basis of scoring positive or negative on their childbirth perceptions, 175 of these mothers were assigned to two cohorts. They were visited at home at 1 month postpartum, where data were collected using self-report.

➤ **Results:** Using multiple logistic regression, greater parenting self-efficacy at 12 to 48 hr after childbirth was predicted by multiparity and single marital status and correlated with positive perception of the birth experience, higher general self-efficacy, and excellent partner relationship. Greater parenting self-efficacy at 1 month was predicted by age ≤30 years and multiparity and correlated with excellent partner relationship and maternal perception of infant contentment.

➤ **Discussion:** Birth perception is a correlate of parenting self-efficacy that is modifiable; therefore, nurses have an opportunity to strive to create a positive birth experience for all women to enhance their early parenting self-efficacy. Nurses can also consider assessing women at risk for suboptimal parenting self-efficacy and intervene through teaching, support, and parenting self-efficacy boosting interventions.

➤ **Key Words:** childbirth perception • parenting • parenting self-efficacy • predictor

Reprinted with permission from *Nursing Research* (2008; 57[4]: 252–259).

Parenting self-efficacy has been identified as one determinant of positive parenting behaviors (Coleman & Karraker, 2003; Sanders & Woolley, 2005). However, there is inconsistent evidence regarding the predictors of parenting self-efficacy, and few studies have investigated this concept in the early postpartum period (Porter & Hsu, 2003; Reece, 1992). With clear evidence about the factors that predict early parenting self-efficacy, nurses will be in a better position to assess for risk of low parenting self-efficacy and intervene appropriately to enhance the transition to parenting.

The purpose of this study, therefore, was to determine the factors predictive of maternal parenting self-efficacy at 12 to 48 hr after childbirth and at 1 month postpartum. The research questions were the following: (a) What are the predictors of parenting self-efficacy at 12 to 48 hr after childbirth? (b) In a subgroup of women with positive and negative childbirth perceptions, what are the predictors of parenting self-efficacy at 1 month postpartum?

Literature Review

Parenting self-efficacy can be defined as a parent's belief that he or she is capable of organizing and executing tasks related to parenting a child (de Montigny & Lacharite, 2005). On the basis of a concept analysis of 60 studies, these authors suggest that parenting self-efficacy research has been plagued by lack of clarity in the definition of this construct. The terms *perceived parenting competence* and *confidence* have been used interchangeably with parenting self-efficacy. These are related, but not identical, concepts. Parenting self-efficacy is more situation specific, whereas confidence is a more stable state of certainty that is not situation dependent. Parenting competence is a judgment held by others, whereas perceived self-efficacy is the parent's own judgment (de Montigny & Lacharite, 2005). Perceived competence is focused on the number of skills a parent has, and, according to Bandura (1997), parents not only require the knowledge of appropriate parenting behaviors and skills but must also believe in their ability to carry out these behaviors to put their knowledge and skills into action.

Although many parents are able to meet the challenges of parenting and derive satisfaction from it, others lack persistence and adequate parenting skills, feel overburdened, and receive little enjoyment. These parents become psychologically unavailable, which can have detrimental effects on their infants' physical, socioemotional, and cognitive development (Coleman & Karraker, 1997). These authors suggest that the self-efficacy construct offers hope in advancing the understanding of varying responses to parenting, and inclusion of cognitive factors rather than just overt parenting may assist in enhancing the explanatory power of theoretical models and the effectiveness of parenting programs.

Efficacious parents work diligently to provide positive experiences for their children and combat risks, even when faced with multiple stressors (Elder, 1995). Those with greater self-efficacy are able to focus their resources toward mastering the situation at hand. A mother who feels efficacious in her parenting is more likely to be successful in establishing a warm and sensitive relationship with her baby and be able to interpret infant signals correctly and respond appropriately (Teti & Candelaria, 2002). Maternal self-efficacy and perceived competence and confidence have been identified as central correlates of adaptation to parenthood, maternal–infant attachment, and satisfaction with parenting and the infant (Coleman & Karraker, 2000; Mercer & Ferketich, 1990, 1994; Reece & Harkless, 1998).

In contrast, persons with low self-efficacy tend to expend energy worrying about negative outcomes, which may undermine their efforts and effectiveness. A mother who feels inefficacious may have more difficulty in handling her baby and be indecisive, insensitive, and awkward (Teti & Gelfand, 1991). Low parenting self-efficacy has been associated with reduced parenting effectiveness, insecure attachment, and increased susceptibility to helplessness (Donovan & Leavitt, 1989; Donovan, Leavitt, & Walsh, 1990; Tucker & Gross, 1997).

The predictors and correlates of parenting self-efficacy and the related constructs of confidence and competence have been investigated in a number of studies. There are inconsistencies in findings, which may be accounted for by differences in construct definition, methodologies, timing of measurements, and tools. For example, some researchers have reported that maternal age does not affect parenting self-efficacy (Mercer, 1986; Pridham, Lytton, Chang, & Rutledge, 1991), whereas Conrad, Gross, Fogg, and Ruchala (1992) found a positive correlation between age and maternal confidence. In contrast, others reported an inverse relationship between age and parenting self-efficacy and competence (Coleman & Karraker, 2003; Tarkka, 2003). Higher maternal education has been associated with increased self-efficacy and competence (Coleman & Karraker, 2000; Mercer, 1986), but no effect has also been reported (Pridham & Chang, 1992; Tarkka, 2003). Higher socioeconomic status has been associated with increased parenting self-efficacy (Coleman & Karraker, 2000; Teti & Gelfand, 1991). In contrast, Tarkka (2003) found no relationship between these two variables. Being married, having a supportive relationship with a mate, and marital quality have been related to higher maternal self-efficacy and competence (Mercer, 1986; Porter & Hsu, 2003). Multiparity has been associated with increased parenting self-efficacy and competence (Pridham et al., 1991; Secco, 2002), whereas other researchers have reported no differences based on parity (Conrad et al., 1992; Tarkka, 2003). Infant temperament has been investigated, with parenting easier infants being associated with higher self-efficacy and competence (Mercer, 1986; Porter & Hsu, 2003). Mothers of infants with colic (Papousek & von Hofacker, 1998) and a difficult temperament (Tarkka, 2003) have demonstrated lower parenting self-efficacy.

Few researchers have examined parenting self-efficacy at 1 month postpartum. Reece (1992) reported that greater parenting self-efficacy at 1 and 3 months was associated with increased confidence in parenting at 1 year. Porter and Hsu (2003) found that prenatal self-efficacy was associated positively with parenting self-efficacy at 1 month in first-time mothers. No reported research has examined the relationship between the childbirth experience and parenting self-efficacy, although studies have demonstrated that a positive experience can influence a woman's self-confidence and self-esteem (Callister, 2004; Simkin, 1991).

To summarize, there is a growing body of literature describing parenting self-efficacy, although lack of theoretical clarity is evident. Greater parenting self-efficacy has been associated with more positive parenting behaviors, but few studies have been conducted on early parenting self-efficacy. The literature provides evidence regarding the predictors and correlates of parenting self-efficacy, but the findings are inconsistent. Research is required to investigate the predictors of parenting self-efficacy, particularly in the early transition to parenting.

Theoretical Framework

The theoretical framework of this study was developed by integrating three self-efficacy theories, hypothesizing that parenting self-efficacy arises from a combination of task-specific, general, and domain self-efficacy, as well as other factors identified in the literature. According to Bandura (1995), self-efficacy is a situation, task-specific attribute enhanced by performance accomplishments (previous successes), vicarious experience, verbal (social) persuasion, and emotional arousal in judging one's capabilities. This framework hypothesized that parenting self-efficacy is influenced by the above factors and may be as specific as self-efficacy in one task of parenting such as breast-feeding or may range over a number of specific parenting tasks. Sherer et al. (1982) defined general self-efficacy as a composite of a person's past experiences with success and failure across a variety of situations, which results in a general set of expectations that a person carries into a new situation.

This is viewed as a relatively stable personality trait. It is hypothesized that a new mother's general self-efficacy will also influence her parenting self-efficacy.

Woodruff and Cashman (1993) hypothesized that domain self-efficacy arises from a larger portion of life events through combined information from several theoretically related or similar experiences. It relates to beliefs about a person's ability in a particular aspect of life rather than a specific task. These authors suggested that domain self-efficacy is broader than task-specific self-efficacy; however, it is not as broad as general self-efficacy. The study framework hypothesized that childbirth and parenting are conceptually related experiences and that a positive childbirth experience has the potential to influence parenting self-efficacy through an increase in domain self-efficacy. The influence of other factors such as age; marital status; parity; education; income; and perception of partner relationship, partner support, and infant contentment on parenting self-efficacy was examined in the framework.

METHODS

Design

This study employed a prospective cohort design. A consecutive sample of 652 new mothers was recruited from hospitals, and a subsample of 175 of these women were assigned to cohorts based on positive or negative childbirth perceptions. Data were collected at 12 to 48 hr after childbirth and at 1 month postpartum.

Setting

The in-hospital recruitment and data collection were conducted on the postpartum units of two general hospitals on Prince Edward Island, Canada. In one hospital, women labor, give birth, and recover in a birthing room and are then transferred to a postpartum unit, where they and their newborns are cared for by separate nurses. The second hospital has birthing suites where women labor, give birth, recover, and have their postpartum stay in one room. Mother and baby are cared for by the same nurse. One-on-one nursing support during active labor is a standard of care in both settings. Data collection at 1 month was completed in the women's homes.

Population and Sample

All women who gave birth on Prince Edward Island from October 2004 to December 2005 were assessed for inclusion, except one woman who gave birth at home and those who were discharged before the research assistants were able to assess them. Women were included if they had a vaginal, emergency cesarean, or planned cesarean birth; were ≥15 years; and were able to read and speak English and provide consent. They were excluded if they had an unresolved serious illness; had received general anesthesia; were leaving the province before 1 month; had given birth to a stillborn infant; had infants who were at <37 weeks' gestation; had infants who weighed <2,500 g; had infants who were multiples; had infants who had major congenital anomalies, traumatic birth injuries, or other serious illnesses; or had infants who were placed in foster care or adopted. Situations in which infants were not well may have created extended separation and maternal guilt, helplessness, anxiety (Bennett & Slade, 1991; Teti, O'Connell, & Reiner, 1996), depression, concerns about their infant, and difficulty expressing affection (Bennett & Slade, 1991), which may have influenced parenting self-efficacy.

Ethics approval for the full study was obtained from four university and hospital research ethics boards. Written, informed consent, obtained in hospital, was reconfirmed prior to the in-home data collection.

Data Collection

Demographic and obstetrical data were recorded from every consenting woman's chart. Parenting self-efficacy; perceptions of the childbirth experience, partner relationship, partner support, and infant contentment; and general self-efficacy were measured through self-report. Research assistants regularly reviewed the patient information kardexes on both units, and women who were eligible were approached within 12 to 48 hr of childbirth. Those who agreed to participate were given the questionnaires to complete and return to the nurses' station in a sealed envelope. The subsample of women assigned to the positive and negative cohorts were contacted at 3.5 weeks postpartum to arrange for a home visit at 1 month. At this time, the parenting self-efficacy questionnaire was read-ministered. If mothers were unable to be contacted after three calls or refused the home visit, they were lost to follow-up. Before initiating the study, a pilot with 30 women was conducted to determine negative and positive cutoff scores for the birth perception scale; these women were not included in the study sample.

Description of Measures

Parenting self-efficacy was measured using the Parent Expectations Survey (PES). This 25-item Likert-type scale was developed by Reece (1992). The original scale was revised by Reece and Harkless (1998), with the addition of 5 items related to affective tasks of parenting. Bandura (1997) suggested that efficacy beliefs should be measured with "items portraying different levels of task demands" that parents rate according to "the strength of their belief in their ability to execute the activity" (p. 43). This scale meets these requirements. The PES includes items about the mother's self-efficacy in her abilities to feed and soothe her infant, meet other nonfeeding needs, and manage her lifestyle. For each item, the woman responds with the number from 0 (*cannot do*) to 10 (*certain can do*) that most closely represents how she feels about herself as a new parent. To score the PES, individual items are summed and divided by 25 to determine the mean PES score, which ranges from 0 to 10. Content validity was established by seven doctorally prepared nurses who rated each item as appropriate or inappropriate, resulting in a 92% agreement on all items. The questionnaire was reviewed also by Bandura, and feedback was obtained from four pediatric and family nurse practitioners (Reece, 1992). Concurrent validity was established using the self-evaluation subscale of the What Being the Parent of a Baby is Like questionnaire (Pridham & Chang, 1989). Predictive validity results showed that self-efficacy at 1 and 3 months was associated with greater maternal confidence and less stress at 1 year. Test-Retest reliability was not calculated due to the theoretical underpinnings that self-efficacy changes over time. Cronbach's alpha has been .90 at 2 to 3 weeks postpartum (McCarter-Spaulding & Kearney, 2001) and .91 at 1 month.

Perception of the childbirth experience was measured, for women giving birth vaginally or by emergency cesarean, using the Questionnaire Measuring Attitudes About Labor and Delivery. This 29-item questionnaire measures attitudes about labor and birth on a 5-point Likert-type scale (Marut & Mercer, 1979). The higher the total score of individual items, the more positively the childbirth experience is perceived, for a possible total score of 29 to 145. The Cronbach's alpha coefficient reliability has ranged from .76 to .87 (Cranley, Hedahl, & Pegg, 1983; Fawcett, Pollio, & Tully, 1992; Marut & Mercer, 1979). Women giving birth by planned cesarean used the Modified Questionnaire Measuring Attitudes About Labor and Delivery. Cranley et al. (1983) adapted the original instrument by replacing the items related specifically to labor with the ones measuring perception of the preoperative experience. This adaptation has been used in several studies, with alpha reliabilities ranging from .84 to .91 (Cranley et al., 1983; Fawcett et al., 1992). In the current study, ongoing scoring and assignment of women to the cohorts was based on the established cut-offs of < and >1 standard deviation from the pilot study mean (negative <87; positive >112).

General self-efficacy was measured using the general self-efficacy subscale of the Self-efficacy Scale (Sherer et al., 1982). This 17-item subscale measures general self-efficacy that is not tied to specific situations or behaviors. Construct validity was assessed by correlating scores with six measures of other personality characteristics related to but not synonymous with self-efficacy (Sherer et al., 1982). Sherer and Adams (1983) reassessed the construct validity with a sample of 101 students, using three other personality scales, and refined the instrument to a 5-point scale from the original 14-point scale. Criterion validity was established with a separate sample of 150 veterans. Sherer et al. (1982) reported the alpha coefficients for the subscale to be .86, and possible scores range from 17 to 85. Single-item ratings from 1 to 10 were used to measure perception of partner relationship, partner support, and infant contentment.

Sample Size Requirements

Calculations were based on an alpha of .05 and a power of .80. To establish the cohorts of women with negative and positive birth perceptions, a subsample of 160 participants (80 per cohort) was required. A total sample of 652 were recruited to obtain the subsample requirements as most women scored neutral on birth perceptions. Ten participants per predictor were required for regression modeling.

Data Analysis

After data entry and cleaning, data were analyzed using SAS Version 9.1. Descriptive statistics were computed to determine the distribution of the variables, assess for outliers, and describe the sample. The distributions of the mean scores for the two parenting self-efficacy variables (after childbirth and 1 month postpartum) were assessed and were skewed negatively; both variables were therefore dichotomized.

Research Question 1 This question was addressed using multiple logistic regression with the full sample (Model 1). Independent variables arose from the theoretical framework and are listed in the maximum models in Table 1. Birth perception was used as a continuous variable as data were available for women having positive, negative, and neutral birth perceptions. Bivariate statistics (*t* tests and chi-squares) were calculated for the independent variables and outcome variables to determine relationships prior to modeling. A maximum model was developed with all independent variables. The variables with *p* values <.05 were kept in the model, and all others were taken out one at a time, starting with the one with the highest *p* value. Each time a variable was removed, the changes in all the remaining beta coefficients were assessed. When a variable coefficient changed by more than 10%, it was placed back into the model. To evaluate the model, continuous variables were assessed for linearity in logit. If a variable was not linear, it was categorized based on its quartiles and clinical judgment and the model was reanalyzed.

Research Question 2 This question was addressed using multiple logistic regression with the subsample of women. Birth perception was a categorical variable in Model 2 because at 1 month, the subsample consisted of women who had positive or negative birth experiences only. The rest of the analyses were identical to those described for Model 1.

TABLE 1 MAXIMUM MODELS		
VARIABLE	PARENTING SELF-EFFICACY AFTER CHILDBIRTH	PARENTING SELF-EFFICACY AT 1 MONTH POSTPARTUM
Maternal age	X	X
Perception of birth experience	X	X
Marital status	X	X
Parity	X	X
Education	X	X
General self-efficacy	X	X
Income	X	X
Partner relationship	X	a
Partner relationship at 1 month	NA	X
Partner support	NA	X
Maternal perception of infant contentment	NA	X

Note. X indicates that the variable was present in the maximum model; a indicates used measurement taken at 1 month; NA indicates that the measurement was taken at 1 month, so it is not applicable after childbirth.

RESULTS

Participant Flow

All 1,442 women who gave birth in a hospital during the study period were assessed for eligibility, except 31 who were discharged early. Of the 1,411 remaining women, 195 were not eligible, and 46% of the eligible women refused participation. The main reasons for refusal included not interested, too busy, disliked surveys, or the partner or woman did not want a home visit. The remaining 652 women participated in the in-hospital data collection. Ninety-one of the 652 women were assigned to the negative cohort; 11 were lost to follow-up ($n = 80$). One-hundred two women were allocated to the positive cohort, of which 7 were lost to follow-up ($n = 95$). Reasons for discontinuing did not differ between the cohorts and included mother not well, too busy, too tired, or moving out of province.

Description of Sample

The sample of 652 mothers ranged in age from 16 to 43 years, with a mean age of 28.4 years. Over half (56.4%) were multiparas. The majority were married or living in a common-law relationship (73.2%), had an adequate income (76.5%), and had some college or university through postgraduate education (76.6%). Almost three quarters (73.3%) experienced a vaginal birth. Approximately one third (31.9%) had attended prenatal classes with the present pregnancy and 36% with past pregnancies, whereas 32.1% had never attended prenatal classes. The subsample of 175 women was not significantly different when compared with the total sample on the major baseline demographics and obstetrical characteristics. There were also no differences between the subsample and the 18 women lost to follow-up.

Research Question 1: Parenting Self-efficacy After Childbirth The Maximum Model 1, presented in Table 1, consisted of eight variables. As shown in Table 2, seven variables plus the intercept remained in the final model. Results indicated that, when controlling for age and income, parity and marital status were predictive of parenting self-efficacy after childbirth, and perception of the birth experience, general self-efficacy, and partner relationship were correlated significantly with parenting self-efficacy. Because the latter three variables were measured at the same time as parenting self-efficacy, predictive ability could not be confirmed, but theoretically these variables are antecedents to parenting self-efficacy. Multiparas were 2 to 5 times more likely to score high on parenting self-efficacy than were primiparas (odds ratio [OR] = 3.35, confidence interval [CI] = 2.18, 5.13). Married women were 29% to 77% less likely to score high than were single women (OR = 0.41, CI = 0.23, 0.71). Women who had high general self-efficacy were 1 to 2.6 times more likely to score high on parenting self-efficacy as compared with those who had low general self-efficacy (OR = 1.72, CI = 1.13, 2.62). Those who perceived their partner relationship to be excellent were 1 to 2.4 times more likely to have high parenting self-efficacy than were their counterparts (OR = 1.60, CI = 1.06, 2.41). Lastly, for every point increase in birth perception, women were 1 to 1.1 times more likely to score high on parenting self-efficacy (OR = 1.04, CI = 1.02, 1.05).

Research Question 2: Parenting Self-efficacy at 1 Month The Maximum Model 2, presented in Table 1, consisted of 10 variables. As shown in Table 2, all variables remained in

TABLE 2	**FINAL MODELS FOR PREDICTORS OF PARENTING SELF-EFFICACY**				
VARIABLE	b ESTIMATE	SE	ODDS RATIO	95% CONFIDENCE INTERVAL	p
Model 1: parenting self-efficacy after childbirth (n = 651)[a]					
Maternal age	−0.30	0.23	0.74	0.48, 1.16	.19
Birth experience	0.03	0.01	1.04	1.02, 1.05	<.00
Marital status	−0.90	0.28	0.41	0.23, 0.71	.00
Parity	1.21	0.22	3.35	2.18, 5.13	<.00
General self-efficacy	0.54	0.21	1.72	1.13, 2.62	.01
Income	0.28	0.28	1.32	0.77, 2.27	.31
Partner relationship	0.47	0.21	1.60	1.06, 2.41	.02
Intercept	−3.19	0.80			
Model 2: parenting self-efficacy at 1 month (n = 162)[b]					
Maternal age	−1.23	0.49	0.29	0.11, 0.76	.01
Birth experience	0.75	0.44	2.12	0.89, 5.07	.09
Marital status	−0.04	0.59	0.96	0.30, 3.06	.95
Parity	0.98	0.50	2.67	1.01, 7.08	.05
Education	0.05	0.61	1.05	0.32, 3.46	.93
General self-efficacy	0.05	0.46	1.05	0.43, 2.60	.91
Income	−0.18	0.57	0.83	0.27, 2.55	.75
Partner relationship at 1 month	1.25	0.59	3.50	1.10, 11.12	.03
Partner support	0.07	0.56	1.07	0.36, 3.21	.90
Maternal perception of infant contentment	1.34	0.43	3.03	1.65, 8.07	.00
Intercept	−0.74	0.68			

[a]One woman did not complete the parenting self-efficacy questionnaire.
[b]Sample size was less than the original 175 due to missing data.

the final model. Results indicated that age and parity were predictive of parenting self-efficacy at 1 month, and perception of partner relationship and infant contentment were correlated significantly with parenting self-efficacy, when controlling for perception of the birth experience, marital status, education, general self-efficacy, income, and partner support. Women who were >30 years old were 24%–89% less likely to score high on parenting self-efficacy than were women who were ≤30 years old (OR = 0.29, CI = 0.11, 0.76). Multiparas were 1 to 7 times more likely to have high parenting self-efficacy than were primip-aras (OR = 2.67, CI = 1.01, 7.08). Women who perceived their infant's contentment to be excellent were 1.7 to almost 9 times more likely to have high parenting self-efficacy than were their counterparts (OR = 3.83, CI = 1.65, 8.87). Lastly, women who perceived their partner relationship to be excellent were 1 to 11 times more likely to have high parenting self efficacy than were those whose partner relationship was not excellent (OR = 3.50, CI = 1.10, 11.12).

DISCUSSION

When comparing the predictors and correlates of parenting self-efficacy after childbirth and at 1 month, there were two similarities and several differences. At both times, multiparity was a strong predictor of parenting self-efficacy. Although the literature is inconsistent regarding this predictor, the current finding has been reported (Pridham et al., 1991; Secco, 2002). This result also supports the theoretical framework, which suggests that self-efficacy is enhanced by performance accomplishments or previous successes (Bandura, 1995). As hypothesized, women who previously have performed parenting tasks successfully feel more self-efficacious in performing the tasks again.

The association between perception of partner relationship and parenting self-efficacy after childbirth and at 1 month has also been reported (Porter & Hsu, 2003; Tarkka, 2003) and also supports the theoretical framework. According to Bandura (1995), self-efficacy is enhanced by verbal (social) persuasion. If a woman believes that her relationship with her partner is good, and if he or she tells her she is a good parent, for example, she may be more likely to have greater parenting self-efficacy.

Parenting Self-efficacy After Childbirth

Single marital status, as a predictor of parenting self-efficacy after childbirth, has not been reported in the literature. In contrast, Copeland and Harbaugh (2004) found perceived parenting competence to be lower in single mothers.

The confirmed relationship between general and parenting self-efficacy after childbirth supports the theoretical framework. As hypothesized, high general self-efficacy influences a woman's self-efficacy in parenting.

The finding that birth perception was correlated significantly with parenting self-efficacy after childbirth has not been reported previously. However, researchers have found that a woman's self-esteem and confidence may be increased by a positive birth experience (Callister, 2004; Simkin, 1991). The current result supports the theoretical framework and suggests that self-efficacy developed in a conceptually related situation, through a positive childbirth experience, enhances a woman's parenting self-efficacy by increasing domain self-efficacy.

Parenting Self-efficacy at 1 Month

Younger age was predictive of parenting self-efficacy at 1 month. The literature is not conclusive about the effect of age on parenting self-efficacy; however, findings of two studies support the current results (Coleman & Karraker, 2003; Tarkka, 2003).

Maternal perception of infant contentment was correlated significantly with parenting self-efficacy at 1 month. Although the directionality of this relationship could not be established due to simultaneous measurement, this relationship has been reported previously (Porter & Hsu, 2003; Tarkka, 2003). A bidirectional relationship is conceivable. If an infant has a difficult temperament and is hard to parent, a mother may feel less efficacious in her parenting and vice versa. On the other hand, a mother who has high parenting self-efficacy may be better able to deal with her infant and perceive the infant as being more content (Teti & Candelaria, 2002).

It is unclear why birth perception did not predict parenting self-efficacy at 1 month. The impact of the birth experience may diminish over time as the woman gains experience in parenting. It is also unclear why general self-efficacy was not predictive of parenting self-efficacy at 1 month. As a mother gains more experience with parenting, her parenting self-efficacy may be influenced less by her general self-efficacy.

In conclusion, the results suggest that the theoretical framework demonstrates beginning empirical adequacy and credibility. As hypothesized, parenting self-efficacy after childbirth was predicted by task-specific, general, and domain self-efficacy; however, the relationships at 1 month were less clear and require further investigation and theory testing. The concept of domain self-efficacy is especially intriguing and requires further development.

The evidence provided by this study has direct clinical implications for the nursing care of childbearing families. In the early postpartum period, nurses can assess women for potential risks for suboptimal parenting self-efficacy based on the predictors and correlates found in this study. Extra teaching and support may benefit those who are at risk for having low parenting self-efficacy. For example, primiparas are more likely to have lower parenting self-efficacy than are multiparas; therefore, nurses can spend time working on areas of concern for them. This includes not only in-hospital teaching but also follow-up in the community. Women who have a poor relationship with their partner also may be at higher risk for having lower parenting self-efficacy; additional support and a parenting self-efficacy boosting intervention may be of help.

Limitations

Forty-six percent of eligible women refused participation. When compared with nonparticipants, the final sample underrepresented cesarean births by 7% and complications by 10.7%. Although it makes sense clinically that these women were less likely to participate, due to the longer recovery time, it is possible that they may have been more negative about their experience, which may have affected the results. As well, the results are generalizable only to Caucasian women who have healthy, term, singleton infants weighing $\geq 2,500$ g and who give birth in an environment where one-on-one nursing support in active labor is the standard of care. They are, however, generalizable across the spectrum of women with respect to parity, marital status, education, and income.

SUMMARY AND CONCLUSIONS

The study findings identify several important predictors and correlates of early parenting self-efficacy. Birth perception is modifiable; therefore, nurses have the potential to create a positive birth experience for all women to enhance their early parenting self-efficacy. They also can consider assessing women at potential risk for suboptimal parenting self-efficacy and intervene through teaching, support, and parenting self-efficacy boosting interventions. The theoretical framework requires further testing for empirical adequacy. Additional research regarding the influence of birth perception on parenting self-efficacy is needed to replicate the current findings and to clarify the diminished relationship at 1 month.

REFERENCES

Bandura, A. (1995). Exercise of personal and collective efficacy in changing societies. In A. Bandura (Ed.), *Self-efficacy in changing societies* (pp. 1–45). New York: Cambridge University Press.

Bandura, A. (1997). *Self-efficacy: The exercise of control.* New York: W. H. Freeman and Company.

Bennett, D. E., & Slade, P. (1991). Infants born at risk: Consequences for maternal post-partum adjustment. *British Journal of Medical Psychology, 64,* 159–172.

Callister, L. C. (2004). Making meaning: Women's birth narratives. *Journal of Obstetric, Gynecologic, and Neonatal Nursing, 33*(4), 508–518.

Coleman, P. K., & Karraker, K. H. (1997). Self-efficacy and parenting quality: Findings and future applications. *Developmental Review, 18,* 47–85.

Coleman, P. K., & Karraker, K. H. (2000). Parenting self-efficacy among mothers of school-age children: Conceptualization, measurement, and correlates. *Family Relations, 49,* 13–24.

Coleman, P. K., & Karraker, K. H. (2003). Maternal self-efficacy beliefs, competence in parenting, and toddlers' behavior and developmental status. *Infant Mental Health Journal, 24,* 126–148.

Conrad, B., Gross, D., Fogg, L., & Ruchala, P. (1992). Maternal confidence, knowledge, and quality of mother-toddler interactions: A preliminary study. *Infant Mental Health Journal, 13,* 353–362.

Copeland, D. B., & Harbaugh, B. L. (2004). Transition of maternal competency of married and single mothers in early parenthood. *Journal of Perinatal Education, 13*(4), 3–9.

Cranley, M. S., Hedahl, K. J., & Pegg, S. H. (1983). Women's perceptions of vaginal and cesarean deliveries. *Nursing Research, 32*(1), 10–15.

de Montigny, F., & Lacharite, C. (2005). Perceived parental efficacy: Concept analysis. *Journal of Advanced Nursing, 49*(4), 387–396.

Donovan, W. L., & Leavitt, L. A. (1989). Maternal self-efficacy and infant attachment: Integrating physiology, perceptions, and behavior. *Child Development, 60*(2), 460–472.

Donovan, W. L., Leavitt, L. A., & Walsh, R. O. (1990). Maternal self-efficacy: Illusory control and its effect on susceptibility to learned helplessness. *Child Development, 61*(5), 1638–1647.

Elder, G. H. (1995). Life trajectories in changing societies. In A. Bandura (Ed.), *Self-efficacy in changing societies* (pp. 46–68). New York: Cambridge University Press.

Fawcett, J., Pollio, N., & Tully, A. (1992). Women's perceptions of cesarean and vaginal delivery: Another look. *Research in Nursing & Health, 15*(6), 439–446.

Marut, J. S., & Mercer, R. T. (1979). Comparison of primiparas' perceptions of vaginal and cesarean births. *Nursing Research, 28*(5), 260–266.

McCarter-Spaulding & Kearney, M. H. (2001). Parenting self-efficacy and perception of insufficient breast milk. *Journal of Obstetric, Gynecologic, and Neonatal Nursing, 30*(5), 515–522.

Mercer, R. T. (1986). *First-time motherhood. Experiences from teens to forties.* New York: Springer.

Mercer, R. T., & Ferketich, S. L. (1990). Predictors of parental attachment during early parenthood. *Journal of Advanced Nursing, 15*(3), 268–280.

Mercer, R. T., & Ferketich, S. L. (1994). Maternal-infant attachment of experienced and inexperienced mothers during infancy. *Nursing Research, 43*(6), 344–351.

Papousek, M., & von Hofacker, N. (1998). Persistent crying in early infancy: A non-trivial condition of risk for the developing mother-infant relationship. *Child: Care, Health and Development Supplement, 24*(5), 395–424.

Porter, C. L., & Hsu, H. C. (2003). First-time mothers' perceptions of efficacy during the transition to motherhood: Links to infant temperament. *Journal of Family Psychology, 17*(1), 54–64.

Pridham, K. F., & Chang, A. S. (1989). What being the parent of a new baby is like: Revision of an instrument. *Research in Nursing & Health, 12*(5), 323–329.

Pridham, K. F., & Chang, A. S. (1992). Transition to being the mother of a new infant in the first 3 months: Maternal problem solving and self-appraisals. *Journal of Advanced Nursing, 17*(2), 204–216.

Pridham, K. F., Lytton, D., Chang, A. S., & Rutledge, D. (1991). Early postpartum transition: Progress in maternal identity and role attainment. *Research in Nursing & Health, 14*(1), 21–31.

Reece, S. M. (1992). The Parent Expectations Survey: A measure of perceived self-efficacy. *Clinical Nursing Research, 1*(4), 336–346.

Reece, S. M., & Harkless, G. (1998). Self-efficacy, stress, and parental adaptation: Applications to the care of childbearing families. *Journal of Family Nursing, 4,* 198–215.

Sanders, M. R., & Woolley, M. L. (2005). The relationship between maternal self-efficacy and parenting practices: Implications for parent training. *Child: Care, Health and Development Supplement, 31*(1), 65–73.

Secco, L. (2002). The infant care questionnaire: Assessment of reliability and validity in a sample of healthy mothers. *Journal of Nursing Measurement, 10*(2), 97–110.

Sherer, M., & Adams, C. H. (1983). Construct validation of the Self-efficacy Scale. *Psychological Reports, 53,* 899–902.

Sherer, M., Maddux, J. E., Mercandante, B., Prentice-Dunn, S., Jacobs, B., & Rogers, R. W. (1982). The Self-efficacy Scale: Construction and validation. *Psychological Reports, 51,* 663–671.

Simkin, P. (1991). Just another day in a woman's life? Women's long-term perceptions of their first birth experience: Part I. *Birth, 18,* 203–210.

Tarkka, M. T. (2003). Predictors of maternal competence by first-time mothers when the child is 8 months old. *Journal of Advanced Nursing, 41,* 233–240.

Teti, D. M., & Candelaria, M. A. (2002). Parenting competence. In M. H. Bornstein (Ed.), *Handbook of parenting* (2nd ed., pp. 149–180). Mahwah, NJ: Lawrence Erlbaum Associates.

Teti, D. M., & Gelfand, D. M. (1991). Behavioral competence among mothers of infants in the first year: The mediational role of maternal self-efficacy. *Child Development, 62*(5), 918–929.

Teti, D. M., O'Connell, M. A., & Reiner, C. D. (1996). Parenting sensitivity, parental depression and child health: The mediational role of parental self-efficacy. *Early Development and Parenting, 5,* 237–250.

Tucker, S., & Gross, D. (1997). Behavioral parent training: An intervention strategy for guiding parents of young children. *Journal of Perinatal Education, 6,* 35–44.

Woodruff, S. L., & Cashman, J. F. (1993). Task, domain, and general efficacy: A reexamination of the Self-efficacy Scale. *Psychological Reports, 72,* 423–432.

Janet Bryanton, PhD, MN, RN, is Associate Professor, School of Nursing, University of Prince Edward Island, Charlottetown, Canada.

Anita J. Gagnon, PhD, MPH, RN, is Associate Professor, School of Nursing, McGill University, Montreal, Quebec, Canada.

Marie Hatem, PhD, MHSA, RN, is Assistant Professor, Faculty of Medicine, University of Montreal, Quebec, Canada.

Celeste Johnston, DEd, MS, RN, is Professor, School of Nursing, McGill University, Montreal, Quebec, Canada.

Accepted for publication February 2, 2008.

Thank you for the funding received for this study to the Canadian Nurses Foundation Nursing Care Partnership Program, Groupe de recherche interuniversitaire en soins infirmiers de Montréal (GRISIM), Isaac Walton Killam Health Centre, University of Prince Edward Island, Children's Health & Applied Research Team, and University of Prince Edward Island School of Nursing. Le Fonds de la recherche en santé du Québec (FRSQ) provided career support to Anita J. Gagnon during the time of this study.

Corresponding author: Janet Bryanton, PhD, MN, RN, School of Nursing, University of Prince Edward Island, 550 University Ave., Charlottetown, Prince Edward Island, Canada CIA 4P3 (e-mail: jbryanton@upei.ca).

APPENDIX B.

Living in a World of Our Own: The Experience of Parents Who Have a Child With Autism

Roberta L. Woodgate
Christine Ateah
Loretta Secco

In this article, we discuss findings of a hermeneutic phenomenological study that sought to describe the experiences of parents who have a child with autism. Qualitative interviews were conducted with parents from 16 families of children with autism residing in a western Canadian province. "Living in a world of our own" emerged as the essence of the parents' experiences. In "living in a world of our own," parents described a world of isolation. Three themes representing the essential challenging elements of the parents' experiences included vigilant parenting, sustaining the self and family, and fighting all the way. Although much is known about the fundamental importance of support to parents of children with chronic conditions and/or disabilities, findings from this study indicate that knowledge has not been adequately transferred to the care of children with autism.

Keywords: autism • children • families, caregiving • parenting • phenomenology

Autism is a complex developmental disorder characterized by a triad of impairments in reciprocal social interaction; communication; and restricted, repetitive, and stereotypic patterns of behaviors, interests, and activities (Committee on Children With Disabilities, 2001). Compared to other developmental deviations such as developmental intellectual impairment, autism manifests itself not in developmental delays but rather in striking deviations in development (Beauchesne & Kelley, 2004). Although the onset of symptoms for most children with autism occurs during late infancy, some children may not display any symptoms until 2 years of age after a period of relatively typical development (Committee on Children With Disabilities, 2001).

Understandably, few disorders can pose a greater threat to the well-being of families than autism (Seltzer, Krauss, Orsmond, & Vestal, 2001). Parents of children with autism are faced with many challenges. Adding to the challenges experienced by parents is that in spite of an early onset, autism often remains undiagnosed until or after late preschool years (Beauchesne & Kelley, 2004). Equally challenging is the intense treatment that requires a combination of strategies (Committee on Children With Disabilities, 2001). Although there is no proven cure for autism, the goal of treatment is to improve the overall functional status of the child by promoting the development of communication, social, adaptive,

Reprinted with permission from *Qualitative Health Research* (2008; 18[8]: 1075–1083).

behavioral, and academic skills as well as lessening maladaptive and repetitive behaviors (Committee on Children With Disabilities, 2001).

In achieving treatment goals, there is growing evidence that treatment should be started before the age of 5. One of the primary components of treatment involves intensive behavioral training based on the applied behavioral analysis (ABA) approach. The aim of training is to reinforce desirable behaviors and decrease undesirable behaviors (Committee on Children With Disabilities, 2001; Pelios & Lund, 2001). Undertaking ABA programming is highly detailed and structured, requiring up to 40 hours per week of one-to-one behavioral training. Despite the professional expertise and guidance provided to parents, a great deal of parental input and commitment is required. In fact, parents have been described as "co-therapists" (Pakenham, Samios, & Sofronoff, 2005). Increasingly, parental and professional (therapeutic and educational) collaboration is being deemed essential, especially in countries (Canada, United States) that are integrating children with autism into regular (full- and part-time) school classes (Bryson, Rogers, & Fombonne, 2003; Committee on Children With Disabilities, 2001).

Research directed at understanding what it is like to be a parent of a child with autism is in its early stages. Primarily, the existing research explores the degree of stress and level of functioning in parents in relation to a variety of factors including coping behaviors (e.g., Hastings et al., 2005; Higgins, Bailey, & Pearce, 2005; Sivberg, 2002), depression (e.g., Dale, Jahoda, & Knott, 2006), and personality and demographic factors (e.g., Duarte, Bordin, Yazigi, & Mooney, 2005). Although this work points to parents experiencing increased stress and the potential for adjustment problems, it is not considered within the context of the family's evolving life experience of children with autism (King et al., 2006). King and colleagues (2006) reinforced that the research tends to adopt a narrow perspective of the child with autism where the child is viewed as a "stressor" testing parents' ability to cope and negatively influencing their psychological well-being.

Although minimal, there is research that seeks to understand the meanings parents assign to having a child with autism. This includes work by Gray who through an ongoing study produced a series of articles about the social experiences of Australian parents of children with autism. Gray focused on describing how parents experienced "normal family life" (1997) and stigma (1993, 2002). "Normal family life" for these parents was not associated with the outward signs of domesticity (e.g., owning a house or holding a job) but was instead linked to factors such as their ability to socialize, the emotional quality of their interactions among family members, and the routines and rituals that comprised their perceptions of what "normal" families do (Gray, 1997). Although most parents with a child with autism felt stigmatized, parents of aggressive children were more likely to experience stigma more acutely than parents of passive children (Gray, 1993, 2002). As a consequence, many parents isolated themselves and their families from social contacts, finding communal encounters burdensome because of the combination of their child's disruptive, antisocial behaviors coupled with a normal appearance (Gray, 1993).

Findings from another Australian study revealed that the lived experience of parenting a child with autism is best characterized as a shrinking nature of the parent's self (less spontaneity, social contact, and having fewer things), where parents felt pulled into a vortex of a restricted and repetitive way of being-in-the-world (Cashin, 2004). On the other hand, King et al. (2006) found through qualitative inquiry that the belief systems of families of children with autism or Down's syndrome changed. Specifically, shifting familial beliefs reinforced that raising a child with a disability can be a life-changing experience that spurs families to examine their belief systems (King et al., 2006). Seemingly a burdensome experience, some parents of children with autism experience positive adaptations in the form of changed worldviews concerning life and disability with the recognition of positive contributions made by their child to themselves, their family, and to society in general.

Despite this increasing understanding of what it is like to be a parent of a child with autism, more research needs to be undertaken that strives to understand, make sense of, and elicit the meaning of childhood autism from the perspectives of parents. The overall purpose of this study was to describe the lived experience of parents who have a child with autism.

METHOD

Design

The methodology of hermeneutic phenomenology, as described by van Manen (1990), was used to address the study's purpose. Hermeneutic phenomenology seeks to "uncover the structure, the internal meaning structures, of lived experience" (van Manen, 1990, p. 10). Foundationally, hermeneutic phenomenology explores the individual's context to capture the essence or the underlying meaning of lived experiences as they are brought to light through the experiences of individuals. The experience needs to be described as well as interpreted to fully understand the meaning of the lived experience.

Setting and Participants

The study was conducted in a city in a province of western Canada. The only legitimate informants in phenomenological research are those who have lived the reality (Baker, Wuest, & Todd, 1992). Therefore, recruitment strategies were directed at selecting individuals who had lived the experience of being a parent of a child with autism. Participants were recruited through a support group whose purpose is advocacy, support, and the facilitation of accessibility to effective treatment.

Twenty-one parents from 16 families of children with autism participated. Sixteen of the 21 parents were mothers, and 5 were fathers, with a total of five couples participating in the study. The parents ranged in age from early 30s to late 40s. Nineteen parents were Caucasian, and 2 were Asian. All parents were married except for one mother who was separated at the time of the interview. Except for 2 parents, all parents had at least one other child in addition to their child with autism.

The children with autism ranged in age from 3 to 9 years, with the children's age of initial diagnosis ranging from 2.5 to 3.5 years. The children with autism were all boys except for one child, which supports current incidence of autism being four times more common in boys than girls (Committee on Children With Disabilities, 2001). The children, as described by the parents, varied in the severity with respect to the degree of impairment in communication, social relations, and repetitive and stereotyped behavior. All the children except for two were involved in ABA training (the number of years and hours per day devoted to the training, structure, and content varied for each child). During the time of the study, funding for families had just been made available from the government to support preschool children in the ABA program. However, only six families qualified for the funding. For the other families, the children were too old or already enrolled in the ABA program with cost incurred by the parents. Additional treatment services for the children included speech therapy, occupational therapy, physical therapy, psychiatric services, respite services, and a child care or teacher's assistant. Funds for these services were also provided by the government but only if parents accessed them through the public health care system. The extent of treatment that the children received was dependent both on what services were available to them and what parents could afford. Parents often sought out private treatment services because of the unavailability of services in the publically funded health care system.

Data Collection

Data collection took place over a 16-month period. All parents participated in audiotaped, open-ended, in-depth qualitative interviews conducted by the first author. Parents were given the option to be interviewed either individually or with their spouse. The open-ended interview method helped to elicit detailed responses deemed significant to the study's purpose (Morse & Field, 1995) but also afforded parents the opportunity to use their own words and talk about what really mattered to them. A minimal number of broad, data-generating questions were asked as recommended in phenomenology (Munhall, 1994; Streubert & Carpenter, 1999; van Manen, 1990). For this study, parents were asked to describe what life was like for them before, during, and after their child was diagnosed with autism. Open-ended probes ("Tell me what happened next?" or "How did that make you feel?") were used as necessary to facilitate parents' telling their stories. In asking the questions, care was taken not to introduce concepts that would have biased parents' responses. Field notes describing the interview context were made. Parents also completed a brief demographic form prior to being interviewed.

Five joint interviews (i.e., involving both parents) and 14 individual interviews were conducted for a total of 19 interviews. The individual interviews all involved mothers, with three of the mothers requiring a second interview. Interview sessions for all parents lasted from 1.5 to 3 hours.

Data Analysis

Data analysis was concurrent with data collection. All interviews and field notes were transcribed using the Microsoft Word word processing program. The transcripts were reviewed repeatedly for significant statements in an attempt to find meaning and understanding through themes. Thematic statements were isolated using van Manen's (1990) selective highlighting approach. In this approach, the search for themes or structures of the experience involved selecting and highlighting sentences or sentence clusters that stood out as thematic of the experience. Notes were made to capture the thematic statements. All phrases, sentence clusters, notes, and textual data were then reduced until essential themes emerged. Essential themes are unique to the phenomenon of parents who have a child with autism and are fundamental to the overall shared description of living the experience. Critical to interpretation was a movement from an understanding of the whole text to more specific parts within the text and then back again to the whole (Benner, 1985). In an effort to be as true to the meanings as possible, descriptions were written and rewritten to include the meaningful themes and to ensure that they were presented as disclosed (van Manen, 1990). Saturation occurred when there was ongoing replication of data concerning the emerging essential thematic elements of the phenomenon under study. Measures to enhance the methodological rigor of the research process were undertaken to include prolonged engagement with participants and data, careful line-by-line analysis of the transcripts, and detailed memo writing (Lincoln & Guba, 1985). Preliminary interpretations were also discussed with participants during and following each interview, which helped to uncover and lend support for the emerging essential themes.

Ethical Issues

Ethical standards were maintained throughout the course of the project by careful attention to issues of recruitment, written consent, confidentiality, anonymity, potential vulnerability, and sensitivity. Ethical approval from a university-based ethical review committee was sought and obtained. The one transcriptionist hired for the project signed a confidentiality agreement.

FINDINGS

This section describes the essence, themes, and subthemes that emerged from the analysis of the experiences of parents who have a child with autism.

The Essence of the Parents' Experiences: Living in a World of Our Own

The essence, "living in a world of our own," ultimately defined what it was like to be a parent with a child with autism. Just as parents described children with autism as "being in their own world," so too did parents experience similar feelings. Parents basically felt that they were now having to "go it alone" in all aspects of their daily lives but especially with respect to dealing with the challenges of parenting and caring for a child. In "living in a world of our own," parents described a world that left them at times feeling isolated. Parents' sense of isolation is described as arising from four main sources.

Society's Lack of Understanding Parents expressed feeling isolated because of what they perceived was a lack of understanding by society of what autism was and what was involved in caring for a child with autism. Despite the challenging nature of autism, parents felt that their suffering was not recognized by others around them but instead was invisible. Parents felt that society placed less value on the lives of the children with autism and felt stigmatized, thereby adding to the feelings of isolation:

> The school is stigmatizing my son. The resource person said I should not expect other kids in Grade 1 to buddy with him. They are saying, "Why would another kid want to play with your kid?"

Missing a "Normal" Way of Life Parents expressed feeling isolated from a "normal" way of life. Many aspects of the parents' life were affected by their child's autism because of the intensive care that their child with autism required. One parent reinforced the impact autism had on his life by stating, "We have no life, we only have a program [referring to the ABA program]!"

Feeling Disconnected From the Family Although parents reinforced that they garnered their major source of support and strength from their family, parents were not immune from experiencing isolation within the family. Most notably was the sense of isolation parents experienced in not always feeling like they were a part of the world that their child with autism lived in. They first experienced this isolation when their child's behavior started to change and during those times when they tried to connect to their child only to have the child resist the parent's getting close to them. Parents on occasion also felt disconnected from their spouses when both experienced different feelings that resulted in their not "always being on the same wavelength" or stage of the autism trajectory. Parents also experienced feeling isolated from those extended family members who seemed to lack an essential understanding of what they were going through and/or failed to be present to provide practical support and assistance.

The Unsupportive "System" The most concerning factor contributing to parents' sense of isolation was the "system." The "system" was defined by parents as a conglomerate of all child-related agencies and institutions (e.g., health care facilities, educational settings) existing to protect and advance the development of the child with autism. Parents described a system that was inaccessible in many ways. The inaccessible system is manifested by having to deal with unsupportive professionals in the system who appeared to lack training in, and knowledge of, autism, along with limited, inadequate, and inappropriate resources deemed necessary in providing support to raising a child with autism. "There are not enough people, there is not enough funding, and so on" were words consistently voiced by parents.

Parents also had experiences of the "system" itself isolating them from their child:

> Maybe my husband would not like me using this word, but really the total brutality of how parents are treated. You are really made to feel like an outsider in your child's life.

Overall, the product of the sense of isolation left parents with a diminished sense of hope.

Parents expressed feeling completely defeated and on their own when they felt that family members, friends, professionals within the system, and others in their lives were not there to support their sense of hope that things would get better for their child.

Themes Supporting the Essence

Three themes supported the essence: (a) vigilant parenting, (b) sustaining the self and family, and (c) fighting all the way. These themes speak to how parents struggled and fought to remove the isolation that they and their children experienced.

Theme 1: Vigilant Parenting

To be able to protect their child with autism from a world that was not always there to support them, parents became superparents completely focused on every aspect of their child's world.

Parents described having to develop sense of heightened watchfulness and preparation for action or, as one parent referred to it, "mental monitoring." The intensive nature of parenting is exemplified by the following:

> Well, it is almost like a home with an alcoholic. You walk around on eggshells because you do not want to possibly upset them in anyway. It is just that you are walking on eggshells 24 hours a day. You are continually trying to teach a child who does not want to learn. During the bad parts it was, we were just drowning in autism.

Although it was not uncommon for the mothers to assume the primary responsibility of the direct treatment for their child, fathers were also involved in some aspect of the direct care in addition to assuming traditional responsibilities. Parents viewed parenting as a team effort and, when sharing their thoughts on parenting during the interviews, often responded in the voice of "we" as opposed to "I." They recognized the importance of standing by and supporting each other even during those times when they had differing perspectives.

In becoming "vigilant," parents adopted three strategies that helped them to protect their children: (a) acting sooner rather than later, (b) doing all you can, and (c) staying close to your gut feelings.

Acting Sooner Rather Than Later This strategy referred to parents' keeping abreast of all aspects of their child's care. Parents described always having to anticipate the next course of action to ensure that their child received the most appropriate and timely treatment. It was important, as one parent expressed, "not to let the window of opportunity pass them by." Parents shared many stories of the great lengths that they went to in order to get the help for their child in a timely fashion:

> They said it would be 6 months to a year to get into speech therapy. And I said, "That is not acceptable." I said, "Get us in as soon as possible, and what is your earliest you can get us in?" And he told me that they occasionally phone parents if

someone is sick or does not show up for an appointment. I said, "Okay, you give me a 30-minute notice, 5-minute notice, I will be there." And we got in, in 3 weeks.

Doing All You Can This strategy referred to parents trying anything and everything to help their child develop to his or her full potential, whatever that potential might be. It was important, as one mother reinforced, "to adopt a try-anything-that-works attitude." "Doing all you can" involved a range of activities for parents from seeking out specialized services for their child, to changing their home environment to enhance the safety and comfort features for their child.

Associated with the do-all-that-you-can approach was the belief that their child had the ability to learn and grow. Parents needed to be committed to advancing their child's potential. Parents also needed to be both flexible and reasonable when considering multiple options and acknowledged that professionals who were also flexible and willing to consider new solutions helped parents to be able to do all that is possible for their child.

Staying Close to Your Gut Feelings This strategy referred to parents' acknowledging and acting on the innermost feelings that they held about their child with autism. Parents reinforced that it was important to trust their "gut feelings" and to persevere in doing what they thought was the best thing for their child and not to be concerned about what others think. The "gut feelings" served as a special source of information for parents that helped them to make decisions about their child's care.

Theme 2: Sustaining the Self and Family

Just as important as it was for parents to protect the child with autism, so too was protecting their own sense of self as well as the family's sense of self. The challenges posed by autism placed parents on guard to the possibility of permanently losing pieces of their self and their family. Parents felt it was important not to let autism get the better of them or their family, or else this would only lead to further isolation. Sustaining the self and family was important to parents in and of itself, but also because parents viewed that a strong sense of self and family would enhance protective measures for the child with autism:

> Everything changes when you find out your child has autism, and you know that you have to be and do this for your children, absolutely that comes first. But you also have to put your own self in perspective because if you are not up to par, then you are not going to help him anyway.

In keeping things together as a person and a family, parents reinforced it was important to (a) work toward a healthy balance, (b) cherish different milestones, and (c) learn to let go.

Working Toward a Healthy Balance "Working toward a healthy balance" referred to parents' recognition of the importance of having a life that is not solely focused on helping their child with autism develop to his or her full potential. Parents needed to create a balance between their focus on parenting a child with autism and all the other aspects in life if they hoped to arrive at a healthy sense of well-being for themselves and their family. In striving for a healthy balance, it was important for parents to step back and acknowledge that they and their children without autism had needs of their own that needed to be met. Although the child with autism required additional parental attention, parents spoke of the need to take time away from all the work that went into parenting a child with autism.

In working toward a healthy balance, parents stressed that it was important to set priorities and concentrate on issues defined as important. As one father noted, it was important "not to sweat the small stuff anymore."

Cherishing Different Milestones In sustaining the self and family, parents expressed the importance of accepting that their child with autism would experience milestones in his or her development differently compared with other same-aged, normally developing children. Despite the differences, parents stressed that these milestones were just as important as the "normal" milestones and that each milestone needed to be celebrated. Cherishing different milestones helped to preserve parents' sense of hope. One mother, in reference to the loss of her son's normal development, expressed,

> I was grieving the loss of my son and looking at this new challenge. I was going to have to deal with this for the rest of my life, and I had no hope, and it is only with minor little accomplishments that my son with autism made that I was able to regain the hope bit by bit.

The minor accomplishments often came about from parent and child working on some aspect of the child's therapy in which a connection was made between the two.

Learning to Let Go "Learning to let go" referred to the parents acknowledging that there were certain situations associated with their child's autism that they could not always change and that in those situations it was important to step back and let things transpire as they naturally would. It was important to recognize that as a parent, one cannot be responsible for everything and to avoid the "what ifs":

> But also we had to realize one of the last two years that our son cannot go past his potential. We ran his program as best as we could, we made sure he had the right staff and supplies, and maybe we did not spend as much time on some things, but we cannot change the past. We did as best as we could. We had to learn to let go.

Theme 3: Fighting All the Way

"Fighting all the away" referred to how parents fought to make the system work for them and their child.

Parents fought to improve the system not only for their own child with autism but for all families who have a child with autism. Parents' altruistic motives were sharpened by their need to prevent other families from experiencing a similar fate of intrusive feelings of isolation. Parents realized that for their voices to be heard, they needed to function as advocates:

> We do not have the strength in numbers, so what we have to do is we have to stay in there advocating for all special needs kids and in our case particularly those with autism. We cannot let the system rip them off.

Parents stressed that in fighting to make the system work, they needed to (a) become more direct, (b) learn all they could, and (c) educate others.

Becoming More Direct To fight all the battles, parents had to change their behavior. Specifically, parents had to precipitously pull themselves together emotionally (to prevent controversy and confrontations) and become more direct in how and what they asked for in relation to support and treatment options for their child with autism:

> I have become more and more straightforward to the point that, I think they are all afraid of me. But it is not my nature, like to be really challenging. I see myself as kind of a shy person, a soft-spoken person.

Learning All You Can Ensuring the effective functioning of the system, parents stressed the importance of learning about every dimension of raising a child with autism. Especially useful sources of information included conversations with other parents of children with autism about a range of issues such as learning how to navigate the system. Another important source was what parents learned from the interactions they had with professionals who were involved in the care of their child. With each professional–parent encounter, parents learned more about how best to respond to the professional so that the professional would listen to them.

However, the most important source of learning was the knowledge they gleaned directly from their child with autism. Parents consistently indicated that they had learned so much from their child, which helped them to become more discerning, understanding, and patient. The intense nature of caring for a child with autism heightened their sensitivity to the behaviors of others and helped them become expert teachers.

Educating Others In making the system work, parents found it was important to educate others about the importance of respecting the child with autism and his or her parents. Parents fought to ensure that friends, professionals, and society in general knew about the unique characteristics of and contributions made to the world by children with autism.

Parents wanted others to realize that parents of children with autism try their best in raising their child and as such should not be judged or blamed for their child's behavior. Parents expressed that professionals needed to be more receptive to both the child and the parent and, more important, advocate with the parent in ensuring that the needs of children with autism are met.

DISCUSSION AND CONCLUSION

The ultimate aim of our study was to gain a better understanding of the lived experience of parents who have a child with autism. In order not to delimit the parents' account of their experiences, we avoided using the word *parenting* in the description of the overall purpose. In doing so, parents shared with us not only aspects of their parenting role but also other aspects of their lives that were central to the autism experience. Findings in our study revealed both similarities to and differences from previous research conducted in the area.

For the Canadian parents in our study, having a child with autism not only affected their parenting role but more to the point defined how they lived in their world. The parents experienced feelings of being in their own world and going it alone to the point that it became the essence of their experience. Gray (1993, 1997) also found a sense of isolation to be a dominant condition in the lives of Australian parents who had a child with autism. However, what was unique in our study was that from the perspectives of the parents, their sense of isolation was found to be mainly the result of external sources (e.g., society's lack of understanding). In contrast, the isolation reported by Gray was more self-imposed in that parents tended to isolate themselves from social contact with the outside world because of the awkward encounters with outsiders.

Another difference noted between our study and Gray's work was how parents dealt with their isolation. Gray (1994) found that parents coped by using a variety of strategies, most notably the use of service agencies (e.g., treatment services, respite services), family support, and social withdrawal. In contrast, parents in our study received a lot of support by valuing any accomplishment that their child achieved. Parents in our study also coped by trying to make changes within the system. They were dissatisfied with the system and fought for their voices to be heard. One possible explanation for the different findings could be that parents in our study were recruited from a support group of families of children with autism, whereas in Gray's work parents were recruited from a treatment center. The parents in our study, although feeling isolated from many external sources, nonetheless had the support from other families of children with autism and might have been encouraged to be advocates for their child.

Similar to the Australian parents in Cashin's (2004) study, parents in our study also experienced a different way of life because of their child's autism. In both studies, the different way of life usually meant having to give up things associated with a "normal" life as well as experiencing changes to their sense of self. However, whereas parents in Cashin's study experienced it as a loss of self to autism, parents in our studied experienced it as a struggle to preserve their sense of self. The parents in our study recognized the potential for a loss of self and family and identified numerous strategies to preserve the self and family. Similar to the families in Gray's (1997) study, parents achieved a sense of normalcy by focusing their energies on maintaining some type of routine family life.

Our study also lends support to the work done by others in the field of parenting experiences of families of children with varying chronic health conditions (Ray, 2002; Rempel & Harrison, 2007). Most notable is the need for parents to develop an increased sense of parenting that is intense in both quality and quantity of behaviors. The fear of "letting the window of opportunity pass them by" combined with an "unsupportive system" where expert professionals lacked knowledge and expertise in dealing with the needs of families greatly contributed to the parents in our study becoming "vigilant." "Vigilant parenting" is similar to Ray's (2002) "parenting plus" and Rempel and Harrison's (2007) "extraordinary parenting." Although these two studies involved parents of children with a variety of chronic conditions (excluding children who had behavioral or developmental disabilities alone), the parents in these studies, similar to our parents, worked hard and did whatever they could to ensure their child's survival and optimal development. In addition, they tried to balance their intense parenting with the need to sustain the self and the family while at the same time deal with "system" problems (Ray, 2002). Recognizing that parents of children with chronic conditions and disabilities experience similar experiences and struggles lends reinforcement for applying similar standards of care specific to how best to support parents regardless of the idiosyncratic nature of the child's condition.

LIMITATIONS AND RECOMMENDATIONS

As in all studies, this research was not without limitations. The cross-sectional nature of the study's design precluded understanding how the perspectives of parents change over time. Other limitations include a sample that lacked cultural diversity and that was mainly composed of mothers. We also recognize that parents in our study worked together in protecting their child with autism and as such, the findings may not reflect the experiences of single parents who lack the support of the other parent in parenting their child with autism. Future work addressing these limitations may result in additional stories of parents of children with autism. Despite the limitations, our findings help to confirm what it is like to be a parent of a child with a chronic condition such as autism, which might help professionals to provide more comprehensive and sensitive care. This study is important in light of the growing number of children diagnosed with autism (Committee on Children With Disabilities, 2001). The meanings parents assigned to their experiences could be used to inform future policy and program development.

Although there has been a dramatially increased understanding within the past two decades of the etiology, diagnosis, and management of autism (Committee on Children With Disabilities, 2001), this study reinforces that there are still gaps between what is done in model autism programs across Canada and the United States and what is generally available for most young children (Bryson et al., 2003; Committee on Children With Disabilities, 2001). A seamless system that will help to foster more enduring relationships between parents and all professionals involved in the care of children with autism should be fostered (Sperry, Whaley, Shaw, & Brame, 1999). Professionals, family, friends, and others in the system who lack an understanding of the impact that autism has on children and parents need to be educated. Professionals caring for families of children with autism should be made cognizant of the concerns and meanings parents assign to their experiences. Sperry and colleagues (1999) also recommended that professionals assist parents in their role of advocator by familiarizing parents with their rights and by helping them to negotiate the service delivery system. Future work may be directed to doing intervention studies that involve the "expert" parent's teaching the professional how to respond to parents of children with chronic conditions and/or disabilities. Given the expertise of parents of children with autism, parents could become invaluable assets in helping professionals understand human relationships and responses.

REFERENCES

Baker, C., Wuest, J., & Todd, A. (1992). Method slurring: The grounded theory/phenomenology example. *Journal of Advanced Nursing, 17*(11), 1355–1360.

Beauchesne, M., & Kelley, B. (2004). Evidence to support parental concerns as an early indicator of autism in children. *Pediatric Nursing, 30*(1), 57–67.

Benner, P. (1985). Quality of life: A phenomenological perspective on explanation, prediction, and understanding in nursing science. *Advances in Nursing Science, 8*(1), 1–14.

Bryson, S., Rogers, S., & Fombonne, E. (2003). Autism spectrum disorders: Early detection, intervention, education and psychopharmacological management. *Canadian Journal of Psychiatry, 48*(8), 506–516.

Cashin, A. (2004). Painting the vortex: The existential structure of the experience of parenting a child with autism. *International Forum of Psychoanalysis, 13*, 164–174.

Committee on Children With Disabilities. (2001). Technical report: The pediatrician's role in the diagnosis and management of autistic spectrum disorder in children. *Pediatrics, 107*(5), e85, 1–18.

Dale, E., Jahoda, A., & Knott, F. (2006). Mother's attributions following their child's diagnosis of autistic spectrum disorder. *Autism, 10*(5), 463–479.

Duarte, R., Bordin, I., Yazigi, L., & Mooney, J. (2005). Factors associated with stress in mothers of children with autism. *Autism, 9*(4), 416–427.

Gray, D. (1993). Perceptions of stigma: The parents of autistic children. *Sociology of Health and Illness, 15*(1), 102–120.

Gray, D. (1994). Coping with autism: Stress and strategies. *Sociology of Health and Illness, 16*(3), 275–300.

Gray, D. (1997). High functioning autistic children and the construction of "normal family life." *Social Science and Medicine, 44*(8), 1097–1106.

Gray, D. (2002). "Everybody just freezes. Everybody is just embarrassed": Felt and enacted stigma among parents of children with high functioning autism. *Sociology of Health and Illness, 24*(6), 734–749.

Hastings, R., Kovshoff, H., Brown, T., Ward, N., Espinosa, F., & Remington, B. (2005). Coping strategies in mothers and fathers of preschool and school-age children with autism. *Autism, 9*(4), 377–391.

Higgins, D., Bailey, S., & Pearce, J. (2005). Factors associated with functioning style and coping strategies of families with a child with an autism spectrum disorder. *Autism, 9*(2), 125–137.

King, G., Zwaigenbaum, L., King, S., Baxter, D., Rosenbaum, P., & Bates, A. (2006). A qualitative investigation of changes in belief systems of families of children with autism or Down syndrome. *Child: Care, Health & Development, 32*(3), 353–369.

Lincoln, Y., & Guba, E. (1985). *Naturalistic inquiry.* Thousand Oaks, CA: Sage.

Morse, J., & Field, P. (1995). *Qualitative research methods for health professionals* (2nd ed.). Thousand Oaks, CA: Sage.

Munhall, P. L. (1994). *Revisioning phenomenology: Nursing and health science research.* New York: National League for Nursing Press.

Pakenham, K., Samios, C., & Sofronoff, K. (2005). Adjustment in mothers of children with Asperger syndrome. *Autism, 9*(2), 191–212.

Pelios, L., & Lund, E. (2001). A selective overview of issues on classification, causation, and early intensive behavioral intervention for autism. *Behavior Modification, 25*(5), 678–697.

Ray, L. (2002). Parenting and childhood chronicity: Making visible the invisible work. *Journal of Pediatric Nursing, 17*(6), 424–438.

Rempel, G., & Harrison, M. (2007). Safeguarding precarious survival: Parenting children who have life-threatening heart disease. *Qualitative Health Research, 17*, 824–837.

Seltzer, M., Krauss, M., Orsmond, G., & Vestal, C. (2001). Families of adolescents and adults with autism: Uncharted territory. *International Review of Research in Mental Retardation, 23*, 267–294.

Sivberg, B. (2002). Family system and coping behaviors: A comparison between parents of children with autistic spectrum disorders and parents with non-autistic children. *Autism, 6*(4), 397–409.

Sperry, L., Whaley, K., Shaw, E., & Brame, K. (1999). Services for young children with autism spectrum disorder: Voices of parents and providers. *Infants and Young Children, 11*(4), 17–33.

Streubert, H. J., & Carpenter, D. R. (1999). *Qualitative research in nursing: Advancing the humanistic imperative* (2nd ed.). Philadelphia: J. B. Lippincott.

van Manen, M. (1990). *Researching lived experience: Human science for an action sensitive pedagogy.* London, Canada: Althouse.

Roberta L. Woodgate, RN, MN, PhD, is an associate professor at the Faculty of Nursing, University of Manitoba, Winnipeg, Manitoba, Canada.

Christine Ateah, RN, PhD, is an associate professor and associate dean, Undergraduate Programs, at the Faculty of Nursing, University of Manitoba, Winnipeg, Manitoba, Canada.

Loretta Secco, RN, MN, PhD, is an associate professor at the Cape Breton University, Nursing Department, Cape Breton University, Sydney, Nova Scotia, Canada.

Authors' Note: *This research was funded by a Sister Bertha Baumann Research Award from St. Amant Centre in Winnipeg, Manitoba, Canada. Dr. Woodgate is supported by a Dorothy J. Lamont Scientist Award, funded by the National Cancer Institute of Canada and the Canadian Institutes of Health Research's (CIHR) Institute of Cancer Research. We would like to thank the families who participated in this study.*

APPENDIX C.
(Continence Care)

Do Catheter Washouts Extend Patency Time in Long-term Indwelling Urethral Catheters?: A Randomized Controlled Trial of Acidic Washout Solution, Normal Saline Washout, or Standard Care

Katherine N. Moore

Kathleen F. Hunter

Rosemary McGinnis

Chasta Bacsu

Mandy Fader

Mikel Gray

Kathy Getliffe

Janice Chobanuk

Lakshmi Puttagunta

Donald C. Voaklander

➢ **Purpose:** Blockage of long-term indwelling catheters with mineral deposit is an ongoing management issue, but evidence on optimal management is lacking. Our purpose was to examine whether catheter washouts prevent or reduce catheter blockage.

➢ **Design:** A multisite randomized controlled trial.

➢ **Subjects and Setting:** Adults with long-term indwelling catheters that required changing every 3 weeks or less, living in the community, and requiring supportive or continuing care were recruited. Participants were randomly assigned to 1 of 3 groups: control (usual care, no washout), saline washout, or commercially available acidic washout solution (Contisol Maelor Pharmaceuticals Ltd, Wrexham, UK).

➢ **Methods:** At baseline visit, the catheter was changed and participants were followed weekly for 8 weeks, with checks for catheter patency and urine pH. Participants randomized to saline or commercial solution had a weekly washout with the appropriate solution. Endpoints were 8 weeks (completion data), 3 or more catheter changes in the 8-week period, or symptomatic urinary tract infection (UTI) requiring antibiotics. The study hypothesis was that catheter life would be extended by 25% in the commercial solution group. It was not possible to blind participants or research nurses to washout versus no intervention, but participants in the saline and washout solution groups were blinded to solution type.

Reprinted with permission from *Journal of Wound Ostomy Continence Nursing* (2009; 36[1]: 82–90).

➢ **Results:** One hundred twelve potential participants were screened; 73 were enrolled, randomized, and included in the final analysis. Of these, 53 completed the full 8 weeks of data collection; 16 terminated early because of 3 catheter changes or self-reported 'UTI'. Other reasons for termination were hematuria, latex sensitivity, deceased/severe illness, or personal choice. Analysis of variance was used to analyze mean differences on demographic variables and mean number of weeks in study. Kaplan-Meier survival curve analysis showed no statistical difference between the groups in time to first catheter change.

➢ **Conclusion:** At this time, the evidence is insufficient to state whether catheter washout with saline or Contisol is more effective than usual care with no washout in preventing blocking. No increased risk of UTI was associated with washout regimes.

INTRODUCTION

Indications for the use of a long-term (>30 days) indwelling catheter are urinary retention or urinary incontinence that cannot be managed by alternative means, management of selected patients receiving palliative or end-of-life care, and prevention of wound contamination (by urine) in patients with pressure ulcers.[1,2] Common complications associated with long-term use of an indwelling catheter include bypassing (leakage around the catheter), irritation of the urethra and bladder neck, urethral erosion or injury, urinary calculi, and potential increased risk of bladder cancer.[3] The most prevalent complications are bacteriuria, urinary tract infection (UTI), and blockage by sediment or crystals.[4,5] Bacterial biofilm colonization increases the risk for catheter encrustation and subsequent blockage, a complication particularly common among people with long-term catheterization. Figure 1 illustrates marked biofilm buildup around a hair nidus at the tip of the indwelling catheter.

Routine catheter washouts with a catheter washout solution are often recommended by nurses and physicians to prevent or reduce blockage events. In Canada, one strategy used by homecare nurses is saline catheter washouts; in the United Kingdom (Contisol), another widely available commercial catheter washout solution (citric acid 3.23%, light magnesium oxide 0.38%, sodium bicarbonate 0.7%, and disodium edetate 0.01%) is frequently used. However, little research exists evaluating washouts, and current evidence is insufficient to determine the clinical effectiveness despite relatively widespread usage.[6]

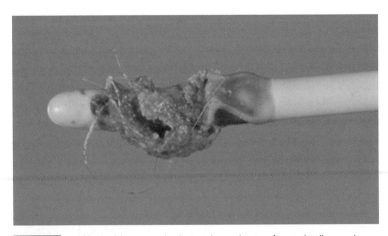

FIGURE 1   Biofilm buildup around a hair nidus at the tip of an indwelling catheter.

Pathogenesis of Bacterial Colonization and Encrustation

When an indwelling catheter is inserted, a biofilm is rapidly formed. Bacteria present in the urine in planktonic form (free living) adhere to and colonize the catheter surface. The biofilm becomes strongly adherent to the catheter surface because the bacteria synthesize a slimy, glue-like substance, called glycocalyx. As a result, bacteria become attached to the biofilm and convert to a sessile form of life.[7-9] When urease-producing bacteria, particularly *Proteus mirabilis*, *Proteus vulgaris*, and *Providencia rettgeri*, are present, urinary pH rises, as ammonia is released from urinary urea due to bacterial enzymic activity. Catheter encrustation occurs when struvite (magnesium ammonium phosphate) crystals and amorphous calcium phosphate deposits precipitate and agglomerate onto the surface catheter and its biofilm.[9-11] Encrustation reaches clinical significance when it obstructs urine outflow through the catheter.

Few studies have examined the prevalence of encrustation in persons with long-term indwelling catheters, but Kunin and associates[12] reported that 40% of a group of 50 participants experienced encrustation with or without subsequent blockage when an indwelling catheter remained in place for 30 days. Similarly, Getliffe[13] reported the rate of encrustation to be as high as 50%.[14] Both researchers note that certain patients are prone to recurrent encrustation while others are catheterized over prolonged periods of time, experience no blockage.

Multiple strategies have been investigated to determine their influence on encrustation. To date, there is no evidence that hydrogel coating,[4,15] catheter coating with silver[16] or antibiotics,[17] composition, or antibiotic use affects the development of encrustations in the long-term catheterized patient.[18] Laboratory-based studies have suggested that silver-coated catheters or the use of catheter valves may have some beneficial effect,[8] but clinical evidence remains unavailable.

Routine washout with normal saline is often used to prevent catheter encrustation and blockage in Canada, but no randomized trials testing normal saline in the clinical setting have been published and laboratory studies have shown equivocal results.[10] Washout with acidic solutions such as Contisol are believed to dissolve crystals by acidifying the urine (temporarily), thus reducing encrustation and potential blockage. Acidic solutions have shown benefits over saline in the laboratory setting,[9,19] but no clinical studies have yet been undertaken.

The 2 currently accepted strategies to manage catheter blockage are replacement of the catheter at set intervals, depending on the "catheter life" of that individual, or regular catheter washouts.[4,20] Removal and replacement removes the catheter, its biofilm and any encrustation. However, patient discomfort and homecare or institutional costs must be considered when frequent replacement of an indwelling catheter is required. The use of washout solutions may help prolong the life of the catheter and reduce concomitant costs to the patient and the healthcare service. The primary aim of our study was to determine the effectiveness of catheter washouts in prolonging catheter patency and thereby reducing the number of catheter changes per month for individuals with long-term indwelling catheters and frequent blockage.

METHODS

Design and Study Participants

This prospective, multisite randomized controlled trial included 3 groups: control (usual care, no washout), saline washout, or commercially available mildly acidic washout solution (Contisol) (Table 1). Patients who resided in a long-term care setting or received homecare and who had a long-term indwelling catheter (defined as indwelling catheterization > 30 days) that was blocking on a regular basis (more than

TABLE 1	DESCRIPTION OF STUDY GROUPS
STUDY GROUP	INTERVENTION
Standard catheter care group	No intervention (no washout)
Saline washout group	Catheter washout weekly with 50-mL sterile normal saline
Contisol washout group	Catheter washout weekly with 50-mL sterile Contisol

once a month) were eligible. Additional inclusion criteria for participants were 18 years or older and sufficiently alert according to the Mini-Mental State Examination (MMSE score > 24) to consent to participation in the study and respond to verbal questions about experiences associated with catheterization or washout. Exclusion criteria included symptomatic UTI, although individuals were eligible for the study following successful treatment of the UTI after a symptom-free period of 14 days. Further exclusion criteria included urethral erosion allowing continuous bypassing (leakage) around urinary catheter; history of bladder cancer, or radiation or interstitial cystitis; impaired renal function as evidenced by a serum creatinine level of 2.0 mg/dL or higher; gross hematuria; or indwelling catheter that was changed less frequently than every 8 weeks. Approval from the 2 joint university and health region research ethics boards overseeing the study sites/agencies was obtained.

Outcomes

The primary outcome variable was mean time to first catheter change. Secondary outcomes included mean urinary pH, incidence of microscopic hematuria and leukocytes, measurement of cross-sectional luminal area of used catheters, and incidence of symptomatic UTI. Symptomatic UTI was defined as having at least 1 of the following signs or symptoms with no other recognized cause: (1) fever ($\geq 38°C$); (2) urgency; (3) dysuria or suprapubic tenderness; (4) hematuria; or (5) positive urine culture ($\geq 100,000$ microorganisms per cc of urine with no more than 2 species of microorganisms).[21]

STUDY PROCEDURES

Randomization

Group assignment was determined by a computer-generated list of random numbers and placed in opaque envelopes marked on the front with participant numbers 1 through 120. The sequentially numbered sealed envelopes were opened by the participant after eligibility was confirmed and the consent form signed. The envelope and assignment were placed in the participant's file. It was not possible to blind the research nurse to the 2 washout solutions because of the nature of the sterile packaging. Nevertheless, every attempt was made to keep the participant unaware of which washout solution was used until the end of the study.

Recruitment and Enrollment

Nurse managers on long-term care units and homecare nurses in the community approached potential participants. The names of those who agreed to have their names released were sent to a private fax number for the study coordinator, who then completed a screening visit to determine eligibility, explain the study, and obtain informed consent. Baseline data collected on initial visit included age, gender, and care setting; medical history including medical diagnoses, current medications, bowel elimination patterns, mobility, cognitive status measured by the MMSE, and urine pH obtained from the newly inserted catheter. The reason for and the length of catheterization were confirmed via interview with the participant or the staff nurse or by review of the participant's medical record. The catheter type and balloon size, history of washout regimen (if any), and the intervals between the last 3 catheter changes were all recorded.

Day 0 (Baseline) was the day of catheter insertion and commencement of data collection. Assessment occurred weekly for 8 weeks, until the end of 3 catheter changes, or a UTI was reported. At each visit, the research RN assessed the participant for evidence of catheter blockage and symptomatic UTI. The participant was asked about discomfort level following catheter change or washout, and a dipstick urinalysis was performed before washout. If catheter blockage occurred or was judged imminent, based on reduced flow rate observed by the participant, the nurse, or the caregiver, bypassing, or large amounts of sediment in the drainage tubing, the catheter was changed as per standard protocol by homecare or nursing home staff. Whenever possible, the catheter was forwarded to the pathology laboratory for slicing and photography. Participants were withdrawn from the study if they developed a symptomatic UTI or were prescribed antibiotics for a suspected UTI.

For participants in the washout groups, products were used according to manufacturer's directions. Both Contisol and saline were provided in sterile, 50-mL single-use containers. For the Contisol washout, the catheter was clamped, disconnected, and both the drainage tube and the catheter end were wiped with an alcohol swab. The nozzle of the container was inserted into the catheter and the contents (50 mL) were gently squeezed by pressing on the base, providing a controlled flow over 60 seconds. The bellows of the container were then allowed to slowly rein-flate, and the flushing action was repeated 5 times. At the next weekly visit, participants were asked to recall whether they experienced any adverse reactions to the catheter washout. For the saline washout, the same procedure was followed (Figure 2).

 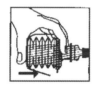

| The nozzle of the container will be inserted into the catheter | The container neck is held between first and second fingers and the bottle squeezed by pressing on the base with the thumb, providing a controlled flow into the catheter without the introduction of excess air. A period of 60 seconds (timed) is recommended. | The solution is retained in the bladder by drawing the clip over the base of the container | On the completion of the 15 minute retention period, the clip will be released. The catheter drainage will be checked for clarity and allowed to drain back into the container. The catheter will then be reconnected to the drainage bag. |

FIGURE 2 Procedure for irrigating with either normal saline or Contisol.

STATISTICAL ANALYSIS

Data were entered into SPSS, Version 14.0 (SPSS Inc, Cary, North Carolina). Randomized groups were compared on baseline characteristics to ensure that groups were balanced. Continuous variables were compared by using analysis of variance and categorical variables were compared by using the chi-square statistic. Kaplan-Meier survival curves were generated for "time to first catheter change" for each randomized group. The log-rank test was used to determine statistical significance between groups. Data were analyzed using an intention-to-treat analysis for the primary outcome variable; that is, the time to first catheter change was recorded as occurring on the date that the participant withdrew from the study.

RESULTS

Participants

One hundred twelve potential participants were screened and 73 enrolled. Fifty-three completed all 8 weeks of the study protocol. Sixteen subjects terminated early because of 3 catheter changes or self-reported UTI. The remaining subjects terminated before completing 8 weeks because of hematuria, latex sensitivity, deceased/severe illness, or personal choice. Table 2 summarizes subject characteristics, diagnosis, and catheter change history. Only the mean number of catheter changes per month prior to enrolling in the study approached statistical significance $(P = .07)$, with those randomized to the Contisol group reporting the most frequent mean number of changes. Figure 3 shows the progress of participants through the study. There were no group differences between terminated participants.

Primary Outcome Variable

At baseline, the mean time between catheter changes was 3.2 (SD = 3.6) weeks $(P = .480)$. The mean time to first catheter change was 4.75 (SD = 2.77) weeks $(P = .642)$ overall and did not differ between groups or within subjects from baseline to endpoint (Table 3, and illustrated in Figure 4). The Kaplan-Meier curves (Figure 5) showing the "survival" time of the first catheters in each group followed each other closely and were not significantly different to each other.

TABLE 2	BASELINE CHARACTERISTICS OF PARTICIPANTS BY GROUP			
	CONTISOL (n = 26)	SALINE (n = 21)	CONTROL (n = 26)	p <.05
Age, mean (SD)	63.92 (17.25)	66.24 (17.38)	68.56 (18.65)	NS
Gender				
Male	13	9	14	NS
Female	13	12	12	
Mini-Mental State Examination score	27.0	27.1	25.7	NS
Baseline weeks between catheter changes prior to enrollment, mean (SD)	2.65 (3.02)	3.09 (4.18)	3.86 (3.53)	NS

Primary diagnosis related to bladder dysfunction: Multiple sclerosis, Other neurological disease, Paraplegia/quadriplegia, Other.

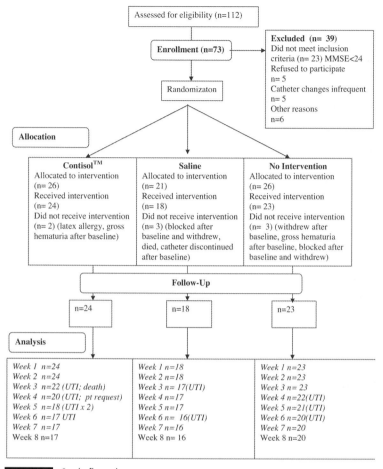

FIGURE 3 Study flow chart.

Secondary Outcome Variables

There were no significant differences between any of the secondary outcome variables. All participants consistently showed microscopic hematuria and leukocytes in the urine.

Two to 3 participants in each group did not complete data collection due to self-reported UTI and initiation of antibiotic treatment, although none met study

TABLE 3 RESULTS BY GROUP	CONTISOL (n = 26)	SALINE (n = 21)	CONTROL (n = 26)	p <.05
Weeks between catheter changes prior to study enrollment	2.65 (3.02)	3.09 (4.18)	3.86 (3.53)	NS
Number of weeks to first catheter change in study, mean (SD)	4.57 (2.61)	5.18 (2.90)	4.55 (2.91)	NS
Number of weeks in study, mean (SD)	5.92 (2.47)	6.45 (2.06)	6.33 (2.33)	NS

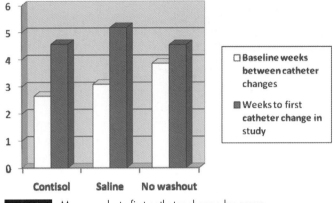

FIGURE 4   Mean weeks to first catheter change by group.

criteria for symptomatic UTI. No adverse events were reported in either of the washout groups. Dipstick urinalysis revealed that 80% of all subjects had positive nitrites on at least 1 occasion. The mean urinary pH was 6.3 (SD = 1.04) (range, 5-8.5) at baseline and did not change over the course of the study. Urinary pH did not correlate with incidence of blocking.

Catheter slicing supported available data that accumulation of biofilm or encrustations begins at the catheter tip, first affecting the eyes and then proceeding down the shaft of the catheter. Slicing did not prove useful in comparing effectiveness of washouts and was discontinued after 50 catheters were sliced. Figure 6 illustrates the cross section of a catheter of a subject randomized to the Contisol group. The percentage of catheters with encrustations was low. The majority were obstructed with heavy accumulation of thick biofilm described by the homecare nurses or the caregiver as common in their clinical experiences in catheterized patents.

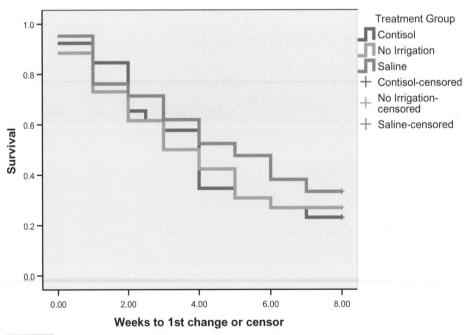

FIGURE 5   Kaplan-Meier survival function (intention to treat).

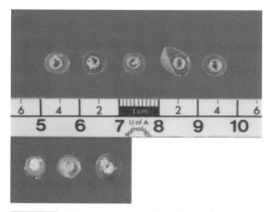

FIGURE 6 The cross section of a catheter of a subject randomized to Contisol Group.

DISCUSSION

Based on our results, evidence is insufficient to state whether catheter washout with saline or Contisol is more effective than usual care with no washout in preventing blocking. In vitro research has supported the concept that washouts with a commercially prepared solution extend the time that the catheter, which is subject to encrustation, remains patent. However, these laboratory findings have not been applied clinically. We evaluated whether washout solutions improved catheter patency in people with recurring catheter blockage in the clinical setting. We found that the mean time until first catheter change was similar between groups (4.75 weeks), and we found no significant differences between groups in secondary outcome variables such as perceived infection, hematuria, and urine pH.

It is important to note that Contisol was developed to address the issue of encrustations rather than biofilm formation in catheters, and in our study, the number of subjects with true encrustations was small. Therefore, our sample was inadequate to test the theory that Contisol is effective against encrustation adherence. However, in homecare in Alberta, saline is used as the solution of choice when catheter washouts are undertaken in catheterized patients. The results of our study suggest that the mechanical action of the saline is inadequate to effectively extend the catheter life. Even when data were combined for both washout groups in which a mechanical advantage of washouts may have been realized, there was no statistically significant difference in patency when catheter life was compared to the no-intervention group. It would thus appear that washouts with any solution may not be an effective measure in extending catheter patency in people in homecare or long-term care when biofilm accumulation results in recurrent blockage.

In Figure 4 it appears as if time between catheter changes was improved compared to baseline, but it must be noted that time was also similarly improved for the control group. The differences may be attributable to participation in the study and the expert care provided by the research nurse. Specifically, the research nurse was able to reassure participants when their catheter appeared to be blocking (but was not blocked) and provide guidance to participants on catheter positioning and fluid intake and generally act as a resource to the homecare nurses.

Initial sample size calculation indicated that 30 participants per group would provide sufficient power to detect a statistically significant difference between groups. This was based on an estimated effect size of 0.20 because no previous published trials existed on which to base our calculations. Consideration after the fact suggests that the difference between groups would be very small, and post hoc power analysis indicated that a minimum of 400 in each group would be required to achieve adequate power. Therefore, obtaining an adequate sample will require a multicenter trial.

We experienced considerable difficulties with recruitment of patients, and the study target numbers fell short within each group. There were also difficulties in maintaining participants in the study mainly for participant-orientated reasons such as ill health. There were no indications that participant dropout was caused by adverse effects related to the washout solutions.

Results of this study raise the question whether more frequent washout with solutions, perhaps twice weekly, would have had a greater impact on catheter patency. Such a question would need to be the basis of a future clinical trial, but the results of such a study must be tempered with knowledge that more frequent washout would add to direct costs of products, impact on the patient, and nursing time.

Concerns over increased risk of UTI when the closed catheter drainage system is broken are often raised by practitioners. However, we found no evidence of an increased risk of UTI in subjects assigned to washout groups (which requires breaking the closed system) compared to normal care.

There were some unexpected findings. For example, catheters were changed by staff when leakage around the catheter (bypassing) occurred, although on slicing and examination of the catheters, it was clear that they were not blocked. As well, perceived symptoms of infection were cloudy urine, bypassing, and urine odor without meeting criteria for infection as established by the National Institute on Disability and Rehabilitation Research.[21] Some subjects had bottles of ciprofloxacin or trimethoprim-sulfamethoxazole in their medicine cupboards, and they self-treated when a UTI was suspected. Others contacted the homecare nurse or the family physician and were started on antibiotics and therefore censored from the study. Such events are of concern, considering the known risk of antibiotic resistance. Despite extensive education of physicians and nurses concerning the risk of antibiotic resistance associated with asymptomatic bacteriuria, changes in practice are not readily apparent. Therefore, further strategies to improve knowledge transfer regarding management of asymptomatic bacteriuria are indicated. Finally, despite multiple participants experiencing difficulty with catheter management over an extended time, few had been referred to a urologist for cystoscopy and evaluation of the bladder for stones or other nidus likely to promote ongoing biofilm development.

Three participants who had an indwelling catheter for over 6 months and were experiencing considerable catheter-related problems had no clear indication why a catheter had been inserted. After discussion with the urology research nurse on the screening visit, they chose to have their catheter removed. In all 3 cases, the individuals were satisfied with the choice and managed well with containment products, toileting, and skin care. Such findings illustrate the importance of documenting the initial indications of catheter use and having adequate communication and appropriate follow-up when patients are discharged from the hospital or an outpatient setting with an indwelling catheter.[22] Limited resources and resource allocation act as incentives to discharge patients from hospital as soon as possible. Insufficient follow-up, exacerbated by a lack of continuity of care and reliance on walk-in clinics, may lead to an increasing number of patients managed with long-term catheterization. Furthermore, as many as 24% of elderly patients who are hospitalized may be catheterized without a clear medical indication.[23] They are frequently unaware of the potential complications of long-term catheterization and may not question the healthcare professionals' decisions.[22] One solution to address the issue of insufficient catheter follow-up is standardizing documentation for catheter insertion, providing better patient education, and ensuring that the catheter is still required at the time of each change.

Dipstick urinalysis revealed that all participants had microscopic hematuria and positive leukocytes; many had positive nitrites, traditional indicators of infection in the noncatheterized individual. These findings indicated that dipstick urinalysis results alone are not useful in confirming a suspected UTI in the patient with an indwelling catheter. The finding of positive nitrites is of interest because laboratory studies have indicated that urine must be accumulated in the bladder for at least an hour to allow nitrates to break down into nitrites in the presence of gram-negative bacteria. Our findings suggest that (1) there is enough residual urine in the bladder of the catheterized patient to allow this chemical breakdown or (2) the nitrite test is not a good indicator of UTI. Further evaluation on the residual urine in the catheterized patient may be worthwhile.

CONCLUSION

Catheter management remains a problematic issue for both the patient and the nurse. Based on results of this study, we are unable to recommend routine catheter washouts in patients who have recurrent catheter blockage. Our findings do not necessarily indicate that catheter washouts with a mildly acidic solution are ineffective. Instead, they reveal that catheter blockage is caused by several factors other than encrustation alone. Therefore, the most strategic approach is individualized catheter changes based on the patient's own pattern of blockage rather than a prescribed regimen.

KEY POINTS

➤ There is inadequate or no evidence to support the use of catheter washouts to decrease the need for frequent catheter changes among individuals with a long-term indwelling urinary catheter.

➤ Our study showed no difference between time to first catheter change between or within groups randomized to 1 of 3 groups: weekly washout with a mildly acidic commercial solution, weekly washout with saline, or no washout.

➤ Individualized catheter change protocols are suggested as one way to manage recurrent catheter blockage.

ACKNOWLEDGMENTS

The study was funded by the Alberta Heritage Foundation for Medical Research and the Canadian Nurses Foundation.

REFERENCES

1. Wong ES. Guideline for prevention of catheter-associated urinary tract infections. *Am J Infect Control.* 1983;11:28–36.
2. *Clinical Fact Sheet: Indwelling Catheter.* Mount Laurel, NJ: Wound, Ostomy and Continence Nurses Society; 2000.
3. Liedl B. Catheter-associated urinary tract infections. *Curr Opin Urol.* 2001;11:75–79.
4. Ackerman RJ, Monroe PW. Bacteremic UTI in older people. *J Am Geriatr Soc.* 1996;44:933–937.
5. Sedor J, Mulholland SG. Hospital-acquired urinary tract infections associated with the indwelling catheter. *Urol Clin North Am.* 1999;26:821–828.
6. Mayes J, Bliss J, Griffiths P. Preventing blockage of long-term indwelling catheters in adults: are citric acid solutions effective? *Br J Community Nurs.* 2003;8:172–175.
7. Fuqua C, Greenberg EP. Self perception in bacteria: quorum sensing with acylated homoserine lactones. *Curr Opin Microbiol.* 1998;1:183–189.
8. Stickler D, Morris N, Moreno MC, Sabbuba N. Studies on the formation of crystalline bacterial biofilms on urethral catheters. *Eur J Clin Microbiol Infect Dis.* 1998;17:649–652.
9. Getliffe KA. The use of bladder wash-outs to reduce urinary catheter encrustation. *Br J Urol.* 1994;73:696–700.

10. Getliffe K. Managing recurrent urinary catheter encrustation. *Br J Community Nurs.* 2002; 7:574, 576, 578–580.
11. Morris NS, Stickler DJ, McLean RJ. The development of bacterial biofilms on indwelling urethral catheters. *World J Urol.* 1999;17:345–350.
12. Kunin CM, Chin QF, Chambers S. Indwelling urinary catheters in the elderly. Relation of "catheter life" to formation of encrustations in patients with and without blocked catheters. *Am J Med.* 1987;82:405–411.
13. Getliffe KA. *Encrustation of Urinary Catheters in Community Patients* [PhD thesis]. Surrey, England: University of Surrey; 1992.
14. Getliffe K. Managing recurrent urinary catheter blockage: problems, promises, and practicalities. *J Wound Ostomy Continence Nurs.* 2003;30:146–151.
15. Hukins DWL, Hickey DS, Kennedy AP. Catheter encrustation by struvite. *Br J Urol.* 1983;55: 304–305.
16. Verleyen P, De Ridder D, Van Poppel H, Baert L. Clinical application of the Bardex IC Foley catheter. *Eur Urol.* 1999;36:240–246.
17. Gray M. Managing urinary encrustation in the indwelling catheter. *J Wound Ostomy Continence Nurs.* 2001;28:226–229.
18. Cox AJ, Harries JE, Hukins DW, Kennedy AP, Sutton TM. Calcium phosphate in catheter encrustation. *Br J Urol.* 1987;59:159–163.
19. Hesse A, Schreyger F, Tuschewitzki GJ, Classen A, Bach D. Experimental investigations on dissolution of incrustations on the surface of catheters. *Urol Int.* 1989;44:364–369.
20. Muncie HL Jr, Hoopes JM, Damron DJ, Tenney JH, Warren JW. Once-daily irrigation of long-term urethral catheters with normal saline. Lack of benefit. *Arch Intern Med.* 1989;149: 441–443.
21. Anonymous. The prevention and management of urinary tract infections among people with spinal cord injuries. National Institute on Disability and Rehabilitation Research consensus statement. January 27–29, 1992. *J Am Paraplegia Soc.* 1992;15:194–207.
22. Potter J. Risks of long-term catheterization in the community—and managing them. *Br J Community Nurs.* 2006;11:370–373.
23. Holroyd-Leduc JM, Sands LP, Counsell SR, Palmer RM, Kresevic DM, Landefeld CS. Risk factors for indwelling urinary catheterization among older hospitalized patients without a specific medical indication for catheterization. *J Patient Saf.* 2005;1:201–207.

Katherine N. Moore, PhD, RN, CCCN, Professor, Faculty of Nursing, University of Alberta, Edmonton, Alberta, Canada.

Kathleen F. Hunter, PhD, RN, NP, Assistant Professor, University of Alberta, Edmonton, Alberta, Canada.

Rosemary McGinnis, MSc, RN, Calgary Health Region Home Care.

Chasta Bacsu, MD, Urology Resident, University of Alberta, Edmonton, Alberta, Canada.

Mandy Fader, PhD, RN, Reader, University College London, London, United Kingdom.

Mikel Gray, PhD, FNP, PNP, CUNP, CCCN, FAANP, FAAN, Nurse Practitioner and Professor, Department of Urology and School of Nursing, University of Virginia, Charlottesville.

Kathy Getliffe, PhD, RGN, NDN, Professor, University of Southampton, Southampton, United Kingdom.

Janice Chobanuk, MN, RN, East Central Health Area, Alberta, Edmonton, Alberta, Canada.

Lakshmi Puttagunta, MD, FRSC, Pathologist, University of Alberta, Edmonton, Alberta, Canada.

Donald C. Voaklander, PhD, Professor, School of Public Health, University of Alberta, Edmonton, Alberta, Canada.

Corresponding author: Katherine N. Moore, PhD, RN, CCCN, Faculty of Nursing, University of Alberta, Edmonton, Alberta, Canada T6G 2G3 (Katherine.moore@ualberta.ca).

Critique of the Study by Moore and Colleagues, "Do Catheter Washouts Extend Patency Time in Long-term Indwelling Urethral Catheters? A Randomized Controlled Trial of Acidic Washout Solution, Normal Saline Washout, or Standard Care"

OVERALL SUMMARY

Overall, the study is important, calling into question the widespread practice of catheter washouts. The study directs the readers to the need for more research into catheter blockage issues and best practice recommendations. The research team is to be commended for pioneering much needed work in this area. A few issues, however, are noteworthy. First, the presence of a theoretical framework to guide this study would have been useful in elucidating some of the unexpected findings. Certain background information such as history of encrustation and blockage according to study groups would have helped to assess group equivalence at the outset of the study. Last, the relative small sample size reduces statistical power— that is the propensity to detect genuine group differences. Nevertheless, this study remains highly relevant to the body of nursing knowledge and for patient care.

TITLE

The title clearly communicates the research question and method. The only concern might be the use of the term "standard care" given that catheter washout is a common practice for catheter management. As stated by the authors, "routine washout with normal saline is often used to prevent catheter encrustation and blockage in Canada…." (p. 83). This statement seems to imply that normal saline washouts are considered usual treatment for prevention of encrustation and blockage of long-term indwelling catheters. A definition of what constitutes "standard care" would have been useful.

ABSTRACT

The article begins with a succinct and thorough synopsis of the study, organized under the headings: Purpose, Design, Subjects and Setting, Methods, Results, and Conclusion. One wonders if the concluding statement should have been "the evidence does not support routine catheter washout with saline or Contisol to prevent or reduce catheter blockage" rather than "the evidence is insufficient to state whether catheter washout with saline or Cortisol is more effective than usual care."

INTRODUCTION

The introduction to this study is divided into two parts. The first consists of introductory paragraphs that are excellent in setting the stage for the study, utilizing literature to describe the indications for and complications of long-term indwelling urethral catheters, routine catheter care practice, and the need for more research that evaluates the clinical efficacy of the rather widespread use of routine catheter washouts. Next, in the "Pathogenesis of Bacterial Colonization and Encrustation" section, the problem and purpose are elaborated through a literature review of the pathogenesis of bacterial colonization and encrustation involving long-term indwelling catheters and current practice in managing encrustation and subsequent catheter blockage.

Problem Statement and Purpose for the Research

The authors clearly explain the purpose of long-term indwelling catheter use and list the problems that may arise. They also describe common practices and recommendation for saline (Canada) and Contisol (UK) washouts. Through this, the problem is well established: catheter blockage is a common problem for patients with indwelling catheters and, despite widespread usage of routine washouts, there is insufficient evidence on the effectiveness of this practice. The authors might have elaborated on the dangers of catheter blockage to further underscore the importance of the research problem. This would further clarify the importance of the research problem.

The study aim or purpose is conveniently placed at the end of the introduction section and serves to effectively transition to the subsequent "Methods" section. The study aim "was to determine the effectiveness of catheter washouts in prolonging catheter patency and thereby reducing the number of catheter changes per month or individuals with long-term indwelling catheters and frequent blockage."

Literature Review

The second part of the introduction involves a more substantial discussion and review of the literature regarding the processes through which catheters may be blocked, as well as strategies use to unblock catheters. Given the significance of encrustation in causing subsequent blockage, comparing the formation of encrustation between the treatment and control groups would have been useful in predicting long-term catheter patency. Ample information is provided on the evidence pertaining to the research problem and its relevance for clinical care.

Hypothesis

The study hypothesis "catheter life would be extended by 25% in the commercial solution group" appears in the abstract. Although not all hypotheses are necessarily grounded in theory, it would have been helpful for the authors to identify the basis for the formulated hypothesis. They state that in vitro studies support the claim that commercial solutions extend catheter life but they do not provide the produced evidence to date.

Framework

Although the authors indicate that the theory of pathogenesis of bacterial colonization and encrustation guides propositions for the study, an encompassing theoretical framework would have been helpful in contextualizing the broader contributions of the study.

METHOD

Research Design

A randomized controlled trial was used to test the efficacy of catheter washouts for extending the patency time of long-term indwelling urethral catheters. The design involved 3 groups: a control group receiving "usual care" with not catheter washout, a treatment group receiving saline washout, and a treatment group receiving catheter washout with a commercial solution (Contisol).

Reliance on a randomized controlled trial is a robust strategy. However, the authors' choice to describe the control group as those participants receiving "usual" or "standard" care is confusing because the authors indicate that common catheter care in Canada includes the use of saline washout. As well, the strength of the RCT lies, in part, in its potential for strong internal validity, meaning that the results unequivocally reflect the effect of the independent variable or intervention. It is unclear whether the groups were equivalent in terms of history of encrustation and blockage. Did the researchers account for this important variable in the composition of the groups? They discussed how encrustation and blockage is dependent upon individual patients; so, were participants equally matched on this variable? Although nurses could not be blind to the washout solutions used, keen attempts were made to ensure that participants were.

The data collection procedure is clearly presented. At the initial visit by the research nurse, baseline data were collected including demographics, care setting, medical history and diagnoses, medications, bowel elimination patterns, mobility, cognitive status as established via Mini-Mental State Examination (MMSE), urine pH, reason for catheter, catheter type, balloon size, washout history, and intervals between last 3 catheter changes were obtained. The day of catheter insertion was considered Day 0 when data collection began with weekly assessments performed over a period of 8 weeks.

The Intervention

The authors describe the content of the intervention, supplementing the description with an effective diagram. The intervention involved participants in the washout groups receiving either saline or Contisol solution as per the manufacturer's directions. This description could have been presented in the study procedures section as one is not intuitively drawn to look for this description in the "Recruitment and Enrolment" section.

Study Sample

Recruitment procedures are clearly described under the "Recruitment and Enrolment" subsection of the "Study Procedures" section. The study sample is described under the "Participants" subheading of the "Results" section. A table summarizes clearly participants' characteristics, diagnosis, and history of catheter changes. As well, a diagram is provided summarizing the progress of participants through the period of study. The sample included 73 participants assigned to the following groups: 26 participants in the intervention group receiving Contisol washout solution, 21 in the intervention group receiving saline washout solution, and 26 assigned to the control group.

The obtained small sample size, however, lowers statistical power and increases risk for Type II error, namely failing to reject a false null hypothesis. A pilot study may have been helpful in estimating effect size and the required sample size.

Validity Issues

Randomization and other means of control inherent in RCT designs enhance internal validity. As mentioned previously although the authors describe how the groups were not significantly different at baseline, it would have been helpful to assess whether groups were equivalent in their history of encrustation.

Measures

Several types of weekly assessments were performed such as extent of catheter blockage, symptomatic urinary tract infection (UTI), participants' discomfort level after catheter changes or the washout procedure, and a urinalysis by dip-stick prior to washout. The authors also describe that, when possible, catheters that were discontinued for blockage or imminent blockage were sent to a pathology lab for slicing and photographs were taken.

The authors identify the primary and secondary outcome variables in a subtitled section called "Outcomes". The authors explain that the primary outcome variable pertains to mean time until first catheter change. The secondary variables include: mean urinary pH, microscopic hematuria and leukocytes, measurement of a cross-section of the lumen of used catheters, and the incidence of symptomatic UTI. Five UTI signs or symptoms are described with participants having at least one of these for being considered as having symptomatic UTI. Outcome measures were justified and relevant as suggested by the literature reviewed. Inclusion of information on the psychometric quality of the measures would have been helpful.

Ethical Aspects

Ethics approval was obtained for the conduct of the study. Authors also mention that once agreeing to take part in the study, participants' names were sent via a private fax number to the study coordinator who, in turn, obtained informed consent at initial visit.

RESULTS

The use of analysis of variance for continuous variables and chi-square statistic for categorical variables are suitable to the study questions. Kaplan-Meier survival curves were created for time to first catheter change and the log-rank test was used to determine statistical significance between groups on the time to first catheter change. The authors state that they used intention-to-treat analysis for those participants who withdrew from the study. The main results were not significant between groups or within subjects. As for the secondary variables, the authors also found no significant differences.

DISCUSSION

The discussion is substantial, balanced, and offers significant insights into the phenomenon of interest. The authors begin with a review of the non-significant findings related to the primary outcome variable of time to first catheter change. The report also provides direction for future research on the topic.

CONCLUSION

The conclusion effectively summarizes the findings and their clinical implications. Again, the recommendation for individualized care due to the variety of factors influencing catheter blockage and/or change is valuable.

GLOBAL ISSUES

The report is very well-written. The study is complex and the chosen design is robust. Authors are to be commended on their use of effective tables and figures to convey their information.

RESPONSE FROM KATHERINE MOORE

Clinical trials involving individuals in long term care are fraught with challenges of comorbid conditions, attrition due to death, differing perspectives by practitioners, and access to participants. Students will have noticed that there are few randomized controlled trials conducted by nurses (or other health care professionals) in areas other than industry-sponsored drug trials. Why is this? We are quick to notice that our practice is not evidence based but when we look for studies to support a particular intervention such as catheter flushing, we find there is only evidence based on laboratory studies. Is a laboratory study enough? As already discussed in this textbook, the answer is "no." Experimental results from a laboratory need to be applied in the clinical area—this is the difference between *efficacy* and *effectiveness*. The example trial on catheter flushing for people with long term indwelling catheters is the first to test the hypothesis that flushing with a mild acidic solution could improve catheter patency and reduce the number of changes required. It has been common practice in some settings to routinely flush yet no one has evaluated whether this is useful; as health professionals, we have an obligation to provide care that is based on evidence. Whilst this study has some limitations which are described in the discussion, one must keep in mind that one study on a topic, no matter how good the trial is, is never enough to base practice changes. What we learn from the study is that staff is inconsistent in its approach to catheter management. This inconsistency certainly interfered with data collection and meant missing data. The next research team who explores this topic can use this study as a guideline to consider design and sample size issues. Last, students may wish to consult the Consort statement for reporting of clinical trials (www.consort-statement.org) as it provides a clear outline of the points to look for when reporting or reviewing trials such as the one above. We thank the reviewers for these insightful comments.

Katherine N. Moore, PhD,
RN, CCCN
Professor, Faculty of Nursing, University of Alberta
Adjunct Professor Faculty of Medicine/Division of Urology

APPENDIX D.
Women and Prostate Cancer Support Groups: The Gender Connect?*

Joan L. Bottorff**
John L. Oliffe
Michael Halpin

Melanie Phillips
Graham McLean
Lawrence Mroz

Abstract

There are more than 100 prostate cancer support groups (PCSGs) in Canada, most of which meet on a monthly basis—yet little attention has been paid to the role of women at these groups. As part of an ongoing ethnographic study of PCSGs, we examined women's motivations for attending the groups, their ways of functioning in PCSGs and the benefits they accrued. Participant observations conducted at 13 British Columbian-based PCSGs and individual interview data from 20 women who regularly attended PCSG meetings were analyzed. Although the groups did not overtly limit women's attendance, the women's decisions to attend and their participation at group meetings were subject to much self-reflection, uncertainty and tension. Motivations to access a PCSG included a desire to support their partners, develop understandings about the illness and disease, and to manage their own experience of prostate cancer. Our analyses revealed that women assume three roles in PCSGs: social facilitator, background supporter and cancer co-survivor. The women reported many interrelated benefits as a result of attending, including information, hope and reassurance, and connecting with other women in similar circumstances. The results from this study reveal how traditional feminine ideals, such as nurturing and caring for the men in their lives, facilitating social connections and the desire to share emotional experiences guided the behaviors. Based on the study findings, we suggest that efforts to support women's involvement in PCSGs are critical to enhancing the effectiveness of the groups for both men and women.
© 2007 Elsevier Ltd. All rights reserved.

Keywords: Prostate cancer • Support groups • Health promotion • Gender roles • Women • Spouses

*This study was made possible by the Canadian Institutes of Health Research (CIHR) (Institute of Gender and Health) (#11R91563), with career support for the second author provided by CIHR Institute of Gender and Health, New Investigator award and the Michael Smith Foundation for Health Research (MSFHR) Scholar award.

**Corresponding author.* Tel.: +1 250 807 9901.

E-mail addresses: joan.bottorff@ubc.ca (J.L. Bottorff), oliffe@nursing.ubc.ca (J.L. Oliffe), halpin@nursing.ubc.ca (M. Halpin), melanie.phillips@nursing.ubc.ca (M. Phillips).

Reprinted with permission from *Social Science & Medicine* (2008; 66: 1217–1227).

INTRODUCTION

Women influence spousal experiences of prostate cancer, and are also significantly affected themselves by living with a partner who has prostate cancer. So much so, that prostate cancer has emerged as a 'couple's illness' (Arrington, Grant, & Vanderford, 2005; Boehmer & Clark, 2001; Soloway, Soloway, Kim, & Kava, 2005) in which the disease, as well as its treatments, challenge gender identities and relations across the entire illness trajectory (Chapple & Ziebland, 2002; Fergus, Gray, Fitch, Labrecque, & Phillips, 2002; Oliffe, 2004, 2005, 2006). In an effort to meet men's diverse needs for information and support with treatment decision making and the management of treatment side effects, prostate cancer support groups (PCSGs) have been established in many western countries. Although a growing body of research on PCSG has begun to document men's experiences, there has been little recognition of the involvement of women in these groups. The purpose of this research and article is to offer understandings about how prostate cancer is situated, and negotiated as a 'couple's illness', by describing women's participation at PCSGs.

BACKGROUND LITERATURE

The experiences of women in relation to prostate cancer have been described in several ways. Gender comparisons, for example, have revealed that men's concerns for maintaining erectile function are not necessarily shared by women, who tend to react more strongly to issues of survival (Harden et al., 2002; Volk et al., 2004). Despite this, and other divergent viewpoints, little attention has been paid to the specificities of gender relations in prostate cancer, especially from the perspectives of women.

Investigations into the way prostate cancer survivors situate their wives have provided some important insights. In the early illness stages of prostate cancer, women have been reported to serve as their husbands' health agents and advocates, seeking knowledge because men find it difficult to process and retain the specific information (Heyman & Rosner, 1996). Women are also recognized as integral to empowering their patient-husbands to regain a sense of mastery and control, and are expected to complement men's coping strategies whilst not indulging their own responses and reactions to the illness (Maliski, Heilemann, & McCorkle, 2001). Such expectations are often implicit, a by-product of men's refusal to communicate to their wives the impact of the illness on their life (Boehmer & Clark, 2001). Some men actively engage in illness minimization strategies (i.e., limiting disclosure) as a way to ameliorate the emotional effect of prostate cancer on the couple, restricting women from engaging in their usual expressive coping styles (Gray, Fitch, Phillips, Labrecque, & Fergus, 2000a). Others have reported that men portrayed their wives as "selfless supporters" with few concerns or needs of their own, and "health monitors" who actively seek diagnostic and prostate cancer treatment information (Arrington et al., 2005).

There is some evidence that women partners experience significant challenges providing support to prostate cancer survivors. Healthy spousal caregivers have been shown to suffer similar distress levels to their patient-husbands diagnosed with prostate cancer and reduced quality of life ratings akin to those of female cancer patients (Hagedoorn, Buunk, Kuijer, Wobbes, & Sanderman, 2000). The empirical support for female spousal caregiver burden and distress has led to a number of recommendations for support interventions to promote positive coping strategies for those providing care (Resendes & McCorkle, 2006). A qualitative study of women partners *(n = 18)* indicated that participants portrayed themselves as a source of support, rather than assuming an active role in the process (O'Rourke & Germino, 2000). In a survey questionnaire study of 66 women partners, researchers described emotional wellness (feelings of anxiety, guilt, concern for partner, etc.) and balance (balancing prostate cancer with their own illness, and schedule, etc.) as the two primary concerns for women (Hawes et al., 2006). In summary, this emerging focus on women's experiences related to prostate cancer demonstrates the usefulness of this line of research, as well as gaps in current understandings.

Cancer Support Groups

Cancer support groups have been responsive to the needs of patients and, as such, are characterized by a variety of structures and processes. In the instance of breast and prostate cancer, support groups have evolved in gender-specific ways and comparisons have revealed important differences in patterns of attendance, group dynamics and spousal involvement (Carlson, Ottenbreit, St. Pierre, & Bultz, 2001; Krizek, Roberts, Ragan, Ferrara, & Lord, 1999). The interactions at cancer support groups also vary between male and female survivors. For example, men have been reported to use selective disclosure strategies in order to maintain normality within their lives and avoid the "double stigma of a life threatening-illness and sexual dysfunction" (Gray, Fitch, Phillips, Labrecque, & Fergus, 2000b, p. 274). Women, on the other hand, assign a high value to emotional and tangible support networks available at breast cancer support groups, whereas men best respond to formal, organized PCSG meetings primarily as a means of accessing information (Gray, Fitch, Davis, & Phillips, 1996; Krizek et al., 1999). Other studies have highlighted the primacy of information in men's prostate cancer experience, rather than the networking and emotional expressivity favored by women who attend breast cancer support groups (Boberg et al., 2003; Breau & Norman, 2003). These trends also held true in a comparison of men's and women's online cancer support groups (Seale, Ziebland, & Charteris-Black, 2006). The differences raise questions about how women participate in PCSGs, and how genders are negotiated and performed in groups predominately made up of men.

The dynamics of PCSGs—particularly in terms of roles, behaviors, and attitudes of women who attend—are poorly understood with only a few studies focusing on women who attend PCSGs. Arrington et al. (2005) conducted an ethnographic study of US-based PCSGs that included partner-orientated meetings. Their findings indicated that the behaviors of women (and men) in support groups were directly influenced by facilitators who utilized strategies such as "topic turning" and "stories of survival and selflessness" to dissuade the emotional elements of the discussion. Instability of the group structure and time constraints was also described as barriers to sharing emotions (Arrington et al., 2005). In an earlier qualitative pilot study conducted in Canada, most women PCSGs interviewees' (n = 21) suggestions for group modifications and future strategies were interpreted to reflect women's disparate needs, including those related to the provision of information (Butler, Downe-Wamboldt, Marsh, Bell, & Jarvi, 2000).

The aim of this study was to explore women's self-perceptions and commentaries about the roles of women who attend PCSGs to add to the emergent body of knowledge related to how prostate cancer is enacted as a couple's illness. The research questions that focused this study were: (a) Why do women attend PCSGs? (b) How do women situate themselves and function at PCSGs? and (c) What benefits do women accrue from participation?

METHODS, PROCEDURES AND PARTICIPANTS

A qualitative ethnographic design including field-work, participant observations and semi-structured interviews was utilized to build contextual understandings about how women situated themselves and perceived their role at PCSG meetings.

Following university ethics approval, the leaders of 13 British Columbian (BC)-based PCSGs were contacted to explain the study and request permission for two trained male researchers to conduct fieldwork and participant observations at one support group meeting. All the groups that were contacted agreed to participate in the study. We were invited to observe designated group meetings, and recruit group members interested in participating in individual interviews to tell us about their experiences of attending PCSGs.

At the PCSG meetings, field notes were made to describe what was observed, paying particular attention to the interactions that directly involved women. At three PCSGs separate men's and women's discussion groups were made available in the second half of the meeting. Participant observations were conducted at two women's sub-groups by a male researcher (the second author) and a female researcher completed observations at the third women's group. At the conclusion of the meeting, the two researchers discussed and compared their observations and preliminary interpretations, and their conversations were digitally recorded and transcribed verbatim. The text data were subsequently discussed amongst the investigative team to inductively develop interpretations and derive category labels to organize the commonly observed behaviors and interactions.

The semi-structured interviews with women who participated in the PCSGs averaged approximately one hour in duration and were digitally recorded and transcribed verbatim. Interview participants received a nominal honorarium ($20) to acknowledge their time and contribution to the study. The transcripts were checked for accuracy and subsequently managed using NVivo™. An inductive approach to data analysis was used in which each participant interview transcript was read multiple times by the researchers, highlighting key phrases, noting ideas and interpretations in the margins (Gambling & Carr, 2004). Data and analyses were discussed by the authors at monthly team meetings and an ethnographic style of coding, categorizing and clustering themes was used to develop our interpretations (Morse & Field, 1995). The data were coded, organized and re-organized several times as sub-categories were developed. Exploration of the relationships between and within sub-categories was explored, and descriptive notes for each of the sub-categories were developed. Data were organized under each category and reviewed, noting the commonalities and differences (Gambling & Carr, 2004). Themes, defined as coherent behavioral and belief patterns identified in participants' accounts (both within and across transcripts) (Morse & Field, 1995; Stenner, 1993), were developed during the analyses, and continued from the outset to the writing up of the study and this article.

Sample

The original sampling strategy was to recruit one woman from each PCSG to participate in the interview component of the study. However, many women were eager to talk with us, and early on we decided to interview as many women as possible. Our final study cohort of 20 women was recruited from 11 PCSGs. We conducted participant observations at a total of 13 PCSGs, all of which had women attendees. The average total number of attendees at each of the 13 PCSG meetings was 31 and on average 7 (23%) were women. Interview participants self-identified as Anglo-Canadian $(n = 14)$ and Northern European $(n = 6)$, ranged in age from 54 to 84 years $(M = 68.5$ years), and most were retired $(n = 15)$. Eighteen of the 20 participants first attended the group within 12 months of their husband's prostate cancer diagnosis and, at the time of interview, had attended group meetings from 6 months to 13 years $(M = 6.5$ years). The interviewee demographic data reflected what was typically observed at the support group meetings. Sixteen participants attended with their husbands, and all the participants' husbands were currently receiving, or had previously received, treatment for prostate cancer.

FINDINGS

Joining a men's group focused on prostate cancer was not straightforward for most of the women. Although the groups did not overtly limit women's attendance, the women's decisions to attend and their participation at group meetings were subject to much self-reflection, uncertainty and tension. Cutting across many of the participant narratives was an undercurrent of anxiety about where exactly women fit in, and what roles were appropriate for them to assume in a men's group. One participant described the anxiety that she and many other women experienced:

> I didn't go [at the beginning] much. I went a couple of times, then I got more involved little by little. I was not sure as a spouse what I was supposed to say because the group was already set up . . . I don't want to say anything sexual about [husband] . . . on the other hand [I was] having a really tough time. (66-year-old, attended with husband for three years)

Although the women were adamant that men needed space to talk about shared concerns, their compelling reasons for attending helped them overcome their hesitations and made it necessary for them to negotiate a place in the group. In the following sections, we describe women's reasons for attending PCSGs and the variety of roles they assumed in the groups. Finally, the women's self-reported benefits of attending PCSGs are presented.

Women's Reasons for Attending PCSGs

Initial attendance at group meetings was prompted by a variety of factors including the advice of health care providers, friends, colleagues at work, other prostate cancer survivors and media announcements about PCSG services. However, the motivations to access a PCSG, and the reasons for continued attendance were often distinctly different.

The diagnosis of prostate cancer was described as a shock by most participants and, not surprisingly, the majority of the women framed their reasons for initially attending PCSGs as a form of support for their husband, as well as to obtain much needed information. Our observations verified this, in that many women attended the group with their husbands, sat next to them during the meetings and supported their participation. Interviewee's explained that taking a "back seat" was intentional because it was after all a "men's group." The women justified their need to support their husbands by emphasizing that it was not always easy to access and understand information about prostate cancer. The PCSGs were, therefore, perceived as a critically important avenue for their husbands to receive relevant information from expert speakers, and an opportunity to hear others' illness stories.

Some women indicated that their husbands would not have attended the group without them. Certain that their husbands needed the information and support of the group, some women even began attending the groups alone, hoping that their participation would convince their husband to attend. One participant recalled an instance when a woman attended a meeting by herself. During the meeting she told the group leader that her husband was reluctant to join the meeting, and was waiting for her in the parking lot to drive her home. Together they went out to the car, and convinced the man to join the group meeting.

The second major motivation for women's attendance at PCSGs was related to their need to understand and manage their own experience of prostate cancer. Many participants admitted that they needed the information to understand the treatments, cope with the inherent uncertainty of the disease and find ways to support and encourage their husbands. A related motivation for initially attending group meetings focused on women's own support needs. A 64-year-old participant, who had been attending group meetings with her husband for one year, explained:

> I went to support my husband because he was newly diagnosed but I was also quite overwhelmed by the amount of information there was . . . So I found that maybe the support group there would be an opportunity to begin to make more sense of . . . the medical aspect of it but also maybe the psychological, also to hear people's stories and then for myself to be able to not only discuss things with my husband but hopefully to discuss things with other women.

In our fieldwork, we observed that some women attended the group without their partners (e.g., because their partners were unwilling to attend) to connect with others and access support. These women were often open about sharing their reasons for attending in the group, even at their first meeting. One woman who came to the group alone gave an emotional explanation in front of approximately 40 other attendees that although she already had information about prostate cancer and knew her husband would not die of the disease, she needed help, support and strategies to deal with his difficulty in coping with the diagnosis.

Women's long-term attendance at the PCSG was motivated by different reasons. Some participants established friendships and connected with others going through similar experiences, and this strongly influenced their resolve to continue attending the group meetings. The desire to "give back" to the group as a couple, and as a woman who had been through the experience of prostate cancer, was also central to many participants' long-term attendance. In particular, women were motivated by their perceptions about the importance of survivor stories for others, especially those attendees who were newly diagnosed. A 75-year-old participant who had attended meetings with her husband for more than a decade explained her commitment to the group:

> I only go with him . . . Every once in a while he would say, "I do not know why I am going anymore." I always come back with, "Well it is for the other fellows that are there, the new people, because you are a survivor." I think it is important for them to hear the survivors . . . I sometimes wonder why we go too, but it is for the others.

Women's Roles in PCSGs

The PCSGs meetings observed in this study revealed a strong orientation to the provision of information as their core business, and women negotiated their place by taking up diverse roles that varied in and across the groups. Some women were purposely inconspicuous whilst others took on roles that were more visible. The three distinct roles that women assumed in the PCSGs, reflected in our observations and supported by interview data, were: social facilitator, background supporter, and cancer co-survivor. It is important to note that these roles were not mutually exclusive or fixed. Rather, our observations and the participants' narratives suggested that these roles shifted over time and were strongly influenced by group composition and dynamics, the length of time they had been in the group, their husband's health status and other events in their everyday lives.

Social Facilitator

This was the most common role assumed by women, and was reflected in many activities that established and sustained social connections for their husbands and themselves, as well as for others who attended the group. The degree of involvement in social facilitation varied from initiating brief informal conversations when welcoming new members and serving refreshments at meetings, to devoting considerable time and energy to arranging special social events (e.g., potluck dinners, annual summer or Christmas parties). We noticed, in particular, how some women who were long-term group members interacted with others, creating a hospitable environment where individuals could socialize with each other prior to and following the formal part of the meeting. These informal interactions provided both men and women with another way to learn about each other and extend their understandings about how prostate cancer was part of their lives. Participants generally downplayed the contributions they made to the social life of the group, explaining that they took on these tasks because they were more experienced than the men, and felt comfortable contributing to the group through these activities. A 67-year-old participant who had attended with her husband for eight years explained that her role was to take care of the "social side of things" and "meet and greet and have a bit of fun with people". Similarly, a 60-year-old participant, who had attended group meetings with her husband for 10 years, explained her substantive role:

> I'm the refreshment lady . . . The tea, coffee, actually I used to make everything at one time . . . they had a meeting, I wasn't there, [laughs] and they voted me to do it [laughter] . . . Because there's a lot of people that didn't want to do it, it doesn't have to be the woman, it could be the guys but they didn't want to do the coffee, 'How much coffee do I put in, how much water do I put in?' you know, and they'd really stress themselves out about it.

In a few instances, the women's "hard work" was acknowledged along with the importance of their contributions to the group. However, a reluctance to take credit for the effectiveness of the groups was evident throughout this and many other women's interviews. At the suggestion of the interviewer, one participant agreed that women might be the "glue" in keeping her particular group together:

> Participant: A lot of women do a lot of hard work in that group . . . his wife has done a tremendous amount of work to keep that place going. She's on the board; she supplies all the fruit and vegetables that are there. She looked after the Christmas party, she does everything.
>
> Researcher: Women might be the glue?
>
> Participant: I think that's very possible. Men tend to be independent people. (64-year-old, attended with husband for 6 years)

Background Supporter

The second role that women fulfilled was that of background supporter for their husband and the group. In this role, women engaged in a range of activities that they perceived to be helpful without drawing attention to themselves, and at the same time respecting and promoting men's ownership of the group. Despite their motivation to support the group, they were careful not to do "too much" because they perceived this as inhibiting men's support for each other.

As a background supporter to their husbands, women typically sat quietly beside their husbands and were observed to speak very little and often not at all during mixed meetings. A 75-year-old participant who had been attending for 12 years explained that she was "just a listener" who simply wanted to "be there" for her husband. Similarly, a new attendee explained that during question time and discussions she remained quiet because her husband was the one who needed to talk:

> I don't get involved with the questioning because its [husband] that has it, and he's the one that knows how he feels so if he has a question he'll ask but I don't really say anything. (65-year-old, attended with husband for 1 year)

Positioning themselves as a background supporter helped the women minimize their anxiety about attending a men's group, and the strategy provided a way to avoid inhibiting men's self-disclosure and talk about ordinarily private issues such as impotence and incontinence. Although the role of background supporter limited women's active participation in group discussions, it sustained their efforts to record, collect and synthesize the information shared at the meetings. We observed many instances when women made extensive notes and took charge of gathering information at the group meetings. As the note-takers, these detailed records not only provided a valuable source of information for future reference and discussion, but also allowed men to maintain their focus on the discussion. Although many women were active consumers of health information, they located their efforts as jointly constructed and/or tailored to the learning styles of their husbands. A 65-year-old participant, who had attended group meetings with her husband for one year, justified her approach to collecting information, by explaining that as a couple, "the more we know about prostate cancer the better we can handle it." Another participant described how she targeted information to her husband, whilst simultaneously addressing her own anxiety:

> I immediately made him a whole page list, things I thought he could, should, would do and so I didn't overwhelm him, I told him what they were [laughing] but, you know, I'm aware that I have to be really careful, I over function pretty quickly so taking care of my own anxiety was important. (64-year-old, attended with husband for one year)

Some participants used the role of background supporter to empower their husbands to take responsibility for their own health. A 73-year-old participant decided to attend meetings occasionally in order to facilitate her husband's ownership and investment in his own health:

> I'm very, very interested in medical and scientific things and research and genetics and so forth. I could have jumped in with both feet, but I sort of thought that this is something that (husband) should do on his own because he'll get more out of it. If he's going to the meetings and then coming home and telling me about them, and I'm asking questions about, you know, what did they say about this and how much of it is genetic? And how much of it is environmental? And, you know, it makes him more interested and it makes him take more responsibility. (Attended occasionally with husband over 10 years)

Some women were also background supporters in how they supported group leaders to meet the diverse needs of attendees. For example, some participants described how they served on the group steering committee. Even though these women had important roles, they downplayed their contributions and consistently located the group leadership as residing exclusively with the men, rather than the women. A 66-year-old participant explained that she routinely telephoned group members to remind them about upcoming meetings; however, she differentiated her assistance from the male "support" in the group:

> When you really think about what the group does, the women would do things like phoning. See that everybody knows. But we are not phoning to see how the guys are and, like, 'tell me your problems.' To me that's not a women's function; the guys are the one's who support the guys. (Attended three years with her husband)

In our fieldwork, we noted that this participant focused on the meeting aesthetics and amenities, and did not initiate conversations with the men (including her husband). However, she actively engaged with the other women at the meeting during the refreshment break as well as by facilitating a separate woman's sub-group in the second hour. So, whilst she was a background supporter in relation to the men at the group, she made significant contributions to supporting other women by listening, talking and advising them outside the confines of the formal mixed meeting.

Cancer Co-survivor

Women also assumed the role of cancer co-survivor in the group by explicitly positioning the experience of prostate cancer as a couple's illness, whether they attended with their husband or on their own. In this role, women were stakeholders and equally entitled to contribute to, as well as receive, the group's support and services. Although observational data indicted their participation mirrored that of the men as they described experiences of treatment[s] and side effects, it also differed in that the women shared their emotions and solicited psychosocial support. Interestingly, when women participated in group meetings in this way, both men and women listened intently. Although the group rarely raised questions about or openly discussed women's emotional experiences with the disease when they brought these experiences forward in mixed groups, nods and silent acknowledgement seem to suggest that these experiences were shared by others. In this way, women appeared to open the door for others to acknowledge a less talked about dimension of prostate cancer. Unlike the other roles, the cancer co-survivor role was not downplayed or muted, rather women were afforded an equal voice and visibility. As one participant pointed out during a support group meeting, "Women realize that it's just not a man's disease, it's their disease too."

The cancer co-survivor role was most often embodied by couples who attended the group meetings together. However, we also observed four PCSG meetings when women attended without their partners and talked openly about the difficulties they were having coping with their husbands' prostate cancer. As active participants, the women's emotional stories generated strong support from both men and women at the group. For example, it was common for experienced group members to "rally around" women in this situation to listen, provide reassurance, and offer assistance. While their husbands had patient-orientated forums to discuss their challenges and difficulties, some women noted that the PCSGs were the only arena for discussing their prostate cancer experiences. As one 59-year-old participant explained, the group support was also distinctly different from that of family and friends:

> I had a need to talk desperately, I had my friends who had empathy and caring but they had no idea what I was going through and if any of them were losing their husbands, they were losing them through divorce not this. As much as your family and friends love you and care about you, often they don't really have the knowledge, this group can give you that knowledge. I believe that the groups can help enormously, emotionally, and I think that emotion plays a huge role in the disease. I think people underestimate the importance of it. (Widow, attended 12 years)

Perceived Benefits

The women reported many interrelated benefits as a result of attending PCSGs, including information, hope and reassurance and connecting with other women in similar circumstances. Many participants perceived that they heard, and had time to understand, "a lot more" about treatments and treatment side effects at the meetings than they could obtain elsewhere. The information was important in helping the women understand "what was going on," as well as the "different experiences" that can occur. One 72-year-old woman who had attended with her husband for one year explained:

> Here were these women who, they were all at different levels and their husband had done it this way and this husband had done it that way and I got to know the difference, what was available, the different procedures that could happen and what the outcomes were for them and, of course, everyone is different but then you hear about it, then you know what the options are.

The topic of prostate cancer was difficult for some couples to talk about; however, women were able to hear the same information that their husbands heard at the meetings, and were privy to the questions that their husbands (and other group members) asked. This provided opportunities to learn about their husband's potential and actual challenges, without having to ask directly. Following the meetings, information presented and issues raised provided a context for continued discussion among couples. In addition, information enabled some participants to monitor, advise and understand their husbands' illness. A 65-year-old participant explained how she used the information collected at the group meetings:

> For me, it's [attending the group] so I understand what he's going through. I can watch for signs if I see anything, I think its really important as a partner to know what's happening with your mate, you know, I think lots of times you can help with, sometimes you might know something that they don't like, for instance, if he's really tired I'll just say, 'Go to bed,' you know, where if you didn't know anything you might resent that. (Attended with husband for one year)

Hope and reassurance were also important benefits. Participants suggested that group discussions gave them optimism about life after diagnosis and/or treatment for prostate cancer, as well as much needed reassurance by talking with long-term survivors. One 64-year-old participant explained how normalizing prostate cancer helped to dissipate the anxiety she and her husband experienced at diagnosis:

> It's less profound kind of symptoms it seems from what we've heard so I think that's helpful, its normalized it in a way, that's a word, having radiation is not necessarily a normal kind of thing but it puts it in a different kind of perspective, here's somebody with radiation eight years ago and he still looks healthy and living a reasonable life. (Attended with husband for one year)

Another interrelated benefit of attending PCSGs came from the friendships with other women who had been through the experience of prostate cancer. Unlike during formal meetings when women spoke very little, we observed many animated, friendly conversations among women during refreshment breaks and sometimes prior to the commencement of the meetings that reflected the close bonds that women developed. The "sisterhood" that emerged enabled many women to feel—often for the first time—that they are not alone in dealing with the disease. Linking with the other women created an extended support network and provided a sense of security and ability to deal with the disease. One participant noted how friendships served to establish her involvement with the group:

> For me, there wasn't a whole lot for me to talk about and I wasn't sure I wanted to talk about it. I didn't ask anybody. I found that there were some of the women I really liked and so I got more comfortable. (66-year-old, attended with husband for three years)

At three PCSGs, meetings were organized to accommodate separate discussion groups for men and women. As such, the women's sub-group discussions were typically held during the second half of the meeting, in a space separate from the men, either behind a partition or in another room. Most women believed that this format fostered more sharing between the men. Furthermore, many participants indicated that their own reservations about talking in the presence of men was addressed with this arrangement. One participant explained:

> It's the fact that women can share with other women what they are feeling or thinking and ask questions, that you would never ask in front of other men. Like, I would never ask certain questions especially if strange men were sitting around. (64-year-old attended with husband for six years)

Establishing parallel women's groups, therefore, also allowed women to talk openly and communicate and receive support from each other. The women's group discussions were characterized by emotive, open dialogue and women were invited to talk about how they were "feeling." The conversations and support were anchored in the solidarity of having shared experiences. One woman contrasted men's and women's talk:

> I think women are much more open than men are. They [men] are very reticent to share, but women are not; they'll share. (72-year-old, attended with husband for five years)

The group facilitated "women speaking from their own experience" [64-year-old, attended with husband for five years] and, as one participant eloquently explained, diverse, multi-dimensional—and often ignored—needs of women who were living with prostate cancer were explicitly addressed in the women's sub-groups:

> The women in the group I learned had such different issues, uh, their husbands were battling disease, and had the doctors to look after them. These women did not have anyone to look after them so to speak and their issues were huge. They ranged from physical, emotional, financial, sexual, the gambit and often they couldn't talk to anyone, their families, friends, they either didn't trust them or just didn't feel comfortable or didn't feel they were given support. (59-year-old widow who attended alone for 12 years)

Some five years later, one participant vividly recalled how the members of the women's group were especially skillful in not overwhelming her with information, but providing much needed hope and reassurance:

> She [another female group member] said, 'You come with me.' And she took me by the arms and took me to the lady's group and sat me at the end of the table. All the other ladies sat down and she sat at the other end of the table and somewhere in the conversation she made the comment, 'We're not going to do all of that, you're only going to have one of those.' And she gave me the lecture, 'We've all been through this, we know how you're feeling and I promise you will come out of it feeling fine. You will come out of this, but we've all been there, so we understand exactly how you feel and you will be fine. YOU WILL BE FINE. Remember they're only going to do one procedure.' Then I...ah...relaxed. It was the best thing that could happen to me. (64-year-old, attended with husband for six years)

In many groups, women also exchanged telephone numbers to forge relationships that were not bound by the limited time frame of the group meeting. Attendance at funerals and support of widows was mentioned by one participant as a regular part of how she helped other women from the group. As such, women experienced a continuum of support—from the intimacy of a group to informal social gatherings—that ensconced them in the group in ways that their own interests were served, and needs met, whilst affirming their place in the couples' illness.

DISCUSSION AND CONCLUSION

The findings of this study highlight women's needs related to prostate cancer, their influence in PCSGs and the important benefits they receive from participating in these groups. The concept of prostate cancer as a couple's illness as previously described (Arrington et al., 2005; Boehmer & Clark, 2001; Soloway et al., 2005) is supported by these findings and extended within the milieu of PCSGs. Although PCSGs are promoted as important sources of information for men in particular, it is clear from the findings in this study that women not only access information at PCSGs, but also receive support from both men and other women going through similar experiences that is otherwise unavailable to them. Thus, the PCSGs that involve women are important in that they locate prostate cancer as a couple's illness, and provide a potential forum for recognizing and addressing the burden of prostate cancer for women.

The women's initial disquiet over what they could say and do at group meetings was a dominant theme in our findings. However, this was often overcome by relying on traditional gendered ideals. Specifically, feminine characteristics of nurturing, caring and compassion were consistently reflected in women's efforts to promote social ease within the group, empower men to legitimately talk about ordinarily taboo subjects and to provide emotional support to other women. Through these gendered activities, women were able to assume peripheral roles that did not challenge men's leadership or the group mandate, while at the same time meeting their needs for information and support.

Although the provision of information is deemed to be a central mission of PCSGs, as reflected by the priority given to biomedical information and survivor testimonials, this study indicates that PCSGs provide an important avenue for health promotion that is dependent on more than information dissemination. Our findings suggest that women play a crucial role in the success of health promotion efforts directed towards men. The women not only actively encouraged their partners to attend the group; but also supported their partners' autonomy in taking responsibility for managing their prostate cancer and overall well being. While respecting the limits of men's talk, the women expanded what men heard about experiences of prostate cancer by openly sharing emotional consequences of the disease for themselves. In this way, the PCSG is a site where women can express themselves in ways that benefit men's understanding of their partners' experience of prostate cancer. The study raises questions about the gendered roles in men's health promotion for future research.

The three roles women took up in PCSGs, social facilitator, background supporter and cancer survivor, have not been previously described. All of these roles are based on traditional ideals of femininity and were instrumental contributions to the functioning and overall effectiveness of the group for both men and women. The identification and descriptions of these roles may be useful for group leaders to facilitate the entry of women to PCSGs and better understand their individual and collective contributions. Importantly, through their involvement in the group, women were able to strengthen their efforts in supporting their husbands in a number of ways. For women, the experiences and questions discussed in the group meetings provided important points of comparison and insights into what their husbands might be experiencing, as well as a stimulus for couple discussions that occurred long after the meetings were over. Because of the potential benefits of connecting with other women through their involvement in PCSGs, further research should focus on evaluating whether benefits are greater in groups that facilitate the formation of a women's sub-group compared to those that do not.

The model on which PCSGs operated women's subgroups deliberately replicated the "Man to Man" support group franchise in the United States (Arrington et al., 2005; *Man to Man*, 1990). It is important to note that no rationale for this format, other than it seemed to work, was offered by the women, and they did not contest this model, but rather confirmed the appropriateness of a man-led group for addressing prostate cancer, and worked hard to function in the group without "taking over the group." In terms of masculinity, many women were complicit in sustaining dominant ideals that men do not easily socialize and talk or connect with others, but sought to remedy this by taking up the aforementioned roles. Such self-positioning was likely influenced by modernist feminine ideals embodied over many years and numerous "social" situations and within the domestic sphere. It is important to acknowledge that many men at PCSGs also broke with masculine ideals in talking publicly about their health and prostate cancer. A study of men's help-seeking behaviors by O'Brien, Hunt, and Hart (2005) confirms that men can triage specific masculine ideals to trump the much cited denial of illness and disinterest in self-health. In the context of PCSGs, our study findings indicated that women are often integral to creating an environment and providing subtle permissions conducive to men privileging their talk as a means to problem solving their health and prostate cancer specific issues.

Our observations that many men attended the PCSGs alone suggest that some women, unlike our study participants, may have been unable to overcome perceived barriers to joining a men's group or believed men needed space to discuss their illness without women being present. It is not unreasonable to expect that other women, whether daughters or female siblings, may have information and support needs similar to those of the study participants. Despite evidence about the prominent role of women partners in prostate cancer, limited dedicated support resources are available to them. As such, PCSGs can offer an important and unique support resource for women. In addition to efforts to promote PCSGs in ways that encourage women to attend, attention to the way support group meetings are structured is an important consideration. It appears that the inclusion of both large group and gender-based sub-group discussions have important benefits for both women and men, and the functioning of PCSGs. Although exclusive reliance on a mixed gender environment may hinder women's ability to communicate with one another, even in PCSG settings where subgroups did not occur, women noted that the presence of other women generally increased their comfort in attending meetings. Clearly, the importance of the opportunity for women to share experiences as partners of men who have prostate cancer should not be ignored. There is potential to create a bond of sisterhood that informs how women interact at PCSGs and in their extended support networks that ultimately will satisfy the needs of many women and concurrently yield benefits to the group as a whole.

The findings of this study are based on PCSGs situated in Western Canada and, therefore, may not be generalizable to other settings where gendered roles may influence the functioning of men's support groups in different ways. Because there is diversity in the way PCSGs function, it is possible that the ways women participated in the groups varied with these differences. It is also important to acknowledge that the interviews with women were conducted by male researchers, and this might have influenced the rather conventional reports of women's roles. Additional research is needed to examine how the roles women assume in PCSGs influence the effectiveness of the groups for both men and women, and if these roles can be extended to other types of health promotion strategies to support men's health.

In conclusion, the findings of this study underline the importance of women's involvement in PCSGs and also illustrates how their participation in PCSGs replicate, and perhaps extend, traditional gender roles where women can implicitly and explicitly look after the health of the men in their lives. By being an intermediary between experts and men who have prostate cancer, women can act as a critically important conduit for men's access and engagement with health messages. The results from this study reveal how traditional feminine ideals—such as nurturing and caring, facilitating social connection and the desire to share emotional experiences—guided the women's roles at PCSGs. Finally, the potential role of PCSGs in providing information and support to women needs to be acknowledged. Our findings suggest that efforts to support women's involvement in the PCSGs are critical to enhancing the effectiveness of PSCGs for both men and women.

REFERENCES

Arrington, M. R., Grant, C. H., & Vanderford, M. L. (2005). Man to man and side by side, they cope with prostate cancer: self-help and social support. *Journal of Psychosocial Oncology, 23*(4), 81–102.

Boberg, E. W., Gustafson, D. H., & Hawkins, R. P., et al. (2003). Assessing the unmet information, support and care delivery needs of men with prostate cancer. *Patient Education and Counseling, 49*(3), 233–242.

Boehmer, U., & Clark, J. A. (2001). Married couples' perspectives on prostate cancer diagnosis and treatment decision-making. *Psycho-Oncology, 10*(2), 147–155.

Breau, R. H., & Norman, R. W. (2003). The role of self-help groups in educating and supporting patients with prostate cancer and interstitial cystitis. *BJU International, 92*(6), 602–606.

Butler, L., Downe-Wamboldt, B., Marsh, S., Bell, D., & Jarvi, K. (2000). Behind the scenes: partners' perceptions of quality of life post radical prostatectomy. *Urologic Nursing: Official Journal of the American Urological Association Allied, 20*(4), 254–258.

Carlson, L. E., Ottenbreit, N., St. Pierre, M., & Bultz, B. D. (2001). Partner understanding of the breast and prostate cancer experience. *Cancer Nursing, 24*(3), 231–239.

Chapple, A., & Ziebland, S. (2002). Prostate cancer: embodied experience and perceptions of masculinity. *Sociology of Health and Illness, 24*(6), 820–841.

Fergus, K. D., Gray, R. E., Fitch, M. I., Labrecque, M., & Phillips, C. (2002). Active consideration: conceptualizing patient-provided support for spouse caregivers in the context of prostate cancer. *Qualitative Health Research, 12*(4), 492–514.

Gambling, L. F, & Carr, R. L. (2004). Lifelines: a life history methodology. *Nursing Research, 53*(3), 207–210.

Gray, R., Fitch, M., Davis, C., & Phillips, C. (1996). Breast cancer and prostate cancer self-help groups: reflections on differences. *Psycho-Oncology, 5*(2), 137–142.

Gray, R. E., Fitch, M., Phillips, C., Labrecque, M., & Fergus, K. (2000a). Managing the impact of illness: the experiences of men with prostate cancer and their spouses. *Journal of Health Psychology, 5*(4), 531–548.

Gray, R. E., Fitch, M., Phillips, C., Labrecque, M., & Fergus, K. (2000b). To tell or not to tell: patterns of disclosure among men with prostate cancer. *Psycho-Oncology, 9*(4), 273–282.

Hagedoorn, M., Buunk, B. P., Kuijer, R. G., Wobbes, T, & Sanderman, R. (2000). Couples dealing with cancer: role and gender differences regarding psychological distress and quality of life. *Psycho-Oncology, 9*(3), 232–242.

Harden, J., Schafenacker, A., & Northouse, L., et al. (2002). Couples' experiences with prostate cancer: focus group research. *Oncology Nursing Forum, 29*(4), 701–709.

Hawes, S., Malcarne, V., & Ko, C, et al. (2006). Identifying problems faced by spouses and partners of patients with prostate cancer. *Oncology Nursing Forum, 33*(4), 807–814.

Heyman, E. N., & Rosner, T. T. (1996). Prostate cancer: an intimate view from patients and wives. *Urologic Nursing: Official Journal of the American Urological Association Allied, 16*(2), 37–44.

Krizek, C., Roberts, C., Ragan, R., Ferrara, J. J., & Lord, B. (1999). Gender and cancer support group participation. *Cancer Practice, 7*(2), 86–92.

Maliski, S. L., Heilemann, M. V., & McCorkle, R. (2001). Mastery of post prostatectomy incontinence and impotence: his work, her work, our work. *Oncology Nursing Forum, 28*(6), 985–992.

Man to Man. (1990). [From American Cancer Society Web Site]. Available from <http://www.cancer.org/docroot/ESN/content/ESN_3_lX_Man_to_Man_36.asp?sitearea=SHR>. Accessed 09.03.07.

Morse, J. M., & Field, P. A. (1995). *Qualitative research methods for health professionals,* (2nd ed.). Thousand Oaks, CA: Sage Publishing.

O'Brien, R., Hunt, K., & Hart, G. (2005). 'It's caveman stuff, but that is to a certain extent how guys still operate': men's accounts of masculinity and help seeking. *Social Science & Medicine, 61,* 503–516.

Oliffe, J. L. (2004). Anglo-Australian masculinities and Trans Rectal Ultrasound Prostate Biopsy (TRUS-Bx): connections and collisions. *International Journal of Men's Health, 3*(1), 43–60.

Oliffe, J. L. (2005). Prostatectomy induced impotence and masculinity. *Social Science & Medicine, 60*(10), 2249–2259.

Oliffe, J. L. (2006). Embodied masculinity and androgen deprivation therapy. *Sociology of Health & Illness, 28*(4), 410–432.

O'Rourke, M. E., & Germino, B. B. (2000). From two perspectives to one choice: blending couple and individual views of prostate cancer treatment selection. *Journal of Family Nursing, 6*(3), 231–251.

Resendes, L. A., & McCorkle, R. (2006). Spousal responses to prostate cancer: an integrative review. *Cancer Investigation, 24,* 192–198.

Seale, C, Ziebland, S., & Charteris-Black, J. (2006). Gender, cancer experience and internet use: a comparative keyword analysis of interviews and online cancer support groups. *Social Science & Medicine, 62*(10), 2577–2590.

Soloway, C T., Soloway, M. S., Kim, S. S., & Kava, B. R. (2005). Sexual, psychological and dyadic qualities of the prostate cancer 'couple'. *BJU International, 95*(6), 780–785.

Stenner, P. (1993). Discoursing jealousy. In E. Burman, & I. Parker (Eds.), *Discourse analytic research: Repertoires and readings of texts in action* (pp. 114–132). London: Routledge.

Volk, R. J., Cantor, S. B., Cass, A. R., Spann, S. J., Weller, S. C, & Krahn, M. D. (2004). Preferences of husbands and wives for outcomes of prostate cancer screening and treatment. *Journal of General Internal Medicine, 19*(4), 339–348.

Joan L. Bottorff, University of British Columbia Okanagan, Faculty of Health and Social Development, 3333 University Way, Kelowna, BC, Canada V1V 1V7

John L. Oliffe, Michael Halpin, Melanie Phillips, Graham McLean, Lawrence Mroz, University of British Columbia, Vancouver, BC, Canada

Available online 27 December 2007

Critique of the Study by Bottorff and Colleagues, "Women and Prostate Cancer Support Groups: The Gender Connect?"

OVERALL SUMMARY

Bottorff and colleagues conducted an important and fascinating ethnographic study. The description of results includes thick, rich descriptions of wives' experiences with Prostate Cancer Support Groups (PCSGs). The study has implications for nurses and other health care professionals involved in the planning and implementation of PCSGs, particularly when considering group membership and spouses' participation. The report could have provided more detail about method, such as strategies used pertaining to data collection and analysis.

TITLE

The title of the article is appealing and 'catchy' which would attract potential readers to learn more about this topic. Key concepts examined in the study are included. However, the title does not allude to the type of research that was conducted (i.e., qualitative). Possibly, the title could have read: "Women's roles in prostate cancer support groups: Exploring the gender connect".

ABSTRACT

The abstract succinctly and clearly summarizes the main features of the study. Bottorff and colleagues describe the research problem, the study purpose, the specific qualitative research design and data collection methods used, and the implications of findings for future work on prostate cancer support groups. More content could have been provided as the abstract was about 243 words and this journal permits 300 words. For example, the abstract could have included more information about the women participating in the study (e.g., wives, daughters, or sisters) and the process of data analysis.

INTRODUCTION

The introduction sets the stage for the study by identifying the problem, articulating the phenomenon of interest, reviewing key points in the literature, and stating the study purpose. However, the study significance and implications are not explicit in this section—instead these are discussed in the conclusion.

Problem Statement

Bottorff and colleagues clearly state at the outset that a cancer diagnosis not only impacts on the lives of individuals diagnosed, but also on the well-being of those close to them, to the point that prostate cancer can be construed as a "couple's illness". In addition, the authors articulate the problem being addressed in the very first paragraph: "Although a growing body of research on PCSG has begun to document men's experiences, there has been little recognition of the involvement of women in these groups." This is a problem that is certainly relevant for health care as nurses and other health care providers often are involved in setting up support groups for individuals touched by cancer.

Literature Review

In the first two paragraphs of the literature review section, Bottorff and colleagues cite relevant the literature regarding the illness experience of wives of men diagnosed with prostate cancer. In addition, the authors discuss studies emphasising differences in behaviour and level of participation of men and women in support groups. This provides a relevant context for the "gender connect" being explored.

There is seemingly a dearth of studies exploring the experience of women attending prostate cancer support groups; however the authors do point out two other qualitative studies conducted in this area. The reader may have gained from more elaboration on these studies' findings to show how the researchers capitalized on these to conceptualize their own study.

Study Purpose and Rationale

At the outset of the report, the purpose of the study is clearly stated "to offer understandings about how prostate cancer is situated, and negotiated as a 'couple's illness', by describing women's participation at the PCSGs". In addition, in the concluding paragraph of background, three research questions are presented: (a) Why do women attend prostate support groups? (b) How do women situate themselves and function at prostate support groups? And, (c) What benefits do women accrue from participation?

Framework

Bottorff and colleagues chose a naturalistic paradigm for their study so that the women could describe and voice their experiences and perspectives. The authors chose ethnography as their methodological approach. This is a good match with the aim of the study that seeks to understand better how prostate cancer is situated and negotiated within couples through describing women's experience in PCSGs participation. The authors chose ethnography for its emphasis on examining the "culture" within PCSGs participation. Although ethnographies are generally thought to be conducted with large communities or broadly defined cultural groupings, it is not uncommon for this approach to be selected to examine concrete or more narrowly-defined groups. A brief definition of this qualitative methodology and rationale for its use might have better orient readers that are less familiar with ethnography.

METHOD

The method section of the report describes how the researchers gained entry into the setting, and processes related to sampling, the actual sample, data collection, and analysis.

Approach

The methods Bottorff and colleagues used to collect and analyze their data were congruent with ethnography through fieldwork and participant observation. In addition, the authors used field notes; a strategy often used in ethnography to record observations and reflects on the data being collected.

Study Sample

The researchers gained access to the support groups through the assistance of 13 leaders of PCSGs in British Columbia. All groups that were contacted agreed to participate in the study. The researchers were fortunate to have the cooperation of these leaders. Initially, Bottorff and colleagues had planned to recruit one woman from each PCSG to participate in an in-depth individual interview. However, the researchers modified their sampling strategy when they realised that many of the women were keen on talking with them. It seems implicit that, at that time, convenience sampling was undertaken and whoever wanted to discuss their experience with the groups was interviewed. It is not uncommon in qualitative research to change aspect of the initial method to respond to the needs of the study, especially if it will contribute more directly to answering the research questions. The eligibility criteria for the study are not provided in the report. However, again, this is not unusual in a qualitative study, as these are kept broad to enhance the breadth of exploration. The main criterion is usually to interview individuals that are most willing to talk to the researchers about their experiences.

The researchers do not specify what criteria they used to decide on the number of interviews or observations to be conducted. Typically, in qualitative research, the principle of saturation is used to guide decisions. However, 20 individual interviews are often considered an adequate sample for ethnography. Demographic information on participants is provided, although additional information about husbands would have been useful.

Data Collection

The researchers explain their overall data collection procedures. Participant observation is often favoured by ethnographers to get to know a culture intimately. A combination of data collection methods is also usually used to comprehensively understand the complexity of groups or culture being studied. Bottorff and colleagues use both participant observation and in-depth individual interviews to obtain different views of women's experiences with PCSGs. The reader senses that the research team 'culturally immersed' itself in PCSGs to obtain comprehensive accounts of women's experience.

Some additional information about the data collection methods used would have been useful. For instance, fieldwork is listed as a separate data collection method and it is not clear what type was conducted by the authors (or if participant observation was the main fieldwork activity). Also, more details could have been provided on duration of focus groups, level of participation of the researcher in the focus groups (e.g., observer only, observer with some participation). The authors emphasise that both male and female researchers completed the observations; however, there is no discussion regarding the implications of this for the data. In ethnography, interviews are often informal or unstructured and include mainly open-ended questions. However, from the report it is unclear who conducted the individual interviews, what was the interviewing process or technique, and what type of questions were asked The length of time spent in data collection is not specified. Although, the authors mention that they conducted 20 interviews in total, lasting on average one hour. It is unclear where these interviews were conducted (e.g., at the hospital, in participants' homes). Interviews were audio-taped and then transcribed verbatim, which helped preserve the richness and accuracy of the data.

Rigour

Regarding enhancement of rigour, Bottorff and colleagues do not have a separate section in their report on this topic, as is the case in an increasing number of qualitative reports, nor do they explain their efforts to ensure trustworthiness. However, we can infer that several methods were used to enhance the trustworthiness, including audio-taping and transcribing the interviews, investigator and method triangulation, and peer debriefing. Additional strategies could have been used (and perhaps they were, but the report does not state this), including member checking and an audit trail.

Ethics

With regard to the ethical aspects of the study, the authors do mention that the study was approved by the university's ethics committee; however, they do not indicate that the participants signed a consent form and that issues of confidentiality or anonymity were addressed.

RESULTS

Bottorff and colleagues describe their process of data management and data analysis in general terms. The authors used an inductive approach to data analysis, which is most appropriate for qualitative inquiry. In addition, the researchers used the increasingly popular qualitative data analysis software NVivo. The authors describe that their analysis followed "ethnographic style" and reference a prominent, experienced qualitative researcher; however, no specific information is presented to illustrate the steps taken for analysis.

Bottorff and colleagues' analysis yields insightful findings on the experiences and roles of women attending a PCSG. Women's experiences with the PCSGs are clearly described and insightful excerpts are chosen to illustrate the main issues identified by the participants. The researchers' discussion of participants' dilemma pertaining to focus group attendance provides a poignant context to keep in mind as findings are reviewed. The researchers then discuss participants' motives for group attendance (e.g., support for their husband, obtain information), their roles in the PCSGs (social facilitator, background supporter, and cancer cosurvivor), and perceived benefits of attending a PCSGs (e.g., hope and reassurance, connecting with other women in similar situations).

DISCUSSION

The main findings are discussed in the concluding section of the report. Bottorff and colleagues begin by summarising key findings emphasising mutual benefits of PCSGs, not only for the men diagnosed but also for the wives. In addition, the authors highlight additional studies reporting on similar findings, such as the work by Arrington et al. (2005) and Boehmer & Clark (2001). However, some of Bottorff and colleagues' findings are new and a major portion of the discussion is spent interpreting and discussing these unique findings using literature on related topics and concepts. For instance, early on in the discussion, the authors contextualise their findings within broader issues related to gender identity and roles, which emphasise how these can be transposed to the social context of PCSGs. A discussion around general gender expectations is useful in providing further insights into issues that influence participants' experiences with support groups. It would have also been interesting to be told of studies in other illness contexts, where support group membership is also found to be related to gender. Likewise, are there studies that have examined interactions with gender mix cancer support groups (e.g., colorectal cancer support groups)? How are the roles identified by the participants in this study similar or different from those identified by wives actively engaged in preserving or promoting their husbands' general health status (e.g., through diet and exercise)? Interestingly, the authors discuss the 'Man to Man' support group franchise and emphasise the lack of evidence for this practice.

Bottorff and colleagues also comment on some of the study limitations, namely the issue of generalizability and how particular PCSGs dyanamics might influence findings. In addition, the authors discuss the implications of the findings for planning and implementating PCSGs. They also suggest areas for future research (e.g., examining how the roles assumed by women in PCSGs influence groups dynamics).

GLOBAL ISSUES

Bottorff and colleagues' report is very well written and well organized. The description of findings is rich and the chosen quotes relevant to the research questions and interpretations. The in-depth exploration of women's experiences provides evidence to guide future planning and implementation of PCSGs.

AUTHORS' RESPONSE TO THE CRITIQUE

We thank the reviewers for their thoughtful comments on this paper. This research was conducted as part of a larger ethnographic study lead by Dr. John Oliffe to examine the role of prostate cancer support groups (PCSGs) in health promotion. Because there are few examples of men's groups that are focused on health issues, we believed there was much to be learned from PCSGs that may be transferable to other areas of men's health. When we started this study we did not realize that women played such an important role in PCSGs. We initially wanted to talk with women to gather their observations and insights into how PCSGs functioned to promote men's health in the context of prostate cancer. However, during the course of conducting this study as we observed women's involvement in the groups, we became more interested in their role in the groups and included direct questions about their experiences in our interviews with them. Adding this line of inquiry to our study proved to be very valuable.

In preparing this manuscript, we attempted to balance the need to include details in each section while being mindful of the space limitations mandated by the journal editors. To privilege the findings through thick description, some information about data collection and analysis were omitted. We included the most pertinent features of the methodological approaches used. Additional details about methods have been provided in other publications from the study (OliffeHalpin, Bottorff, Hislop, McKenzie, & Mroz, 2008; Oliffe, Gerbrandt, Bottorff, & Hislop, in press; Oliffe, Ogrodnickzuk, Bottorff, Halpin, & Hislop, in press). The PCSG members welcomed us into their groups. Although our role in the groups primarily involved in observation, we were drawn into informal discussions with participants as the group came together and during coffee breaks. Initially, we thought it would be important to have male research assistants attend all of the PCSGs to conduct observations and interviews with the men, and to have a female research assistant conduct interviews with women. However, there were times when this was not possible because of the availability of research staff and other logistical issues. We found that the information that was shared by the women was consistently rich regardless of the interviewer's gender. Because the data collection occurred over a period of 18 months, we were able to verify interpretations from on-going analysis in subsequent interviews and participant observations. In effect, this allowed us to continually verify findings as we conducted this project.

We believe that the findings of this study are very interesting and could be discussed in relation to a range of other studies and theoretical issues. In the discussion section of the manuscript we made decisions about what we wanted to highlight and the possible implications of the findings. The reviewers raise other topics that could have been discussed in relation to the findings. In our opinion, this is a good sign in that the findings raised additional questions and prompted readers to think about gender roles in new and novel ways.

Joan L. Bottorff, R.N., Ph.D.
Professor, University of British Columbia Okanagan,
Faculty of Health and Social Development

John L. Oliffe, R.N., Ph.D.
Associate Professor, University of British Columbia

REFERENCES

Oliffe, J. L., Halpin, M., Bottorff, J. L., Hislop, T. G., McKenzie, M., & Mroz, L. (2008). How prostate cancer support groups do and do not survive: British Columbian perspectives. *American Journal of Men's Health, 2*(2), 143–155.

Oliffe, J., Gerbrandt, J., Bottorff, J. L., & Hislop, T. G. (in press). Health promotion and illness demotion at prostate cancer support groups. *Health Promotion Practice*.

Oliffe, J., Ogrodnickzuk, J., Bottorff, J. L., Halpin, M., & Hislop, T. G. (in press). Connecting humor, health and masculinities at prostate cancer support groups. *Psycho-oncology.*

Index

Page numbers in bold indicate glossary entries.